Emergency Psychiatry

PRINCIPLES AND PRACTICE

Second Edition

Emergency Psychiatry
PRINCIPLES AND PRACTICE

EDITORS

Rachel Lipson Glick, MD
Clinical Professor, Emerita
Department of Psychiatry
University of Michigan
Ann Arbor, Michigan

Scott L. Zeller, MD
Vice President, Acute Psychiatry
Vituity
Emeryville, California
Assistant Clinical Professor of Psychiatry
University of California-Riverside
Riverside, California

Jon S. Berlin, MD
Clinical Professor
Department of Psychiatry & Behavioral Medicine;
Department of Emergency Medicine
Medical College of Wisconsin
Milwaukee, Wisconsin

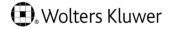. Wolters Kluwer

Philadelphia • Baltimore • New York • London
Buenos Aires • Hong Kong • Sydney • Tokyo

Acquisitions Editor: Chris Teja
Development Editor: Ariel S. Winter
Editorial Coordinator: Ashley Pfeiffer
Editorial Assistant: Brian Convery
Marketing Manager: Gretchen Hauselt
Production Project Manager: Kim Cox
Design Coordinator: Teresa Mallon
Illustrator: Jennifer Clements
Manufacturing Coordinator: Beth Welsh
Prepress Vendor: TNQ Technologies

2nd edition
Copyright © 2021 Wolters Kluwer.

9 8 7 6 5 4 3 2 1

Printed in China

Library of Congress Cataloging-in-Publication Data

ISBN-13: 978-1-975113-68-1

Cataloging-in-Publication data available on request from the Publisher.

shop.lww.com

Foreword

The practice of emergency psychiatry involves expertise in multiple domains. Psychiatrists who work in this field must have knowledge about general medicine, emergency medicine, trauma, and acute care. They must also be familiar with the culture of law enforcement and the legal system, as well as an understanding of politics and bureaucracy. In addition, they must be well trained in the rapid assessment of mental illness, substance abuse, and addiction. Emergency psychiatry involves making quick decisions about very sick patients utilizing existing systems of care.

Emergency psychiatry also deals with patients that reflect some of our biggest social problems including homelessness, violence, suicide, and criminal behavior. Therefore, education in emergency psychiatry is now more important than ever. Professionals in any field who encounter individuals in crisis need to understand the importance of being trauma-informed, how de-escalation and calming can be superior to coercion, and that negative and aggressive behaviors may be due to treatable symptoms, rather than character flaws.

This second edition of *Emergency Psychiatry: Principles and Practice* is a welcome and much-needed new book that will assist everyone, from beginning students to accomplished experts, in the multiple aspects of emergency psychiatry. I thank Drs Glick, Zeller, and Berlin for their continued dedication to providing education about the intricate, fascinating, and truly necessary modern practices of emergency psychiatry.

Renée L. Binder, MD
Professor and Director of Psychiatry and Law Program
Associate Dean for Academic Affairs
University of California,
San Francisco School of Medicine
Past President, American Psychiatric Association

Preface

The response to the first edition of *Emergency Psychiatry: Principles and Practice* has been very positive. Thousands of copies have been sold, and feedback indicates the book has become a cornerstone for education and training in emergency psychiatry around the world. Yet over the past 10 years, there have been significant advances and changes in perspectives around crisis and emergency mental health care. The number of patients presenting to emergency departments in crisis has continued to grow (1), while the number of patients being held in emergency departments waiting for transfer to inpatient psychiatric units has risen to levels which are, at times, catastrophic (2). Clearly, it was time to revise and update our textbook.

Since the publication of our first edition, emergency psychiatry has moved closer to becoming a well-established subspecialty. More providers, both psychiatrists and emergency physicians, are focusing their careers on the treatment and understanding of behavioral emergencies, with more emphasis on outcomes research to establish best practices (3). Emergency psychiatry fellowship programs and tracks within psychiatry residencies have been developed. The National Update on Behavioral Emergencies (NUBE) conference, sponsored by the American Association for Emergency Psychiatry, attracts clinicians, administrators, and researchers from around the world for its yearly multiday conference (4).

More hospitals and healthcare institutions have created separate Psychiatric Emergency Services (PESs) (5,6), and crisis stabilization units (CSUs) are becoming a standard component of many mental health systems (7,8). On-demand telepsychiatry is emerging in scores of locations (9-11), beaming into hospital emergency departments which formerly could not hope for prompt psychiatric consultations. It is truly an era of incredible progress and growth in emergency psychiatry, and we are optimistic about the direction our subspecialty is moving.

Much work, however, remains to be done. To cite just a few problematic areas: One, too many healthcare systems and government organizations continue to operate on the premise that inpatient psychiatric hospitalization is the only option for patients with high-acuity psychiatric symptoms. This belief exists despite a consensus among emergency psychiatrists that prompt acute care in the emergency setting is often sufficient to stabilize conditions without the need for inpatient admission. Nonetheless, there remains a need for more good data and outcomes research on this topic. Two, many, perhaps even the majority of, medical emergency departments persist in using coercive interventions such as physical restraints and forcibly injected antipsychotics or sedatives as a routine treatment for agitation or psychosis, rather than as a last resort only after more collaborative interventions have failed. Three, there remains a pervasive stigma against serious mental illnesses, with insufficient recognition by numerous first responders and healthcare professionals that psychiatric emergencies are no less optional, urgent or distressing than "real" medical emergencies like chest pain and asthma attacks. Four, emergency psychiatrists still need more tools with which to evaluate and treat the most serious disorders—as some patients persist in resisting engagement, certain psychiatric conditions are refractory to treatment, and safety net mental health systems struggle to provide adequate disposition options for the small but labor-intensive subset of people with severe mental illness who do not respond to assertive community treatment, residential options, or intermittent episodes of acute care.

Bearing all this in mind, we have attempted to assemble the most relevant, up-to-date and evidence-based information for this second edition of *Emergency Psychiatry: Principles and Practice*. We have recruited many of the leaders in the field to serve as section editors and authors. We have reorganized the book into six sections: Models and Standards of Patient Care, Research, and Education; General Principles of Care; Staffing and Support; Common Presenting Problems; Special Populations; and Policy and Special Topics.

The first section includes a new chapter which addresses the issue of psychiatric boarding, the practice of holding psychiatric patients in the ED for hours to days with little or no treatment until an inpatient bed can be found. A separate chapter focused on standards and quality of care is also included.

In the second and fourth sections, we have presented general principles and then specific approaches to common problems seen in psychiatric emergency care. We have aligned the approach to agitation with Project BETA (12) recommendations and have assured that each chapter includes evidence-based management and treatment.

Section three covers staffing and support and adds a chapter on staffing models to updated chapters on peer and consumer input and involvement as well as inclusion of the family in crisis care. An expanded section on special populations covers children and adolescents, pregnancy, geriatrics, and the developmentally disabled among others from the first edition, but also adds up-to-date information about the approach to several additional groups who are being seen in emergency mental health settings in increasing numbers, including college students, transgender people, prisoners, and immigrants and refugees.

Finally, we end with a section on Policy and Special Topics, such as legal issues that emergency mental health providers must be aware of, emergency telepsychiatry, best practices for working with police and law enforcement, crisis phone services, and disaster psychiatry.

We anticipate that this Second Edition will be useful and timely for our readers. We have endeavored to provide the information clinicians and trainees in emergency psychiatry will find helpful to guide their clinical care, but also have included concepts and ideas for medical leaders when considering program development and policy issues along with administrators and others in the community. Our goal is to continue to expand the science, understanding, and best practices of our still relatively young discipline. Seeing the accomplishments of the past ten years, we can only imagine what the next decade might bring to the spectrum of crisis and emergency mental health care. We sincerely hope that this textbook will provide a solid foundation for readers for years to come.

REFERENCES

1. Weiss, A. J., Barrett, M. L., Heslin, K. C., et al. Trends in Emergency Department Visits Involving Mental and Substance Use Disorders, 2006-2013. https://www.hcup-us.ahrq.gov/reports/statbriefs/sb216-Mental-Substance-Use-Disorder-ED-Visit-Trends.pdf. Accessed February 17, 2019.
2. Nolan, J. M., Fee, C., Cooper, B. A., Rankin, S. H., Blegen, M. A. (2015). Psychiatric boarding incidence, duration, and associated factors in United States emergency departments. *Journal of Emergency Nursing, 41*(1), 57–64.
3. Boudreaux, E. D., Allen, M. H., Classeen, C., et al. (2009). The psychiatric emergency research collaboration-01: Methods and results. *General Hospital Psychiatry, 31*(6), 515–522.
4. https://www.emergencypsychiatry.org/. Accessed February 17, 2019.
5. Lee, T. S., Renaud, E. F., Hills, O. F. (2003). Emergency psychiatry: An emergency treatment hub-and-spoke model of psychiatric emergency services. *Psychiatric Services, 54*, 1590–1594.
6. Allen, M. H. (1999). Level 1 psychiatric emergency services. The tools of the crisis sector. *Psychiatric Clinics of North America, 22*(4), 713–734.
7. Wolff, A. (2008). Development of a psychiatric crisis stabilization unit. *Journal of Emergency Nursing, 34*, 458–459.
8. Heyland, M., Emery, C., Shattell, M. (2013). The living room, a community crisis respite program: Offering people in crisis an alternative to emergency departments. *Global Journal of Community Psychology Practice, 4*(3), 1–8.
9. Narasimhan, M., Druss, B. G., Hockenberry, J. M., et al. (2015). Impact of a telepsychiatry program at emergency departments statewide on the quality, utilization, and costs of mental health services. *Psychiatric Services, 66*, 11. http://ps.psychiatryonline.org/doi/pdf/10.1176/appi.ps.201400122.
10. Southard, E. P., Neufeld, J. D., Laws, S. (2014). Telemental health evaluations enhance access and efficiency in a critical access hospital emergency department. *Telemedicine Journal and e-Health, 20*, 664–668.
11. Telepsychiatry program eases patient crowding in the ED, expedites mental health services to patients and providers. *ED Management.* 2013, 25, 121–124.
12. Holloman, G. H., Zeller, S. L. (2012). Overview of project BETA: Best practices in evaluation and treatment of agitation. *Western Journal of Emergency Medicine, 13*(1), 1–2.

Contributors

Marc E. Agronin, MD
Affiliate Associate Professor
Department of Psychiatry and Neurology
University of Miami Miller School of Medicine
Miami, Florida

Carlos Almeida, MD
Assistant Clinical Professor
Faculty
Department of Psychiatry
NYU-Langone
New York, New York

Manuel G. Alvarez Romero, BA
Research Coordinator,
Department of Emergency Medicine
University of Arkansas for Medical Sciences,
Little Rock, Arkansas

Margaret E. Balfour, MD, PhD
Associate Professor
Department of Psychiatry
University of Arizona
Tucson, Arizona

Jon S. Berlin, MD
Clinical Professor
Department of Psychiatry & Behavioral Medicine
Department of Emergency Medicine
Medical College of Wisconsin
Milwaukee, Wisconsin

Bernard Biermann, MD, PhD
Clinical Assistant Professor
Department of Psychiatry
University of Michigan
Ann Arbor, Michigan

Renée L. Binder, MD
Professor and Director of Psychiatry and Law Program
Associate Dean for Academic Affairs
University of California, San Francisco School of Medicine
Past President, American Psychiatric Association

Katrina A. Bozada, MD
Clinical Instructor
Department of Psychiatry
University of Michigan
Ann Arbor, Michigan

Flávio Casoy, MD
Private Practice
New York, New York

Jamie C. Cerny, BA
Senior Business Analyst
Department of Acute Psychiatry
Vituity Practice Management
Emeryville, California

Thomas Chaffee, MD
Resident
Department of Psychiatry
University of Michigan
Ann Arbor, Michigan

Ann L. Christiansen, MPH
Health Director/Health Officer
North Shore Health Department
(Previously Employed at) Medical College of Wisconsin
Milwaukee, Wisconsin

Lee Combrinck-Graham, MD
Medical Director
Life Bridge Community Services
Bridgeport, Connecticut

Julia C. Cromwell, MD
Instructor
Department of Psychiatry
Harvard Medical School
Boston, Massachusetts

Glenn W. Currier, MD, MPH
Professor and Chair
Department of Psychiatry
USF Morsani College of Medicine
Tampa, Florida

Robert N. Cuyler, PhD
President
Clinical Psychology Consultants Ltd, LLP
Houston, Texas

Ronald J. Diamond, MD
Professor Emeritus
Department of Psychiatry
University of Wisconsin
Madison, Wisconsin

John Draper, PhD
Executive Director
National Suicide Prevention Lifeline
New York, New York

Ken Duckworth, MD
Assistant Professor
Department of Psychiatry
Harvard Medical School
Boston, Massachusetts

Jonathan G. Dunlop, MD, JD
Fellow in Forensic Psychiatry
Program in Psychiatry, Law and Ethics
University of Michigan
Ann Arbor, Michigan

Carla D. Edwards, MSc, MD, FRCP(C)
Assistant Clinical Professor
Department of Psychiatry and Behavioral Neurosciences
McMaster University
Hamiliton, Ontario, Canada

Shami Entenman, MD
Resident Physician
Department of Psychiatry
University of Michigan
Ann Arbor, Michigan

Laura Erickson-Schroth, MD, MA
Assistant Professor
Department of Psychiatry
Columbia University Medical Center
New York, New York

Bruce Fage, MD
Resident Physician
Department of Psychiatry
University of Toronto
Toronto, Ontario

Avrim B. Fishkind, MD
General Manager-Psychiatry
SOC Telemed
Houston, Texas

Cecilia M. Fitz-Gerald, MD
Resident Physician
Department of Psychiatry
University of Texas Southwestern Medical Center
Dallas, Texas

Kaitlyn Garcia, MD
Resident Physician
Department of Psychiatry
The University of Toledo
Toledo, Ohio

Marina Garriga, MD
PhD Candidate
Department of Medicine
University of Barcelona
Barcelona, Spain

Rachel Lipson Glick, MD
Clinical Professor, Emerita
Department of Psychiatry
University of Michigan
Ann Arbor, Michigan

Joseph S. Goveas, MD
Associate Professor
Department of Psychiatry and Behavioral Medicine
Medical College of Wisconsin
Milwaukee, Wisconsin

Benjamin T. Griffeth, MD
Associate Professor
Department of Psychiatry
University of South Carolina School of Medicine
Greenville, South Carolina

Jon E. Gudeman, MD
Emeritus Professor of Psychiatry
Department of Psychiatry
Medical College of Wisconsin
Milwaukee, Wisconsin

Rahael Rohini Gupta, MD, MS
Resident Physician
Department of Psychiatry
UCLA
Los Angeles, California

Stephen W. Hargarten, MD, MPH
Professor of Emergencey Medicine
Department of Emergency Medicine
Medical College of Wisconsin
Milwaukee, Wisconsin

Herbert J. Harman, MD
Regional Director, Psychiatry
Vituity
Emeryville, California

Harold H. Harsch, MD
Professor
Department of Psychiatry and Behavioral Medicine
Medical College of Wisconsin
Milwaukee, Wisconsin

Mark J. Hauser, MD
Instructor, Part Time
Department of Psychiatry
Harvard Medical School
Boston, Massachusetts

Erin J. Henshaw, PhD
Associate Professor
Department of Psychology
Denison University
Granville, Ohio

Alison M. Heru, MD
Professor of Psychiatry
Department of Psychiatry
University of Colorado Denver
Denver, Colorado

Victor Hong, MD
Assistant Professor
Department of Psychiatry
University of Michigan
Ann Arbor, Michigan

Lucy A. Hutner, MD
Co-Founder, Phoebe
New York, New York

Gregory L. Iannuzzi, MD
Resident Physician
Department of Psychiatry and Behavioral Neurosciences
University of South Florida Morsani College of Medicine
Tampa, Florida

Edward M. Kantor, MD, DFAPA, MD, PA, EMT-P
Residency Program Director, Associate Professor
Department of Psychiatry and Behavioral Sciences
Medical University of South Carolina
Charleston, South Carolina

James. N. Kimball, MD
Associate Professor
Department of Psychiatry and Behavioral Medicine
Wake Forest School of Medicine
Winston-Salem, North Carolina

Kelley-Anne C. Klein, MD
Assistant Professor
Department of Psychiatry
University of Vermont
Burlington, Vermont

Robert Kohn, MD, MPhil
Professor
Department of Psychiatry and Human Behavior
Brown University
Providence, Rhode Island

Sara A. Kohlbeck, MPH
Assistant Director
Comprehensive Injury Center
Medical College of Wisconsin
Milwaukee, Wisconsin

Kimberly Kulp-Osterland, DO
Acting Director of Psychiatry and Medical Services
Center for Forensic Psychiatry
State of Michigan Department of Health and Human Services
Saline, Michigan

Joe Kwon, MD
Assistant Professor
Department of Psychiatry
University of Texas Southwestern
Dallas, Texas

Katherine G. Levine, MD
Assistant Professor
Department of Psychiatry and Behavioral Medicine
Medical College of Wisconsin
Milwaukee, Wisconsin

Jodi Lofchy, MD, FRCPC
Associate Professor
Department of Psychiatry
University of Toronto
Toronto, Ontario

Karen M. Lommel, DO, MHA, MS
Department Chair
Department of Psychiatry & Emergency Medicine
USC-School of Medicine Greenville
Greenville, South Carolina

Sheila M. Marcus, MD
Professor
Department of Psychiatry
University of Michigan,
Ann Arbor, Michigan

Cheryl McCullumsmith, MD, PhD
Professor and Chair
Department of Psychiatry
University of Toledo College of Medicine and Life Sciences
Toledo, Ohio

Hunter L. McQuistion, MD
Clinical Professor
Department of Psychiatry
NYU School of Medicine
New York, New York

Lyle Barnes Montgomery, MD
Psychiatrist
SOC Telemed
Reston, Virginia

Joshua C. Morganstein, MD
Associate Professor/Assistant Chair
Department of Psychiatry
School of Medicine
Uniformed Services University
Bethesda, Maryland

Gillian Murphy, PhD
Director-Standards, Training & Practices
National Suicide Prevention Lifeline
New York, New York

Anthony T. Ng, MD
Assistant Professor
Department of Psychiatry
Uniformed Services University of Health Sciences
Bethesda, Maryland

Sarah A. Nguyen, MD
Assistant Professor
Department of Psychiatry
University of Conneticut School of Medicine
Farmington, Connecticut

Joshua Niclas, MD, PhD
Staff Psychiatrist
Pscyhiatric Emergency Services
Contra Costa Regional Medical Center
Martinez, California

Ilana Nossel, MD
Assistant Professor of Clinical Psychiatry
Department of Psychiatry
Columbia University
New York, New York

Charles F. Palmer, MD
Resident Physician
Department of Psychiatry
Medical Univerity of South Carolina
Charleston, South Carolina

Nicole S. Parrish, MD
Resident Physician
Department of Psychiatry and Behavioral Medicine
PRISMA Health/USC
Greenville, South Carolina

Jagoda Pasic, MD, PhD
Professor of Psychiatry
Department of Psychiatry and Behavioral Sciences
University of Washington
Seattle, Washington

Gonzalo Perez-Garcia, MD
Medical Director-Emergency Psychiatry
SOC Telemed
Houston, Texas

Debra A. Pinals, MD
Clinical Professor of Psychiatry
Department of Psychiatry
University of Michigan
Ann Arbor, Michigan

Justo E. Pinzón, MD
PhD Candidate
Department of Medicine
University of Barcelona
Barcelona, Spain

Divy Ravindranath, MD, MS, FACLP
Clinical Associate Professor (Affiliated)
Department of Psychiatry
Stanford University School of Medicine
Palo Alto, California

Priyanka P. Reddy, DO
Psychiatry Resident
Department of Psychiatry
University of Michigan
Ann Arbor, Michigan

Janet S. Richmond, MSW, LICSW
Associate Clinical Professor
Department of Psychiatry
Tufts University School of Medicine
Boston Massachusetts

Ron C. Rosenberg, MD
Attending Psychiatrist
Department of Psychiatry
Lenox Hill Hospital
New York, New York

John S. Rozel, MD, MSL
Associate Professor of Psychiatry and Adjunct Professor
of Law
University of Pittsburgh
Pittsburgh, Pennsylvania

Leigh J. Ruth, MD
Assistant Professor
Department of Psychiatry and Behaviroal Neurosciences
University of South Florida
Tampa, Florida

Lucas Andrew Salg, MD
Chief Resident
Department of Psychiatry
University of Colorado
Aurora, Colorado

Scott A. Simpson, MD, MPH
Assistant Professor
Department of Psychiatry
University of Colorado School of Medicine
Aurora, Colorado

Eva Solé, MD
PhD Candidate
Department of Medicine
University of Barcelona
Barcelona, Spain

Mina R. Spadaro, MSN, RN, PHN
Corporate Director of Behavioral Health
Department of Clinical Operations
Prime Healthcare Services
Ontario, California

Susan Stefan, MPhil, JD
Visiting Professor of Law
University of Miami School of Law
Coral Gables, Florida

Theodore A. Stern, MD
Ned H. Cassem Professor of Psychiatry in the field of
* Psychosomatic Medicine/Consultation*
Department of Psychiatry
Harvard Medical School
Boston, Massachusetts

Victor G. Stiebel, MD
Clinical Assistant Professor
Department of Psychiatry
University of Pittsburgh
Pittsburgh, Pennsylvania

Anderson E. Still, MD
Attending Psychiatrist
Department of Child and Adolescent Psychiatry and
* Behavioral Sciences*
Children's Hospital of Philadelphia
Philadelphia, Pennsylvania

Alan C. Swann, MD
Pat R. Rutherford Jr. Chair, Professor and Vice-Chair for
* Research*
Department of Psychiatry
University of Texas
Medical School
Harris County Psychiatric Center
Houston,Texas

Tony Thrasher, DO, DFAPA
Assistant Clinical Professor
Department of Psychiatry and Behavioral Medicine
Medical College of Wisconsin
Milwaukee, Wisconsin

Howard D. Trachtman, BS, CPS, CPRP, COAPS
Executive Team, MBRCC
Department of Psychiatry
Boston Medical Center
Boston, Massachusetts

Samidha Tripathi, MD
Assistant Professor
Department of Psychiatry
University of Arkansas for Medical Sciences
Little Rock, Arkansas

Eduard Vieta, MD, PhD
Professor
Department of Medicine
University of Barcelona
Barcelona, Spain

Jennifer G. Votta, DO
Clinical Instructor
Department of Psychiatry
University of Michigan
Ann Arbor, Michigan

Ryan C. Wagoner, MD
Assistant Professor
Department of Psychiatry
University of South Florida
Tampa, Florida

Michael Wilson, MD, PhD
Assistant Professor
Department of Emergency Medicine
UAMS
Little Rock, Arkansas

Van Yu, MD
Clinical Assistant Professor
Department of Psychiatry
NYU Medical Center
New York, New York

Paul Zarkowski, MD
Clinical Assistant Professor
Univeristy of Washington
Seattle, Washington

Scott L. Zeller, MD
Vice President, Acute Psychiatry
Vituity
Emeryville, California
Assistant Clinical Professor of Psychiatry
University of California-Riverside
Riverside, California

Leslie Zun, MD, MBA
Professor
Department of Emergency Medicine
Chicago Medical School
North Chicago, Illinois

Acknowledgments

JOINT EDITOR ACKNOWLEDGMENT

The editors wish to acknowledge a number of people who have helped make this textbook become a reality. First, we want to thank Chris Teja, Acquisitions Editor at Wolters Kluwer, who asked us to update our original text. Without his encouragement, we would not have embarked on this project. We also want to thank others from the Wolters Kluwer team including our Development Editor, Ariel S. Winter, and our Editorial Coordinator, Ashley Pfeiffer. Both have put up with answering to three lead editors and have worked with us to manage the process of editing, and moving to production, over 50 chapters written by almost as many authors, each with their own idiosyncrasies and ideas, all while pushing us to keep on a strict timeline. Others to mention are our design team, Teresa Mallon (Design Coordinator) and Jennifer Clements (Illustrator) as well as our production team led by Kim Cox (at Wolters Kluwer) and Soundararajan Ramkumar (at TNQ Technologies) and Wolters Kluwer Marketing Team.

We want to thank our five Section Editors, Drs Victor Hong, Cheryl McCullumsmith, Divy Ravindranath, Jack Rozel, and Scott Simpson. Without their help, we are not sure if we could have completed this second edition. We also appreciate the hard work all of our authors have done for this project. Without their expertise and willingness to contribute, we could not have compiled a comprehensive text of emergency psychiatry.

We again want to acknowledge the American Association for Emergency Psychiatry (AAEP) and its founders and officers. If this group had not existed, we would never have met, nor would we have realized that psychiatrists around the country are doing this work, often in isolation. AAEP continues to be a professional home for those of us who do emergency psychiatry work. This project would not have been possible without contributions from many of our AAEP colleagues.

We also gratefully acknowledge our families for putting up with us while we worked on this project.

We thank each other for being great partners and for helping each other get the job done.

Finally, we especially want to thank our psychiatric emergency service colleagues, and all of our patients and their families. Without what they have taught us, none of us would be emergency psychiatrists.

RLG, SLZ, and JSB

DR GLICK'S ACKNOWLEDGMENTS

As I prepare to retire after 30 years of work in Emergency Psychiatry, there are many mentors and colleagues for me to thank. Drs George Tesar and Doug Hughes first introduced me to this important work. Drs Michael Allen, Glenn Currier, Seth Powsner, Anthony T. Ng, Joseph J. Zealberg, Peter L. Forster, and Ricardo Mendoza, all past presidents of AAEP, have been invaluable sources of information and support. Many others who have become involved with AAEP more recently, including Drs Jack Rozel, Tony Thrasher, Leslie Zun, Margie Balfour, and Victor Stiebel, have also influenced and enriched my work, and I thank them for this. Several colleagues from the Academy of Consult Liaison Psychiatry special interest group in emergency psychiatry also deserve mention and thanks, including Drs Scott Simpson, Cheryl McCullumsmith, Karen Lommel, and Mary Jo Fitz-Gerald.

I also want to thank Dr Jon Berlin and Dr Scott Zeller, my editing partners on this book and my close friends in emergency psychiatry.

Without their support and involvement this book would not have been written and edited. They have each taught me so much and without them my career in emergency psychiatric work would not have been as fulfilling or as much fun. I also want to thank Dr Avrim Fishkind, another close friend and a co-editor on the first edition of this text. He helped with the initial planning of this second edition, and even though he had to step away from the project because of other commitments, his advice and counsel helped with the development of this book.

A big thanks is also owed to John Kettley, Dr Victor Hong, and the rest of the faculty, staff, and residents at Michigan Medicine where I have practiced emergency psychiatry since 1991. Michigan Medicine's PES has gone from a part-time service staffed by social workers with one interview room where fewer than 3,000 adult patients were seen each year to a full-service, 24/7 emergency department with five interview and three observation rooms, its own nursing staff, and full-time physician presence now seeing over 8,000 patients of all ages each year. I have been privileged to help with and watch this maturation, learning a tremendous amount about systems of health care along the way. I also want to thank the hundreds of families and patients I have seen through the years. You are the reason I do this work.

Finally, I thank my mother, Dr Marilyn Heins, who tells me that I make it look easy to have both a successful career and family, but doesn't seem to realize that I learned how to do this from her. And my husband, Gary, and children, Hannah and Jeremy. I celebrate all of your successes and think I am so lucky to have such a wonderful family.

DR ZELLER'S ACKNOWLEDGMENTS

A very heartfelt thank you to all my colleagues at the physician partnership Vituity, the first large medical group in the United States to embrace Emergency Psychiatry and to recognize the important role of integrating behavioral health into the acute care spectrum of medicine. A special thanks to the visionary Dr Prentice Tom, Vituity Chief Innovation Officer, whose out of the box thinking first brought me into the Vituity organization, which was then known as CEP America. And to the Vituity leadership which has been so nurturing and supportive to our Psychiatric Emergency Medicine Practice Line: CEO Dr Imamu Tomlinson, President Dr Theo Koury, Chief Strategy Officer Dr Denise Brown, Chief Operating Officer Dr David Birdsall, Chief Medical Officer Dr Gregg Miller, and Chief Transformation Officer Dr Rick Newell, as well as Executives Leslie Anglada, Andrew Smith, Erin Hyatt, Mitch Cohen, and Michael Harrington.

Tremendous thanks to my Acute Psychiatry teammates Dr Herb Harman, Sumter Armstrong, and Kimberly Lopez, as well as everyone who has worked alongside us at Vituity to develop our fantastic psychiatry practice, now in so many hospitals across the country. It is an honor to be part of such a terrific group of people; I wish I could name you all!

So much of what I know in Emergency Psychiatry came from the many years of working at the Alameda Health System, especially the John George Psychiatric Hospital; thanks to all the physicians, clinicians, nurses, administrators, patients, and others there for teaching me so very much.

Thanks also to all the marvelous people at the American College of Emergency Physicians, especially Dr Mike Gerardi, Dr Sandy Schneider, and Loren Rives, who have embraced Emergency Psychiatry as an essential part of their specialty, and whose support has truly led to incredible advancements and advocacy in recent years, not the least of which has been the creation of the national Coalition on Psychiatric Emergencies.

But biggest thanks of all go to Dr Rachel Glick, Dr Jon Berlin, and Dr Avrim Fishkind. The four of us have done remarkable things together over the past 20 years. It's a privilege to know you and to work with you, but the best thing of all is to have you as friends. I will always treasure the memories with you, individually and collectively.

DR BERLIN'S ACKNOWLEDGEMENTS

I owe so much to so many—teachers, colleagues, patients, students, analysts, family, and friends. At the risk of leaving someone out, it is a pleasure at least to mention a few.

Thanks to Rachel for once again spearheading this project and keeping us all on track with her unfailingly positive attitude; to Scott for his preternatural energy and willingness to take on any extra assignment; and to our superb group of subspecialist contributors. I hope the opportunity for them to concentrate their subject and put their stamp on it offers some kind of meaningful recompense. This book is their book.

Trailblazer Michael Weissberg introduced me and my classmates to emergency psychiatry in our residency at the University of Colorado Health Sciences Center 40 years ago, when the field was still in its infancy. It was an exciting time. He was figuring things out one day and teaching them the next. Almost 20 years later, when I left a private practice in rural Nebraska and returned to an urban "psych ED" setting, I discovered that emergency cases had multiplied in the interim but also that excellent people around the country had been busy advancing this young discipline. Pioneers of the American Association for Emergency Psychiatry, they helped to bring me up to speed: Michael Allen, Glenn Currier, Peter Forster, Jorge Petit, Janet Richmond, Rachel Glick, Scott Zeller, Tony Ng, and Avrim Fishkind. Since then, new blood continues to strengthen and stimulate us: Kim Nordstrom, Les Zun, Jack Rozel, Margie Balfour, Scott Simpson, Seth Powsner, Victor Stiebel, and Mike Wilson, to name just a few.

The chapter "Types of Initial Psychiatric Interviews in Emergency Settings" sums up, and, to a certain extent, extends my 12 years of writing on the subject. I began to put words to the page relatively late in life, but a topic like the interview draws on so many different cognitive, affective, and experiential components and is already so well-traversed in the literature that a long gestation period might not be unreasonable.

My ideas are not brand new, but I may have applied and combined existing ideas in new ways. The educated reader will easily recognize my many influences. Every author needs at least one keen reviewer; I've been lucky to have three. Drs Glick, Fishkind, and Ron Diamond all read critically and helped me better understand what it was that I was trying to say. Rachel made very useful editorial recommendations for this current chapter. She also kindly suggested that this second edition of *Emergency Psychiatry* reproduce "Interviewing for Acuity and the Acute Precipitant" from the first edition as a companion piece to the new interview chapter.

Thanks of a different order are required for the chapter on psychiatric patient boarding in the ED. To my PES compadres, Scott and Avrim, who instilled in me the belief that every psychiatric emergency service (PES) systems problem has a solution. To my friend and colleague, Stephen Hargarten, who was Chair of Emergency Medicine at the Medical College of Wisconsin while I lived and worked through a major boarding crisis. He welcomed me into the EM world, brought perspective and humor, and unobtrusively had my back as the boarding crisis reached its climax. To Peter Brown at the Institute for Behavioral Health Improvement, for sharing his invaluable idea of applying Don Berwick's principles of medical system change to emergency psychiatry. To one of our associate editors, Divy Ravindranath, for the deft writing advice on my sections of this chapter, improving both clarity and style. Finally, deep gratitude to my coworkers in the Milwaukee County Crisis Service, an unforgettable band of brothers and sisters.

A book on psychiatry, if it is to be any good, must have as its backdrop a sense of what matters most in this world. I am lucky to know a host of people who represent life at its best: most particularly, my son, Jesse, and, my vision of loveliness, Susan.

Rachel L. Glick
Scott L. Zeller
Jon S. Berlin

Table of Contents

PART I

Models and Standards of Patient Care, Research, and Education

Section Editor: Divy Ravindranath

Delivery Models of Emergency Psychiatric Care

Scott L. Zeller, Jamie C. Cerny

"If you're having a psychiatric emergency, please hang up and dial 911, or go to your nearest emergency room." Virtually everyone interacting with mental health providers or systems has heard some variation of this voice message. When an individual experiencing a psychiatric crisis follows these instructions, the result can vary widely depending on geography. This chapter will explore the varied models and approaches to emergency psychiatric interventions now prevalent across the United States.

The volume of Emergency Department (ED) visits has continued to rise in recent years in the United States; furthermore, one in eight ED visits now involves a behavioral health emergency (1). From 2006 to 2014, the rate of ED visits for mental health/substance abuse diagnoses increased by 44%, and out of all diagnosis types, ED visits with a diagnosis of suicidal ideation increased the most—by a staggering 414% (2).

According to the US Federal Emergency Medical Treatment and Labor Act (EMTALA), patients with acute psychiatric conditions rendering them either a danger to themselves, or a danger to others, are considered to have emergency medical conditions (EMCs), legally equivalent, in terms of hospital responsibilities, to serious physical ailments. As such, patients with psychiatric EMCs cannot be discharged until they are considered to be stable and safe, with no further emergent dangerousness (3). Thus, all psychiatric emergencies at hospital EDs must be fully assessed, and treated as necessary, with appropriate and secure dispositions; those whose psychiatric EMC remains unstable must either be admitted for inpatient care or transferred to an appropriate facility.

Patients who present to the ED with the mental health and substance abuse complaints are 2.5 times as likely to be admitted as those with purely physical problems (4). Furthermore, the overall number of psychiatric inpatient beds in the United States dropped by 95% from 1955 to 2005 (5). With an increasing number of psychiatric emergency patients and a decreasing number of inpatient psychiatric beds, the tradition of EDs admitting all acute psychiatric patients for inpatient care has become unmanageable. This often leads to long hours of "boarding" in the ED (see Boarding chapter), with distressed, untreated patients waiting for an elusive bed to open up. Clearly, alternatives to the traditional paradigm are needed, and by this necessity, a number of approaches have been developed. This chapter outlines these alternative models of psychiatric care that focus on initiation of treatment in the emergency setting, rather than the inpatient setting.

GOALS OF PSYCHIATRIC EMERGENCY TREATMENT

Although a variety of methods have evolved to address psychiatric crises in emergency settings, all are based on similar aims for the evaluation and treatment of these conditions. These objectives can be summed up into what are known as the "Six Goals of Emergency Psychiatry" (6):

1. Exclude medical etiologies of symptoms and ensure medical stability
2. Rapidly stabilize the acute crisis
3. Avoid coercion
4. Treat in the least restrictive setting
5. Form a therapeutic alliance
6. Formulate an appropriate disposition and aftercare plan

Exclude Medical Etiologies for Symptoms and Ensure Medical Stability

Because many medical conditions can present with symptoms that appear similar to endogenous psychoses, mania, or other acute psychiatric states, it is essential that medical etiologies be ruled out prior to commencing psychiatric treatment. A significant number of patients who present to emergency settings with apparent psychiatric disorders have acute medical illnesses either coexisting or at the root of their symptoms (7); failure to recognize these conditions can lead to serious morbidity (8,9). For example, a mistaken diagnosis of psychosis in a patient suffering from an intracranial bleed, thyroid storm, or toxic delirium can place the patient at serious, perhaps, life-threatening risk. Even commonplace medical issues in psychiatric patients, such as diabetes, hypertension, and alcohol withdrawal, can have severe sequelae if not properly addressed.

At the very least, psychiatric emergency programs need to have access to patient evaluations by a qualified medical professional, along with the measurement of vital signs, prior to commencement of psychiatric treatment. Simple on-site testing methods such as pulse oximetry, fingerstick glucose, and breathalyzers can prove invaluable.

Rapidly Stabilize the Acute Crisis

Once a patient's medical stability has been ensured, emergency psychiatry programs need to focus on prompt stabilization of the acute crisis. Every effort should be made to ensure safety and prevent danger to self and others, while simultaneously working to alleviate the patient's suffering. This includes timely triage and defined levels of staff observation based on the degree of acuity, including ligature-safe environments as appropriate.

It is not uncommon in many acute care settings for emergency psychiatry patients to experience very long waits for evaluation and treatment, while other "more urgent" medical patients get more immediate assistance. And indeed, it can be difficult for many caregivers to recognize that the distress of a psychiatric crisis can be, in a way, just as crippling as more obvious conditions such as asthma attacks or motor vehicle accidents. Some

ED staff have even been heard to say that because there are no blood tests or X-rays that show psychiatric illness, it is hard to compare mental health symptoms with more straightforward medical cases.

Yet there is another very common symptom that virtually everyone has experienced, that also cannot be detected on blood tests or X-rays, and that is "pain." And thus, teaching healthcare personnel to think of psychiatric emergencies as analogous to their "worst headache ever"—something they can all relate to—helps them to empathize with the severity of the psychiatric emergency and understand that the patient is truly agonizing and needs relief as soon as possible.

Avoid Coercion, Treat in the Least Restrictive Setting, Form a Therapeutic Alliance

Practitioners in the emergency setting may be the first contact a patient will have with mental health care. A bad experience during this initial mental health contact may lead to long-term problems in which consumers might fear, distrust, or dislike psychiatrists and other behavioral health providers. Such issues might interfere with the consumer's desire to obtain help, continue in treatment, or willingness to take medications. So, during the early phases of psychiatric illnesses, even brief interactions can have enduring implications for a patient's long-term wellness.

In realizing this, it is extremely important that emergency professionals work with patients in a supportive and compassionate manner, creating with the patient what is known as a *therapeutic alliance*. A therapeutic alliance might be most simply described as a collaborative, supportive relationship between a patient and a clinician. Rather than the professional acting excessively authoritative or giving the patient orders, a therapeutic alliance should instead involve clinicians' attempts to bond and empathize with patients, as well as treat them as partners in healing and recovery. This can lead to a working relationship with shared responsibility for achieving treatment goals in the acute setting and often results in better outcomes. Results of studies have shown that the quality of the therapeutic alliance is a significant factor in predicting the likelihood of a patient becoming violent during psychiatric hospitalizations. In one predictive model, the quality of the therapeutic alliance was able to predict 78% of aggressive behavior in patients (10).

Working with a therapeutic alliance mindset also means avoiding *coercion*—the use of force or threats to make patients do things against their will. In emergency psychiatry, avoiding coercion includes the administration of oral medications willingly via informed consent, as opposed to forcible injections; verbal de-escalation of agitated individuals to calmness, instead of imposing physical restraints; and little or no infringement on a patient's rights when possible. Treating in the least restrictive level of care is another means of avoiding coercion.

The more restrictive the level of care, the more there is a propensity for a coercive experience and thus less opportunity for a therapeutic alliance. Examples of levels of mental health care from most to least restrictive include physical restraints and/or seclusion rooms, locked clinical settings and involuntary inpatient units, and then voluntary, unlocked facilities. The least restrictive settings are outpatient clinics where patients are free to come and go as they wish. Most individuals will do best in the appropriate level of care that is least restrictive; thus avoiding hospital admissions, when possible, can be quite advantageous for patients.

Collectively, therapeutic alliance, avoiding coercion, and least restrictive settings are part of a *trauma-informed* approach to emergency psychiatric care. A substantial percentage of patients experiencing a mental health crisis have experienced trauma in their lives, more so than the general population (11,12). Given this, services for all patients should be provided in a manner that supports wellness and healing, and limits the opportunity for *retraumatization*. Retraumatization can occur when treatment in an emergency setting resurfaces feelings and issues from past traumatic episodes an individual has experienced. Occurrences common in emergency settings that might cause retraumatization can include physical restraints, forcible injections of medication, restriction of movement, and harsh or condescending interactions or orders from staff.

Appropriate Disposition and Aftercare Plan

In emergency psychiatry, the duties of the treating professional are not complete merely with cessation of the presenting crisis. It is strongly recommended that a patient be provided with appropriate postdischarge care plan. This includes appointments (when possible) with outpatient providers, referral to mental health clinics and/or substance abuse treatment programs, and instructions about what to do if crisis symptoms recur. Frequently, assistance with housing may be a part of the aftercare plan, as might be coordination of arrangements with loved ones or caregivers.

Appropriate aftercare planning can be of substantial benefit to the long-term stability of patients and help prevent recidivism. Individuals who do not have an outpatient appointment after discharge are two times more likely to be psychiatrically hospitalized in a year than patients who went to at least one outpatient appointment (13).

Simply put, the main goals in the evaluation and treatment of patients in mental health crises are to ensure medical stability, evaluate for safety, relieve the patient's distress as quickly as possible in a noncoercive, supportive, collaborative manner, and get the patient to the least restrictive environment with a safe and well-communicated discharge plan, that will help individuals to avoid a return to crisis-level symptoms.

MODELS OF CARE

This section will review the most prominent paradigms of psychiatric emergency care, evaluating the pros and cons of each, and will include a discussion of several innovative and alternative models, which have evolved more recently. The reader should recognize that there are multiple iterations and combinations between the various prototypes, and no academic description could possibly reflect each site in complete accuracy, yet the following will endeavor to describe the general attributes of the main models of care.

Mental Health Consultants in Medical Emergency Department

It is recognized that some EDs have little or no opportunity for emergency psychiatric evaluation and treatment beyond what can be provided by the general medical ED professional on duty. But in those settings that do have access to separate psychiatric personnel, the use of a mental health professional to consult on patients within the general ED population is likely the most utilized emergency psychiatry care approach in the United States (14). With this model, psychiatric patients enter the ED and are triaged alongside patients with general medical complaints; all receive a medical screening examination (MSE) by a licensed independent provider. If a psychiatric intervention is deemed necessary, a request will be made for a mental health consultant to assess the patient. Most commonly, the consultant is not on duty within the ED but arrives from another location, typically another area of the hospital, on-call from the community, or, in some cases, via a municipal or regional mobile crisis team or assessment team.

The preferred professional level for such consultants is psychiatrists, but often these may be psychologists, social workers, or other mental health clinicians. Some facilities even employ psychiatric technicians or other practitioners with less than master's level training to perform consultations; the use of these less clinically qualified personnel has been described as an "insufficient" level of care for those in psychiatric crisis (15).

The requested consultant will typically perform an assessment and may recommend a course of treatment, but most commonly his or her role is to make a determination as to the need for psychiatric hospitalization (as opposed to discharge). However, the attending ED physician remains the clinician ultimately responsible for the patient's care in this model and, in most systems, is also the one who will make the final decision as to disposition—in some cases, even overruling the mental health consultant's recommendations.

Pros and Cons: This design may be useful in EDs that encounter relatively few psychiatric patients in crises, such as smaller community or rural hospitals, where the census is insufficient to justify round-the-clock on-site mental health personnel or a separate site for psychiatric patients. A benefit of the model is that comorbid medical issues will be addressed while the patient is in the ED, which allows for the treatment of medically compromised patients who might

otherwise exceed the capability of a psychiatric-only program. This model is also typically the least expensive option for many hospitals, as no separate infrastructure for the psychiatric patient is needed.

However, because the consultant is often not on-site when the consult is requested, patients may wait hours before the consultant arrives, occupying valuable space in the ED and impacting throughput. Also, during this time, there is frequently no treatment being provided (16). Furthermore, patients who are in the midst of a severe psychiatric emergency may further decompensate or become agitated in the chaos of the ED, especially when untreated, and this may lead to an increase in the level of care required for them (17).

One of the most noteworthy shortcomings of this model is that disposition decisions are typically made as the result of a "snapshot" at the time of the initial consultation. This will not allow, for example, the opportunity to see if the patient might soon show a good response to medications or detoxify or have a change in perspective or otherwise improve enough for clinicians to consider changing the disposition plans. The ability to "observe and reevaluate later" is present in several of the other models, and those using this strategy appropriately will often have better diversion rates from hospitalization as a result (17).

If the consultant is not a psychiatrist or licensed prescriber, another major issue in this model may be that he or she cannot make medication or other physical care recommendations. In that case, the burden falls upon the ED physician to determine the course of treatment—often with little guidance or expertise to prescribe challenging psychopharmacologic regimens. As a result, too often a patient might receive little more than sedation during his or her ED stay. Also, nonpsychiatrist consultants may also lack the expertise to rule out organically caused symptoms that mimic psychiatric emergencies, such as delirium (18).

An additional concern about using nonphysicians for psychiatric consultations is that such consultants might be viewed as "lesser authorities" by some emergency medicine physicians, who may thus feel justified in exerting undue influence on the consultant toward certain dispositions. This can happen even with the common practice of using psychiatry residents to do ED psychiatric consults because the physicians in training may be understandably anxious about countermanding an ED attending-level physician's opinion.

There are EDs where the mental health consultation is provided by a visiting "intake" team from an area inpatient psychiatric facility. The impartiality of decisions by such teams may come into question, as there are perverse financial incentives for their employers regarding admissions, especially for those patients with attractive private insurance reimbursement potential.

Another compelling drawback of the consultant model is that medical ED staff may not be sufficiently trained to intervene with psychiatric emergencies and may actually exacerbate patients' symptoms with excessive coercion, or by misunderstanding the needs of a person in crisis. Further, there have been instances where staff can be disdainful, condescending, or even derisive to these patients, seemingly from a mindset that the psychiatric afflictions are not "real" emergencies or perhaps should be the lowest priority for care. This phenomenon is considered part of the "stigma" of psychiatric illness that patients have referred to in their complaints about treatment in medical EDs (19).

Telepsychiatry

The newest version of the consultant model is the telepsychiatry model—accessing a psychiatrist via telemedicine. Most commonly, this service is provided in the ED via an "on-demand" format; the ED only requests a consultation when necessary, and then will access an off-site mental health professional consultant via video teleconferencing (20). Online consultants are able to perform face-to-face assessments and make recommendations on treatment and disposition; efficacy, safety, and patient satisfaction have been shown to be roughly equivalent to interactions with a psychiatrist in the same room (21). The use of telepsychiatry consultants is rapidly expanding, acting as either a complementary service when on-site clinicians are unavailable or as the sole source of ED psychiatric consultations. It has been successfully utilized in EDs across the state of South Carolina for several years (22) and is now available from multiple provider groups in most parts of the United States (23).

Pros and Cons: Studies to date demonstrate that telepsychiatry in the ED can substantially reduce ED crowding and delays in care, while improving access and timeliness of psychiatric interventions (24,25). Shortcomings of ED telepsychiatry consultation may be the significant dollar charge per consult, and the difficulties, time delays, and costs in credentialing large groups of providers in each individual hospital when the service is provided by a large, external telepsychiatry team. As telepsychiatry is often only a single video consultation without a later follow-up, frequently the recommendations are limited and do not afford the opportunity for the consultant to suggest treatment in the ED and then personally reassess to determine effects or improvement. An additional drawback is that consulting telepsychiatrist may not be well informed about local resources that can impact recommendations for disposition.

Dedicated Mental Health Wing of Medical Emergency Department

In this model, the ED has a separate area or room specifically for patients experiencing psychiatric emergencies. Typically, this area might be more relaxing and less chaotic than the main ED, and there may be staff members assigned who are knowledgeable in psychiatric care, especially psychiatric nurses, and possibly including social workers, therapists, and even on-site psychiatrists. As the patient is still located within the ED proper, the patients will remain under the supervision of the emergency medicine attending physician, and involved professional staff in this wing may have simultaneous responsibilities in other areas of the ED or hospital.

Pros and Cons: These specialized sections for psychiatric emergencies tend to be more therapeutically appropriate for individuals in crisis, particularly when the staff is well trained to manage such patients; there may be dimmed lighting, soothing music, and artwork or color schemes conducive to calming. Patients will often have the opportunity for longer stays than in the consultant model because they are not taking up beds allocated for traditional medical patients in the primary ED. The longer stays may allow time for healing, detoxification, and medications to become effective, each of which might improve the chances for a patient to avoid inpatient hospitalization. In addition because this area is part of the ED, medical emergency personnel are nearby and any medical concerns can be dealt with quickly and efficiently, including differential diagnosis cases where psychiatric versus neurologic conditions need further determination. This arrangement thus permits psychiatric treatment to commence for patients with serious medical comorbidities, who might otherwise be considered medically unsuitable for stand-alone psychiatric programs.

However, while this separate area of the ED has its benefits, it certainly also has its potential drawbacks. For one, despite its focus and adaptation for psychiatric care, it is still in the midst of the bustling ED, with its cacophony of loud noises, hectic personnel activity, sirens, and enigmatic machinery that can interfere with healing and increase anxiety. For the crisis patient, being separated from the main areas of the ED may lead to further marginalization or ostracization, along with lack of confidentiality, as other medical and nursing staff (and even other patients) might quickly identify the separated individuals as "the psych patients." Some EDs even dress their psychiatric patients in distinctive, different-colored gowns from the general population, with the idea being that this will assist the staff in recognizing "where patients belong" and help prevent elopements; however, this has often resulted in serious stigma, as others in the ED quickly recognize "that color means a psych patient"—and it may be completely unnecessary with more modern options such as video monitoring or electronic wristbands (26). Finally, on occasion, owing to a high census in the general ED population, these psychiatric wings of the ED might be turned into "float" areas where nonpsychiatric emergency patients will be housed, which may interfere or lead to less specialized care for the psychiatric patients.

Distinct Psychiatric Emergency Programs

Distinct Psychiatric Emergency Programs come in many shapes, sizes, and abbreviations. Names for these facilities include Emergency Psychiatric Assessment Treatment and Healing (EmPath) units, Psychiatric Emergency Services (PES), Psychiatric Urgent Care Centers (PsyUCC) and Crisis Stabilization Units (CSU), among other monikers. These programs can be part of a hospital campus, or completely free-standing and independent, and can vary in operations from simple screening processes and short-term interventions all the way up to comprehensive emergency psychiatric and medical diagnostic evaluation and treatment centers. Some sites even serve as the nexus of the region's acute mental health system, additionally housing such offerings as mobile crisis teams, outpatient clinics, and day treatment centers (27). Some wide-ranging Psychiatric Emergency Programs have even been described as comparable for psychiatric care to a Level 1 trauma facility for emergency medical care (28).

Rather than attempt an all-encompassing overview of these varied Distinct Psychiatric Emergency Programs, we will describe the basic models in order, from those with the lowest acuity capability and capacity to the most comprehensive and high-acuity sites. It should be understood that these descriptions are an attempt to categorize widely diverse operations, and there may be considerable overlap between the models suggested here at any particular site. For as it is often said about emergency psychiatry programs, "When you've seen one, you've seen one."

Psychiatric Urgent Care/Voluntary Crisis Centers

PsyUCC may be found as part of a community mental health clinic or may be stand-alone programs funded by the local behavioral health agency. Some psychiatric hospitals have urgent-care drop-in units where patients might predominantly be screened for possible hospitalization on-site, but the service may also offer referrals to outpatients or medication refills for lower-acuity individuals.

These walk-in care centers may be beneficial for several reasons, especially from the patient point of view. They are usually voluntary-only (meaning no patients held on involuntary psychiatric detention) and tend to focus on empathetic crisis counseling rather than acute medical interventions, so patients may feel they are in a more comfortable and supportive situation, without the stigma they may experience at a larger ED. The personnel are often therapists and social workers rather than nurses and doctors, although many of these programs also have access to prescribers to help clients obtain short-term medications or medication refills.

However, most urgent care centers will exclude individuals who are presently dangerous to self or others, have a history of dangerous behavior, or who are acutely hallucinating, medically compromised, intoxicated, or in substance withdrawal. Patients in those circumstances, which tend to be a substantial percentage of the overall urgent-needs behavioral health patients in a region, will still need to go to an ED or a PES for a higher level of care, or the center itself may have to call 911 or summon police should these more-acute patients present at the site. This can limit the overall effectiveness of these programs in reducing ED utilization for acute psychiatric conditions.

Crisis Stabilization Units

The concept of a "crisis stabilization unit" (CSU) has garnered varied meanings in different parts of the United States. Depending on location, a CSU could be anything from a hospital-based outpatient department to a community counseling "drop-in" center to a 30-day "halfway house"–style residential program (29,30). California's Medicaid Code defines a CSU as an outpatient "… service lasting less than 24 hours, to or on behalf of a beneficiary for a condition that requires more timely response than a regularly scheduled visit. Service activities include but are not limited to one or more of the following: assessment, collateral and therapy." (31). Sometimes a CSU aligned with this California description is referred to as a "23-hour program."

Most commonly across the United States, a CSU is a community-based, drop-in program with a focus on crisis intervention and primarily serving lower-acuity patients. This model often functions to provide more prompt access to counseling than a patient's regular provider can offer, or perhaps delivering brief respite from stressors or living situation issues, rather than as a site for active, high-acuity psychiatric intervention. Higher-acuity patients are more commonly referred out for psychiatric hospitalization; in some cases, the design of these programs even calls for immediate referral for hospitalization, perhaps even by contacting police or 911, as part of the CSU's paradigm for patients presenting with highly acute symptoms.

Many CSUs strive to create an environment that is more "homelike" than a typical hospital or ED, with comfortable furnishings and a setting that appears more like a clubhouse or hotel lobby than a clinic. It is believed that by making the treatment area a more welcoming, "less-restrictive" venue, patients will feel less stigma and anxiety, and be more relaxed, which will allow for calming and healing. A good example of this is with the "Living Room" concept, where in addition to the homelike setting, an emphasis is placed on using peer support specialists (recovering mental health patients who have specialized training to work on-site in therapeutic and supportive roles) with individuals in crisis (32).

EmPath Units

EmPath units are a more recent development—a hospital-based program that combines the calming and comfortable 23-hour short-term setting of the community CSU with the capacity and capability to work with higher-acuity patients, including those under both voluntary status and involuntary psychiatric detention, who otherwise would be relegated to hospital EDs or psychiatric inpatient units. EmPath units allow for hospital EDs to quickly medically screen individuals experiencing a psychiatric emergency, and then immediately move medically appropriate patients into the more therapeutic EmPath setting, where psychiatric assessment and treatment can take place, with the objective of prompt stabilization and avoiding inpatient hospitalization when possible.

The acronym "EmPath" stands for "Emergency Psychiatric Assessment, Treatment, and Healing" unit. Accordingly, the objectives of this unit are closely tied to the "Six Goals" of emergency psychiatry previously outlined. Whereas the "dedicated mental health wing" is often more of an observation unit, or even limited to a "boarding" section where psychiatric patients await transfer to an inpatient hospital bed or other dispositions, in the EmPath unit, attention is paid to medical stability along with prompt, trauma-informed evaluation and treatment, and constant noncoercive reassessment of an individual's condition by the unit staff, who are engaging via therapeutic alliance, with the aim of a disposition to the least restrictive setting (33).

EmPath units differ from the "dedicated mental health wing of the ED" in that EmPath units are discrete programs, completely separate from the ED, operating in an alternate location of the hospital (or even on a different campus) with a goal of quickly evaluating and then treating a patient for up to 24 hours. Whereas the ED wing will usually be staffed by ED team members and the patients remain under the jurisdiction of the ED emergency medicine attending, an EmPath unit is typically a thoroughly independent operation, with its own personnel, who are responsible for all of the assessment, treatment, and disposition of patients. However, an EmPath unit may not have a licensed independent medical provider on duty on-site at all times (though a psychiatrist will be available around the clock via telepsychiatry or on-call), and thus an EmPath unit, to be compliant with federal EMTALA laws, will be unable, in most designs, to accept presentations directly from the community or police. The most common EmPath unit model has all patients receiving a MSE at a general ED to rule out or stabilize nonpsychiatric EMCs and, once cleared, promptly transferred to the EmPath unit for psychiatric evaluation.

In an EmPath unit, patients are not relegated to individual rooms or isolated "beds" but are treated concurrently in a large room known as the "milieu." Here, each patient will be allowed to choose a "sleeper chair" or recliner, which can be folded flat for a nap or set up as a chair to facilitate group or individual therapy. There is ample room to move about and no requirement to stay in a certain location as would happen in a general ED, which can help to relax patients who lessen symptoms by walking or pacing around or who benefit from feeling less confined. Some EmPath units feature outdoor areas or gardens to further allow patients a spot for peacefulness and recovery.

To assist with the overall philosophy of a calming, restorative environment that encourages meeting individual needs, rather than coercion, patients are able to access food, beverages, and linens for themselves without asking permission from staff. And rather than the staff being behind a walled-off nursing station, professionals are interspersed with the patients in the milieu and thus will quickly recognize when a patient might need additional assistance. Unlocked "Calming Rooms" are available for individuals who might benefit from a period of privacy (34).

Because of the unit design and the overall focus on avoiding coercion, EmPath units have reported dramatically lower incidence of physical restraints, aggression, and assaults than more traditional units or EDs, even with a highly acute patient population under evaluation for dangerousness to self and/or others (35). While some might question placing such individuals at risk into a common room rather than isolation, this group setting has been demonstrated to encourage interpersonal engagement and respect and gives patients the feeling they have caring human contact rather than facing their troubles alone, with resulting positive outcomes (35). As in some CSUs and Urgent Care programs, peer support specialists are commonly also part of EmPath unit staffing, further enhancing the opportunity for therapeutic engagement.

Pros and Cons: A key part of the EmPath unit philosophy is that all newly arriving patients will receive an evaluation by a psychiatric provider as quickly as possible, with medications starting immediately when indicated. Ensuring that upsetting symptoms are assessed and treated promptly will further reduce patient distress and improve the chances for stabilization within the 24-hour limit. EmPath units have successfully reported diversion from inpatient hospitalization in more than three-quarters of high-acuity patients treated (35).

EmPath units can be very effective in reducing their affiliated ED's overcrowding and shortening its throughput times, especially in those that follow the model of "accepting all the ED's medically clear psychiatric patients promptly." However, their design still requires patients to be evaluated in a medical ED before transfer to the EmPath unit, and so this design still makes demands on the medical ED, and there can be limits on overall utilization. Thus, for regions with a high volume of psychiatric emergency patients daily, it may be justified to consider a completely independent PES program.

Psychiatric Emergency Services

As opposed to an EmPath unit, which pre-screens its patients and whose medical clearance is done prior to referral, a PES program is a distinct, ED-like operation that is solely dedicated to managing and treating psychiatric emergencies and can accept patients directly from the field via police or ambulance, or self-presentation (36). A PES is "EMTALA-compliant," meaning it is a receiving facility with a physician or other licensed independent professional on duty at all times, that is open for emergency care. In this regard, a PES can even be considered a specialized, mental health ED roughly analogous to a Level I trauma center (37).

Like many CSUs and EmPath units, under the most common definitions, a PES is considered an emergency outpatient program that is permitted to treat patients up to a maximum of 23 hours, 59 minutes; any patients needing care beyond 24 hours should be admitted to an inpatient psychiatric hospital.

PES programs typically can provide psychiatric evaluations and treatment for both voluntary patients and those individuals under involuntary psychiatric legal detentions. The designs can span from fully locked, partially locked, or completely unlocked facilities, depending on each unit's policies and obligations. PES may vary greatly depending on scope of practice and exit resources, with some sites also offering such services as detox centers, crisis counseling, drop-in medication clinics, long-term or short-term housing referrals, site-based mobile crisis units, partial hospitalization, day treatment, and intensive outpatient case management (22).

Yet despite the numerous differences between PES programs, there can be many commonalities as well. PES programs usually consist of full-time staff dedicated to and trained for psychiatric emergencies, including psychiatrists, psychiatric nurses, therapists, social workers, and mental health technicians. Evaluation, medical screening, diagnosis, and treatment can all be initiated quickly on-site; the more prompt the interventions, the greater the possibility of stabilization within 24 hours and avoidance of hospitalization (17).

One of the chief advantages of a PES, as it can accept individuals directly from the community, is that patients can bypass the entire process of going to a separate general medical ED first. This subjects patients to less stress, delays, stigma, confusion, and redundancy, while allowing for prompt initiation of psychiatric care with knowledgeable personnel and in the appropriate setting. This paradigm also can mean substantial cost savings to the overall system, by reducing expensive visits to multiple locations and avoiding costly and time-consuming interfacility transfers, and it significantly reduces medical ED crowding and improves throughput, in that most psychiatric patients in such systems will be at the appropriate site from the beginning rather than adding to medical ED censuses.

PES programs can be located near hospital EDs, elsewhere on hospital campuses, or even as stand-alone operations outside of hospital grounds. Many PES programs are directly affiliated with medical EDs or inpatient psychiatric hospitals, but neither of these is a requirement (15).

Pros and Cons: It is likely true that the great majority of emergency psychiatric patients can be stabilized, to the point of no longer requiring an acute or hospital level of care, in less than one day (38). With a focus on prompt interventions, and with a philosophy of attempting stabilization for up to 24 hours prior to making a decision on hospitalization, it is not uncommon for PES programs to divert patients from hospital stays in 75% or more of their cases (39). This not only can lead to better outcomes for patients, but can help preserve the limited numbers of available inpatient psychiatric beds for those individuals for whom there is truly no alternative.

The main drawback of PES programs is, given their 24/7 operational demands, that they may be much more expensive to operate than the other emergency psychiatry models; the expenditures required will usually mean that a PES should only be considered in systems with a volume of psychiatric emergencies in excess of 3,000 patients per year (23). Constructing a de novo PES facility can also be a costly undertaking, even if just remodeling an already existing physical plant—as there is a need for adequate space for patient care, along with enough room for staff, administration, registration, and billing personnel; even once constructed, there are still all the ongoing budgetary issues associated with operations of a distinct program (40). Another issue is the difficulty in recruiting and maintaining adequate and proper staffing around the clock. This can be challenging for these facilities, as it is not uncommon for busy and demanding crisis programs to experience a high degree of employee turnover (40).

Furthermore, because PES programs are EMTALA-compliant, patients must receive a MSE and be stabilized to the point that they are no longer a danger to themselves or others before a discharge can occur, or they must be admitted to an inpatient hospital. As noted before, psychiatric emergencies involving dangerousness qualify as EMCs under EMTALA. But it is important to note that although a PES must do a screening examination for medical concerns, it is not required to provide such services as advanced life support; EMTALA recognizes the existence of specialty emergency centers with limited capabilities and permits transports from such sites to higher-level-of-care EDs (3). Thus, despite having 24-hour physicians on duty, PES programs that are not colocated with a medical ED will typically not have the capability to stabilize serious medical conditions. A PES such as this will thus necessitate acute medical conditions be stabilized elsewhere prior to arrival and will need to rapidly transport outpatients with medical emergencies arising or arriving on-site to a medical ED, even calling 911 in urgent situations.

Regional Dedicated Psychiatric Emergency Services Programs

Presently, most PES programs in the United States have a limited catchment area or are part of a specific medical center. However, there are a number of "Regional Dedicated Psychiatric Emergency Services" programs—which accept all emergency psychiatric patients from a defined widespread geographic area, directly from the field. Such programs also have a collaborative relationship with a number of otherwise-unaffiliated EDs, as the higher-level-of-care ED transfer destination for all their psychiatric emergency patients (41).

This regional design allows for a shorter duration of "boarding times" of psychiatric patients in medical EDs. One regional PES showed more than an 80% improvement over comparable boarding time state averages—remarkably, for an overall "cost per patient" less expensive than the average price tag of that same patient languishing those same hours in a medical ED, merely waiting for a disposition, when little or no psychiatric care is occurring (39). And because of the ability to bypass general EDs and present directly to the regional PES, the number of psychiatric emergencies evaluated in the area medical EDs are a much smaller percentage of the total that would be seen in systems without a regional PES (39). As such, it not only allows for patients to receive treatment in an appropriate setting much more quickly but also reduces ED crowding and overall expenditures that are incurred by areas with high censuses and lengthy boarding times.

Alternative Crisis Options

In addition to the emergency psychiatry models outlined above, there are several other alternative strategies for assisting those in psychiatric crisis that are typically off hospital grounds; these include mobile crisis teams and acute diversion units such as crisis respite and crisis residential housing.

Mobile Crisis Teams

Mobile crisis teams are usually comprised of mental health professionals who travel via car or van to the site of a patient in crisis, instead of having police or emergency providers bring the patient to a fixed site. Mobile teams are found in many communities around the United States and can provide a wide range of on-site crisis intervention, de-escalation, and conflict resolution services, as well as assistance with housing and access to more permanent care (42). Some systems have police summon mobile teams as a consultation for possible involuntary psychiatric detentions, while others may ride along with specially trained police units known as Crisis Intervention Teams (CIT). Because mobile crisis teams are more focused on intervening in emerging situations in the field, they are not a replacement for ED or PES services, but they can often help resolve a patient's crisis without having to transport to a treatment center. Mobile crisis teams can be invaluable assistance for solving problems where they occur and in the prevention of unnecessary ED presentations (43).

Acute Diversion Units/Crisis Respite/ Crisis Residential Housing

Residential programs (sometimes called Acute Diversion Units or ADUs) are community-based facilities that are often in actual private houses, allowing the care to take place in a setting that is comfortable and integrated into the outside world. These can be ideal for patients who would normally be thought to require several days of intensive mental health care but are eager to engage in treatment, willing to participate in groups and activities, and have not reached a level of acuity or dangerousness that would necessitate hospitalization. Given the nonclinical setting, much of the stigma and difficulties some patients associate with hospitalization can be mitigated. Most commonly, these programs will take in 8 to 16 patients at a time for up to a maximum of 2 weeks (44), but some will accept individuals for 30 days or even longer (45). Most ADUs require a prescreening from an ED or PES, but some may also accept patients from mobile crisis units or other community providers.

SUMMARY

With the number of psychiatric emergencies on the rise, EDs often find themselves inundated with sufferers of psychiatric crises. The needs of this population can often surpass most general medical ED personnel's expertise and capability and will thus require more specialized interventions. While psychiatric consultation, including that done via telemedicine, can work well in EDs with a low volume of psychiatric crises, areas with a higher census of psychiatric emergencies will serve their population best by developing urgent care alternatives such as Crisis Centers, CSUs, EmPath units, and/or PES facilities. Surprisingly enough, although these emergency psychiatry programs can seem expensive when viewed in isolation, they can actually provide much-needed, targeted, immediate, and appropriate care for patients in crisis. This will actually save systems substantial dollars in other ways, by reducing ED utilization, eliminating boarding, and improving throughput times, all while successfully diverting patients away from unnecessary, highly restrictive and costly hospital inpatient admissions.

REFERENCES

1. Weiss, A. J., Barrett, M. L., Heslin, K. C., & Stocks, C. (2016). *Trends in emergency department visits involving mental and substance use disorders, 2006–2013*. Retrieved July 5, 2018, from https://www.hcup-us.ahrq.gov/reports/statbrieds/sb216-Mental-Substance-Use-Disorder-ED-Visit-Trends.pdf.
2. Moore, B. J., & Owens, P. L. (2017). *Trends in emergency department visits, 2006–2014*. Rockville, MD: HCUP Statistical Brief #227 [Internet]; Retrieved from http://www.hcup-us.ahrq.gov/reports/statbriefs/sb227-Emergency-Department-Visit-Trends.pdf.
3. Department of Health and Human Services, Centers for Medicare and Medicaid Services. (2010). *State operations manual. Appendix V. Emergency Medical Treatment and Labor Act (EMTALA) Appendix V. interpretive guidelines – responsibility of medicare participating hospitals in emergency cases*. Retrieved from https://www.cms.gov/Regulations-and-Guidance/Guidance/Manuals/Downloads/som107ap_v_emerg.pdf.
4. Owens, P. L., Mutter, R., & Stocks, C. (2007). *Mental health and substance abuse-related emergency department visits among adults*. Retrieved July 5, 2016, from http://www.hcup-us.ahrq.gov/reports/statbreifs/sb92.pdf.
5. Torry, E. F., Entsminger, K., Geller, J., et al. (2008). *The shortage of public beds for mentally ill persons*. Retrieved July 5, 2018, from http://www.treatmentadvocacycenter.org/storage/documents/the_shortage_of_publichospital_beds.pdf.
6. Holloman, G. H., & Zeller, S. L. (2012). Overview of project BETA: Best practices in evaluation and treatment of agitation. *Western Journal of Emergency Medicine, 13*(1), 1–2.
7. Chennapan, K., Mullinax, S., Anderson, E., et al. (2018). Medical screening of mental health patients in the emergency department: A systematic review. *Journal of Emergency Medicine, 55*(6), 799–812. doi:10.1016/j.jemermed.2018.09.014.
8. Citrome, L. L., Holt, R. I., & Zachry, W. M. (2007). Risk of treatment-emergent diabetes mellitus in patients receiving antipsychotics. *Annals of Pharmacotherapy, 41*, 1593–1603.
9. Kar, S. K., Kumar, D., Singh, P., & Upadhyay, P. K. (2015). Psychiatric manifestation of chronic subdural hematoma: The unfolding of mystery in a homeless patient. *Indian Journal of Psychological Medicine, 37*(2), 239–242.

10. Beauford, J. E., McNiel, D. E., & Binder, R. L. (1997). Utility of the initial therapeutic alliance in evaluating psychiatric patients' risk of violence. *American Journal of Psychiatry, 154,* 1272–1276.

11. Kessler, R. C., McLaughlin, K. A., Green, J. G., et al. (2010). Childhood adversities and adult psychopathology in the WHO World Mental Health Surveys. *British Journal of Psychiatry, 197*(5), 378–385.

12. Khalifeh, H., Moran, P., Borschmann, R., et al. (2015). Domestic and sexual violence against patients with severe mental illness. *Psychologie Medicale, 45*(4), 875–886.

13. Nelson, E. A., Maruish, M. E., & Axler, J. L. (2000). Effects of discharge planning and compliance with outpatient appointments on readmission rates. *Psychiatric Services, 51,* 885–889.

14. Zeller, S. L. (2010). Treatment of psychiatric patients in emergency settings. *Primary Psychiatry, 17,* 35–41. Retrieved from http://primarypsychiatry.com/treatment-of-psychiatric-patients-in-emergency-settings/.

15. Fishkind, A. B., & Berlin, J. S. (2008). Structure and function of psychiatric emergency services. In Glick, R. L., Berlin, J. S., Fishkind, A. B., & Zeller, S. L. (Eds.). *Emergency psychiatry: Principles and practice* (pp. 9–23). Philadelphia, PA: Wolters Kluwer Health/Lippincott Williams & Wilkins.

16. Hoot, N. R., & Aronsky, D. (2008). Systematic review of emergency department crowding: Causes, effects, and solutions. *Annals of Emergency Medicine, 52,* 126–136.

17. Zeller, S. L. (2013). Psychiatric boarding: Averting long waits in emergency rooms. *Psychiatric Times, 30*(11). Retrieved from http://www.psychiatrictimes.com/psychiatric-emergencies/psychiatric-boarding-averting-long-waits-emergency-rooms.

18. Flaherty, J. A., & Fichtner, C. G. (1992). Impact of emergency psychiatry training on residents' decisions to hospitalize patients. *Academic Medicine, 67,* 585–586.

19. Neauport, A., Rodgers, R. F., Simon, N. M., Birmes, P. J., Schmitt, L., & Bui, E. (2012). Effects of a psychiatric label on medical residents' attitudes. *International Journal of Social Psychiatry, 58,* 485–487.

20. Yellowlees, P., Burke, M. M., Marks, S. L., Hilty, D. M., & Shore, J. H. (2008). Emergency telepsychiatry. *Journal of Telemedicine and Telecare, 14,* 277–281.

21. Seidel, R. W., & Kilgus, M. D. (2014). Agreement between telepsychiatry assessment and face-to-face assessment for emergency department psychiatry patients. *Journal of Telemedicine and Telecare, 20,* 59–62.

22. Narasimhan, M., Druss, B. G., Hockenberry, J. M., et al. (2015). Impact of a telepsychiatry program at emergency departments statewide on the quality, utilization, and costs of mental health services. *Psychiatric Services, 66*(11), 1167–1172. Retrieved from http://ps.psychiatryonline.org/doi/pdf/10.1176/appi.ps.201400122.

23. Butterfield, A. (2018). Telepsychiatric evaluation and consultation in emergency care settings. *Child and Adolescent Psychiatric Clinics of North America, 27*(3), 467–478.

24. Southard, E. P., Neufeld, J. D., & Laws, S. (2014). Telemental health evaluations enhance access and efficiency in a critical access hospital emergency department. *Telemedicine Journal and e-Health, 20,* 664–668.

25. Telepsychiatry program eases patient crowding in the ED, expedites mental health services to patients and providers. *ED Management.* (2013), *25,* 121–124.

26. Macy, D., & Johnston, M. (2013). Using electronic wristbands and a triage protocol to protect mental health patients in the emergency department. *Journal of Nursing Care Quality, 22,* 180–184.

27. Lee, T. S., Renaud, E. F., & Hills, O. F. (2003). Emergency psychiatry: An emergency treatment hub-and-spoke model of psychiatric emergency services. *Psychiatric Services, 54,* 1590–1591, 1594.

28. Allen, M. H. (1999). Level 1 psychiatric emergency services. The tools of the crisis sector. *Psychiatric Clinics of North America, 22,* 13–34, vii.

29. Adams, C. L., & El-Mallakh, R. S. (2009). Patient outcome after treatment in a community-based crisis stabilization unit. *The Journal of Behavioral Health Services & Research, 36,* 396–399.

30. Wolff, A. (2008). Development of a psychiatric crisis stabilization unit. *Journal of Emergency Nursing, 34,* 458–459.

31. Barclays Official California Code of Regulations. Title 9: Rehabilitative and Developmental Services. Division 1: Department of Mental Health. Chapter 11: Medi-Cal Specialty Mental Health Services. §1810.210: Crisis Stabilization.

32. Heyland, M., Emery, C., & Shattell, M. (2013). The living room, a community crisis respite program: Offering people in crisis an alternative to emergency departments. *Global Journal of Community Psychology Practice, 4*(3), 1–8.

33. Zeller, S. L. (2018). What psychiatrists need to know: Patients in the emergency department. *Psychiatric Times, 35*(8), 1–3.

34. Miller, V. (2018). UI Hospitals debuts more help for mental health patients – new "stabilization unit" eases long waits in the emergency room. *Iowa Gazette*, 9–10.

35. Zeller, S. L. (2017). EmPath units as a solution for ED psychiatric patient boarding. *Psychiatry Advisor*. Retrieved February 9, 2019, from http://www.psychiatryadvisor.com/practice-management/EmPath-mental-health-crisis-management-emergency-department-setting/article/687420/.

36. Allen, M. H., Forster, P., Zealberg, J., & Currier, G. (2002). *Report and recommendations regarding psychiatric emergency and crisis services. A review and model program descriptions*. Washington, DC: American Psychiatric Association Task Force on Psychiatric Emergency Services. Retrieved from https://www.psychiatry.org/File%20Library/Psychiatrists/Directories/Library-and-Archive/task-force-reports/tfr2002_EmergencyCrisis.pdf.

37. Allen, M. H., & Currier, G. W. (1999). Medical assessment in the psychiatric emergency service. *New Directions for Mental Health Services*, (82), 21–28.

38. Wilson, M. P., & Zeller, S. L. (2012). Introduction: Reconsidering psychiatry in the emergency department. *Journal of Emergency Medicine, 43*, 771–772.

39. Zeller, S. L., Calma, N., & Stone, A. (2014). Effects of a dedicated regional psychiatric emergency service on boarding of psychiatric patients in area emergency departments. *The Western Journal of Emergency Medicine, 15*, 1–6.

40. Fishkind, A. B., Zeller, S. L., & Snodgress, M. (2008). Administration of psychiatric emergency services. In Glick, R. L., Berlin, J. S., Fishkind, A. B., & Zeller, S. L. (Eds.). *Emergency psychiatry: Principles and practice* (pp. 497–512). Philadelphia, PA: Wolters Kluwer Health/Lippincott Williams & Wilkins.

41. Intriguing model significantly reduces boarding of psychiatric patients, need for inpatient hospitalization. *ED Management*. (2015), 27, 1–5.

42. Muehsam, J. P. (2018). Association between clinical observations and a mobile crisis team's level of care recommendations. *Communications Mental Health Journal*, 1–7.

43. Fahim, C., Semovski, V., & Younger, J. (2016). The Hamilton mobile crisis rapid response team: A first-responder mental health service. *Psychiatric Services, 67*(8), 929.

44. Patel, R. M. (2008). Crisis residential settings. In Glick, R. L., Berlin, J. S., Fishkind, A. B., & Zeller, S. L. (Eds.). *Emergency psychiatry: Principles and practice* (pp. 393–412). Philadelphia, PA: Wolters Kluwer Health/Lippincott Williams & Wilkins.

45. Chafetz, L., & Collins-Bride, G. (2017). Primary care for mentally ill adults in acute residential treatment facilities. *Issues in Mental Health Nursing, 38*(10), 791–797.

2

Boarding of Psychiatric Patients in the Emergency Department: Flow, Throughput, and Systemic Change

Jon S. Berlin, Scott L. Zeller

Given their Emergency Medical Treatment and Active Labor Act (EMTALA) requirement to evaluate and stabilize everyone who presents for care, hospital emergency departments (EDs) have always placed a premium on effective flow of patients from their front door to discharge; any program with inefficiency and delays will soon become fraught with overcrowding and unhappy customers. But, for all the efforts by EDs to maximize patient movement, even the most exemplary facilities could not have been prepared for the dramatic increase of mental health emergencies coming to EDs in the past decade, a deluge that shows no signs of abating. Psychiatric emergency presentations in the United States increased to 44.1% from 2006 to 2014 alone, with a remarkable 414% jump in the number of suicidality cases treated in EDs over that period (1). This massive influx has been overwhelming for many centers, and too often the result has been high numbers of psychiatric patients wedged into EDs, waiting for evaluations or dispositions for significant periods of time, a phenomenon commonly referred to as psychiatric patient "boarding" (2).

Presently, psychiatric patient boarding is an unfortunate situation that arises in over 90% of US hospital EDs on a regular basis (3). Individuals suffering a psychiatric emergency or crisis—whether transported by first responders or seeking help on their own—commonly find the only possible destination in their community to be the local hospital ED. Yet these EDs frequently are ill-equipped, in terms of staff and physical space, to intervene effectively with mental health patients.

Thus, far too often, little is offered in the way of actual treatment: care plans are limited to isolation (often with a sitter), sedation, physical restraint, boarding, and transfer to a psychiatric facility.

A frequently suggested culprit for the boarding problem is the dwindling number of psychiatric inpatient beds nationwide while behavioral emergency cases have increased. But this is an oversimplified analysis that has led to an impractical call for reopening, or opening more, psychiatric hospitals and inpatient beds to solve the boarding dilemma. True, more beds are needed in some regions. But as a sole solution, this approach perpetuates an incorrect mantra about psychiatric crisis that it is one of the few medical emergencies for which hospitalization should be the default approach to care. It also results in far too many patients being unnecessarily hospitalized at a very restrictive and expensive level of care.

Unfortunately, with transfer to an inpatient bed as the ultimate goal, extended boarding has become a regular occurrence. The average boarding time for a psychiatric patient—defined as from the time he is considered medically clear for transfer or inpatient admission to the moment he finally departs the ED—can run between 7 and 34 hours across the country, although in some outlier cases delays have even persisted for weeks (4,5).

Boarding creates a host of problems: It can detract resources from an ED's ability to care for its other patients. It can lead to unsafe patient care conditions in which psychiatric illness can escalate, resulting in poorer outcomes and increased difficulty arranging transfers. It can result in an increase in patient walkouts, medical errors, and negligence claims. It is expensive—one study estimated the average cost to an ED to board each psychiatric patient to be $2,264 (2). It may be viewed as an infringement of a patient's legal right to treatment, exposing the hospital to problems with litigation and accreditation. In 2014, the State of Washington outlawed boarding of involuntary patients and established the requirement that ED patients awaiting disposition receive active evaluation and treatment appropriate to their condition (6,7). In 2014 and 2015, The Joint Commission issued Quick Safety alerts regarding the care of boarded patients and ways to reduce the boarding of psychiatric patients (8,9).

Healthcare systems have already confronted scarce medical/surgical beds in general hospitals by expanding outpatient and ambulatory services in nonpsychiatric medical specialties (10). A similar approach can be taken in psychiatry, expanding capacity in emergency and outpatient levels of care.

Indeed, studies and clinical experience have found that with prompt intervention, sixty to eighty percent of psychiatric emergencies can be resolved in less than 24 hours, without the need for inpatient admission (11-14). The stumbling block in the past has been lack of swift access to onsite psychiatric consultation and discharge planning.

ED boarding does not only occur with psychiatric patients. There can be a shortage of hospital beds in other medical specialties, such as intensive care (15). But ED staff tend to be less well-versed in psychiatric care than in other specialties, so much so, in fact, that it is not uncommon to hear ED personnel refer to psychiatric cases as "nonmedical" (16).

What constitutes a boarding *crisis* per se is subjective. By definition, boarding is never a good situation, even for one patient, and it may be onerous enough for that one person to consider it a crisis. From the ED perspective, most sites are able to absorb and withstand a finite number of boarding cases. The emergency medicine (EM) ethos is to be adaptable and creative. However, when the frequency, severity, and duration of boarding cases increase to the point of dominating the ED environment, when the situation negatively impacts staff morale and effectiveness, and when there is no relief in sight, at that point the term "boarding crisis" begins to be invoked.

Another marker is when the media takes notice. In recent years, many major newspaper and television outlets have featured prominent stories on this troubling new phenomenon (17-19).

Compared to EDs, psychiatric emergency services (PESs) tend not to have the same institutional knowledge of flow and throughput. Yet lately PESs have begun to experience their own unmanageable patient surges and boarding dilemmas (20,21). Moreover, whenever PES boarding is severe enough to cause ambulance and squad car diversion, boarding is likely to overflow to affiliated EDs. Thus, while it is correct to expect the creation of a PES to relieve pressure on the emergency medical system, with regard to continuous improvement of clinical process, PESs cannot afford to be complacent about boarding either.

An analysis of boarding typically identifies areas of concern that are both internal and external to an ED's function. While the creation of a PES might be the single most cost-effective solution for a city or region with a serious boarding problem, there is a wide range of possible improvements that can be made. Meanwhile, individual hospital EDs often find that the initial impetus for upgrading local psychiatric emergency services must come from within the ED itself.

BRIEF LITERATURE REVIEW

There has been a progression in the literature on boarding over the last 2 decades. Stefan's landmark book in 2006 detailing various challenges of psychiatric care in the ED accurately describes boarding but does not focus on it (22). Bender, Pande, and Ludwig produced an extensive literature review on psychiatric boarding for the US Department of Health and Human Services in 2008 (13). Alakeson, Pande, and Ludwig followed this with "A plan to reduce emergency room 'boarding'..." in 2010 (14). Nicks and Manthey wrote on the impact of boarding in the ED in 2012 (2). Zeller, Calma, and Stone published on the beneficial effects of a dedicated regional PES on boarding in 2014 (12). The following year the American College of Emergency Physicians, in collaboration with the Operations Workgroup of the Coalition on Psychiatric Emergencies, created a white paper on practical solutions to boarding (23). This effort included lessons from the Alameda model, the Banner model, and the Milwaukee boarding project. In 2018, the board of the American Psychiatric Association (APA) approved an APA resource document on "Psychiatric Boarding of Mentally Ill Patients in Emergency Departments" (24). The lead article of a recent issue of the *New England Journal of Medicine* is a cautionary tale about the negative impact of psychiatric bed shortages on medical decision-making. It describes the case of a disabled and severely disturbed ED patient and implies that staff's intense aversion to boarding him led them to "demedicalize" his psychiatric illness and excessively abbreviate his treatment (25). Brown, Buttlaire, and Phillips describe a systematic approach to improving ED process and flow for psychiatric patients (26). Their account is an excellent companion piece to our section below on Internal Approaches.

REDUCTION OF BOARDING

A comprehensive plan to reduce boarding focuses on three areas: reducing input, improving throughput, and facilitating output. Making an impact on input and output involves collaboration with external community partners. But an ED is in the strongest position to influence others when it improves its own process first. We begin with a discussion of necessary internal changes.

Internal Approaches

Medical directors of PESs in the United States report being able to appropriately avoid hospitalization in a high percentage of their cases (12,27). In our experience, they achieve a much higher rate of diversion than is typical for psychiatric emergencies seen in EDs, and of course this reduces the number of patients waiting for beds. Therefore, EDs with boarding should consider the concepts, approaches, and experience that inform PES clinical practice.

A Subcategory of Medical Emergency

The majority of individuals experiencing a psychiatric crisis do not need high-acuity, nonpsychiatric, emergency medical care. They need psychiatric emergency care and can best be treated in a center specializing in emergency psychiatry and mental health. However, these centers are not ubiquitous, and most psychiatric emergencies in this country present first to an ED. When they do, psychiatric

and mental health specialists embedded in the ED should be the ones taking care of them. Unfortunately, these personnel are usually unavailable as well. The preferred specialty resources for real-world EM professionals exist more in theory than practice. It therefore becomes EM's mission to take care of these individuals themselves.

Psychiatry is a branch of medicine, and psychiatric emergencies are a subcategory of medical emergencies. They are only distinguishable as one type of medical emergency, just as "cardiac" and "surgical" are each one type. They may be more unique in some ways than the other types, but they are not nonmedical. In the context of the present discussion, therefore, it is a bit cumbersome to specify whether the medical emergencies one is referring to are "psychiatric" or "nonpsychiatric," but it is necessary.

The medical side of psychiatry is no more hypothetical than the humanistic side of nonpsychiatric medicine. New developments in psychiatric genetics, biochemistry, and neurophysiology appear almost daily. EM educators and directors are equally clear about their goals for trainees and staff. Most, if not all, emergency medicine textbooks have chapters on psychiatric emergencies (28). In the preface to the first edition of his distinctive textbook, Zun notes that "expertise in management of behavioral emergencies is just one of several proficiencies expected of emergency care providers, regardless of their training or access to specialty consultants" (29).

The EMTALA legislates this expectation. It defines Emergency Medical Conditions as "acute symptoms of sufficient severity (including severe pain, psychiatric disturbances and/or symptoms of substance abuse) such that the absence of immediate medical attention could reasonably be expected to result in - (i) Placing the health of the individual... in serious jeopardy" (30). EMTALA adds that, in the case of psychiatric emergencies, if an individual expressing suicidal or homicidal thoughts or gestures is determined dangerous to self or others, he would be considered to have an Emergency Medical Condition (31).

The mind-brain duality in psychiatry, and the corollary medical/nonmedical continuum in mental health, can be somewhat confusing. The analogous terminology for alcohol detoxification helps to clarify it: Lesser degrees of alcohol abuse and dependence are often handled in facilities referred to as "social detox," which is considered a "nonmedical" setting. The cases are uncomplicated and involve little or no physical dependence on alcohol. Somewhat more serious cases, with moderate physical dependence, require nursing care and medication protocols. The programs and facilities that treat them are referred to as "medically enhanced detox." Finally, the most severe cases—for example, delirium tremens—require intravenous medications and fluids, cardiac monitoring, and daily or more frequent medical decision-making. These interventions, which usually take place on a medical unit, fall under the heading of "medical detox."

In a similar way, less severe degrees of mental health crisis such as a flare up of long-standing auditory hallucinations might be managed in a counseling center or a subacute "nonmedical" facility. Mental health staff in the facility may also be "nonmedical." They may encourage a patient to take his medication, making the program "medically enhanced," but they themselves may have a theoretical orientation for working with clients that in their minds (staff and clients) is decidedly "nonmedical."

On the other hand, the most serious psychiatric emergencies, such as a bipolar disorder with the triad of manic psychosis, treatment refusal, and physical violence, need an ED, preferably a PES with an adjacent or neighboring ED. Attempts to address the treatment refusal and violence will be based on a psychological and behavioral approach, while the management of the mania itself will usually involve medication and therefore be considered biological or medical.

Types of Boarding Cases

How should EM providers best focus their efforts? What are the conditions and interventions that alternatively facilitate or impede a speedy transition through the ED? One good place to start is with an analysis of actual ED cases that end up boarding. The ED is a safety net. Therefore, given the assumption that many of these patients do not need a psychiatric inpatient bed, or did not when they arrived, the particular makeup of this cohort will reflect gaps in mental healthcare specific to one's own location or locale.

There are a number of clinical scenarios, each offering lessons about how to improve ED throughput:

1. *Nonemergency.* A verbal outburst at home in the heat of the moment, or a life crisis of some kind; an evaluation by someone in the community whose tolerance of risk is too low, for example, someone who mistakenly equates all types of suicidal ideation with high suicide risk. Any of these could result in a mental health hold that might safely be discontinued. The initial hold may or may not have been necessary to provide brief containment and galvanize therapeutic changes in the environment. Regardless, a reevaluation combined with a beneficial brief intervention can turn a boarding case into an outpatient case.

2. *Resolved emergency.* An individual arrives in a state of crisis that was initially serious enough to warrant hospitalization, and possibly involuntary detention, but has since abated. For example, the crisis may have been a bout of alcohol-induced suicidality or a maladjustment to a life stressor (an adjustment disorder) that spontaneously resolved. The individual needs a reevaluation to confirm the improved condition, brief intervention, and help with linkage to community resources.

3. *Exaggerated or feigned symptoms; frequent visitors.* EM staff are accustomed to seeing individuals who present with a malingered chief complaint that claims to require hospitalization. Sometimes they are also frequent visitors, well-known to staff. But staff may not have sufficient experience with such conditions and want psychiatry to make the call. What the patient really does need is not always that obvious. On occasion, an admission or extended ED/PES stay should be considered: the patient is unknown to the system, it is time for a careful inpatient reevaluation, the patient may actually be experiencing a worse-than-usual crisis, or the outpatient providers feel completely at a loss and request assistance. These same considerations often apply to frequent visitors. More commonly, the patient does need to be discharged, but first needs an evaluation, brief intervention, possibly a curbside consult, good documentation, teamwork with outpatient staff, and management by a practitioner with decent risk tolerance and equanimity in handling a patient's displeasure.

4. *Intermediate crisis.* An individual presents to an ED for a moderate degree of crisis. It may be psychotic agitation in the context of previously diagnosed mental illness, along with a voluntary request for treatment. It may be a flare up of severe and persistent suicidality. These are cases that PESs treat as a time-sensitive emergency in the making and often successfully discharge after a short stay. ED staff, however, tend to give them a low priority. The person's psychiatric distress is not overt. He is not acting out so he is triaged to wait. ED staff lack the training and the protocol to do some basic things that are helpful: offer him the comfort of a safe and welcoming area, tell him when he can expect to be seen, inquire how long he can wait to be seen, and what he needs in the meantime. Typically, without these calming measures, this patient will escalate, sometimes to the point of no longer being cooperative or voluntary. He may shut down or try to elope. He may become so much sicker that security or the police needs to be called, and he ends up on emergency detention. If there are no beds in the community, what started out as a case that could have been handled with an intermediate ED stay and release becomes a boarding case.

5. *High-acuity, possible iatrogenic escalation.* This scenario is similar to the ones in #4, except that the person is often on a mental health hold and is more seriously suicidal or agitated. If staff with prescriptive authority and good verbal de-escalation skills engage him at the front door, he might respond to noncoercive de-escalation (32-34). Depending on the severity of his condition, he might still require admission to a psychiatric facility, but if a physical confrontation is avoided, the options for disposition increase: more facilities will be willing to consider taking him. If he engages in treatment and becomes a voluntary patient, possibly making the emergency detention unnecessary, this may increase the disposition options even further. He might become appropriate for a nonhospital, community-based facility. On the other hand, if he is not approached skillfully or in a timely manner, he could easily end up in restraints. This increases boarding time as well as the demands on staff.

6. *Special populations.* Pediatric, geriatric, veterans, homeless, developmentally disabled, substance use, med-psych: Specialized programming and staff exist for the psychiatric treatment needs of each of these populations, and different regions of the country may have different ratios of disease burden and different gaps in the continuum of care. An analysis of the types of boarding cases in one's own ED can direct initiatives for development of internal program tracks, along with targeted hiring and training of staff.

7. *Needs hospitalization.* Very high risk for harm to self or others, treatment-refractory psychiatric illness (35) (frequent visitors often fall into this category), unsuccessful ED and community-based crisis interventions, new-onset psychosis, and special population cases which must have a specialty bed, such as a child: When psychiatric beds are unavailable, these are examples of conditions for which it will be very difficult to avoid boarding. However, the same types of internal improvements in the ED for the other conditions discussed can mitigate iatrogenic complications for these cases, as well as expenditure of staff time and energy during an extended boarding stay.

Provide Treatment

*Treatment **versus** triage.* Historically, busy EM practitioners have limited their role with psychiatric problems to triage and assessment: Perform the nonpsychiatric medical tasks and decide whether to admit to psychiatry or not. Admission secures the psychiatric consultation they need, and as long as there are sufficient beds, this approach works (though it may not work at all for the patient when the admission is only expedient for the practitioner). When the beds are insufficient and when back-end resources in general are inadequate, boarding begins to occur. Addressing these internal problems requires attention to these two components: embrace of psychiatric cases as worthy of one's full attention and close inquiry into one's boarding cases for trends in the cases that might be finessed into a nonadmission with the right approach. The third component is to *shift out of a triage mode into a treatment mode.*

Allen articulated the usefulness of this idea for emergency psychiatry over 20 years ago (36), before the boarding crisis. The inspiration draws on the therapeutic energy of EM. When an asthma patient presents in the ED with acute bronchospasm, breathing treatment accompanies evaluation and the hoped-for disposition is discharge home. Similarly, when a patient with schizophrenia presents with command hallucinations to harm himself, the default mode should be evaluation and treatment, not hospitalization. A good intervention in the ED may be all the person needs.

Specifically, one needs to establish a working alliance; conduct a sensitive but focused interview; elicit from the individual what he thinks is the problem and what he thinks he needs; collaborate on a treatment plan, including appropriate and timely medication; address nonpsychiatric medical questions; enlist other staff to assist as needed; reevaluate the patient periodically as treatment is in progress; obtain collateral history, in order to marshal social supports and determine a reasonable end point for acute care; and finally, if moving toward discharge, engage or reengage the individual with outside treatment providers. One must also be prepared for ambiguity and intense emotions, on both sides of the interaction. The skill set for this case is different than that required for other cases in medicine, such as acute bronchospasm, but not completely different. The steps to take follow the same iterative process of all clinical medicine: gather data, interpret and synthesize the data into an assessment, and decide on current and future interventions, both diagnostic and therapeutic.

Treatment is important for another reason: to prevent decompensation of the patient during their stay in the ED. Psychiatric conditions are fluid and changeable. A patient who is calm and agreeable to voluntary hospitalization in a private facility may become impatient and leave the ED or become agitated and require a more complicated disposition. Therefore, with rare exception, initiating appropriate medication and other treatment is virtually always recommended.

Early intervention protocols for acute psychiatric emergencies bring the idea of treatment versus triage to the ED's front door (37). They have yet to be as codified as the protocols for myocardial infarction, stroke, and sepsis, but they are under construction, and they should in time prove to be just as useful. One of the main ones will be based on the set of principles for de-escalation of agitation. These are critical to better flow and better outcomes. In some cases, they can make the difference between successful treatment and release versus additional escalation, coercive measures, and boarding. Another emerging protocol addresses evaluation and management of the patient with suicidal concerns (38-41). It, too, promotes active treatment, as well as psychoeducation, risk reduction strategies, and safe release to community treatment and supports for patients who are no longer a high risk after ED interventions. Active treatment is the guiding principle of a new framework proposed for early intervention in the ED with opiate use disorders. They consider initiation of buprenorphine. The target of the authors' approach is the opioid crisis, not boarding, but the idea is the same (42). Similarly, for select cases of alcohol dependence, one might consider initiating long-acting intramuscular naltrexone.

Iterative process refers to the repeating three-part process in clinical care of gathering data, interpreting and synthesizing the data, and intervening. It is another way of emphasizing the treatment component of emergency care. In an emergency, initial interventions based on preliminary findings are often needed immediately. This remains a key concept in EM. For example, in the case of the severely injured patient, start with tourniquets and antifibrinolytic therapy (43). Once the patient is stabilized, additional data are gathered, the assessment is refined, and the treatment becomes more targeted. This is a schema that encourages ED staff to integrate treatment with evaluation. It also implies the need to see patients more than once during an episode of care as needed, thereby increasing the chances of disposition to a lower level of care. For example, the schizophrenia patient with command hallucinations may improve significantly in the ED with medicine, nourishment, and emotional support. Repeat evaluation is often not performed when working in a triage mode; it is essential in the treatment mode.

The idea of iterative process also inspires success with some of the patients who are high utilizers of the emergency system. ED staff should try to string together the results of an individual's multiple visits, leading to a cumulative effect of therapeutic engagement and ultimately the transition of his therapeutic alliance away from the ED to an outpatient provider.

Turning an acute patient into an outpatient. Adapted from the overall operational goal that Sederer describes for psychiatric inpatient treatment (44), this concept of turning an acute patient into an outpatient applies equally well to psychiatric emergency care, allowing for the fact that, in the case of inpatient admissions, the ED only initiates the transformation. Nevertheless, this is a powerful idea that integrates the various aspects of an evaluation and gives direction to the entire team. It can motivate uncooperative patients who feel locked up to work with us once they realize their goal of freedom is shared. It also promotes a partnership with outpatient providers that in the long run pays multiple dividends.

Consider the classic emergency, a police mental health hold. It has three parts: (1) acute psychiatric illness or substance disorder, (2) high risk for harm to self or others, and (3) inability or unwillingness to cooperate with voluntary treatment (45). Each of these elements exists on a spectrum of severity, and each of them will hopefully be ameliorated to some extent: symptoms treated, risk reduced, and engagement achieved. The elements are semi-independent variables; their positive and negative fluctuations are usually linked. When their collective improvement is sufficient, the patient's acuity and risk can be reassessed, and a referral to outpatient care starts to make sense.

A good illustration of all the treatment principles highlighted thus far is the case of bipolar disorder with manic psychosis, treatment refusal, and physical violence. At the outset, we introduce ourselves and ask the person what he wants and needs and typically he says, I want to get out of here. We say, excellent, let's start the process of your getting out of here—it just has to be safe to go. What do you need when you're feeling like this? Once he realizes we want what he wants, with one reasonable condition, safety, he may be willing to do what it takes to be less symptomatic and less dangerous. He may ask for medicine and try to control his anger. Beyond holding out for a reasonable amount of improvement, we may not have to force him to do anything. He may become an equal partner in treatment. Depending on the rapidity of his response to somatic therapy, the relative dangerousness of his preadmission behavior, and the readiness of the outpatient setting, it is conceivable he could become appropriate for nonadmission and a careful discharge from the ED or PES. At the very least, his ED course and inpatient stay will have been given a strong, positive impetus.

Risk tolerance. The final step in deciding if a person is ready for discharge involves risk assessment and risk tolerance: Is he safe to go? This is the bottom line, as one can only hope for persistent improvement in symptoms and engagement in treatment after discharge from the ED. Both of these conditions are highly desirable for discharge and are factors indicating lower risk. But in and of themselves, they are not essential for discharge. What is essential is that the patient is not an acute danger to himself or others on leaving the ED, in other words, that he does not have an emergency medical condition.

Unfortunately, as crucial as this concept of risk is to moving people out of the ED, there is some murkiness to it. Beyond the wording of acute dangerousness, there is no universally accepted statement that spells out the cutoff point between admission and discharge. There is no universally accepted instrument or tool for stratifying a person's risk. Nor is there universal agreement as to whether one should even declare an opinion on a patient's degree of risk. Community standards exhibit some regional differences, and risk assessment remains a clinical judgment. Nonetheless, most practitioners would agree that dangerousness is a quality that exists on a spectrum from low to high, and most emergency practitioners would be comfortable with setting a high bar for involuntary hospitalization. Combining their respective psychiatric and legal perspectives, Berlin and Stefan defined the admission criterion based on dangerousness as "high, short-term risk for serious harm [to self or others]" (46).

This statement distinguishes probability, time frame, and severity: high risk from low and moderate risk, short-term risk from long-term risk, and serious harm from less-than-serious harm. For example, a patient in the ED might be a high short-term risk for scratching her wrist. Given multiple risk factors, she might also pose a high long-term risk for suicide. But given engagement in intensive outpatient therapy and an absence of major current stressors, this woman might present a moderate short-term risk for suicide. She might therefore be appropriate for nonadmission, brief treatment, and discharge home.

There are also individuals with chronically high suicide risk that may be considered for discharge. Careful evaluation, emergency treatment of acute issues, and consultation with outpatient providers are all necessary. These cases are not automatic admissions. They may have a history of multiple hospitalizations and may have been told more than once that they have reached maximum hospital benefit. They challenge emergency practitioners to exercise nuanced judgments regarding their current crisis, demanding a balance between inadequate risk tolerance and excessive risk tolerance. In his discussion of severe personality disorders, Kernberg writes, "Sometimes the acceptance of a chronic risk of suicide is the price of outpatient treatment…" (47).

Increasing staff's risk tolerance to an appropriate level requires training, mentoring, experience, and clinical maturation. There is a typical progression in psychiatric residency training. For example, when faced with a well-known antisocial patient malingering dangerousness, first-year residents are uncertain how to proceed; second-year residents err on the side of safety and admit; third-year residents realize they can discharge, perhaps after staffing the case and having security stand by; and fourth-year residents ask the question, Why is this person here today and not another day, and what does he really need? Psychiatrists without previous experience with these cases can make this transition in a PES in 6 to 12 months' time.

There is variation in risk tolerance between different practitioners based on temperament, experience, and recent exposure to negative outcomes or malpractice litigation. There are also regional differences based on tradition, recent history of publicized bad outcomes, and the availability of intensive outpatient care and intermediate housing resources.

Specialty staff. EDs looking to upgrade their psychiatric services to deal with boarding should bring on staff with emergency psychiatric and mental health expertise. Typically, EDs start by adding a psychiatric nurse or social worker, then psychologist, then psychiatric evaluator, sometimes via telemedicine. As an ED's psychiatric volume increases, the next step might be to carve out space for an emergency psychiatry section in the ED. This is often designated as an observation area, partly for billing and coding purposes, but it is really a brief treatment unit with the goals of evaluation, engagement, and active intervention. The term "observation" is characteristic of an earlier time when the importance of treatment from the start was underappreciated.

Placing mental health and psychiatric staff in the ED serves a dual purpose of adding expertise for direct patient care and providing consultation and education to nonmental health staff on their own cases. This fits with the emphasis on integrated care (48).

External Approaches
Psychiatric Emergency Services

Ultimately, there is only so much that EDs can do themselves to facilitate the appropriate flow and throughput of psychiatric cases. When a region reaches a volume of 15 or 20 psychiatric emergencies cases a day, or 500 to 600 a month, the next step is to think about establishing a PES. Having enhanced their influence by making good-faith efforts to maximize the psychiatric pathways in their own operations, ED leaders play an important role in advocating for the creation of this new community resource.

A PES may be attached to an ED, in close proximity to an ED, or geographically remote. While several medical centers had developed separate PESs prior, the PES concept was more broadly accepted after the New York State in the 1980s created the model of an integrated, multicomponent service, the comprehensive psychiatric emergency program (CPEP)(49). Many variations have been created since. To function optimally, they all require a multidisciplinary team with expertise in psychiatric and nonpsychiatric medical emergencies. The full-fledged model includes a psychiatric ED, observation area, crisis mobile team, crisis line, urgent care clinic, and community-based crisis beds. But other very useful models exist. One is a streamlined version that includes only a combination psychiatric ED and 24-hour brief treatment/observation area. Originally called the Alameda model, now known better as an EmPATH Unit (Emergency Psychiatry Assessment, Treatment and Healing Unit), it has made a positive impact on boarding.

There are other ideas external to the functioning of the ED or PES, for example, providing real-time psychiatric consultation to first responders in the field (police, paramedics) by means of mobile crisis workers, either in person or real-time virtual staff via tablets and videoconferencing. One can also enhance a community's outpatient network and subacute crisis system. All of these strategies help an ED at the front end and back end: they address psychiatric emergencies before they reach the ED, and they increase a community's holding capacity: the ability to engage and treat referrals from the ED after discharge.

Depending on the specifics of each region, creation of additional psychiatric inpatient beds may be necessary. But they should not be the default boarding solution. There are three reasons for this: One, in most cases, enhancements in the emergency portion of the continuum of care mitigates boarding dramatically. Two, creating beds poses significant political and financial hurdles. Three, when inpatient bed creation does need to be part of a community's solution, one should have exhausted other methods first and have data to support the recommendation.

When faced with a boarding crisis, a community should look at three steps or processes: formal collaboration, a paradigm shift for data, and key metrics. These become especially important when a city is trying to establish the need for a PES or to solve a boarding crisis in a locale that already has a PES.

Collaboration

The most important first step for making systemic change in healthcare is developing a collaborative effort. Berwick writes, "To whatever degree these aims [of systemic change] are within our reach as a system, not one of them is within the grasp of any individual or group acting alone"(50).

Boarding crises typically generate as much heat as light. In searching for causes, there is a universal tendency toward blame, and all of the different stakeholders in the system come under attack, for predictably stereotyped shortcomings, including EDs, community providers, psychiatrists, private psychiatric hospitals, public hospitals, community-based crisis centers, law enforcement, jails, mental health courts, managed care, healthcare policy makers, families, patients, and legislators who make commitment laws.

Instead, an affected region should convene a task force composed of representatives from each of these groups and begin to gather data on the actual causes of boarding in their community and the potential solutions, as Milwaukee did in the mid-2000s (the Milwaukee Project is discussed in the next two sections). Blaming is discouraged. Members then begin to realize how multifactorial the boarding problem is, and how each stakeholder group might do something to help. There are typical causes of boarding, but there may be also regional particulars. For example, some states have cut bed capacity more drastically and with less forethought than others. To a certain extent, a city or a state may be able to learn from the example of other cities or states, but it should also study its own data. Inevitably, a combination of internal factors of the emergency system and external factors in the surrounding system is identified.

Paradigm Shift for Data

Given its safety net function, the ED is a "room with a view" (51). It not only sees unpreventable emergencies, it sees individuals who might have been better treated in another setting, had that setting been resourced properly. Emergency practitioners may not like what they see, but, in a boarding crisis, the key paradigm shift is to *welcome* boarding cases for what they tell us about the gaps in our mental healthcare systems. This is not to say that boarding is good. On the human and operational level, boarding cases are extremely undesirable. But they are full of useful information, and the etiology of boarding in each one should be analyzed, cataloged, trended, and reported out to the task force. Making this shift in attitude is the first step to achieving a comprehensive and systemic approach. Data are critical.

Milwaukee had a boarding crisis from 2004 to 2008. It started following the closure of three private psychiatric units in 2003 and the closure of the academic regional medical center's three inpatient units a few years before that. Unsurprisingly, there was a call for the reopening of some kind of inpatient psychiatric beds, either privately or in the county facility. A superficial review of the literature on boarding revealed a similar perspective that deinstitutionalization was to blame, and, therefore, the solution must be to reverse the process. Policy makers knew that the creation of a PES could also solve a boarding problem, but in this case, Milwaukee already had a PES, and the budget did not permit the creation of a second one.

However, as the actual data of the boarding cases were analyzed, other solutions presented themselves. The PCS (as it was known in Milwaukee, for Psychiatric Crisis Service) was sending out its crisis mobile team to assist EDs with their boarding patients. These teams, which consisted of psychiatric nurses and social workers, discovered that their evaluations and interventions, after being staffed by telephone with a PCS psychiatrist, could achieve a satisfactory disposition for thirty percent of boarding cases. Thirty percent could go home from the ED. There were 1,460 boarding cases in 2007 and approximately 438 patients that were considered subacute or nonacute. These were in addition to the several thousand subacute cases that were coming directly to PCS every year and going home from PCS after evaluation and treatment. Such numbers strongly suggested that a community-based, subacute crisis center staffed by midlevel practitioners would relieve significant pressure on the EDs and PCS. One seven-bed facility was created and jointly funded by the county and the private hospitals. It proved so successful that a second, identical, 12-bed facility was created.

At the time of this writing, Milwaukee now has 27 community-based, subacute crisis beds. Their success depends on the existence of higher-end hospital beds and a safety net PCS, but they have been a key addition to the spectrum of care that targeted a segment of the population identified in the analysis of boarding data.

In a similar way, the Milwaukee PCS analyzed the disposition of boarding cases once they were received on transfer from neighboring EDs, including cases that had been evaluated in person by the mobile team but not recommended for discharge. In a certain percentage of those, it was determined that the obstacle to discharge had been the appropriate caution of the midlevel practitioners. This led to the decision to add a PsyD psychologist to the mobile team with more experience, authority, and tolerance of risk.

One-sixth of the boarders transferred to PCS could be discharged following active psychiatric management and a one or two night stay in the nine-bed observation/brief treatment unit. As this unit was operating at full capacity and unable to accept all referrals, it was decided to open nine more observation/brief treatment beds rather than to reopen county psychiatric hospital inpatient beds.

Finally, data on some of the boarding patients in Milwaukee *were* revealing the need for more acute inpatient beds. But a careful analysis of the characteristics of those patients showed that, apart from being on a mental health hold, most were indistinguishable from the usual private hospital cases. This led PCS to reach out to the local private hospitals and persuade them to accept mental health hold cases from PCS that were within the private sector's clinical capability. Despite the closure of private psychiatric units, there were still some unfilled private beds. PCS staff rigorously painted an accurate picture of the patients they sought to transfer and agreed to accept back anyone that was not a good fit. One private hospital tested out these referrals; the return rate was less than one percent. Eventually all of the hospitals came on board. When PCS found that the work of arranging these referrals took up too much psychiatry time, it hired psychiatric nurses to be full-time transfer coordinators.

These and other measures, such as PCS psychiatrists providing telephone consultation on boarding cases to their fellow attending EM physicians; CIT training for the police; daily PCS medical director review of every boarding case; and increasing the psychiatrist-patient ratio in PCS and the observation unit—all contributed to a resolution of the boarding crisis by 2009. Boarding as a phenomenon did not entirely disappear, but diversion of new patients brought by police did, and the system crisis had been resolved, at least for several years to come.

Key Metric

Berwick describes the motivational power of plotting measurements related to aims over time (50, p. 82). The third key feature of the Milwaukee project was the use of a single, publicly held chart that plotted total boarding numbers over time (See Figure 2.1). As members of the task force worked together to solve the boarding problem, they came to view the boarding number as a quality indicator of the region's overall mental healthcare system—across private, academic, and public sectors and across the continuum of care from outpatient to inpatient. The graph clearly illustrated a success that everyone shared in.

Median boarding times were also monitored and reported out quarterly. They ranged from 6.0 to 14.3 hours, with infrequent cases lasting over 24 hours (See Figure 2.2).

Boarding in Milwaukee started in April 2004. The graph was created in 2007 at the height of the crisis, when boarding increased exponentially and PCS was so crowded that for the first time in its history, there were times it had to divert police drop-offs.

PCS tracked all cases waiting in EDs for transfer to PCS and referred to them internally as waitlisted cases (See y-axis notation in Figure 2.1). However, as PCS was the one designated receiving center for all of the mental health holds in the county, the patients on the PCS waitlist and the patients boarding in the nine local EDs and hospitals were synonymous. Boarding in PCS itself was negligible, due to the community's willingness to accept its decision not to exceed safe capacity.

CONCLUSION

Psychiatric patient boarding in EDs is a multifactorial problem requiring a multifactorial solution. Improvements should begin with a focus on internal ED operations, then expand outwards to the community at large. When a boarding problem in a community reaches crisis proportions, the single most cost-effective solution is an expansion of psychiatric emergency services, culminating in the creation of a specialized PES. Many patients with acute symptoms respond favorably to a welcoming and safe environment that provides brief (24-72 hours), focused care. Prompt assessment and treatment in the emergency setting can result in a high rate of appropriate hospital diversion. However, emergency services must remain alert to the danger of bed shortages adversely affecting medical decision-making; staff can become too aggressive in their diversion efforts.

Regardless of the role that deinstitutionalization plays in creating boarding problems, creation of new inpatient beds is usually not

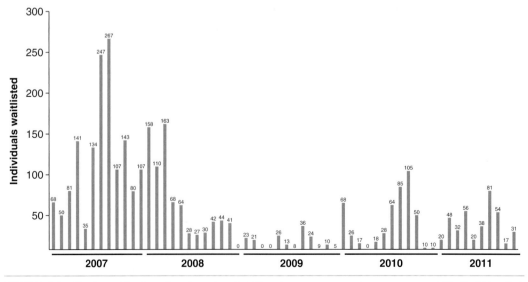

FIGURE 2.1 • Total psychiatric patient boarding in Milwaukee emergency departments and Medical Hospital. Cases per month from Jan 2007-Oct 2011.

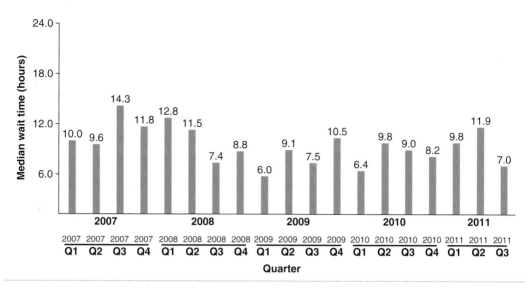

FIGURE 2.2 • Psychiatric patient boarding: Median wait time.

necessary. However, this is not meant categorically: it depends on the particulars of the individual community, and there is no substitute for studying one's own data for insight. Communities are more likely to take the trouble to perform a detailed analysis when boarding problems occur despite the existence of a PES.

Emergency practitioners must make a variety of paradigm shifts to improve the internal operation of their own service and become a part of a system-wide solution. These include understanding that psychiatric problems are medical problems, implementing protocols and actions that promote early treatment, appropriately increasing risk tolerance, and appreciating that boarding cases contain useful information about the problems in the mental health system. As a collaborative approach is developed, boarding crises will resolve, and a community will come to regard their boarding numbers as a valuable quality metric of its healthcare system.

REFERENCES

1. Moore, B. J., Stocks, C., & Owens, P. L. (September 2017). *Trends in emergency department visits, 2006–2014. HCUP statistical brief #227*. Rockville, MD: Agency for Healthcare Research and Quality. Retrieved February 16, 2019, from https://www.hcup-us.ahrq.gov/reports/statbriefs/sb227-Emergency-Department-Visit-Trends.pdf.

2. Nicks, B. A., & Manthey, D. M. (2012). The impact of psychiatric patient boarding in emergency departments. *Emergency Medicine International, 2012*, Article ID 360308.

3. American College Of Emergency Physicians. (2008). *ACEP psychiatric and substance abuse survey*. Irving, TX: American College of Emergency Physicians.

4. Weiss, A. P., Chang, G., Rauch, S. L., et al. (2012). Patient and practice-related determinants of emergency department length of stay for patients with psychiatric illness. *Annals of Emergency Medicine, 60*(2), 162–171.e165.

5. Tuttle, G. A. (2008). *Access to psychiatric beds and impact on emergency medicine*. Chicago, IL: Council on Medical Service, American Medical Association.

6. Bloom, J. D. (2015). Psychiatric boarding in Washington state and the inadequacy of mental health resources. *Journal of the American Academy of Psychiatry and the Law, 43*(2), 218–222.

7. Appelbaum, P. S. (2015). "Boarding" psychiatric patients in emergency rooms: One court says "No more". *Psychiatric Services, 66*(7), 668–670.

8. *Care of psychiatric patients boarded in EDs*. Joint Commission. Quick Safety-Issue One, (April 2014).

9. Alleviating, E. D. (December 2015). *Boarding of psychiatric patients*. Joint Commission. Quick Safety-Issue Nineteen.

10. Beans, B. E. (2016). Experts foresee a major shift from inpatient to ambulatory care. *P&T, 41*(4), 231–237.

11. Currier, G. W. & Allen, M. H. (2003). Organization and function of academic psychiatric emergency services. *General Hospital Psychiatry, 25*, 124–129.

12. Zeller, S., Calma, N., & Stone, A. (2014). Effects of a dedicated regional psychiatric emergency service on boarding of psychiatric patients in area emergency departments. *Western Journal of Emergency Medicine, 15*(1), 1–6.

13. Bender, D., Pande, N., & Ludwig, M. (October 29, 2008). *A literature review: Psychiatric boarding*. U.S. Dept of Health and Human Services. Retrieved November 19, 2018, from http://aspe.hhs.gov/daltcp/reports/2008/PsyBdLR.pdf.

14. Alakeson, V., Pande, N., & Ludwig, M. (2010). A plan to reduce emergency room "boarding" of psychiatric patients. *Health Affairs, 29*(9), 1637–1642.

15. Al-Qahtani, S., Alsultan, A., Haddad, S., et al. (2017). The association of duration of boarding in the emergency room and the outcome of patients admitted to the intensive care unit. *BMC Emergency Medicine, 17*(1), 34.

16. Gerdtz, M. F., Weiland, T. J., Jelinek, G. A., et al. (2012). Perspectives of emergency department staff on the triage of mental health-related presentations: Implications for education, policy and practice. *Emergency Medicine Australasia, 24*, 492–500.

17. Scutti, S. (January 4, 2019). *ERs "flooded" with mentally ill patients with no place else to turn*. CNN.com. Accessed February 9, 2019.

18. Morris, N. (May 19, 2018). *Suicidal? Be prepared to wait for care*. WashingtonPost.com. Accessed February 9, 2019.

19. Gold, J. (April 13, 2011). *Mentally ill languish in hospital emergency rooms*. NPR.org. Accessed February 9, 2019.

20. Simpson, S. A., Joesch, J. M., West, I. I., & Pasic, J. (2014). Who's boarding in the psychiatric emergency service? *Western Journal of Emergency Medicine, 15*(6), 669–674.

21. Hsu, C. C., & Chan, H. Y. (2018). Factors associated with prolonged length of stay in the psychiatric emergency service. *PLoS One, 13*(8). doi:10.1371/journal.pone.0202569.

22. Stefan, S. (2006). *Emergency department treatment of the psychiatric patient*. New York, NY: Oxford University Press, Inc.

23. Practical Solutions to Boarding of Psychiatric Patients in the Emergency Department. (2016). *Product of American College of emergency physicians & operations Workgroup 3 of Committee on psychiatric emergencies*. PracSolutionsPsychiatricBoardIP_081116.pdf; http://www.macep.org/Files/Behavioral%20Health%20Boarding/Practical%20Solutions%20to%20Boarding%20of%20Psych%20Patients%20in%20EDs.pdf. Accessed February 12, 2019.

24. Nordstrom, K., Berlin, J., Nash, S., Shah, S., Schmelzer, N., & Worley, L. (2019). Boarding of Mentally Ill Patients in Emergency Departments, American Psychiatric Association: Resource Document. *Western Journal of Emergency Medicine, 20*(5), 690–695.

25. Braslow, J. T., & Messac, L. (2018). Medicalization and demedicalization–A gravely disabled homeless man with psychiatric illness. *The New England Journal of Medicine, 379*(20), 1885–1888.

26. Brown, P., Buttlaire, S., & Phillips, L. (2013). Improving emergency department process and flow. In Zun, L., Chepenik, L. G., & Mallory, M. S. (Eds.), *Behavioral emergencies: A Handbook for the emergency physician*. Cambridge: Cambridge University Press.

27. Personal communications at meetings of the American Association for emergency psychiatry, 2000-2017.

28. See Cameron's, Tintinalli's, Oxford's.

29. Zun, L. S., Chepenik, L. G., & Mallory, M. S. (2013) *Behavioral emergencies for the emergency physician* (p. xiii). Cambridge: Cambridge University Press.

30. 42 CFR § 489.24(b) 2010 Amendment to the emergency medical treatment and active labor Act (EMTALA).

31. Emergency Medical Treatment and Labor Act (EMTALA). Centers for Medicare and Medicaid Services. Retrieved February 9, 2019, from http://www.cms.gov/Regulations-and-Guidance/Legislation/EMTALA/index.html.

32. Richmond, J. S., Berlin, J. S., Fishkind, A. B., et al. (2012). Verbal de-escalation of the agitated patient: Consensus statement of the American association for emergency psychiatry project BETA Workgroup. *Western Journal of Emergency Medicine, XIII*(1), 17-25.

33. Fishkind, A. (2002). Calming agitation with words, not drugs. *Current Psychiatry, 1*(4), 32–39.

34. Berlin, J. S. (2017). Collaborative de-escalation. In Zeller, S. L., Nordstrom, K. D., & Wilson, M. P. (Eds.), *The diagnosis and management of agitation*. Cambridge: Cambridge University Press.

35. Gudeman, J. E., & Shore, M. F. (1984). Beyond deinstitutionalization: A new class of facilities for the mentally ill. *The New England Journal of Medicine, 311*(13), 832–836.

36. Allen, M. H. (1996). Definitive treatment in the psychiatric emergency service. *Psychiatric Quarterly, 67*, 247–262.

37. Tucci, V., Ahmed, S. M., Hoyer, D., & Moukaddam, N. (2017). Management of psychiatric emergencies in free-standing emergency departments: A paradigm for excellence? *Journal of Emergencies, Trauma, and Shock, 10*(4), 171–173.

38. Fleischmann, A., Bertolote, J. M., Wasserman, D., et al. (2008). Effectiveness of brief intervention and contact for suicide attempters: A randomized controlled trial in five countries. *Bulletin of the World Health Organization, 86*(9), 703–709.

39. Boudreaux, E. D., Camargo, C. A., Jr., Arias, S. A., et al. (2016). Improving suicide risk screening and detection in the emergency department. *American Journal of Preventive Medicine, 50*(4), 445–453.

40. *Caring for Adult patients with suicide risk: A Consensus guide for emergency departments: Quick guide for Clinicians.* Suicide Prevention Resource Center (SPRC). (2013). Retrieved from http://www.sprc.org/sites/default/files/EDGuide_quickversion.pdf.

41. Boudreaux, E. D., Larkin, C., Kini, N., et al. (2018). Predictive utility of an emergency department decision support tool in patients with active suicidal ideation. *Psychological Services, 15*(3), 270–278.

42. D'Onofrio, G., McCormack, R. P., & Hawk, K. (2018). Emergency departments—A 24/7/365 option for combating the opioid crisis. *The New England Journal of Medicine, 379*(26), 2487–2490.

43. King, D. R. (2019). Initial care of the severely injured patient. *The New England Journal of Medicine, 380*, 8763–8770.

44. Sederer, L. I. (1991). *Inpatient psychiatry: Diagnosis and treatment* (3rd ed.). Baltimore: Lippincott Williams & Wilkins.

45. Wisconsin Statutes: Emergency detention, chapter 51.15(1).

46. Berlin, J. S., & Stefan, S., Discharge of the emergency patient with risk factors for suicide: Psychiatric and legal perspectives. In Zun, W. (Ed.), *Behavioral emergencies for the healthcare provider* (2nd ed.). Nordstrom: Cambridge University Press. In press.

47. Kernberg, O. F. (1984). *Severe personality disorders: Psychotherapeutic strategies* (p. 261). Binghamton, NY: Vail-Ballou Press.

48. Joseph, R., Kester, R., O'Brien, C., & Huang, H. (2017). The evolving practice of psychiatry in the era of integrated care. *Psychosomatics, 58*(5), 466–473.

49. *Annual Report to the Governor and Legislature of New York State on Comprehensive Psychiatric Emergency Programs.* New York State Office of Mental Health. (2012). Retrieved February 12, 2019, from https://www.omh.ny.gov/omhweb/statistics/cpep_annual_report/2012.pdf.

50. Berwick, D. M. (2004). *Escape fire* (p. 33). John Wiley & Sons, Inc.

51. Asplin, B. R. & Knopp, R. K. (2001). A room with a view; on-call specialist panels and other health policy challenges in the emergency department. *Annals of Emergency Medicine, 37*, 500–503.

3

Quality Improvement in Emergency Psychiatry: The Path to Better Outcomes and Care Standards

Margaret E. Balfour

Have you ever been annoyed at how long it takes to get something done in your emergency department (ED)? Have you found yourself asking "Why do we do it this way – isn't there a better way?" Have you gotten so fed up with a ridiculous form that you just went ahead and made a better one for you and your colleagues to use? If so, then this chapter is for you.

Have you been asked by an administrator to explain how the psychiatric emergency service provides value to the organization? Have you wondered whether the psychiatric emergency service is doing a good job? How it compares to other similar services? If so, then this chapter is for you.

All of these are addressed by quality measurement and quality improvement (QI). This is a topic oft expected to be dull and dry, but when done well, QI can be rewarding and even fun. QI can improve care for the patients we serve, engage staff in improving their daily work lives, and provide a way to see the results of the hard work we do. Furthermore, despite the important role that crisis and emergency psychiatric services play in the healthcare system, there are currently no national standards for the provision of these services. A first step in the development of such standards is to consistently measure the quality and outcomes of the care we provide.

The purpose of this chapter is to make QI more accessible to clinicians working in emergency psychiatry or behavioral health crisis settings, guide service line leaders in developing QI

programs for crisis and psychiatric emergency services, and lay the foundation for the development of national standards by defining a common framework to measure outcomes.

A BRIEF HISTORY OF QUALITY IMPROVEMENT IN HEALTH CARE

The scientific approach to QI in medicine can be traced as far back as Florence Nightingale's groundbreaking statistical analysis of the relationship between hygiene and mortality among soldiers wounded in the Crimean War in the 1850s (1). However, the importance of QI did not come to the full attention of the US healthcare industry until a series of landmark reports published in 2000-2001 by the Institute of Medicine (IOM, since renamed the National Academy of Medicine). *To Err is Human* (2) exposed the troubling state of American health care, specifically the 45,000 to 100,000 annual deaths linked to preventable medical errors. A follow-up report entitled *Crossing the Quality Chasm* (3) concluded that health care lagged behind other industries in terms of quality and safety by at least a decade and stated that "fundamental, sweeping redesign of the entire health system" was needed rather than incremental or piecemeal attempts at addressing the problem. Together, these works heralded a national call to action and laid out a framework for health care to begin to systematically approach quality and safety as a priority (Table 3.1).

TABLE 3.1 Defining Quality

The Institute of Medicine (IOM) defined quality and safety and identified six aims to guide healthcare organizations in their improvement efforts.	
Quality: The degree to which health services for individuals and populations increase the likelihood of desired health outcomes and are consistent with current professional knowledge.	**Safety:** Freedom from accidental injury when interacting in any way with the healthcare system.

Six Goals for Improvement:

1. **Safe:** avoiding injuries to patients from the care that is intended to help them
2. **Effective:** providing services based on scientific knowledge to all who could benefit and refraining from providing services to those not likely to benefit
3. **Patient-centered:** providing care that is respectful of and responsive to individual patient preferences, needs, and values and ensuring that patient values guide all clinical decisions
4. **Timely:** reducing waits and sometimes harmful delays for both those who receive and those who give care
5. **Efficient:** avoiding waste, including waste of equipment, supplies, ideas, and energy
6. **Equitable:** providing care that does not vary in quality because of personal characteristics such as gender, ethnicity, geographic location, and socioeconomic status

Building on this work, the Institute for Healthcare Improvement (IHI) introduced the concept of the "Triple Aim," challenging healthcare systems to pursue three aspirational goals: improving the experience of care, improving the health of populations, and reducing per capita costs of health care (4). More recently, it has been recognized that achievement of these aims requires a healthy and engaged workforce, resulting in the addition of a Fourth Aim focused on improving the work life of clinicians and staff (5). Subsequent work by the IOM, IHI, and other key organizations such as the Centers for Medicare and Medicaid Services (CMS), the Joint Commission (TJC), and CARF International have further advanced the field of QI in health care. All have recognized a need to learn from and adapt advances in QI from other high reliability fields such as manufacturing and aviation, which are discussed later in this chapter (Table 3.2).

MEASURING QUALITY

Quality measurement is often considered a necessary evil that one must undertake in order to meet regulatory requirements (and to get paid, as value-based contracting gains popularity). However, when designed and used effectively, quality measures reflect something more fundamental—they are the incarnation of value.

"Value" in this context has two meanings. The first is straightforward. Are we achieving the outcomes important to key stakeholders? The second has a more philosophical and soul-searching implication. Most of us went into health care with a desire to make meaningful contributions to society, and quality measurement provides a way to determine whether or not we are achieving this goal. Are we living up to our organization's core values—eg, if we say we value patient-centered care, are we living up to that? The ability to measure adherence to core values has implications for both the health of the organization and the individuals working within it. Tangible results ascribe meaning to the hard work put in day after day, which can contribute to the Fourth Aim's goal of creating "joy of work."

Furthermore, measuring quality outcomes in a systematic way is critical to improvement—both in terms of improving quality at the point of care and for informing research that advances the field as a whole. As Lord Kelvin famously said, "If you cannot measure it, you cannot improve it."

TABLE 3.2 Healthcare's Quadruple Aim

1. Improving the patient's experience of care (including both patient satisfaction and clinical quality)
2. Improving the health of populations
3. Improving the per capita costs of health care
4. Improving the work life of clinicians and staff (including joy and meaning in work)

Measurement and Standards in Emergency Psychiatry

As of this writing, there are no national standards for either the provision or measurement of emergency psychiatric or behavioral health crisis services. Because these services are financed almost exclusively by Medicaid and other local funds, they are primarily regulated at the state level. Thus, there is no national consensus on even the terminology for various types of crisis services much less what their outcomes should be. Even when healthcare services are federally regulated, behavioral health is often overlooked in quality measurement systems. For example, the Hospital Consumer Assessment of Healthcare Providers and Systems (HCAHPS), a patient satisfaction survey required by Medicare for all hospital inpatients, excludes patients with psychiatric diagnoses. Similarly, the Health Information Technology for Economic and Clinical Health Act (HITECH Act) provided financial incentives for healthcare organizations to demonstrate "meaningful use" of electronic health records (EHRs) to improve quality outcomes but excluded psychiatric facilities.

Fortunately, there is increasing interest in developing the needed standards for these critical services. The Interdepartmental Serious Mental Illness Coordinating Committee (ISMICC), an advisory committee created by the 21st Century Cures Act, recommended the development of national standards for crisis services in its 2018 report (6). Professional organizations, including the American Association for Emergency Psychiatry (AAEP), are in the process of developing guidelines and standards of care for patients in acute mental health or substance use crisis. One of AAEP's member organizations, Connections Health Solutions, has developed a draft set of crisis core measures—Crisis Reliability Indicators Supporting Emergency Services (CRISES) (7). The CRISES measures are in use at six crisis programs in Arizona and have been adopted by programs in other states as well.

Aligning Measures With Values

The CRISES framework (Figure 3.1) was constructed by adapting QI tool called a critical-to-quality (CTQ) tree. This tool is designed to help an organization translate values and customer needs into discrete measures (8). When building a CTQ tree, the first step is to define the value we are trying to accomplish, in this case "Excellence in Crisis Services." The next step is to define the key attributes that comprise this value. CRISES values were defined as timely, safe, accessible, least restrictive, effective, consumer/family centered, and partnership. These are consistent with the Institute of Medicine's six aims for quality health care: safety, effectiveness, equity, timeliness, patient-centeredness, and efficiency (3) while also focusing attention on goals unique to the behavioral health crisis setting. The final step is to define discrete metrics that reflect the CTQ tree key attributes.

Choosing Metrics

Whether building the CRISES measurement framework from a CTQ tree or selecting metrics for a QI project, it is important to understand various types of measures and when their application is most effective to support improvement efforts. Dr. Avedis Donabedian—an early pioneer of quality measurement in health care—developed the commonly used structure-process-outcome model: (9).

1. *Structure:* the environment in which care is delivered. Metrics may describe organizational structure, resources, or staffing (eg, whether or not the ED is staffed with a psychiatrist on-site).

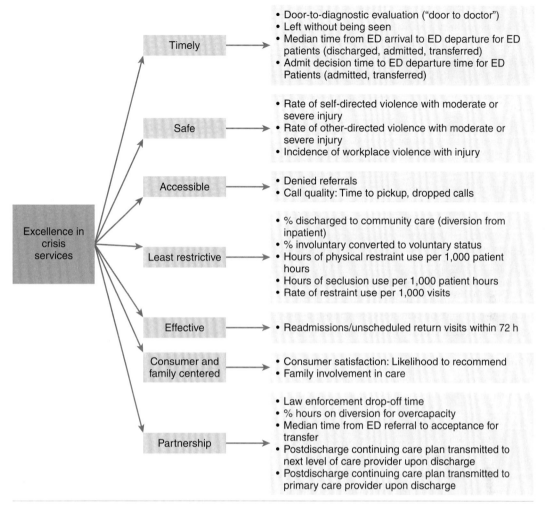

FIGURE 3.1 • CRISES metric framework. A critical-to-quality (CTQ) tree is used to translate values into discrete metrics. ED, emergency department.

2. *Process:* the techniques and processes used to deliver care. Metrics may describe the use of screening tools (eg, percentage of ED patients screened for suicide risk) or how quickly a specific intervention is completed (eg, door-to-doctor time).
3. *Outcome:* the result of the patient's interaction with the healthcare system (eg, injury, death, quality of life, change in symptom rating scales, readmissions).

Different types of measures are appropriate for different settings and purposes. Outcome measures are the most desirable. However, sometimes it is not feasible to collect outcome data,

or it is not within the scope of an organization to change an outcome on its own, thus a process metric is more appropriate.

Many frameworks exist to inform the selection and implementation of individual quality measures. A simple and straightforward approach was described by Hermann and Palmer (10) which requires that measures are meaningful, feasible, and actionable. Some key considerations regarding each of these requirements are outlined below.

Meaningful: Does the measure reflect a process that is clinically important? Is there evidence supporting the measure? Compared to other fields, there is a less robust evidence base for behavioral health measures, so we must often rely on face validity or adapt measures for which there is evidence in other settings. For example, some of the CRISES metrics are adapted from existing core measures for EDs and inpatient psychiatric units. When possible, measures should be selected or adapted from measures that have been endorsed by organizations that set standards for quality measurement such as the National Quality Forum (NQF), CMS, TJC, Agency for Healthcare Research and Quality (AHRQ), etc. Most of these organizations maintain online databases of measures available for use or adaptation.

Feasible: Is it possible to collect the data needed to provide the measure? If so, can this be done accurately, quickly, and easily? Data must be produced within a short timeframe in order to be actionable. An organization's quality department staff should be able to spend most of its time addressing identified problems rather than performing time-consuming manual chart audits. With the advent of EHRs, it is now possible to design processes that support automated reporting, making it feasible to quickly obtain data that were previously too complex or labor intensive to collect via chart abstraction.

Actionable: Do the measures provide direction for future QI activities? Are there established benchmarks toward which to strive? Are the factors leading to suboptimal performance within the span of control of the organization to address? For example, a behavioral health crisis program is in a position to identify many problems in the community-wide system of care (such as lack of housing or ineffective outpatient follow-up after discharge). Crisis programs can be instrumental in collaborating with system partners to help fix these larger issues (11). However, the crisis program's own core measures must be within its sphere of influence to improve, otherwise there is the tendency to blame problems on external factors rather than focus on the problems it can address.

Finally, it is important to disseminate metrics in a way that is useful to the end user. Different types of stakeholders will have different needs. A Quality Improvement Committee may need a detailed scorecard showing many different metrics, while executive leaders may need an abbreviated list of key performance indicators. Table 3.3 shows an example list of key performance indicators in use at Connections Health Solutions that is shared with executive leadership and external stakeholders.

IMPROVING QUALITY

The terms quality assurance (QA), compliance, QI, performance improvement (PI), and quality management are often used interchangeably. For the purposes of this chapter, the following definitions are used:

Quality assurance (QA) is the process of specifying quality and performance standards and then ensuring that those standards are met. These standards may be developed internally or via external professional or regulatory organizations. In the latter case, QA is closely tied to regulatory compliance. To ensure standards are met, QA activities employ tools such as chart audits, inspections, and data reports. When performance on a certain process is out of compliance, solutions focus on the individuals responsible for the process, via corrective action or education.

Performance improvement (PI) is the process of continuously studying and improving processes in order to improve outcomes and reduce errors. Performance targets may be set internally, via regulatory agencies, or by seeking input by customers and stakeholders. In contrast to the QA focus on individual performance, PI focuses on systemic problems and uses tools that help identify and improve processes that need fixing. When an error occurs, PI asks: Why *couldn't*—rather than why *didn't*—staff do their job? PI activities often seek input and participation of individual workers in improvement projects and thus can positively affect organizational culture as well.

An organization needs both QA and PI for a comprehensive approach to quality. CMS defines the marriage of Quality Assurance and Performance Improvement (QAPI) as "the coordinated application of two mutually reinforcing aspects of a quality management system: Quality Assurance and Performance Improvement. QAPI takes a systematic, comprehensive, and data-driven approach to maintaining and

TABLE 3.3 Example Key Performance Indicators

Metric	CRISES Domain	Target	Relevance
Urgent care clinic: Door-to-door **length of stay**	Timely	2 h	Patients get their needs met quickly instead of going to an emergency department or allowing symptoms to worsen.
23-hour observation unit: **Door-to-doctor time**	Timely	90 min	Treatment is started early, which results in higher likelihood of stabilization and less likelihood of assaults, injuries, and restraints.
23-hour observation unit: **Community disposition rate**	Least restrictive	65%	Most patients are able to be discharged to less restrictive and less costly community-based care instead of inpatient admission.
Hours of **restraint and seclusion use** per 1,000 patient hours	Least restrictive	0.46 (R) 0.35 (S)	Despite receiving highly acute patients directly from the field, restraint rates are below the Joint Commission national average for inpatient psychiatric units, without the use of security.
Law enforcement drop-off **Police turnaround time**	Partnership	10 min	If jail diversion is a goal, then police are customers too and crisis services must be quicker and easier to access than jail.
Patient satisfaction: **Likelihood to recommend**	Partnership	85%	Even though many patients are brought via law enforcement, most would recommend our services to friends or family.
Readmissions/return visits within 72 h	Effective	3%	People get their needs met in our program and are connected to effective aftercare. A multiagency collaboration addresses the subset of people with multiple return visits.

improving safety and quality while involving all caregivers in practical and creative problem solving" (12). Organizations with QAPI programs in early development often focus heavily on QA and compliance, while more mature organizations have distinct compliance, QA, and PI functions. The terms Quality Improvement (QI) or Quality Management (QM) are sometimes used as shorthand to refer to the full spectrum of QAPI activities. In this chapter, QAPI is referred to as QI.

QUALITY IMPROVEMENT METHODS

Many of the QI methods used in healthcare settings are based on process improvement methods initially developed for the manufacturing industry in the early to mid-20th century. Much of this work was pioneered by American statisticians Walter Shewhart and W. Edwards Deming.

While working as an engineer at Bell Laboratories, Shewhart pioneered the concept of statistical process control (13), in which performance is measured over time using "control charts" or "run charts" to indicate whether a process is working stably and reliably (Figure 3.2). Both Shewhart and Deming contributed to the development and dissemination of the now ubiquitous PDSA (Plan-Do-Study-Act cycle) (14). This four-step process begins with identifying a problem and designing an improved process to address it (plan), followed by testing the new process (do), analyzing results to determine how well it worked (study), and deciding whether to continue with the new process (act) or start a new cycle. These simple yet effective methods can be adopted in any healthcare setting with a minimum amount of technical training.

Dr Deming went on to develop more advanced QI frameworks that have since been adapted to many industries (15). He first introduced QI concepts to the Japanese manufacturing industry during post-WWII rebuilding efforts. Over the next 50 years, these methods were widely adopted

and further developed into quality management frameworks such as the Toyota Production System, Lean (the implementation of the Toyota Production System in the United States), and Six Sigma (developed by Motorola and refined by General Electric).

Today, Lean (16) and Six Sigma (17) are widely used in healthcare settings. A detailed description of these frameworks is beyond the scope of this chapter, but briefly Six Sigma focuses on reducing variability and error, while Lean focuses on reducing waste, defined as anything "nonvalue added" to the customer, such as time spent waiting (18). This is naturally appealing to fast-paced healthcare settings and thus many implementations of Lean have been in EDs (19) including crisis/psychiatric emergency settings (20). Both Lean and Six Sigma emphasize the need for teamwork, participation of front-line staff in QI activities, standardized protocols, and data-driven decision-making.

Although both QI and research employ many tools for data analysis and outcome measurement,

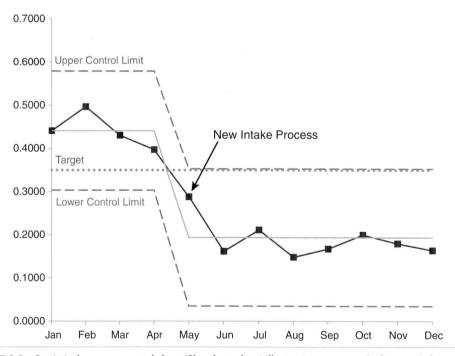

FIGURE 3.2 • Statistical process control chart (Shewhart chart) illustrating a process before and after a quality improvement intervention. The graph depicts improvement in the seclusion rate (hours of seclusion per 1000 patient hours) at the Urgent Psychiatric Center in Phoenix, Arizona. Upper and lower control units are 3 standard deviations above and below the mean. After the intervention, performance is significantly improved (consistently below the lower control limit), so updated control limits are set for the new process. To compare performance with external benchmarks, the Joint Commission's national average for inpatient psychiatric units is plotted as a target.

they are distinct processes (21). Research expands the general body of knowledge regarding evidence-based care, and it is by necessity slow and methodical. In contrast, QI is rapid and iterative. It focuses on applying what is already known to solve or improve complex real-world problems. Many interventions may be tried in rapid succession or at the same time. Results are measured quickly, and modifications are immediately applied and reanalyzed as needed. Both have value in improving health care, and both are publishable.

SO YOU WANT TO TRY QUALITY IMPROVEMENT?

Training: It is important to note that *anyone* can participate in QI activities regardless of training. That said, there are many training programs in QI methods for those wishing to expand their knowledge, including formal certifications reflecting increasing levels of expertise known as "belts" (eg, green belt, black belt). It is increasingly common for healthcare organizations to offer their own in-house training programs as well. The depth and quality of these training programs (even the formal certifications) can vary widely. A good barometer of the quality and utility of a program is whether it requires the completion of a final QI project. The project, even when supervised by an online mentor, gives the learner invaluable practical experience in applying QI concepts and tools in a real-world setting.

Teams: QI is meant to be performed in teams. If possible, at least one member of the team should have training in QI methods and serve as a facilitator. The other key roles do not require formal training and should include clinical leaders, staff who work in the process of interest on a day-to-day basis, and a sponsor. The sponsor might not participate in all of the meetings but serves as a champion and liaison to higher level organizational leaders who can make decisions and allocate resources for the project.

FOCUS-PDSA: The FOCUS-PDCA model (22) is a simple framework used in many healthcare organizations. It requires only a team, some basic data collection capabilities, and the desire to improve something. There are numerous online worksheets to help guide a team through the process. The basic elements are below:

FOCUS on what to improve.

- *F = Find a process to improve*
- *O = Organize a team that knows the process.* Be sure to include front-line staff who work in the process on a daily basis
- *C = Clarify current knowledge of the process.* Map the process to learn how it works in real life, and, importantly, determine how to measure whether or not it is working well
- *U = Understand causes of variation in the process.* Identify the root causes that keep the process from giving you the desired results
- *S = Select the intervention.* Develop an intervention to fix one of the root causes you identified in the previous step

PDSA: Use the PDSA cycle to perform a series of small pilots so that the intervention can be tested and adjusted before being implemented on a large scale.

- *P = Plan.* Determine how you will implement the intervention and how you will measure the outcome. How will you know if you were successful?
- *D = Do.* Implement the intervention and collect outcome data
- *S = Study.* (Sometimes called C for Check.) Examine the results Compare the actual outcome to the expected outcome. Summarize lessons learned
- *A = Act.* Decide whether adopt the change, abandon it, or tweak it by performing another PDSA cycle

Most importantly, have fun!

REFERENCES

1. Kudzma, E. C. (2006). Florence Nightingale and healthcare reform. *Nursing Science Quarterly, 19*(1), 61–64.
2. Institute of Medicine. (2000). *To err is human: Building a safer health system*. Washington, DC: The National Academies Press.
3. Institute of Medicine. (2001). *Crossing the Quality Chasm: A new health system for the 21st century*. Washington, DC: The National Academies Press.
4. Berwick, D. M., Nolan, T. W., & Whittington, J. (2008). The triple aim: Care, health, and cost. *Health Affairs, 27*(3), 759–769.
5. Bodenheimer, T., & Sinsky, C. (2014). From triple to quadruple aim: Care of the patient requires care of the provider. *Annals of Family Medicine, 12*(6), 573–576.

6. Interdepartmental Serious Mental Illness Coordinating Committee. (2017). *The way forward: Federal action for a system that works for all people living with SMI and SED and their families and caregivers.* North Bethesda, MD: SAMHSA.

7. Balfour, M. E., Tanner, K., Jurica, J. S., Rhoads, R., & Carson, C. A. (2016). Crisis Reliability Indicators Supporting Emergency Services (CRISES): A framework for developing performance measures for behavioral health crisis and psychiatric emergency programs. *Community Mental Health Journal, 52*(1), 1–9.

8. Lighter, D. E. (2013). *Basics of health care performance improvement: A lean six sigma approach.* Burlington, MA: Jones and Bartlett Learning.

9. Donabedian, A. (2002). *An introduction to quality assurance in health care.* New York, NY: Oxford University Press.

10. Hermann, R. C., & Palmer, R. H. (2003). Common ground: A framework for selecting core quality measures for mental health and substance abuse care. *Psychiatric Services, 53*(3), 281–287.

11. Balfour, M. E., Zinn, T., Cason, K., Fox, J., Morales, M., Berdeja, C., & Gray, J. (2018). Provider-payer partnerships as an engine for continuous quality improvement. *Psychiatric Services, 69*(6),623–625.

12. Center for Medicare and Medicaid Services. (2016). *QAPI description and background.* Retrieved from https://www.cms.gov/Medicare/Provider-Enrollment-and-Certification/QAPI/qapidefinition.html.

13. Shewhart, W. A., & Deming, W. E. (1986). *Statistical method from the viewpoint of quality control.* Mineola, NY: Dover Publications.

14. Deming, W. E. (1991). *Out of the crisis.* Cambridge, MA: Massachusetts Institute of Technology Center for Advanced Engineering Study.

15. Womack, J. P., & Jones, D. T. (1996). *Lean thinking: Banish waste and create wealth in your corporation.* New York, NY: Simon & Schuster.

16. Womack, J. P., Byrne, A. P., Fiume, O. J., Kaplan, G. S., & Toussaint, J. (2005). *Going lean in health care. IHI innovation series white papers.* Cambridge, MA: Institute for Healthcare Improvement.

17. Lighter, D. E. (2013). *Basics of health care performance improvement: A lean six sigma approach.* Burlington, MA: Jones and Bartlett Learning.

18. Joosten, T., Bongers, I., & Janssen, R. (2009). Application of lean thinking to health care: Issues and observations. *International Society for Quality in Health Care, 21*(5), 341–347.

19. D'Andreamatteo, A., Ianni, L., Lega, F., & Sargiacomo, M. (2015). Lean in healthcare: A comprehensive review. *Health Policy, 119*(9), 1197–1209.

20. Balfour, M. E, Tanner, K., Jurica, J. S., Llewellyn, D., Williamson, R. G., & Carson, C. A. (2017). Using lean to rapidly transform a behavioral health crisis program: Impact on throughput and safety. *Joint Commission Journal on Quality and Patient Safety, 43*(6), 275–283.

21. Moses, J. (2015). *What's the difference between research and QI? IHI open school.* Cambridge, MA: Institute for Healthcare Improvement.

22. American College of Cardiology. (2013). *Introduction to quality improvement and the FOCUS-PDSA model.* ACC Clinical Toolkits. Retrieved from https://cvquality.acc.org/clinical-toolkits/qi-toolkit.

4

Research in the Psychiatric Emergency Setting

Manuel G. Alvarez Romero, Samidha Tripathi, Michael Wilson

AN EMERGENCY PSYCHIATRY RESEARCH PROPOSAL

The difficulties in conducting good clinical research in the general or psychiatric emergency department (ED) include insufficient training, insufficient time, insufficient funding, and challenges obtaining informed consent (1). Emergency providers face an additional challenge of vastly variable pathology, time pressure, and a heterogeneous case mix. Patients also present at unscheduled times, at times out of regular "business hours," thereby making patient recruitment and data collection more difficult (2). ED clinicians often face pressure to disposition patients quickly. Finally, staff rotation and ethical issues related to informed consent also pose challenges in getting a project "off the ground." Despite all these difficulties, it is indeed quite possible to do good ED research, and this chapter will hopefully serve as a good introduction to this process (3).

A COMPREHENSIVE RESEARCH PROTOCOL

A study protocol is a detailed presentation of both the study design and implementation. In other words, it determines how the research question will be answered. The key components of a protocol include(4):

1. The research question
2. Significance of the study (or the importance of the question)
3. Hypothesis (or the predicted outcome)
4. Setting (or the location of the study)
5. Methodology (selection of subjects, sampling, study design, data collection, and statistical analysis)
6. Ethical considerations (informed consent and Institutional Review Boards)
7. Funding source
8. Pilot data
9. Timeline

These key components will be discussed in the following sections of this chapter. We will also discuss two important processes that occur after the conclusion of a study: dissemination and translation of research findings. Lastly, we will highlight some recent notable articles in the field of emergency psychiatry research.

THE RESEARCH QUESTION

The first step necessary for conducting any research (including in the ED) involves formulating an interesting question. This often comes from critical thinking, ongoing clinical practice, continued medical education, extensive reading, and/or academic involvement. An interesting question that is both feasible and well-defined can make writing the protocol easier, enable focused data collection, and facilitate improved interpretation of conclusion and results. A mnemonic to consider while formulating a question is FINER, which stands for feasible, interesting to the investigator, novel, ethical, and relevant (5).

Research supervision is the key to success during this process, as turning a research question into a detailed protocol is a learned skill. Supervisors can provide constructive feedback, anticipate potential hurdles, and mentor for academic advancement. In addition to developing a protocol, knowledge of available institutional resources and funding opportunities is essential in bringing the project to fruition. The number of research articles within the field of emergency medicine has increased in recent periods and funding can be limited (6).

SIGNIFICANCE OF THE STUDY

The significance of a study has implications for a variety of study components including the establishment of funds, interpretation of data, dissemination of information, and translation of findings. As such researchers must adequately explain why it is important to answer their research question in the first place. A significant or notable research question will capture the attention of those in charge of funding sources and can increase the probability that the study will obtain the necessary level of financial support (5). It will also set the ground for novel findings which many other researchers will want to learn about and apply to their research. Moreover, these novel findings will lead clinicians to translate them into clinical practice.

HYPOTHESIS

Researchers can use their knowledge of the literature in order to predict the outcome of their study before any data are collected. This prediction or hypothesis requires reasoning through already known information and applying it in a different perspective. In addition, the formulation of a hypothesis serves as a measure of the testability of a research question (7). If a research question is too broad then formulating a valid, testable hypothesis will be extremely difficult if not impossible. Generally, researchers attempt to determine if there is a significant difference between groups. In such cases, studies establish both a null hypothesis and an alternative hypothesis (8). A study's null hypothesis states that the measured outcome does not actually differ between study groups whereas the alternative hypothesis states that the measured outcome does differ between these groups.

SETTING

The location of a study mainly depends on the research question that researchers must answer. Therefore, research questions pertaining to emergency psychiatry require an emergency setting such as an ED with significant psychiatric cases. Importantly, the unique circumstances and variability of patient demographics in EDs must be considered when drafting a research protocol. Many of these patients may be in distress from their illness and may therefore be unable to appropriately assess the situation and make an informed decision about their participation in a research study (9,10).

METHODOLOGY

Selection of Subjects and Sampling

Participant selection and retention may lead to bias in the design, thus complicating interpretation of the results. The inability to recruit patients may lead to small sample sizes which reduce the precision of findings. Thus, both participant selection and retention are particularly important when designing clinical research so researchers should establish a plan for addressing these potential problems before they occur. For example, selection bias can be minimized through the use of randomization or by simply including all patients who meet the eligibility criteria for the study. Small sample sizes can be addressed by closely examining the inclusion/exclusion criteria for the study, by expanding enrollment hours or by including a second site. Inclusion of multiple sites typically involves collaboration (11). Collaborating with other research teams increases the number of potentially eligible patients in the study population, which can then increase the number of study enrollments.

Study Design

The type of research design necessary for obtaining the appropriate information in any sort of research project ultimately depends on the data collection strategies that researchers intend to utilize. As such, researchers must determine whether their project will require the use of randomization procedures, the collection of data over different periods of time, the blinding of certain steps to researchers, or other factors. Once all these factors have been proposed and reviewed by the research team, a flowchart may be constructed in order to visualize and further demonstrate how data will be collected and processed throughout the study. This helps avoid any disagreements among researchers later regarding an aspect of the study.

Data Collection

After completing all the preparation involved in a study, researchers need to shift their focus to collecting the information necessary to answer their research question. Everyone involved in the collection of data must already be properly trained before they can reliably collect data. This training standardizes the way in which each researcher follows the research protocol as well as records information. Importantly, frequent inspection or review of the team's work will allow for any necessary feedback regarding possible protocol deviations.

Data can be collected in a variety of ways depending on the type of study. Some possible data collection tools include surveys, model algorithms, behavioral assessments, and vital sign monitors. The type of data collection tools ultimately determines the way in which the data will be analyzed and interpreted.

Statistical Analysis

The next critical step in the research process involves closely examining all the data collected in order to observe patterns and make conclusions. This step is typically referred to as data analysis. Although commonly paired with statistics, data analysis does not necessarily involve this step as data may be presented descriptively by creating tables, charts, diagrams, or any other helpful methods of display. Collaboration with senior colleagues may be quite helpful during this process, as investigators must determine whether the patterns in the data justify their interpretations.

Once the appropriate tests and tools are used to understand the collected data, it becomes important to make sure that the figures and the wording of the text used for presenting the results can be understood by a range of individuals. This consists of determining the appropriate vocabulary level required for people with different educational backgrounds to understand the data, analyses, and conclusions.

Providing readers with the information necessary for evaluating the reliability of the data obtained in a study may also improve the understanding of conclusions. It may appear to be counterintuitive, but some researchers fail to report all the relevant data obtained throughout their research project. In fact, lack of comprehensive

reporting is so common that standards for reporting of various types of studies have been recommended by the scientific community. For example, in diagnostic studies, investigators should adhere to the Standards for Reporting of Diagnostic Accuracy (STARD) which is a 30-item checklist covering recommendations about the reporting of eligibility criteria for participation, the demographic background of participants, and the implications of the results (12,13). Similarly, the Preferred Reporting Items for Systematic reviews and Meta-Analyses (PRISMA) recommend standards for reporting systematic reviews and meta-analyses (14). The PRISMA checklist contains 27 items covering details from structuring of the abstract and title to reporting of statistics, although not all items may be relevant to each particular manuscript.

Another important function for research articles is to inform other academics in the scientific community about the advancement in knowledge that studies have yielded. Therefore, effective communication also becomes important in achieving this task. Including as much information as possible about the methodology used in a particular study allows others in the field to form their own conclusions. Reports have previously suggested the need to facilitate the learning of methods among researchers (15). Publishing methods used in a study allows other researchers to build upon those methods to enhance research approaches that can further improve medical care.

ETHICAL CONSIDERATIONS

Informed Consent

Evidently, the planning required in any research study involves a significant amount of both time and effort. Nevertheless, this process allows researchers to think about the entire course of a study. A critical factor to consider in this process and one which has caused some level of difficulty within emergency psychiatry research involves the informed consent process.

Prompted in part by the atrocities of World War II and other flagrant abuses of human rights, it is now generally accepted that any patient approached for enrollment in a study has the right to make an informed decision about their participation, ie, informed consent. This has sometimes created a tension in ED research, as for instance, patients who have had severe trauma, cardiopulmonary arrest, or other life-threatening illnesses cannot reasonably provide consent for study participation.

Given that such research is societally valuable, ethicists and regulators have developed well-accepted methods as an alternative to direct patient consent, in order to permit participation in research (16). Ethically and legally, alternatives to direct consent of the patient should never be utilized if the patient is able to provide consent themselves. In some studies, informed consent is obtained from a surrogate or someone responsible for the patient's health instead of from the patient (17,18). Such an alternative method of consent takes place when a patient is considered medically incapacitated and thus unable to make an informed decision about participation in a study. However, this method requires the presence of a surrogate at the time of consent which may not always be possible.

An approach that has been used in order to address this concern involves the use of a process that authorizes an Exception from Informed Consent (EFIC) (19). This method allows researchers to enroll patients in studies if no surrogate decision-maker is present and if the condition is so life-threatening that care cannot be withheld while obtaining consent (for instance, research on cardiopulmonary resuscitation or CPR). This option is restricted to certain situations, such as those in which patients have a life-threatening condition, there is already no effective treatment, and there is absolutely no other way in which informed consent can be obtained (20,21).

The regulations that federal agencies have placed on the use of these alternative approaches to informed consent have significantly changed over time (22-24). As such, some research teams have found it more challenging than others to use these alternative approaches. Federal agencies have even taken contradictory positions when it comes to conditions that must be treated urgently but are not traditionally considered life-threatening, such as agitation. Some studies, such as Martel et al (2005) which examined agitation in a population of predominantly alcohol-intoxicated patients, have been allowed to proceed

with an EFIC waiver. However, other studies have had to rely on other alternatives. As a possible alternative, Cole et al (2018) investigated the concept of *preconsent* in which patients are asked to provide informed consent for treatment that they presently do not need, but could benefit from, during a subsequent visit to the ED. In this case, informed consent is obtained before a patient meets the inclusion/exclusion criteria for a study. However, the results obtained using this particular approach suggest that it may not be a particularly efficient alternative to traditional informed consent.

Additional studies—namely randomized clinical trials—regarding agitation in the emergency setting could allow for a significant improvement in the treatment of these patients as well as their after-visit outcomes (25). Using the information that has already been obtained, researchers have proposed various ways in which physicians could address agitation in EDs (26). Further evidence in this field of research could potentially lead to the national standardization of procedures used to treat the medical concerns of agitated patients.

Other factors to consider when designing a study within emergency psychiatry research include the benefits and risks associated with experimental interventions. In other words, studies must comply with several ethical principles so that certain participants are not placed in a disadvantaged situation compared to other participants (27). This is critical when considering randomized clinical trials. If researchers are attempting to test various interventions in the emergency setting in order to determine the most effective approach, then there must not already be an effective intervention available in such a setting that could be used to help those potential study participants.

Institutional Review Boards

Before collecting any sort of data for their project, researchers must also submit their research plan along with any other relevant documents, including informed consent and Health Insurance Portability and Accountability Act of 1996 (HIPAA) Research Authorization forms, to the Institutional Review Board (IRB) (28). The IRB is a group of individuals at a research facility who have been tasked with reviewing and approving or disapproving all research projects that involve human subjects. The quantity and quality of information that the IRB needs in order to evaluate a research plan depends on the type of study that researchers are planning to complete. In some instances, this process may require a review of the research plan by a few members of the IRB whereas, in other instances, it may require a full IRB review. One of the crucial factors used in determining the level of review required involves the potential risks that participants may encounter as a result of study procedures. The length of this review process will also vary depending on how well researchers can address the concerns raised by the IRB. Among the many research factors that the IRB will consider are ethicalness, feasibility, necessity, and level of preparedness (28).

Although obtaining approval from the IRB may require a significant amount of work and time before even beginning to collect data, this process ensures that any potential areas of concern are addressed before recruiting participants. Researchers are able to improve upon their research plan through this process. For example, they can more thoroughly think about why the information they plan to obtain is important, plan how participant information will be stored and used, and determine potential unintended consequences of participation. The IRB may reject a research proposal if no new knowledge will result from the study, researchers do not have an acceptable plan for handling the data collected, or there are too many risks for participants.

FUNDING SOURCE

In most research, a funding source becomes an essential component to success. The level of financial support necessary for a study will depend on the resources needed to collect data. There are numerous sources of funding that researchers can take advantage of, but they all require a significant amount of effort and these efforts are not always successful. Adequate funding can be obtained from private donors, charities, commercial companies, health institutions, and a variety of other sources (4). At times funding sources can set specific guidelines for

how their funds may be used (29). Historically, the inability to provide the necessary level of support has set barriers for investigators with a desire to conduct research in the field of emergency medicine. Collaboration across research institutions has the potential to significantly improve the quality of research by exchange of knowledge and understanding the appropriateness and influence of findings (30).

PILOT DATA

Other logistical issues such as funding, data collection, support staff, or whether the project can be completed within the designated time frame should also be addressed before beginning a new research project. A pilot study to assess the methodology of the proposed study is often considered before a larger study is initiated. The role of a pilot study is not to answer the research question but rather test the feasibility of implementation (4).

After approval from the Institutional Review Board, which marks the completion of a crucial step in any research study, collecting the necessary information becomes the next priority. The techniques used for data collection will primarily depend on the resources available and the study design agreed upon.

TIMELINE

Researchers will expect their studies to obtain information that can improve the quality of care for patients. Establishing specific goals throughout a study allows researchers to remain on track to finishing their study on time. It is quite possible to encounter unforeseen problems while conducting the study, but nevertheless, the research protocol must be followed with measures in place to avoid decreasing the quality of the study in any way. Therefore, preventing a study's quality from deteriorating over time will ensure reliability of the results as well as the ability for the information that it provides to translate into clinical practice (31).

Providing an adequate training schedule to clinical researchers can help with data collection within the predetermined time window while adhering to predetermined standards (32).

TRANSLATING RESEARCH INTO CLINICAL PRACTICE

Clinical research studies aim to have an important impact on the broader community by providing results that may improve the care of patients. At times, this particular step of translating research lies beyond the capabilities of individual investigators. In other words, senior investigators may not be the ideal people for implementation of study recommendations, and this important step is often left to clinicians. There are several reasons as to why this is the case, including an investigator's incomplete understanding of the clinical setting, financial concerns, and a lengthy process for institutional changes. It is also the case that clinicians are directly impacted by the implementation of new processes, so they are often more suitable to complete this translational process. The field of dissemination and implementation has been able to improve the techniques used to incorporate knowledge from research studies into techniques used in the medical field (33). Additionally, researchers have developed models over time and used them to facilitate this important process (34,35). These models can even be used to identify facilitators as well as barriers for implementing major research findings in the clinical setting. Therefore, those seeking to implement evidence must determine the model which will work best in those particular cases.

NOTABLE ARTICLES IN EMERGENCY PSYCHIATRY RESEARCH

Despite the lengthy and sometimes challenging process involved when conducting research in the emergency setting, the results obtained at the end of a study in this field of research make this process well worth the time for researchers. In recent years, researchers have been able to study various possible ways in which medical treatment can be improved upon in the emergency setting. These notable findings have the potential for establishing specific recommendations for improvements in the field of emergency psychiatry. Considering the limited amount of time that emergency providers have for assessing and treating any patient, any improvements to medications, screening, interventions, or other treatment options can lead to better long-term outcomes for patients. Some of these notable findings are summarized in the following paragraphs.

D'Onofrio et al (2015), for instance, examined the expected outcome of various possible interventions for opioid dependence in the emergency setting (36). In an attempt to improve outcomes for patients with opioid use disorder (OUD), researchers evaluated three possible interventions in the emergency setting. The randomization involved in their study design allowed researchers to obtain three groups with fairly similar demographic characteristics and other clinical characteristics. Within this study design, researchers were then able to assess the efficacy of these interventions in encouraging patients to seek treatment for their OUD. These researchers concluded that starting buprenorphine-naloxone treatment, a form of medication-assisted treatment, in the emergency setting is not only feasible, but it also results in better outcome for these patients than screening and referral alone.

Another serious psychiatric problem, which is often managed by EDs, consists of treating and preventing future suicide attempts. In a National Institutes of Health (NIH)-funded multicenter trial, Miller et al (2017) analyzed the rates of suicide attempts among three cohorts of patients who received different interventions with sequential phases of the study (treatment as usual or TAU, universal screening + TAU, and universal screening + brief intervention + TAU) (37). After quantifying the number of suicide attempts made by participants up to 1 year after their ED visit, these researchers concluded that patients who obtained a professional suicide screening in the ED, were given additional discharge resources, and received follow-up calls for several weeks were less likely to attempt suicide compared to patients who received no intervention for reducing suicide attempts during their ED visit.

From time to time, it also becomes necessary for experts in any field of research—in this case, emergency psychiatry research—to complete a systematic review of the most important and groundbreaking studies that have profoundly advanced the knowledge of the field. Within emergency psychiatry research, such comprehensive articles allow researchers to better understand where the field has come from as well as the direction in which is it headed (38). The level of analysis and recommendations that some of these systematic reviews provide can offer solutions to ongoing problems in emergency psychiatry or motivate further research studies. A review by Chennapan et al (2018) focused on research articles that examined approaches for providing medical screenings to psychiatric patients in the emergency setting. In their review, the authors considered various studies into the medical screening of psychiatric patients including nonrandomized studies which are usually not included in systematic reviews. The authors' level of analysis allowed them to make numerous recommendations for the field of emergency psychiatry, some of which focused on considering the age of a patient and the specific details of their psychiatric condition. These recommendations allow for a more focused medical screening as any case involving a psychiatric patient can be completely different than the next one.

CONCLUSIONS

Although conducting clinical research studies requires an immense amount of effort and dedication, the ability to positively impact clinical practice makes this a promising and rewarding process. Collaborations among investigators and research sites can have a meaningful impact on the spread of scientific advancements. Research approaches and methods continue to improve and this has the potential for establishing new paths in research.

REFERENCES

1. Kelley, W. N., & Randolph, M. A. (Eds.). (1994). *Careers in clinical research: Obstacles and opportunities*. Washington, DC: National Academies Press.
2. Tandberg, D., & Qualls, C. (1994). Time series forecasts of emergency department patient volume, length of stay, and acuity. *Annals of Emergency Medicine, 23*(2), 299–306.
3. Wilson, M. P., Guluma, K. Z., & Hayden, S. R. (Eds.). (2015). *Doing research in emergency and acute care: Making order out of chaos*. Oxford: Wiley-Blackwell.
4. Good, A. M. T., & Driscoll, P. (2002). Clinical research in emergency medicine: Putting it together. *Emergency Medicine Journal, 19*(3), 242–246.
5. Cummings, S. R., Browner, W.S., & Hulley, S. B. (1988). Conceiving the research question. In Hulley, S. B., & Cummings, S. R. (Eds.), *Designing clinical research* (pp. 12–17). Baltimore, MD: Williams and Wilkins.
6. Wilson, M. P., & Itagaki, M. W. (2007). Characteristics and trends of published emergency medicine research. *Academic Emergency Medicine, 14*(7), 635–640.
7. Mosier, J. M., & Rosen, P. (2015). Aspects of research specific to acute care. In Wilson, M. P., Guluma, K. Z., & Hayden, S. R. (Eds.), *Doing research in emergency and acute care: Making order out of chaos* (pp. 3–6). Oxford: Wiley-Blackwell.
8. Garg, M., Harrigan, R., & Gaddis, G. (2015). Basic statistics: Sample size and power: How are sample size and power calculated? In Wilson, M. P., Guluma, K. Z., & Hayden, S. R. (Eds.), *Doing research in emergency and acute care: Making order out of chaos* (pp. 183–190). Oxford: Wiley-Blackwell.
9. Mader, T. J., & Playe, S. J. (1997). Emergency medicine research consent form readability assessment. *Annals of Emergency Medicine, 29*(4), 534–539.
10. Schmidt, T. A., Salo, D., Hughes, J. A., et al. (2004). Confronting the ethical challenges to informed consent in emergency medicine research. *Academic Emergency Medicine, 11*(10), 1082–1089.
11. Hopper, A., & Wilson, M. P. (2015). How to complete a research study well and in a minimum of time: The importance of collaboration. In Wilson, M. P., Guluma, K. Z., & Hayden, S. R. (Eds.), *Doing research in emergency and acute care: Making order out of chaos* (pp. 167–171). Oxford: Wiley-Blackwell.
12. Bossuyt, P., Reitsma, J., Bruns, D., et al, for the STARD Group. (2015). STARD 2015: An updated list of essential items for reporting diagnostic accuracy studies. *Clinical Chemistry, 61*, 1446–1452.
13. Gallo, L., Hua, N., Mercuri, M., Silveira, A., & Worster, A., for Best Evidence in Emergency Medicine. (2017). Adherence to standards for reporting diagnostic accuracy in emergency medicine research. *Academic Emergency Medicine, 24*(8), 914–919.

14. Moher, D., Liberati, A., Tetzlaff, J., Altman, D. G., & PRISMA Group. (2009). Preferred reporting items for systematic reviews and meta-analyses: The PRISMA statement. *PLoS Medicine, 6*(7), e1000097.

15. Supino, P. G., & Richardson, L. D. (1999). Assessing research methodology training needs in emergency medicine. *Academic Emergency Medicine, 6*(4), 280–285.

16. Martel, M., Sterzinger, A., Miner, J., Clinton, J., & Biros, M. (2005). Management of acute undifferentiated agitation in the emergency department: A randomized double-blind trial of droperidol, ziprasidone, and midazolam. *Academic Emergency Medicine, 12*(12), 1167–1172.

17. Chan, E. W., Taylor, D. M., Phillips, G. S. A., Castle, D. J., Knott, J. C., & Kong, D. C. M. (2011). May I have your consent? Informed consent in clinical trials – Feasibility in emergency situations. *Journal of Psychiatric Intensive Care, 7*(2), 109–113.

18. Miller, S. S., & Marin, D. B. (2000). Assessing capacity. *Emergency Medicine Clinics of North America, 18*(2), 233–242.

19. Klein, L., Moore, J., & Biros, M. (2018). A 20-year review: The use of exception from informed consent and waiver of informed consent in emergency research. *Academic Emergency Medicine, 25*(10), 1169–1177.

20. Dickert, N. W., Mah, V. A., Baren, J. M., Biros, M. H., Govindarajan, P., Pancioli, A., … Pentz, R. D. (2013). Enrollment in research under exception from informed consent: The Patients' Experiences in Emergency Research (PEER) study. *Resuscitation, 84*(10), 1416–1421.

21. Dickert, N. W., Scicluna, V. M., Baren, J. M., Biros, M. H., Fleischman, R. J., Govindarajan, P. R., … Pentz, R. D. (2015). Patients' perspective of enrollment in research without consent: The patients' experiences in emergency research-progesterone for the treatment of traumatic brain injury study. *Critical Care Medicine, 43*(3), 603–612.

22. Brown, J. (2006). The spectrum of informed consent in emergency psychiatric research. *Annals of Emergency Medicine, 47*(1), 68–74.

23. Cole, J. B., Klein, L. R., Mullinax, S., Nordstrom, K. D., Driver, B. E., & Wilson, M. P. (2018). Study enrollment when "pre-consent" is utilized for a randomized clinical trial of two treatments for acute agitation in the emergency department. *Academic Emergency Medicine*, 26(5), 559–566.

24. Silbergleit, R., Biros, M. H., Harney, D., Dickert, N., & Baren, J., on behalf of the NETT Investigators. (2012). Implementation of the exception from informed consent regulations in a large multicenter emergency clinical trials network: The RAMPART experience. *Academic Emergency Medicine, 19*(4), 448–454.

25. Mullinax, S., Shokraneh, F., Wilson, M. P., & Adams, C.E. (2017). Oral medication for agitation of psychiatric origin: A scoping review of randomized controlled trials. *Journal of Emergency Medicine, 53*(4), 524–529.

26. Wilson, M. P., Pepper, D., Currier, G. W., Holloman, G. H., & Feifel, D. (2012). The psychopharmacology of agitation: Consensus statement of the American Association for Emergency Psychiatry Project BETA Psychopharmacology Workgroup. *West Journal of Emergency Medicine, 13*(1), 26–34.

27. World Medical Association. (2013). World Medical Association Declaration of Helsinki: Ethical principles for medical research involving human subjects. *JAMA, 310*(20), 2191–2194.

28. Rafi, N., & Snyder, B. (2015). Ethics in research: How to collect data ethically. In Wilson, M. P., Guluma, K. Z., & Hayden, S. R. (Eds.), *Doing research in emergency and acute care: Making order out of chaos* (pp. 45–51). Oxford: Wiley-Blackwell.

29. Dezman, Z. D. W., & Hirshon, J. M. (2015). How do I write a grant? In Wilson, M. P., Guluma, K. Z., & Hayden, S. R. (Eds.), *Doing research in emergency and acute care: Making order out of chaos* (pp. 247–251). Oxford: Wiley-Blackwell.

30. Aghababian, R. V., Barsan, W.G., Bickell, W.H., et al. (1996). Research directions in emergency medicine. *Annals of Emergency Medicine, 27*(3), 339–342.

31. Grol, R., & Grimshaw, J. (2003). From best evidence to best practice: Effective implementation of change in patients' care. *The Lancet, 362*(9391), 1225–1230.

32. Bounes, V., Dehours, E., Houze-Cerfon, V., Valle, B., Lipton, R., & Ducasse, J. L. (2013). Quality of publications in emergency medicine. *American Journal of Emergency Medicine, 31*(2), 297–301.

33. Bernstein, S. L., Stoney, C.M., & Rothman, R. E. (2015). Dissemination and implementation research in emergency medicine. *Academic Emergency Medicine, 22*(2), 229–236.

34. Stiell, I. G., & Bennett, C. (2007). Implementation of clinical decision rules in the emergency department. *Academic Emergency Medicine, 14*(11), 955–959.

35. Tabak, R. G., Khoong, E. C., Chambers, D. A., & Brownson, R. C. (2012). Bridging research and practice: Models for dissemination and implementation research. *American Journal of Preventive Medicine, 43*(3), 337–350.

36. D'Onofrio, G., O'Connor, P. G., Pantalon, M. V., Chawarski, M. C., Busch, S. H., Owens, P. H., … Fiellin, D. A. (2015). Emergency department-initiated buprenorphine/naloxone treatment for opioid dependence: A randomized clinical trial. *JAMA, 313*(16), 1636–1644.

37. Miller, I. W., Camargo, C. A., Jr., Arias, S. A., Sullivan, A. F., Allen, M. H., Goldstein, A. B., … Boudreaux, E. D., for the ED-SAFE Investigators. (2017). Suicide prevention in an emergency department population: The ED-SAFE study. *JAMA Psychiatry, 74*(6), 563–570.

38. Chennapan, K., Mullinax, S., Anderson, E., Landau, M. J., Nordstrom, K., Seupaul, R. A., & Wilson, M. P. (2018). Medical screening of mental health patients in the emergency department: A systematic review. *Journal of Emergency Medicine, 55*(6), 799–812.

5

Education and Training in the Psychiatric Emergency Service

Bruce Fage, Jodi Lofchy

Psychiatric emergency services (PESs) are well-established educational sites for many training programs (1). Programs may capitalize on the numerous educational opportunities provided within a PES by cultivating a supportive and enriching educational experience for trainees. As the emergency department can be both exciting and stressful, effective supervision and adequate training are critical to empowering students to take advantage of the educational potential of this environment, and mastering the core psychiatric skills needed for the acute care setting. PESs need to promote quality educational experiences to encourage interest in psychiatry and emergency psychiatry as a career choice. No other environment offers trainees the fast-paced excitement and clinical challenges of the PES, with access to high volume work in a collaborative and multidisciplinary setting. This chapter reviews educational activities within the PES, rotations for residents and medical students, clinical placements for allied healthcare professionals, and continuing PES education. In the PES, everyone has something to learn and something to teach.

Using a PES as a clinical teaching unit has many advantages (2). The PES offers the best place to observe acute psychopathology, the effects of acute pharmacologic intervention, and the effects of crisis intervention counseling. It is an excellent setting for trainees to observe and perform numerous assessments to develop rapid assessment skills and to learn to provide multiple treatment modalities in a crisis setting. A PES provides frequent opportunities for exposure to the medicolegal aspects of psychiatry, including consent, capacity, and laws involving involuntary assessment and treatment. Trainees observe firsthand the effects of the psychosocial determinants of health when assessing PES patients and routinely see patients with severe and persistent mental illness, a group that highlights the limits of our medical knowledge and healthcare system. Trainees learn to use collateral sources of information, to become familiar with community resources, and to make rapid treatment decisions with limited information. In addition, the PES is an excellent setting for trainees to begin to work as members of multidisciplinary teams.

There are also challenges to using the PES as an educational site. The PES is an environment with at times a fast pace, unpredictable patient load and service demands, and potentially unclear role for trainees who may be continuously rotating through different clinical environments. These factors can lead to considerable stress for trainees, especially with overnight call duties in a busy PES. Frequent expressions of anger or suicidal and homicidal ideation by patients may be difficult for trainees to experience, or patients may be intolerant of trainees' limited skills. Trainees must cope with patients who harm themselves or engage in violence toward others and face the potential for medicolegal liability. Seeing primarily refractory to treatment patients can be discouraging and skew a new trainee's impression of psychiatry. Trainees may find disposition decisions difficult or the excess time dealing with third-party insurers frustrating (3). Finally, trainees may need time to acculturate and integrate into established and tightly knit teams, and service demands may limit the opportunities for didactic teaching and direct supervision.

PSYCHIATRY RESIDENT TRAINING

All psychiatry residents can expect to perform assessments within the emergency setting during their training (1). Although patients with agitation, suicidal ideation, and other crises are most commonly seen within PESs, they can present in any psychiatric setting. Therefore, all psychiatrists in training should become competent and comfortable in managing crisis situations (4). Residency training programs must promote the care of patients in crisis as valuable and educational and not as simply a necessary service obligation.

The Accreditation Council for Graduate Medical Education (ACGME) includes training in emergency psychiatry as a requirement for psychiatry residents (5). Specifically, emergency psychiatry must be conducted in an organized and supervised PES that is separate from outpatient requirements. On-call experiences must not be the only exposure to emergency psychiatry, and residents must obtain experience with triaging emergency psychiatric patients and the assessment and management of psychiatric crisis.

The American Association for Emergency Psychiatry (AAEP) has developed detailed training objectives (4) that expand on the ACGME requirements just described. These have been adapted to the ACGME competencies (6) format and are listed in Table 5.1.

Many residency programs are affiliated with a comprehensive PES that offers an excellent setting in which to develop emergency psychiatry skills. Residents can work with members of the PES team who demonstrate interviewing and patient management skills and provide support as residents develop clinical skills with PES patients. Residents may provide emergency consultations to patients within a general emergency department or stand-alone psychiatric emergency department. However, high volumes in the emergency department may make lengthy psychiatric assessments challenging and can adversely affect the training experience of psychiatric residents working alone (7).

Other training sites for emergency psychiatry experiences include ambulatory urgent care clinics and mobile crisis services (8). Models for ambulatory urgent care vary widely but generally include time-limited rapid follow-up care with a psychiatrist and possibly other mental health clinicians. If trainees are working in both the emergency department and an associated urgent care service, there may be the opportunity to follow patients throughout the psychiatric crisis and

provide treatment beyond the one-time emergency department intervention. Cross-sectional assessments are limited in their ability to provide trainees an opportunity to develop a fulsome understanding of an individual, and urgent care services may prove useful in adding depth to the educational experience by introducing the resident to models of brief crisis therapies. If available, working with a mobile crisis service may provide trainees an opportunity to work with outreach teams to provide emergency support in a more naturalistic setting.

The ACGME does not specify the duration for training in emergency psychiatry but does stress that on-call duties alone are insufficient for learning the requisite crisis-related skills and knowledge. The AAEP recommends a 2-month rotation (4). The Royal College of Physicians and Surgeons of Canada (RCPSC), the national accrediting body for psychiatry in Canada, mandates a minimum of 1 month of emergency psychiatry within the first year of training (9). Certainly, it is advantageous for residents to become familiar and comfortable with the PES setting and patient population during a daytime core rotation before assuming on-call responsibilities. Daytime rotations provide the opportunity for much closer supervision than is generally available on-call, plus there may be more clinical staff on duty, other mental health services are available for referrals or information, and residents are less stressed and better rested than during an overnight shift. A daytime rotation in a PES allows residents to progress from assisting with assessments to performing interviews independently with immediate supervision over the course of a rotation (10).

Clinical supervision for residents learning emergency psychiatry is crucial. All cases need to be reviewed with an attending psychiatrist, especially for junior trainees. Direct observation of assessments is ideal but may be impractical in the fast-paced environment of the PES. Strategies to ensure residents are developing good clinical skills include observing part of an interview, having an off-duty psychiatrist observe the resident and provide feedback on his or her clinical skills once disposition has been arranged, and having PES clinicians involved in providing some feedback on interviewing or patient management

TABLE 5.1 Training Objectives

By the completion of a residency program, a psychiatric resident will be able to demonstrate the following competencies.
Patient care
Residents must be able to provide patient care that is compassionate, appropriate, and effective for the assessment and management of patients seen within a psychiatric emergency service (PES).

This includes the following skills:

I. Prioritization skills

Given the responsibility of running a PES, residents will:

A. Triage patients presenting to the PES with acute psychiatric illness, symptoms, or distress, recognizing patients whose needs take priority

B. Attend to the most distressed patients first

C. For each patient, recognize and attend to emergent needs for medication, seclusion, restraint, searches, or monitoring

D. Refer patients whose psychiatric symptoms are due to a medical illness promptly for appropriate medical care

II. Patient assessment and management skills

Within the limitations of time and resources in the PES, given a patient with acute psychiatric illness, symptoms, or distress

A. Perform an assessment including:

1. A rapid, focused psychiatric interview to obtain all necessary data
2. An appropriately detailed mental status examination
3. A physical examination, as appropriate
4. A risk assessment for suicidal and homicidal ideation
5. Establishing a therapeutic alliance
6. Demonstrating respect and empathy for the patient
7. Adjusting the detail of the assessment to the needs of the patient and situation
8. Obtaining collateral information (from family, other caregivers, old charts, etc.) when necessary (ie, almost always)
9. Ordering laboratory investigations and medical consultation, when appropriate
10. Documenting the assessment accurately and legibly

B. Once an emergency psychiatric assessment has been completed, integrate the information by:

1. Stating a differential diagnosis
2. Stating a preferred diagnosis
3. Describing a brief biopsychosocial understanding of the patient and the current situation
4. Using this brief biopsychosocial understanding to develop a treatment plan
5. Explaining the factors used to reach the decisions that guide the treatment plan
6. Documenting the proposed treatment plan

C. Using the assessment, diagnosis, and biopsychosocial understanding of an emergency psychiatric patient, initiate emergency management and treatment by:

1. Providing appropriate feedback, counseling, and information to the patient and support persons
2. Giving further instructions to staff to ensure the safety of the patient and staff (eg, use of seclusion, restraint, searches, observation, etc.)
3. Ordering appropriate emergency medications
4. Ordering appropriate monitoring of the patient
5. Demonstrating compassion and respect for the patient's dignity
6. Demonstrating verbal and nonverbal skills to de-escalate high-tension situations

(Continued)

TABLE 5.1 Training Objectives   (Continued)

   D. Given a completed emergency psychiatric assessment, diagnosis, and biopsychosocial understanding, make recommendations for further treatment as appropriate by:
      1. Justifying the need for inpatient treatment
      2. Selecting appropriate outpatient treatment
      3. Explaining treatment recommendations to third-party payers
      4. Communicating (verbally and/or in writing) the assessment findings and patient's needs to inpatient and outpatient treatment facilities
      5. Including social and family supports in treatment plans
      6. Recommending relevant community resources to the patient
      7. Performing short-term crisis-oriented therapy when appropriate
      8. Initiating psychopharmacologic treatments, when appropriate
III. Crisis telephone call skills
   Given a crisis phone call, respond appropriately by:
   A. Listening carefully
   B. Remaining calm
   C. Counseling the caller appropriately
   D. Notifying community resources (police, outpatient therapist, etc.) as needed
IV. Child and adolescent emergency psychiatric skills
   Given a child or adolescent with a psychiatric emergency, perform an assessment, integrate the information, and manage the patient appropriately by:
   A. Utilizing a developmental approach
   B. Including a review of the child's intellectual and emotional functioning and his or her social, interpersonal, educational, and physical functioning
   C. Obtaining a history of recent events, trauma, drug use, and maladaptive behavior
   D. Assessing family structure and relationships, and the supports and capacities of the family or agency who protects and cares for the child
   E. Demonstrating all the skills and competencies listed for adult patients

Medical knowledge

  I. Knowledge areas essential to the PES include the following problems and diagnoses:
   A. Suicidal ideation
   B. Homicidal ideation
   C. Acute psychosis
   D. Acute intoxication and withdrawal
   E. Substance abuse and dependence
   F. Concurrent disorders
   G. Psychiatric illness with medical symptoms
   H. Medical illness with psychiatric symptoms
   I. Depression
   J. Anxiety
   K. Acute exacerbation of chronic psychosis
   L. Personality disorders (especially borderline and antisocial)
   M. Side effects of psychopharmacologic agents
   N. Acute bereavement
   O. Acute psychic trauma
   P. Drug seeking
   Q. Malingering or factitious disorder
   R. Victims of domestic abuse
   S. Situational problems, especially family, vocational, or scholastic

TABLE 5.1 Training Objectives   (Continued)

II. Residents must have and demonstrate knowledge of medicolegal issues relevant to emergency psychiatry by:
   A. Stating local laws on involuntary commitment
   B. Describing the process of finding a patient incompetent to consent/refuse treatment
   C. Stating local laws regarding public intoxication
   D. Stating local laws on confidentiality in emergency psychiatry, describing specific exceptions to confidentiality, including the reporting of child abuse/neglect, elder abuse, domestic violence, and unsafe driving

Practice-based learning and improvement

Residents must be able to investigate and evaluate their patient care practices and appraise and assimilate scientific evidence to improve their patient care practices. Residents are expected to:
A. Exhibit the ability to critically self-evaluate their psychiatric emergency skills and demonstrate improvement as a result of such evaluations
B. Incorporate material discussed in supervision within the PES into clinical work

Interpersonal and communication skills

Residents must be able to demonstrate interpersonal and communication skills that result in effective information exchange by teaming with patients, their patients' families, and professional associates.
   I. Within an emergency setting, residents are expected to communicate effectively by:
   A. Obtaining the background and reasons for all consultation requests
   B. Providing timely, helpful recommendations to the referring physician after completing a consultation, as requested
   C. Communicating recommendations (written and/or verbal) to other clinics and agencies clearly and specifically
   D. Completing required documentation accurately, coherently, legibly, and on time
   II. Given the responsibility of running a PES, the resident will manage the patients, staff, and trainees by:
   A. Obtaining a summary of patients currently in the PES at the beginning of each shift
   B. Providing a summary of patients currently in the PES for the incoming staff at the end of each shift
   C. Collaborating appropriately with staff
   D. Delegating tasks appropriately to staff and trainees
   E. Supervising and teaching trainees and staff as appropriate
   F. Contacting physician backup when indicated

Professionalism

Residents must demonstrate a commitment to carrying out professional responsibilities, adherence to ethical principles, and sensitivity to a diverse patient population. Within a PES, residents are expected to:
A. Demonstrate professional attitudes to colleagues, supervisors, team members, and trainees, including respect
B. Honor professional obligations and responsibilities
C. Perform and complete assessments and other responsibilities within the limitations of time, energy, space, and resources of the PES
D. Maintain a positive attitude
E. Demonstrate flexibility in managing a heavy workload
F. Remain calm in stressful situations
G. Demonstrate an awareness of one's own reactions to crisis situations and to specific types of patients

(Continued)

TABLE 5.1 Training Objectives   (Continued)

Systems-based practice
Residents must demonstrate an awareness of and responsiveness to their community's system of mental healthcare. Residents are expected to: A. Describe the role of the local emergency psychiatric services within the community's mental healthcare network B. Describe community- and hospital-based services that PES patients may need and utilize

Adapted by permission from Springer: Brasch, J., Glick, R. L., Cobb, T. G., et al. (2004). Residency training in emergency psychiatry: A model curriculum developed by the Education Committee of the American Association for Emergency Psychiatry. *Academic Psychiatry, 28*(2), 95–103. Copyright © 2004 Academic Psychiatry.

techniques. Maximum educational benefit is obtained when the resident receives supervision and feedback about an emergency psychiatric consultation in a timely fashion (11). Information about the outcome of an emergency department consultation in both the short and long term provides additional educational value and opportunity for self-appraisal (11).

On-call work in a PES or as a consultant to a general emergency department may be a substantial part of a resident's experience in emergency psychiatry. On-call duty is rich with clinical material and challenging work but can be occasionally lonely (7). As key providers of healthcare services, it is critical for the PES to provide a supportive environment and on-call supervision that enables residents to focus on clinical duties and perform competently outside of regular working hours. There is growing recognition that residents, supervisors, and health systems all play a role in fatigue risk management. The ACGME duty hour requirements limit the amount of time a resident can work to 80 hours per week, averaged over a 4-week period (including on-call responsibilities). Duty periods cannot be longer than 16 hours in the first year of training, and 24 hours in years thereafter (12). In 2013, a pan-Canadian National Steering Committee on Resident Duty Hours reviewed the available evidence and made a number of recommendations about the management of fatigue-related risk that move beyond simply considering consecutive and total hours worked (13). Residents have a dual role as learners and service providers and play a vital role in a healthcare system that is collectively responsible for 24/7 care.

Ideally, there should be graduated responsibility for on-call duties in a PES throughout the residency. In a number of American and Canadian training programs, first year residents have graduated responsibility and senior resident support during the first part of their call experience written in to their collective agreement and terms of employment (14). In some settings, it may be possible to have an on-call team that includes junior and senior residents as well as clinicians and medical students. An on-call team enables junior residents to provide patient care and learn from the senior resident, while the senior resident can focus on triage and patient management issues. A system of graduated responsibility may be especially helpful for less experienced trainees who are still developing their professional identity and may be questioning their own competence, particularly during stressful clinical situations (15).

Assessment of resident performance in the PES may be challenging if acuity or volumes are high. With multiple opportunities for assessment, assessments may need to be focused and specific. Owing to the volumes, complexity, and interprofessional nature of the work environment, the PES provides an excellent opportunity for assessment of more than just straightforward clinical skills. Different approaches to the evaluation of resident performance in the PES have been used. One strategy is to have residents keep a "logbook" to record all patients seen on-call, which can be incorporated into an evaluation and review (4). Review of a written assessment note can provide some feedback to residents and emphasize the importance of effective documentation in the PES.

Handover, or the transfer of clinical information and patient responsibility from one provider to another, is a daily procedure in the PES. Most commonly, structured handover between the day team and on-call team will occur at the end of the day and again at the end of the overnight call shift. Informal handover between providers may happen several times a day (16). Though handover may provide opportunities for a fresh perspective on patient care, these transitional times are high-risk points in patient care where errors can occur. The PES provides several opportunities for trainees to practice this critical professional skill and implement best practices. Strategies for effective handover include having a designated face-to-face meeting that minimizes interruptions and distractions and encouraging trainees to ask clarifying questions of their supervisors despite the possible presence of hierarchies within the medical system. The use of a structured handover tool has been shown to reduce rates of medical errors and adverse events (17). Tools such as the SBAR model—Situation, Background, Assessment, and Recommendations—can provide a structure to guide the team through the discussion of several potentially complex patients (18).

As on-call work may constitute a significant amount of a resident's PES clinical experience, developing a mechanism to provide some feedback about on-call performance should be considered. A meaningful approach to feedback for residents is to monitor actual clinical outcomes, such as changes in patient care and admission rates from the emergency department (19). Systems must be in place to provide feedback and remediation to residents who need extra support to achieve the requisite competencies. Programs developing an evaluation system for residents in the PES may want to consult Epstein's review of assessment in medical education, which outlines the strengths and limitations of many evaluation methods (20).

PESs can also offer elective experiences to residents. Core rotations enable residents to develop sound clinical skills in assessing and managing patients within the PES. Electives can be tailored to a resident's interest and offer opportunities to develop team management skills or to focus on some aspect of administration or a continuous quality improvement project.

Residents in other specialties can benefit from a rotation through a PES (21,22). In fact, Weissberg (21) surveyed program directors and found that over half felt that emergency psychiatry skills would be useful in their specialty, but only one-third offered their residents any training in a PES. In particular, residents in emergency medicine benefit from developing competency in rapid assessment, diagnosis, and acute intervention strategies through a rotation in the PES. Emergency medicine residents can be exposed to effective strategies within a PES for managing unusual and challenging behaviors. The Emergency Medicine Core Content Task Force has identified a number of psychobehavioral disorders that emergency medicine trainees are expected to recognize and manage (23). Emergency medicine residents may wish to adapt the training objectives in Table 5.1 to ensure they develop the required competencies for their specialty.

Though fellowship opportunities for additional training in emergency psychiatry do exist, the majority of emergency psychiatrists do not pursue formal additional training. The American Board of Psychiatry and Neurology does not recognize emergency psychiatry as a subspecialty, and jobs in emergency psychiatry are readily available for recent graduates, so few organized fellowship programs are currently available. The lack of fellowships is reflected in the finding that only about 10% of PES medical directors have fellowship training in emergency psychiatry (1). Instead, senior residents may do electives prior to completing their residency and beginning clinical work in a PES. Senior psychiatrists practicing emergency psychiatry can offer mentorship to support newly trained psychiatrists interested in a career in emergency psychiatry. These informal alliances need to be encouraged and supported. Fellowships in subspecialties such as addictions and consultation-liaison often include clinical experiences in a PES.

MEDICAL STUDENTS AND OTHER TRAINEES

The PES offers an excellent training setting for medical students because of the wide range of patient presentations and opportunities to observe and participate in the assessment and care of many acutely ill patients during a short rotation.

Both elective and core rotations can be useful for medical students. Consideration should be given to combining PES core or elective rotations with other clinical settings for the medical student trainee, as the prevalence of acutely unwell patients is not representative of all of psychiatry, and learners may not spend sufficient time working with one particular patient to observe significant improvement. If programs use the PES for on-call experiences for medical students, it is critical that close supervision be provided in order to ensure these junior learners have the opportunity to ask questions, reflect, and debrief appropriately. The opportunity for medical students to observe psychiatrists showing compassion and providing emergency treatment while integrating medical, pharmacologic, and psychiatric data will allow trainees to appreciate the skills of an acute care interventional psychiatrist which may be contrary to many students' expectations. The skills acquired and knowledge learned in a PES will be of benefit to all physicians, regardless of specialty choice.

The PES can be a valuable training site for students in other disciplines, such as nursing, social work (24), or paramedic programs. Placements for nursing and other allied health professionals can expose trainees to career opportunities they may not have considered. Some programs may have allied health professional students on a regular basis and can develop special educational opportunities and training expectations for them. For programs with infrequent elective students, the training objectives in Table 5.1 can be adapted on an individual basis.

It is critical to emphasize safety issues early in a rotation for medical students and other trainees and to make safety a priority. The PES milieu must convey a commitment to safety by ensuring that safety procedures are clear to all staff. Nonviolent crisis intervention training is important for residents and clinical staff, and discussion of the strategies used to manage agitated patients is beneficial for all trainees.

EDUCATIONAL ACTIVITIES WITHIN THE PSYCHIATRIC EMERGENCY SERVICE

Academic PESs need to provide a structured educational program to ensure that core knowledge, skills, and attitudes are acquired by residents, medical students, and other trainees. Structured

didactic sessions can be helpful for junior learners who may have limited experience in the PES, and the PES provides an opportunity for senior learners to practice their own teaching skills. Although case-based teaching is highly beneficial, core topics specific to PES work can also be presented to residents in an organized manner. Programs may include emergency psychiatry seminars on specific topics in the academic half-day program for residents or incorporate the topics into presentations on related subjects (eg, covering the acute presentation of mania in a talk on mood disorders). Table 5.2 contains a recommended list of core topics. In addition to learning about risk factors for suicide and assessment strategies, residents may benefit from a seminar in which they explore and discuss their own personal attitudes and beliefs about suicide (25). Many of these topics are appropriate for discussions and interactive learning methods where trainees have a chance to reflect and debrief on their own experiences and reactions to challenging cases. Lofchy (26) has described the successful use of standardized patients (either live or on video recordings) to teach key components of interviewing skills in the PES, providing an opportunity to practice sensitive interviewing with respect to agitation, suicide risk assessments, and patients with personality disorders. Some of these topics will be of use to all medical professionals and can be included in the didactic sessions provided to clinical clerks during their psychiatry rotation.

Depending on the needs of the clinical site, morning report may have an educational component. Reviewing the patients seen or currently in the service offers an opportunity to discuss management strategies, differential diagnoses, and offer teaching points. Although this may feel like a natural opportunity for learning when the team is gathered together, on-call residents may have been working for significant periods of time with no breaks and may not benefit from lengthy teaching sessions that are unrelated to the patient care provided overnight. Daytime staff may want to begin seeing the patients needing reassessment or new consultations (27). Table 5.3 presents the characteristics of ideal morning rounds.

Large academic PESs may offer regular clinical teaching rounds to trainees and staff. Rounds can be used to review interesting cases, relevant research articles, or psychotherapy techniques

TABLE 5.2 Essential Topics for Seminars in Emergency Psychiatry

Introduction and overview of emergency psychiatry
Suicide risk assessment and intervention
Violence risk assessment
Assessment and management of agitation
Management of the borderline personality disorder patient in crisis
Homelessness and the emergency department
Concurrent disorders in the emergency department
Medicolegal issues (consent and capacity, confidentiality, involuntary hospitalization)
Identifying and reporting abuse of children, women, and the elderly
The decision-making process and documentation in the psychiatric emergency service
Psychiatric presentations of medical disorders
Models of psychotherapy in the emergency department

Data from Dr. Jodi Lofchy, Curricular Lead, University of Toronto PGY1 Emergency Psychiatry curriculum; Brasch, J., Glick, R. L., Cobb, T. G., et al. (2004). Residency training in emergency psychiatry: A model curriculum developed by the Education Committee of the American Association for Emergency Psychiatry. *Academic Psychiatry, 28*, 95–103.

in the PES, among other topics. The case of the week-type sessions, where an interesting case is presented each week in an engaging, interactive manner through role play, debate, or game models, has been a very successful approach with trainees and teams in a number of settings. Programs have offered medical students opportunities to see emergency patients in crisis follow-up, teaching the valuable skills that will be of use as primary care physicians (28). Such innovative teaching approaches can be highly beneficial to the knowledge base and staff morale in a PES despite the substantial time and effort they require.

CLINICAL STAFF EDUCATION

In general, academic PESs are staffed by trained professionals including psychologists, master's-level nurses, social workers, and licensed counselors (1). For many frontline staff, the PES offers clinical opportunities and challenges not available in other settings. The expectations of clinical staff vary by site, with some PESs expecting clinicians

TABLE 5.3 Recommended Key Attributes of Morning Rounds

Morning Rounds Should
• Be resident driven • Include contributions from all crisis team members • Balance teaching and patient care • Build confidence in all team members • Improve diagnostic and management skills in the biopsychosocial realms • Make efficient use of time • Involve a clear understanding of roles • Acknowledge the resident's fatigue and level of training

Reprinted with permission of the American Association of Emergency Psychiatry, from Mitchel, R., Coxon, C., Baxter, et al. (2001). Evaluation of psychiatry residents' emergency morning round experiences: A continuous quality improvement approach. *Emergency Psychiatry, 7*(1), 11–13.

to act independently, and others providing close supervision and limited responsibilities, which will affect the initial training provided. Some programs include a period during which the new staff shadow a more experienced staff member, learning needed skills and knowledge without having significant clinical responsibility. An effective orientation program needs to cultivate attitudes of respect and dignity for patients to ensure these core values are reflected in the care given throughout the PES.

Continuing education for frontline staff is important to maintain skills and interest in the specialty. Organizations for crisis workers or counselors may offer annual conferences, and staff need to be supported to attend. Nonviolent crisis intervention training with annual updates is critical to ensure consensus in the use of physical restraints and management strategies for agitated patients. Specialized training in an area such as crisis intervention counseling, dialectical behavior therapy, motivational interviewing, or concurrent disorders treatment adds intellectual challenges for staff and deepens the resources in the PES, benefiting patient care. For more on PES staff education see Chapter 15.

SPECIAL EDUCATIONAL OPPORTUNITIES

Emergency psychiatry is an important subject for continuing medical education (CME), especially because the requisite knowledge and skills have expanded over the past few decades. Programs should consider offering educational activities to upgrade the skills of faculty who take call for the PES, especially if they rarely or never work in the PES. Faculty may be reluctant to acknowledge their own discomfort with handling psychiatric emergencies, which may affect the supervision they provide on-call. Locally provided CME sessions can focus on subjects such as on-call medical emergencies or management of the borderline patient. Other topics can include faculty development seminars on clinical supervision and telephone supervision of house staff. Educational opportunities for psychiatrists practicing emergency psychiatry are relatively limited, though several professional conferences offer ongoing education.

As patients may present to the emergency department with undifferentiated general medical and psychiatric conditions, it is important that PES psychiatrists maintain their core medical skills (1). Patients may have a primary psychiatric concern but a concurrent medical issue that may or may not have been recognized by the emergency physician. Agitation can have a broad differential diagnosis, and the primary cause of a psychiatric presentation may not be clear. It is critical that PES staff are aware of symptoms of clinical toxidromes and the possibility of delirium so that medical support can be accessed if needed.

One crucial component of the educational program for all trainees is a system of notification, support, and debriefing following a patient's death by suicide, an experienced assault, or another critical incident within the PES. The PES medical director must ensure all trainees involved are promptly contacted and be available or arrange immediate debriefing and ongoing support. The death by suicide of a patient may cause substantial distress (29).

FUTURE DIRECTIONS

Educational programs in emergency psychiatry serve several functions. They provide essential training in the skills and knowledge needed by all medical professionals. A good experience in the psychiatric emergency setting as a junior resident can be a powerful recruitment tool for a possible career focus after residency. Well-developed, structured training programs in emergency psychiatry will encourage residents to view the PES as an opportunity for challenging clinical work, and develop an appreciation for the skills and knowledge necessary to practice acute care psychiatry (4).

Currently there is a mismatch between increasing numbers of PESs requiring psychiatrists with specialized skills and a lack of fellowship opportunities in which psychiatrists can refine and develop PES expertise. Additional advanced educational opportunities for residents and psychiatrists interested in PES work are necessary to continue to develop the field of emergency psychiatry.

The skills and knowledge learned in a PES will be of benefit to all healthcare trainees, regardless of future profession. Residents may not intend to work in a PES or other resource-rich environment after completing their training. However, the rapid assessment and decision-making skills required for PES work are crucial skills for all psychiatrists to learn so that they are prepared to handle crises in any mental health setting (7).

In a Canadian context, the Royal College of Physician and Surgeons of Canada is embarking on a multiyear transformational change initiative entitled Competence By Design, signaling a shift from traditional or time-based medical education to competency-based medical education (CBME) (30). Educators are now tasked with designing and implementing a new curriculum that aligns with this new framework, utilizing the attainment of specific educational objectives, rather than time, as the benchmark for promotion through a training program. The transition to CBME offers an opportunity for educators to critically reflect on the skills necessary for the practice

of emergency psychiatry. Similarly, the ACGME has implemented the use of competency-based training through a framework of milestones specific to each discipline (31). Though not specific to emergency psychiatry, many of the ACGME milestones for psychiatry are applicable to the emergency setting, and the milestones recognize the importance of knowing how to assess and manage psychopathology in this setting. Using the entrustable professional activity (EPA) and milestone framework, a group of Canadian emergency psychiatric educators has developed a list of core emergency psychiatry content appropriate for residents in the foundational stage of training (30). Figure 5.1 provides an example of how this content is broadly structured.

It is an exciting time to be an educator in the field of emergency psychiatry. Programs and hospitals are creating settings where teams can treat acutely ill patients in safe, well-designed, and appropriately staffed units. Ongoing educational programs utilizing

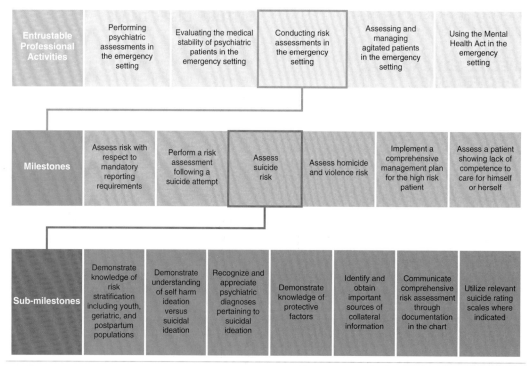

FIGURE 5.1 • Entrustable professional activities and milestones for a foundational emergency psychiatry experience. (Reprinted by permission from: Springer Nature, Academic Psychiatry, Fage, B., Abadir, A., Boyle, M., et al. (2017). Competency-based medical education: Objectives for a foundational emergency psychiatry experience. *Academic Psychiatry*. doi:10.1007/s40596-017-0799-9, Copyright 2017.)

innovative approaches with simulation and case-related teaching help to decrease anxiety and increase comfort in a fast-paced environment with unstable patients who require assessment throughout the day and night. With the advent of CBME and further postresidency subspecialization, an opportunity arises to best define the essential components required to practice safely and competently in the PES.

ACKNOWLEDGMENTS

The authors wish to acknowledge the work done by Dr. Jennifer S. Brasch on this chapter in the first edition of Emergency Psychiatry.

REFERENCES

1. Currier, G. W., & Allen, M. (2003). Organization and function of academic psychiatric emergency services. *General Hospital Psychiatry, 25*(2), 124–129.
2. Thienhaus, O. J. (1995). Academic issues in emergency psychiatry. *New Directions for Mental Health Services, 67,* 109–114.
3. Herman, J. B. (1995). Managed care and residency training in psychiatry. *Harvard Review of Psychiatry, 2,* 290–292.
4. Brasch, J., Glick, R. L., Cobb, T. G., et al. (2004). Residency training in emergency psychiatry: A model curriculum developed by the Education Committee of the American Association for Emergency Psychiatry. *Academic Psychiatry, 28,* 95–103.
5. Accreditation Council for Graduate Medical Education. *ACGME Program Requirements for Graduate Medical Education in Psychiatry.* Retrieved September 10, 2018, from https://www.acgme.org/Portals/0/PFAssets/Program Requirements/400_psychiatry_2017-07-01.pdf.
6. Accreditation Council for Graduate Medical Education. *ACGME Outcome Project: General competencies.* Retrieved from http://www.acgme.org/outcome/comp/compFull.asp#1.
7. Weinerman, R., Leichner, P. P., & Harper, D. W. (1982). Filling the need for emergency psychiatrists: Is better education the answer? *Hospital and Community Psychiatry, 33,* 35–37.
8. Zealberg, J. J., Santos, A. B., Hiers, T. G., et al. (1990). From the benches to the trenches: Training residents to provide emergency outreach services—A public/academic project. *Academic Psychiatry, 14*(4), 211–217.
9. Royal College of Physicians and Surgeons of Canada. (2015). *Specialty training requirements in psychiatry.* Retrieved September 12, 2018, from http://www.royalcollege.ca/rcsite/documents/ibd/psychiatry_str_e.
10. Brasch, J. S., & Ferencz, J. C. (1999). Training issues in emergency psychiatry. *Psychiatric Clinics of North America, 22*(4), 941–954.
11. Hnatko, G. (2002). *Emergency psychiatry goals and objectives.* Edmonton: University of Alberta, Department of Psychiatry. UAH RTC 01/03/2002.
12. Accreditation Council for Graduate Medical Education. (2011). *Common program requirements.* Retrieved September 12, 2018, from https://www.acgme.org/Portals/0/PDFs/Common_Program_Requirements_07012011[2].pdf.
13. National Steering Committee on Resident Duty Hours. (2013). *Fatigue, risk, and excellence: Towards a pan-Canadian consensus on resident duty hours.* Ottawa, ON: The Royal College of Physicians and Surgeons of Canada.
14. PARO-CAHO Collective Agreement. *Attachment 29-PGY1 Call Schedule.* Retrieved September 12, 2018, from http://www.myparo.ca/attachments/#attachment-29-8211-pgy1-call-schedule.
15. Borrell-Carrio, F., & Epstein, R. M. (2004). Preventing errors in clinical practice: A call for self-awareness. *Annals of Family Medicine, 2,* 310–316.
16. Canadian Medical Protective Agency (CMPA) Good Practices Guide. *Section 3: Handover.* Retrieved November 27, 2018, from https://www.cmpa-acpm.ca/serve/docs/ela/goodpracticesguide/pages/communication/Handovers/safer_handovers_through_structured_communications-e.html.
17. Starmer, A. J., Sectish, T. C., Simon, D. W., et al. (2013). Rates of medical errors and preventable adverse events among hospitalized children following implementation of a resident handoff bundle. *JAMA, 310*(21), 2262–2270.
18. Thomas, C. M., Bertram, E., & Johnson, D. (2009). The SBAR communication technique. *Nurse Educator, 34*(4), 176–180.
19. Dawe, I. (2004). Emerging trends and training issues in the psychiatric emergency room. *The Canadian Journal of Psychiatry, 49,* 1–6.
20. Epstein, R. M. (2007). Assessment in medical education. *The New England Journal of Medicine, 356,* 387–396.
21. Weissberg, M. P. (1990). The meagerness of physician training in emergency psychiatric intervention. *Academic Medicine, 65,* 747–750.

22. Weissberg, M. P. (1991). Emergency psychiatry: A critical educational omission. *Annals of Internal Medicine, 114*(3), 246–247.

23. Accreditation Council for Graduate Medical Education. (2005). *Model of the clinical practice of emergency medicine*. Retrieved from http://www.acgme.org/acWebsite/RRC_110/110_clinModel.pdf.

24. Walsh, S. F. (1985). The psychiatric emergency service as a setting for social work training. *Social Work in Health Care, 11*, 21–31.

25. Shea, S. C. (1999). *The practical art of suicide assessment* (pp. 109–123). New York, NY: John Wiley and Sons.

26. Lofchy, J. (1997). The use of standardized patients in the teaching of emergency psychiatry. *Emergency Psychiatry, 3*(4), 78–79.

27. Mitchel, R., Coxon, C., Baxter, et al. (2001). Evaluation of psychiatry residents' emergency morning round experiences: A continuous quality improvement approach. *Emergency Psychiatry, 7*(1), 11–13.

28. Lofchy, J. (2003). The clerk crisis clinic: A novel educational program. *Academic Psychiatry, 27*(2), 82–87.

29. Ruskin, R., Sakinofsky, I., Bagby, R. M., et al. (2004). Impact of patient suicide on psychiatrists and psychiatric trainees. *Academic Psychiatry, 28*(2), 104–110.

30. Fage, B., Abadir, A., Boyle, M., et al. (2017). Competency-based medical education: Objectives for a foundational emergency psychiatry experience. *Academic Psychiatry*, *42*(4), 519-522. doi:10.1007/s40596-017-0799-9.

31. Accreditation Council for Graduate Medical Education and the American Board of Psychiatry and Neurology. (2015). *The psychiatry milestone project*. Retrieved September 12, 2018, from https://www.acgme.org/Portals/0/PDFs/Milestones/PsychiatryMilestones.pdf?ver=2015-11-06-120520-753.

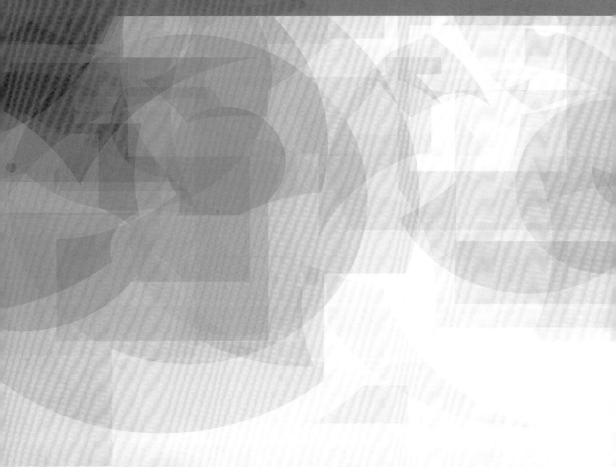

PART II

General Principles
of Care

Section Editor: John S. Rozel

6

Prehospital and Emergency Medical Services Psychiatry Care: Overview and Challenges

Charles F. Palmer, Edward M. Kantor

Prehospital and emergency medical services (EMS) emergency psychiatry may be one of the least defined areas in the emergency care world, as it crosses disciplines, professionals, agencies, and systems. This chapter is intended to provide a broad overview, using the literature when available, but defaulting to consensus expert opinion to provide a complete picture. In order to highlight the range and diversity of prehospital emergency mental health concepts, we describe several well-regarded examples where collaborative psychiatric and behavioral health support has been integrated successfully around the United States, highlighting typical roles, and problems commonly encountered.

Even though there are a few long-standing examples of psychiatrists actively involved in the emergency care of patients with mental illness outside of the hospital, there is yet to be a standardized role or a consistent presence beyond traditional public mental health or fee-for-service medical systems. Some notable examples do exist, where psychiatrists have made inroads into interprofessional and collaborative care through specialized emergency mental health services, collaboration with crisis teams and law enforcement, and telehealth.

Collaborative mental health care is evolving as a viable, team-based approach to care, with the psychiatrist often leading or augmenting a team of other providers. Although a long-standing practice in community mental health systems, mainstream health care is beginning to embrace the concept more fully with the expansion of telehealth practice. EMS frequently utilize emergency physicians to develop protocols and provide

field supervision through radio telemetry, telephone, and other means to basic and advanced responders in the field. Even though emergency department (ED) visits account for 10% to 40% of patient encounters (1), the amount of psychiatric training in emergency medicine (EM) residency programs remains low. And although basic mental health issues are covered in emergency medical technician (EMT) and paramedic training for first responders, the depth and in-training exposure have not evolved much since the 1970s (2).

The next few years will hopefully clarify whether this is due to a lack of interest on the part of the profession, the relative high cost of a psychiatrist compared to other mental health professionals and paraprofessionals, or the organizational divide where prehospital public mental health systems are embedded into a nonmedical paradigm. Even without direct care roles, there are a number of settings and scenarios where psychiatrists could prove useful and facilitate higher-quality care to patients during behavioral emergencies outside of the hospital or emergency department setting.

PREHOSPITAL MENTAL HEALTH

It is not an exaggeration to say that numerous governmental and quasigovernmental groups are involved in prehospital emergency psychiatric situations, often by default, and sometimes under protest. Behavioral events often arise without much warning, and in many cases, the initial response comes from the closest available service, such as law enforcement, EMS, or fire service units and personnel. First responders are not extensively trained to manage behavioral emergencies, mental illness, or crisis intervention. Specialized response personnel, equipment, and strategies for dealing with persons in mental health emergencies are few and far between, even with the emergence of model programs in the last 25 years. Until such time as communities embrace a more trauma-informed and patient-centered response scenario, it is not unreasonable to expect all emergency personnel to have awareness and basic competence in evidence-driven strategies for managing behavioral emergencies, minimizing risk to patients, responders, and other bystanders. Prehospital behavioral emergencies are true emergencies until proven otherwise—no different than more traditional somatic complaints such as chest pain or shortness of breath, with the risk of significant morbidity and mortality if ignored.

Much like the rest of EMS, when a call comes in with limited information, services are dispatched to match the expected issue as much as possible. Avoiding escalation and unnecessary injuries or even death in the management of prehospital behavioral emergencies is certainly preferable and possible much of the time. A combination of improved training, coordinated response guidelines, and interagency cooperation has the potential to improve consistency in care for the most seriously ill patients.

LAW ENFORCEMENT

Although law enforcement officers (LEOs) are not typically thought of as mental health workers, it is estimated that up to 10% of police contact with the public involves persons with serious mental illness (3). The level of training provided to those who handle behavioral complaints varies widely by region, funding, and form of government. Though mental health is a component of most basic officer training and recertification, and several systems identify officers for additional training, few utilize an infrastructure where these trained behavioral specialists are integrated and available consistently in patrol operations.

There have been a number of criminal justice system efforts to improve law enforcement's interface with persons with mental illness. One of the more widely utilized and well-established trainings is the Crisis Intervention Team (CIT) model, originally developed in Memphis in 1987 as a collaboration between a police officer and a psychologist. Also known as the "Memphis model," this program identified police officers who had shown effective interpersonal styles and an interest in the subject to the point that the CIT operational group was a coveted appointment, with selection for the program in Memphis considered an honor. CIT officers completed approximately 40 hours of training, including supervised field work, which when fully qualified allowed them to diffuse volatile situations, often redirecting persons with mental illness toward treatment over jail or criminal charges. Well-integrated and utilized CIT-trained officers demonstrated more positive patient outcomes over typical strategies, with reduced arrests, increased safety, improved consumer feedback, and increased diversion from the criminal justice system into mental health services. CIT program implementation continues to spread rapidly in regions throughout the United States (3). Another program, Mental Health First Aid (MHFA) for Public Safety, is an 8-hour course designed to train LEOs and first responders basic techniques for de-escalation during behavioral disturbances. MHFA has been shown to increase knowledge and decrease stigma, as well as to increase support for mental health treatment (4). The success of programs such as CIT and MHFA is dependent upon a number of core elements beyond just training alone (5).

A critical issue encountered by LEOs is how to determine the ultimate disposition for persons exhibiting behavioral change; whether an individual will be brought to the hospital, left at a "drop-in" center, community mental healthcare centers, or jail. This is dependent on any number of factors—whether a patient's behavior is correctly interpreted as being due to mental health problems; officer knowledge about possible destinations; the makeup of the health system; officer incentives; and even convenience. Long waits in emergency departments taking officers from street duties often shift toward the most expeditious option, regardless of clinical appropriateness from a psychiatry perspective. Standardized and connected systems of care with community agreements and increased training for nonmedical personnel would greatly improve the outcomes of mental health patients who end up inappropriately in the custody of law enforcement, the custody of local jails, as opposed to receiving the care to improve the underlying mental illness.

EMERGENCY MEDICAL SERVICES/PARAMEDICS

Paramedics often are the first responders to behavioral emergencies. They are expected to be able to de-escalate a situation, to appropriately diagnose and treat any emergent medical problems that may be present, and to deliver patients safely to an emergency department for full workup and treatment. However, the role of the paramedic is expanding in terms of treatment of behavioral emergencies as systems continue to develop. In the most effective models, there is typically the possibility of diversion to a community-based or specialized behavioral health center which may cut down on the utilization of traditional EDs and lengthy patient boarding while waiting for an inpatient bed. The prerequisite to utilize these destinations is that patients need to be confirmed to have no medical causes of behavioral disturbance, which becomes the responsibility of the EMS provider (6). Various systems throughout the United States and other countries have shown this to be a possible and much improved system, with increased efficiency, patient satisfaction, and provider satisfaction (7-9). Specialized training for paramedics varies from none, with only the addition of a standardized protocol, to up to 200 didactic and 128 clinical hours (7,10). Regardless of the amount of additional training, results from these programs have been nearly universally positive, suggesting that a global shift to these models could be beneficial.

PROVIDER PERCEPTIONS

It is important to understand EMS provider perception of mentally ill persons as it is likely to impact the care that these patients receive. EMS providers as a whole feel unprepared with too little training (11), with other studies showing that 75% to 90% of EMS lack any mental health-specific training at all and have limited departmental guidelines (12). Research has also found that some providers think that mental health emergencies are "not real emergencies," with lower acuity than other types of calls and believe that EMS usage of these patients is inappropriate. Many providers feel like a "street-level social worker," which they believe to be outside the scope of their job (11). Opinions on how to remedy this problem vary, from the discussion of better patient triage, more mental health training for paramedics, and a broader array of community mental health service availability to calls for an increased focus in changing mental health policy over improving provider skills (13).

PHYSICIANS IN PREHOSPITAL EMERGENCY PSYCHIATRY

Rarely will a psychiatrist be the planned first responder in the prehospital setting. Although there are many examples of physicians augmenting major responses in mass casualty and disaster situations (8), resource allocation (availability and cost) has limited use in most cases. This is true for psychiatry as well. The relative shortage of psychiatrists combined with cost tends to limit widespread utilization. Physician extenders including EMTs and paramedics have become the backbone of the EMS system, whereas counselors (licensed professional counselor [LPC]), social workers, and paraprofessionals are more typical in community mental health systems. Much as the EM physician takes a medical command and consultative role in EMS, psychiatrists can facilitate care provision as part of interprofessional teams in prehospital emergency mental health care.

Most evidence-driven and model programs providing comprehensive crisis care have utilized psychiatrists this way. Programs such as Montgomery County Emergency Services (MCES) outside of Philadelphia has been in operation since 1974 (14). In addition to a full spectrum of emergency mental health services, from initial assessment, acute hospitalization, crisis stabilization, and jail diversion services, the program integrates mental health ambulances and transport services in cooperation with regional law enforcement and EMS. Safe and medically based transport for behavioral health is an ongoing and evolving controversy in the field. In many states, the civil commitment process requires or defaults to law enforcement transport between facilities which has resulted in civil rights complaints, worsening stigma and delays in care. Uniquely, one credible alternative to the CIT model, MCES also provides ongoing support and training to the multitude of small law enforcement agencies and correctional facilities in the region, training officers in therapeutic intervention and assessment, but also supporting them in on-scene engagement and transportation to appropriate treatment. This often involves working with care providers and interested parties throughout the region, such as hospitals, community mental health, EMS, law enforcement, and policy makers (15), working as a point of contact to create an effective system that is utilized appropriately through interagency agreements and protocols. It requires intentional cooperation and ongoing communication but is one proof of concept that could be adopted more broadly.

Although it may be inefficient for psychiatrists to be a direct part of a first response team, it can be very helpful to serve in a consultative role, advising on medical screening needs for patients, facilitating treatment and disposition at local hospital or community mental health center or detox facility, and consulting with complex and ethical dilemmas arising out in the field (16). The physician can either be on call to receive questions from EMS providers on the fly or use telehealth to assess patients themselves from a centralized location. Although there are a number of examples of psychiatrists using telehealth, especially for consultation to EDs in regions where there is a shortage of mental health professionals, examples of use in the prehospital arena are limited.

If serving in a prehospital consultation role, psychiatrists should be familiar with prehospital medicine as there are numerous instances where decisions in care are different than that in a clinical setting. Additionally, many psychiatrists may be unfamiliar with the complexities and realities of prehospital care, such as understanding their local system and the array of treatment dispositions, acceptance criteria for patients to certain locations, and regionally specific mental health laws.

PREHOSPITAL INTERVENTIONS

Behavioral emergencies are true emergencies. If mismanaged, they can result in serious harm to the patient and/or responders. Alterations in behavior and thinking can arise from many causes. Though some conditions are thought of as "purely psychiatric" or idiopathic, many are the result of or are co-occurring with metabolic, traumatic, infectious, vascular, or toxic insults to the brain. As with all areas of EM, initial screening and stabilization is vital to prevent missing disease with the potential to cause serious harm or death. This requires a careful history and directed physical examination pertinent to the situation. Just as in the ED itself, accurate interpretation and response to behavioral emergencies (including agitation) is of critical importance in prehospital evaluation and interventions with patients experiencing acute behavioral change. In many cases, patients are not suffering from a primary psychiatric illness. Many acute and subacute medical conditions can manifest as violence or agitation, or present with what are typically thought of as psychiatric symptoms. Whether the first contact is law enforcement, an EMT paramedic, or a physician, close attention should be paid to the context and evolution of the behavior.

Before engagement, the immediate environment should be assessed for hazards. Based on the information gleaned from dispatch, it may be prudent to wait for additional staff or police. Many jurisdictions send a fire or rescue unit (and/or police) along with EMS for all calls suggestive of violence or self-harm, or if specific information about the scene, individual, or circumstances is known. Though most persons with mental illness are not violent, behavioral emergencies and crisis scenarios in general increase the likelihood of impulsive behaviors. As in all prehospital emergencies, the scene should be surveyed to ensure that entering and approaching the patient is safe, and that no environmental hazards or weapons are involved. It is helpful to have other members of the team utilize on-scene informants who can provide additional information and perspective about the event, and round out the medical history for comorbid medical conditions, allergies, medications likely taken, substance use, as well as past history of similar events, or other mental conditions.

Understanding the onset and course of the behavioral change will help determine the likelihood of a nonpsychiatric cause and direct the level of initial screening to facilitate triage for the next steps in care. Although a known psychiatric history may help lead the responder to believe the current event is related, that alone does not guarantee it is the cause of the current presentation. Exploring the recent course of the patient's symptoms, including the timing and rapidity of onset as well as aggravating and alleviating symptoms, also guides next steps in care. If a similar episode occurred in the past, the surrounding events and the outcome as well as treatment successes and failures will all help lessen the impact of the current episode and ideally lead to earlier recovery. If present, substances of abuse or withdrawal, alcohol use and withdrawal, prescribed medications, and supplements are all known to be associated with a host of behavioral and psychiatric symptoms and help define the immediate and intermediate care needs.

DIFFERENTIAL DIAGNOSIS

When encountering a person exhibiting behavioral changes in the field, the assessing party should try to rapidly form a differential diagnosis, ruling in or out common and rare but serious presentations of illness and toxidromes. Neglecting to do so can lead to poor outcomes that were likely avoidable. Patient demographics affect risk and likelihood of many behavioral syndromes and should be considered; age, race, ethnicity, and gender can all change the direction of an assessment. For example, a 45-year-old experiencing hallucinations for the first time with an otherwise negative psychiatric history would be an unlikely candidate for sudden-onset schizophrenia and more likely result from exposure to substances, suggesting a need for a more comprehensive medical assessment, compared

to a patient who is known to have stopped prescribed antipsychotic medications for a long-standing illness. Still, there is a high medical illness burden among persons living with chronic mental illness.

There are a wide range of general medical conditions associated with behavioral presentations. Maintaining a high index of suspicion, that allows for additional assessment when indicated, facilitates the treatment of reversible causes and preventing serious harm or death.

Some common examples include:

Hypo/hyperglycemia: Hypoglycemia has long been known to cause behavioral disturbance masquerading as psychosis and agitation. The cause is thought to be neuroglycopenia frequently compounded with catecholamine release and is commonly caused by skipping meals or by overdosing on insulin or sulfonylurea drugs, alcoholism, or more rarely, pancreatic adenoma (17-20). Hyperglycemia has less commonly been reported as a cause of agitation, but it is speculated that elevations in cortisol levels could cause the effect (21). Typically, in cases of high or low blood sugar, correction of the abnormality either through IV dextrose or insulin therapy will lead to resolution of symptoms over the course of 24 to 48 hours.

Hypoxia: Hypoxia can be provoked by a general illness, such as chronic obstructive pulmonary disease (COPD) or asthma; respiratory depression (especially after drug use); or misuse

---

 CASE STUDY 6.1

EMS responded to a 75-year-old female living at an assisted care facility. One hour ago, she was combative with staff and appeared to be suffering from hallucinations, calling staff "Gestapo" and demanding that she be freed from the prison cell they were keeping her in. Upon arrival at the scene, a history of the present illness was ascertained from a caretaker at the facility. When she did not come to breakfast in the morning, staff came to check on her and found her in her present state. The caretaker noted that the patient had been feeling "under the weather" for the past 2 days but was otherwise healthy,

with a history of hypertension and depression that was controlled with hydrochlorothiazide (HCTZ) and amitryptyline. When the team tried to talk to the patient, she was somnolent but aroused as they took vital signs, finding her normotensive and nonfebrile but mildly tachycardic. She was not oriented to person, place, or time, and appeared to think that her great uncle was in the room. The patient was brought to the ED without issue and after testing found to have a urinary tract infection. Her symptoms resolved within hours after she was treated with antibiotics.

of medical equipment. Ischemic stroke also causes cerebral hypoxia due to defective oxygen delivery (22). Hypoxia causes decreased neurotransmission, which can lead to agitation, anxiety, hallucinations, and aggressive behavior. Resolution of hypoxia will resolve these symptoms but can have lasting sequelae based on the degree, time, and mechanism of hypoxia.

Nonconvulsive status epilepticus: Neurologists speculate that in the cases of seizure-provoked hallucinations and violent behavior, the epileptic focus exerts a positive effect in producing these experiences. Furthermore, seizures with these effects have been localized to the limbic system, possibly creating a loss of inhibitory control (23,24). Symptoms with an epileptogenic focus can usually be resolved quickly with benzodiazepines and antiepileptic drug treatment. In a prehospital setting, patients with known seizure history, suspicion of alcohol or sedative withdrawal, recent strokes, or use of medications that lower the seizure threshold or recovering from a recent viral illness may be at higher risk and merit additional consideration.

Hyperthyroidism: Graves disease and toxic nodular goiter are common causes of hyperthyroidism and well known to cause symptoms of mania, delirium, and psychosis, with delusions and hallucinations common. These symptoms are thought to be mediated by direct T3 receptor stimulation in the limbic system or through excess catecholamine production (25). Typically, behavioral symptoms begin to appear when thyroid disease is quite severe and are usually treated with antithyroid drugs and antipsychotics, followed by thyroid ablation (26).

Delirium: Delirium is a common overlay precipitated by a wide array of medical conditions and is often multifactorial in origin. It is characterized by changes in sensorium that fluctuate over short periods of time, often with sudden bizarre or violent behavior, hallucinations, and hyperactivity. Drug intoxication and substance withdrawal are common precipitating factors. Fatalities mainly occur because of complications from the underlying illness, though the delirium itself complicates care through limited communication, agitation, and resulting use of physical or chemical restraint. Delirium complications may often affect the delivery of necessary nursing and medical assessment and intervention. Care needs to be taken with these patients and treatment should be prompt (27).

Other conditions with behavioral manifestations that should be considered in the course of assessment include neuroleptic malignant syndrome, serotonin syndrome, dementia, infection, and drug intoxication and/or withdrawal (Figure 6.1). Once again, a thorough history dictates the need for further examination, observation, and laboratory testing. Individual patient demographic and population factors are integral to accurate diagnosis and treatment. In the absence of reliable patient history, additional assessment with laboratory screening and medical monitoring may be required before considering transportation to a freestanding crisis unit outside of a medical facility. These situations will require further medical screening and stabilization, historically referred to as "medical clearance." Because crisis care and available emergency mental health services vary so extensively between communities across the United States, there is rarely a one-size fits all, consistently agreed upon standard between EM and mental health providers. Yet there is probably consensus that a lack of a continuum of mental health services plays a role in ED overuse for medical screening and management of psychiatric emergencies, that if addressed earlier or differently could decrease overcrowding and boarding of patients with mental illness in emergency department settings.

Ideally, a fingerstick glucose measurement, pulse oximetry, and vital signs would be obtained in the field on all patients with behavioral change as soon as practical in order to help determine the etiology of the agitation and to quickly treat potentially reversible conditions. Nonmedical mental health providers may miss or be over cautious in referring patients with behavioral symptoms to the emergency department. More specific field-based care may be appropriate through local EMS protocols, real-time consultation with medical command in the field, and after arrival at the ED.

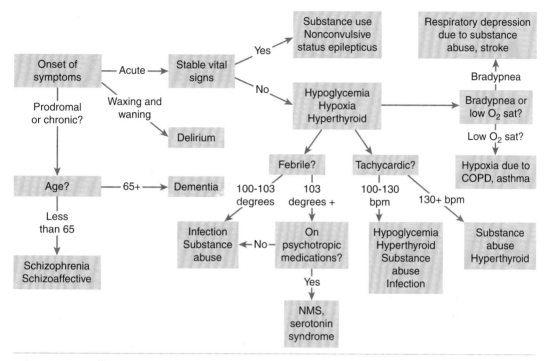

FIGURE 6.1 • Differential diagnosis of psychotic symptoms. COPD, chronic obstructive pulmonary disease; NMS, neuroleptic malignant syndrome.

TREATMENT

Nonpharmacological

Initial approach in the field may be dictated by local protocols. A designated responder would begin with rapport building and verbal de-escalation by using a calm, nonthreatening tone and an honest, straightforward, and supportive approach. Conveying a desire to help and exploring the individual's concerns without

 CASE STUDY 6.2

EMS responded to a call regarding a 21-year-old man on a campus of the local university who was extremely agitated. Upon arrival at the scene, the patient was in his dormitory room, where he had been locked by his frightened roommate. Through the door, the patient could be heard screaming, making loud noises, and banging against the walls. It was exam week, and both the patient and roommate had been in the room studying practically all day, until over the course of a half hour the patient started talking nonsensically, tearing up paper, banging on the desk, and finally pulling at the roommate's shirt. At that point, the roommate left the room, sealed the door, and called 911. The roommate was unaware of any medical issues that the patient suffered from, and

he had no known past psychiatric history. When the paramedics entered the room, the patient was noncommunicative requiring restraint. He was noted to be tremulous and diaphoretic and seemed to have lost some coordination. He was given intramuscular ketamine with rapid sedation following administration. Vital signs showed tachycardia to 130 bpm, and rapid blood glucose screen returned a level of 15 mg/dL. The patient was given 50% IV glucose in the ambulance and came out of sedation with no agitation. He continued to receive IV glucose in the hospital and had returned to normal mental status 3 hours later. After a thorough history was taken, he was determined to be a type 1 diabetic who had not eaten breakfast or lunch after his morning dose of insulin.

judgment or condescension is an almost universally accepted approach to initial engagement. Listening and focusing on patient concerns is likely to be more effective than screening checklists. Still, thoughts of self-harm, suicide, or violence should be elicited as early as possible and can help guide next steps in the intervention and prevent harm to all involved. The presence or likelihood of a weapon should be established as soon as possible. Though there are many models of initial approach in crisis, the American Association for Emergency Psychiatry (AAEP) Best Practices for the Evaluation and Treatment of Agitation (Project BETA) describes four main objectives: ensuring the safety of the patient and others in the area; helping the patient manage emotions and regain behavioral control, avoiding use of restraints, and avoiding coercive interventions. There are 10 verbal domains of verbal de-escalation (Table 6.1). For more in-depth information on this subject, the interested reader is recommended to read the consensus statement of the AAEP Project BETA de-escalation workgroup (28).

Psychological first aid is another excellent resource for de-escalation purposes, especially in the disaster or crisis scenario. This resource suggests enlisting the help of family or friends to calm the patient, moving them to a quiet place, or if they present no immediate danger to themselves or others, giving the patient some time to process before intervening but still remaining available (29). If verbal de-escalation fails or there is imminent risk precluding the use of de-escalation, restraints may be used. Restraints can aid in giving time to produce a diagnosis and to determine the most effective treatment. However, they should be used with a plan for removal as soon as possible, especially if parenteral or IM pharmacological methods for sedation are successful (30). Furthermore, if medications are thought to be safe and can be administered without resorting to restraints, the use of restraints should be avoided.

Pharmacological

If verbal de-escalation and restraint fail to relieve agitation, pharmacological intervention is likely indicated. In the prehospital setting, EM guides the response with first-generation antipsychotics (haloperidol and droperidol), benzodiazepines (midazolam and lorazepam), and more recently, ketamine. Though only recently receiving approval as an emerging option for treatment resistant depression, ketamine's use in emergency medical care for agitation has evolved to be more common, often independently from psychiatric practice. Recent literature compares ketamine to other agents in terms of safety, adverse events, incidence of necessity for airway management, and time to sedation (31). More information is needed on

TABLE 6.1 Ten Domains of De-escalation

1. Respect personal space
2. Do not be provocative
3. Establish verbal contact
4. Be concise
5. Identify wants and feelings
6. Listen closely to what the patient is saying
7. Agree or agree to disagree
8. Lay down the law and set clear limits
9. Offer choices and optimism
10. Debrief the patient and staff

Adapted with permission from Fishkind, A. (2002). Calming agitation with words, not drugs: 10 commandments for safety. *Current psychiatry*, 1(4), 32–39. Retrieved June 13, 2011, from https://www.mdedge.com/psychiatry/article/66121/calming-agitation-words-not-drugs-10-commandments-safety.

the cognitive and emotional sequelae after the acute event in order to recommend this as a common intervention.

Ideally, forced medication IM/IV would be utilized after other methods of intervention have failed and only in the setting of dangerousness and not for convenience or facilitating routine treatment. Most oversight agencies such as CMS and The Joint Commission involved in healthcare accreditation as well as state mental health regulations require patient consent for treatment, and in the absence of informed consent also require imminent dangerousness in order to treat involuntarily. Whenever possible, standard practice dictates the least restrictive intervention and promotes patient participation and choice in treatment decisions, even when decision-making capacity may be partially affected by an individual's mental illness. Oral medication would typically be considered as an option before parenteral administration, and a number of antipsychotic and other anxiolytic medications are available as disintegrating tablets with a fairly quick onset of action.

Haloperidol is one of the most common first-generation, nonphenothiazine antipsychotics used in prehospital care and most providers have some familiarity. Droperidol, which is more sedating but in the same class, has a much shorter half-life (2.5 vs 14+ hours). For this reason, droperidol has gained favor among EMS and emergency physicians, but it is less than ideal for psychiatry. There are anecdotal reports of more akathisia after droperidol use which could affect how an individual sees medication and affect future participation in treatment. Even if successful in the moment, how initial treatment impacts longer-term care has to be considered. When compared with midazolam, droperidol was found to have fewer adverse effects, shorter time to sedation, and decreased necessity for resedation (32). Haloperidol compared with midazolam had similar results, with low incidence of adverse effect in both medications, but a shorter time to sedation with midazolam (33). Practical concerns might limit use of midazolam and droperidol in psychiatric settings because of a lack of advanced life support backup, and a need to consider these medications as a form of "chemical restraint" as the primary reason for administration is behavioral control and not treatment of underlying illness.

Several second-generation antipsychotics have proven efficacy in agitation, and in the context of a chronic psychotic illness have the benefit of moving toward stabilization of the underlying condition. Risperidone and olanzapine have oral disintegrating tablet forms that can be offered as initial oral alternatives prior to considering IM injection or forced medication. Ziprasidone and olanzapine are available in intramuscular formulations as well and have the advantage of more benign side-effect profiles and less oversedation than first-generation antipsychotics, while proving equally as potent.

Loxapine, a first-generation antipsychotic, now has a new inhaled formulation approved by the FDA in 2012. This method of delivery has the benefit of ease of administration, possibly avoiding an IM medication, but requires patient cooperation and could be an option offered as one of several alternatives to choose from. Inhaled loxapine has an onset of effect within 10 to 20 minutes, making it much more rapid than even IM antipsychotic agents. Its side-effect profile is mild, with dizziness, sedation, and throat irritation commonly reported. However, it carries a black box warning for bronchospasm for which patients must be carefully monitored, especially with preexisting pulmonary conditions, and providers need to be prepared for possible intubation (34-36). Even though available for over 6 years, few psychiatrists or ED providers have experience in its use to date, probably due to a combination of factors—availability, cost, and required additional staff time and protocols to ensure safety. Ideally, antipsychotics started in an emergency setting would be one acceptable to the patient and likely to be continued as part of their ongoing management.

Psychiatry as a field is less familiar with medications that originated as anesthetic agents or have less ongoing psychiatric benefit in the continuum of care. Several require advanced airway management backup and would be likely restricted to settings with advanced life support capabilities. However, compared to other drug classes, ketamine achieves most rapid time to sedation at 4 to 5 minutes compared to haloperidol and droperidol at 17 minutes and midazolam at 14 minutes. However, ketamine is associated with an increased risk of complications when compared to haloperidol: hypersalivation was most common, as well as emergence reaction, vomiting, and laryngospasm. Possibly owing to these complications, intubation rate was 35% higher (37). However, duration of mechanical ventilation tended to be brief (38), and it was found to have a comparable on-scene time when compared with haloperidol, suggesting that monitoring for adverse events does not take significantly longer (39). In general, the safety profile of ketamine is good; risks include rise in blood pressure due to catecholamine release (infrequently a major risk with this patient population) and increased intraocular pressure. Emergence reaction, consisting of hallucinations and agitation when recovering from sedation, is seen in up to 30% of patients but can be managed with IV or IM midazolam (40). Because benzodiazepines are limited by dose-limiting respiratory depression and possible oversedation, and first-generation antipsychotics tend to have a delayed onset of action with potential for dystonic reaction, ketamine has shown to be a good alternative. It is relatively efficacious and safe for the majority of patients, and it offers an advantage over other choices in terms of rapid onset of action, minimal incidence of oversedation, and wide therapeutic window (40,41).

However, in general, prehospital settings are much less controlled than the ED and the variables unpredictable. Avoiding a scenario where intubation is necessary for airway control due to sedation is a more desirable goal. Replacing risky and invasive interventions with others such as de-escalation and utilization of medications agreed to by patients can lower costs, improve safety, and ideally engender a longer term therapeutic alliance and adherence.

CONCLUSIONS

Our fee-for-service infrastructure tends to support episodic care as opposed to ongoing patient management (ie, treating illness rather than promoting wellness). Crisis MH care continues to occur often in the highest cost ED and hospital settings in the absence of viable alternatives. Budgets are separate; leadership reports to different organizations; providers often do not have direct relationships. All these serve as systemic barriers to change. Ironically, it may be the insurers who in their goals

of cost-effective care may force systems toward alternative and more effective, yet lower cost, models that more traditional clinical organizations have been reluctant to embrace on their own.

The expansion of telehealth in psychiatry creates new opportunities for out-of-hospital and community collaboration and support by mental health to first responders and police. There are now multiple locations which have been utilizing telehealth creatively to support hospital EDs without psychiatrists and to provide earlier treatment for patients boarding in emergency departments pending the availability of inpatient psychiatric care. In many cases, these collaborations have decreased length of stay and avoided the need for inpatient hospitalization. At the same time, there has not been an expansion of outpatient MH services, long-term care residential treatment programs, or Medicaid.

Even so, there are shining examples of creative, evidence-based, and outcome-driven services that have sustained and thrived over decades. These strong and effective services are effective at least in part because of strong individual relationships between providers and local leadership. Each trust and ensures that the other will do their part without fear of one taking fiscal advantage of the other. Creating incentives to cooperate, work together, and plan comprehensive programs will require greater advocacy, sustained local interest, and significant effort on the part of highly motivated advocates and organizational leaders who are empowered to support cross-system cooperation.

REFERENCES

1. Zun, L. (2016). Care of psychiatric patients: The challenge to emergency physicians. *The Western Journal of Emergency Medicine, 17*(2), 173–176.
2. Samuels, D. J. (1996). *Emergency medical technician-basic: National standard curriculum.* United States Department of Transportation, National Highway Traffic Safety Administration. Retrieved September 25, 2019, from http://www.nhtsa.gov/people/injury/EMS/pub/emtbnsc.pdf.
3. Watson, A. C., & Fulambarker, A. J. (2012). The crisis intervention team model of police response to mental health crises: A primer for mental health practitioners. *Best Practices in Mental Health, 8*(2), 71.

4. Wong, E. C., Collins, R. L., & Cerully, J. L. (2015). Reviewing the evidence base for mental health first aid: Is there support for its use with key target populations in California? *RAND Health Quarterly, 5*(1), 19.

5. Randolph DuPont, P., Major Sam Cochran, M. S., & Sarah Pillsbury, M. A. (2007). *Crisis Intervention Team core elements.* The University of Memphis.

6. Chennapan, K., et al. (2018). Medical screening of mental health patients in the emergency department: A systematic review. *Journal of Emergency Medicine, 55*(6), 799–812.

7. Creed, J. O., et al. (2018). Acute crisis care for patients with mental health crises: Initial assessment of an innovative prehospital alternative destination program in North Carolina. *Prehospital Emergency Care, 22*(5), 555-564.

8. Pajonk, F. G., et al. (2008). Psychiatric emergencies in prehospital emergency medical systems: A prospective comparison of two urban settings. *General Hospital Psychiatry, 30*(4), 360–366.

9. Paton, F., et al. (2016). Improving outcomes for people in mental health crisis: A rapid synthesis of the evidence for available models of care. *Health Technology Assessment, 20*(3), 1–162.

10. Cheney, P., et al. (2008). Safety and compliance with an emergency medical service direct psychiatric center transport protocol. *American Journal of Emergency Medicine, 26*(7), 750–756.

11. Prener, C., & Lincoln, A. K. (2015). Emergency medical services and "psych calls": Examining the work of urban EMS providers. *American Journal of Orthopsychiatry, 85*(6), 612–619.

12. Rees, N., et al. (2014). Perceptions of paramedic and emergency care workers of those who self harm: A systematic review of the quantitative literature. *Journal of Psychosomatic Research, 77*(6), 449–456.

13. Ford-Jones, P. C., & Chaufan, C. (2017). A critical analysis of debates around mental health calls in the prehospital setting. *Inquiry, 54.* doi:10.1177/0046958017704608.

14. Law enforcement training [cited December 04, 2019]. Retrieved from http://www.mces.org/pages/cjs_lawenf.php.

15. Murdock, R. (2017). *Case study: Transporting behavioral health patients to an alternate destination.* EMS Reference.

16. Brenner, J. M., et al. (2018). The ethics of real-time EMS direction: Suggested curricular content. *Prehospital and Disaster Medicine, 33*(2), 201–212.

17. Budner, L. J. (1997). Behavioral effects of hypoglycemia. *Journal of the American Academy of Child & Adolescent Psychiatry, 36*(12), 1651–1652.

18. Lortie, G., & Laird, D. M. (1957). Hypoglycemia simulating psychoses. *The New England Journal of Medicine, 256*(25), 1190–1192.

19. Singh, S. K., et al. (1994). Acute psychotic disorder and hypoglycemia. *Indian Journal of Psychiatry, 36*(2), 93–94.

20. Malouf, R., & Brust, J. C. (1985). Hypoglycemia: Causes, neurological manifestations, and outcome. *Annals of Neurology, 17*(5), 421–430.

21. Sahoo, S., Mehra, A., & Grover, S. (2016). Acute hyperglycemia associated with psychotic symptoms in a patient with type 1 diabetes mellitus: A case report. *Innovations in Clinical Neuroscience, 13*(11-12), 25–27.

22. Suslo, R., et al. (2015). Hypoxia-related brain dysfunction in forensic medicine. *Advances in Experimental Medicine and Biology, 837*, 49–56.

23. Elliott, B. (2009). Psychosis and status epilepticus: Borderland or hidden cause? *Epilepsia, 50*(Suppl. 12), 70–72.

24. Lopez Arteaga, T., et al. (2013). Nonconvulsive status epilepticus and psychotic symptoms: Case report. *Rivista di Psichiatria, 48*(3), 268–270.

25. Snabboon, T., et al. (2009). Psychosis as the first presentation of hyperthyroidism. *Internal and Emergency Medicine, 4*(4), 359–360.

26. Brownlie, B. E., et al. (2000). Psychoses associated with thyrotoxicosis - 'thyrotoxic psychosis.' A report of 18 cases, with statistical analysis of incidence. *European Journal of Endocrinology, 142*(5), 438–444.

27. Gill, J. R. (2014). The syndrome of excited delirium. *Forensic Science, Medicine and Pathology, 10*(2), 223–228.

28. Richmond, J. S., et al. (2012). Verbal de-escalation of the agitated patient: Consensus statement of the American Association for Emergency Psychiatry Project BETA De-escalation Workgroup. *Western Journal of Emergency Medicine, 13*(1), 17–25.

29. Brymer, M., Jacobs, A., Layne, C., et al. (2006). *Psychological first aid: Field operations guide* (2nd ed.). National Child Traumatic Stress Network and National Center for PTSD. Retrieved September 25, 2019, from https://www.ptsd.va.gov/professional/treat/type/PFA/PFA_V2.pdf.

30. Allen, M. H., et al. (2005). The expert consensus guideline series. Treatment of behavioral emergencies 2005. *Journal of Psychiatric Practice, 11*(Suppl. 1), 5–108; quiz 110-2.

31. Mankowitz, S. L., et al. (2018). Ketamine for rapid sedation of agitated patients in the prehospital and emergency department settings: A systematic review and proportional meta-analysis. *The Journal of Emergency Medicine, 55*(5), 670–681.

32. Page, C. B., et al. (2018). A prospective before and after study of droperidol for prehospital acute behavioral disturbance. *Prehospital Emergency Care, 22*(6), 713–721.

33. Isenberg, D. L., & Jacobs, D. (2015). Prehospital agitation and sedation trial (PhAST): A randomized control trial of intramuscular haloperidol versus intramuscular midazolam for the sedation of the agitated or violent patient in the prehospital environment. *Prehospital and Disaster Medicine, 30*(5), 491–495.

34. San, L., et al. (2018). PLACID study: A randomized trial comparing the efficacy and safety of inhaled loxapine versus intramuscular aripiprazole in acutely agitated patients with schizophrenia or bipolar disorder. *European Neuropsychopharmacology, 28*(6), 710–718.

35. Zun, L. S. (2018). Evidence-based review of pharmacotherapy for acute agitation. Part 1: Onset of efficacy. *Journal of Emergency Medicine, 54*(3), 364–374.

36. Cester-Martínez, A., et al. (2017). Inhaled loxapine for the treatment of psychiatric agitation in the prehospital setting: A case series. *Clinical Practice and Cases in Emergency Medicine, 1*(4), 345–348.

37. Cole, J. B., et al. (2016). A prospective study of ketamine versus haloperidol for severe prehospital agitation. *Clinical Toxicology, 54*(7), 556–562.

38. Cole, J. B., et al. (2018). A prospective study of ketamine as primary therapy for prehospital profound agitation. *American Journal of Emergency Medicine, 36*(5), 789–796.

39. Burnett, A., et al. (2015). The administration of prehospital ketamine for chemical restraint does not prolong on-scene times compared to haloperidol based sedation. *Australasian Journal of Paramedicine, 12*(1).

40. Linder, L. M., Ross, C. A., & Weant, K. A. (2018). Ketamine for the acute management of excited delirium and agitation in the prehospital setting. *Pharmacotherapy, 38*(1), 139–151.

41. Cousins, R., et al. (2017). It's time for EMS to administer ketamine analgesia. *Prehospital Emergency Care, 21*(3), 408–410.

7

Nursing Emergency Psychiatry Triage Process

Mina R. Spadaro

Triage is broadly defined in health care as the sorting of patients based on the urgency for care. Psychiatric nursing triage takes this a bit further and can be defined as a clinical process conducted to assess and categorize the urgency of psychiatric emergency conditions. The core function of triage for a psychiatric emergency is to conduct a risk assessment that determines the nature and severity of the presenting problem and identifies how urgently intervention is needed. Most importantly, psychiatric nursing triage aims to determine if a patient is at immediate risk of harming themselves or others. There is significant variation in how this type of triage is conducted and is dependent on the structure of the psychiatric emergency setting. However, there are three core elements that are essential to appropriately triaging a psychiatric emergency: identification of the patient's risk for self-harm or suicide potential, risk for violence or aggression, and level of agitation.

The psychiatric nurse triage process initiates the emergency treatment of a patient experiencing a psychiatric medical emergency. In many settings, this occurs after a patient has been medically evaluated to rule out medical etiologies for the patient's psychiatric symptoms (also known as medical clearance), whereas in others, the psychiatric triage and "medical clearance" process may proceed simultaneously in the emergency setting (1). Individually, the psychiatric nursing process of emergency triage is a clinical procedure to rapidly assess and identify patient needs.

A psychiatric triage nurse performing the triage of a psychiatric medical emergency plays a critical role in the clinical workflow by collecting, organizing, and communicating the information collected through the triage process. This establishes the clinical foundation and framework for the patient's treatment. Equally important, the psychiatric triage nurse establishes the foundation for how the patient experiences the treatment encounter. Psychiatric triage nurses accomplish this by how they approach the patient and manage the process, how well they communicate to the other members of the clinical team, how well they memorialize their finding in the medical record, and their ability to establish trust with the patient during the triage process. Patients themselves have reported the most positive interactions with emergency staff were when they felt they were respected, were listened to appropriately, and were treated in a timely fashion (2).

In addition to all this, psychiatric nursing triage prioritizes interventions based on level of severity identified at the time of triage. It is recommended that nurses utilize evidence-based screening and assessment tools to determine the patient's level of risk and overall acuity. The patient's presenting risk and acuity is then used to determine the level of urgency for timing of treatment interventions.

There is not one uniformly accepted triage scale used to classify the triage level of a psychiatric emergency medical condition. The Emergency Severity Index (ESI) used for the triage of acute physical conditions in many emergency department (EDs) does not fit well for a psychiatric medical emergency because it is designed for more traditional medical emergencies, and thus not equipped to properly measure the urgency of a psychiatric emergency medical condition (3). However, there are evidence-based assessment tools that can be used individually or in combination to develop standardize a triage protocol for psychiatric emergencies. For example, there are evidence-based tools such as suicide risk screens and assessments, violence risk assessments, and agitation scales that can be combined into a triage protocol, which will be discussed later in this chapter. Another option is use of one of the emerging tools such as the Canadian Triage and Acuity Scale (CTAS, Press, 2019), the Crisis Triage Rating Scale (CTRS) (4), or the Australasian mental health triage scale (5) to develop an effective clinical workflow for triage of psychiatric emergencies.

A complicating factor is that accepted standards for measurement are problem-specific and lack uniform scoring. Individual evidence-based screening tools or assessments, such as for suicide, violence, or agitation, each have a different methodology for scoring the level of risk that tools are measuring (6). Whereas triage scales such as Triage Assessment System (TAS) (7) or CTRS use descriptors consistent with triage scales used for emergency medicine for classifying and sorting patients, such as, "high risk," "medium risk," or "low risk," or "immediate," "emergency," "urgent," "semiurgent," or "nonurgent," and these descriptors then influence the level of resources and services provided (8–11).

The Australasian mental health triage scale not only sorts patients into "emergency, urgent, semiurgent, or nonurgent" based on behavioral presentation but also places specific time to treatment goals for each category (10 minutes, 30 minutes, 1 hour, and 2 hours, respectively) (5).

In general, subspecialty triage processes are essential to creating high-quality patient outcomes and require a holistic well-rounded framework to successfully assess patient treatment needs and risk. More specifically, the process of psychiatric nurse triage prioritizes three critical areas of risk screening and contextualizes information for handoff to other professionals. Although the scoring and classifications may not be uniform, each tool places a patient somewhere on a continuum from high to low risk for self- or other harm. The psychiatric triage nurse needs to synthesize and analyze this information to establish an immediate plan of care.

Patients who present at very high acuity in any of these three areas, such as extreme aggression or delirium, may need immediate intervention by the treatment team, which pushes the completion of the full triage assessment to a later time. But a patient who triages at lower risk may be able to remain cooperative through the triage process and also allow for a subsequent full-comprehensive psychiatric nursing assessment, which eliminates the need to hand off to another colleague for to continue the intake process. Especially when there are time constraints or staffing limitations, often the psychiatric triage nurse and admitting nurse can be the same person, and the triage and comprehensive assessment can be combined into one process.

For a psychiatric nurse to effectively triage a patient experiencing a psychiatric emergency medical condition, the psychiatric nurse needs not only competence but confidence in their ability to effectively collect and analyze significant amounts of information in a very short period of time. This requires the nurse to have strong interpersonal and psychiatric nursing assessment skills. An attempt to form a therapeutic relationship with the patient should be initiated during the triage process. The psychiatric triage nurse must balance the complexity of the rapid triage process with therapeutic aspects such as compassion and empathy.

In order to accomplish this, nurses need to be conscious about their nonverbal behaviors and mode of communication during their interaction with the patient, avoiding the appearance of disdain, sarcasm, indifference, or belittling of the sincerity or severity of the patient's symptoms. Instead, if the nurse can perform the triage assessment in a supportive, caring therapeutic fashion, then a level of trust can be established with the patient.

A key element in establishing a therapeutic relationship and creating trust is a nonjudgmental approach. One way for the nurse to successfully remain objective throughout this process is understanding that the mind does not always clearly distinguish between physical or emotional pain. It can be as difficult for a patient to control their reaction to emotional pain as it is for them to control their reaction to physical pain. Many outward symptoms are consistent between physical and emotional pain: changes in mood, tearfulness, restlessness, etc., can be seen in a patient who is in either type of pain (12).

Another important element of psychiatric triage is the nurse's ability to effectively de-escalate a patient. Patients who present with a psychiatric emergency may have waited longer than a patient with a physical medical emergency and be frustrated, irritable, or frightened; any of these emotions can quickly magnify into agitation. A psychiatric triage nurse who can de-escalate and calm an arriving patient showing any signs of emotional instability or agitation, and establish a positive therapeutic relationship during the initial interaction with the patient, will be most likely to lay the foundation for safe, successful, and effective treatment of the patient (13).

NURSING PSYCHIATRIC EMERGENCY TRIAGE PROCESS

The goals of triage are to determine the nature of the psychiatric emergency, including immediate safety concerns (eg, suicidality or violence), need for immediate interventions, and the likely next appropriate level of treatment or supervision while in the emergency setting. The triage process includes pretriage data collection, engagement in a collaborative discussion with the patient focusing on the presenting problem, nonverbal assessment, screening, and/or assessment of patient risk for suicide, self-harm, violence, or grave disability.

Pretriage

In pretriage, the psychiatric triage nurse reviews the patient's medical records and relevant current or historical information that might provide insight into the patient's current presentation. When possible, the psychiatric triage nurse should identify family members, support individuals, or other informants who may be able to provide relevant information about the patient's illness. It is also helpful if there is a treating provider or outpatient psychiatrist who can supply information that may be relevant to the current presentation and how it differs from the patient's baseline. Gathering relevant information prior to engaging in the triage interview can help the nurse to determine the accuracy of the patient-reported history, particularly if the patient is agitated, psychotic, or cognitively impaired, or otherwise might have difficulty communicating accurate information.

Triage Initiation

In the beginning of the psychiatric nursing triage process, the nurse should introduce themselves to

the patient and their purpose for interacting with the patient. For example, "Hello, Mr. Smith, I am Nurse Triage from Behavioral Health and I am here to talk to you about how you're doing. Is it alright if I call you Mr. Smith?" This is a good time to start creating a trusting relationship through respectful interaction. For example, ask the patient permission for talking to them "Is it alright if I spend a few minutes talking to you?" and "Do you mind if I sit down?"

To start this part of the discussion, it helps to make a positive statement and then ask the question in context. For example, "Mr. Smith, I am here to help you and would like to try to do that. Can you tell me what is going on that brought you here today?" It is critical to allow the patient time to respond to the questions they are asked. Additionally, when the patient responds favorably, providing positive responses or saying "Thank You" at the appropriate times during the conversation, trust and respect are built. This also provides the opportunity to assess the patient's nonverbal aspects, by observing their gestures and physical responses to questions and interventions.

During the initiation phase of triage, the presenting problem should be explored, and, if possible, this presenting concern should be discussed. The psychiatric triage nurse should collect and synthesize data associated with the current presentation, for example, when the symptoms started, if there are any specific triggers that occurred prior to current crisis, history regarding substance abuse, and any recent changes in medication. Collections of this basic information about the presenting psychiatric emergency allows the psychiatric triage nurse to bring the presenting crisis and the risk potential together to formulate a strong triage assessment, a starting point for care.

Often the interview is much more effective if the patient can talk freely and the psychiatric triage nurse listens, with the nurse only asking questions to fill in the information gaps. The listening process provides additional time for assessment of nonverbal communication. If the patient is agitated or distressed and unable to engage in the needed exchange for triage, the triage process should be postponed until the patient is able to participate. However, even highly agitated patients can benefit from the triage process, especially when it includes de-escalation techniques and the calming effects of establishing a therapeutic relationship (14).

Triage Assessment of Nonverbal Presentation

Nonverbal communication constitutes an important part of the overall communication process; it strengthens and reenforces verbal messages and information communicated. Within the context of psychiatric nursing emergency triage process, nonverbal communication constitutes a critical element for gathering relevant clinical information. The psychiatric triage nurse should start assessing these nonverbal aspects as soon as the interaction with the patient begins. Nonverbal communication can reveal a wide range of information about the patient, including diagnostic information and the potential for violence (15). Clinically relevant nonverbal findings include appearance, facial expressions, restlessness, tension, eye contact, posture, quality of speech, affect, and other observable information, which provides valuable clues to the overall severity of illness and degree of crisis the patient is experiencing.

The psychiatric triage nurse should prioritize the assessment of agitation based on verbal and nonverbal cues alike throughout the assessment. A common mistake that is made during the psychiatric nursing triage process is inadvertently creating additional tension and therefore increasing or creating agitation in the patient (16). The psychiatric triage nurse will need to use good clinical judgment in timing when and how they collect the needed information. If the initial interview questions create a negative reaction in the patient, the nurse needs to remain calm, supportive, and communicate in noncoercive, nonconfrontational ways. Agitation is a primarily nonverbal assessment and an observable indication of potentially violent behavior. There can be verbal indicators, but if they are inconsistent with the nonverbal communication, verbal information may not be reliable.

Triage Assessment of Risk

The psychiatric nursing triage process assesses the level of patient agitation first, in order to determine if the patient can safely complete the triage assessment without immediate intervention. If

the patient is calm and cooperative enough to be further assessed, then the other risk areas should be prioritized. All patients presenting with behavioral health chief complaints should be screened for suicide risk, which can often be accomplished with a simple two-question process; if the two-question patient screen is positive, the evaluation tool will then lead to a more comprehensive suicide risk assessment. Contemporary regulatory standards in the United States now require that standardized and evidence-based suicide assessments be utilized, such as the Columbia Suicide Severity Rating Scale (C-SSRS), Patient Health Questionnaire (PHQ-9), Suicide Behaviors Questionnaire-Revised (SBQ-R), or another standardized tool (7,17).

The suicide risk assessment used should then assist the staff to stratify the level of suicide risk potential for each individual screened as high, medium, or low (The Joint Commission, 2018). Each level of risk is required to have specific interventions and levels of observation assigned to that risk classification. The purpose of risk specific interventions is to ensure safe treatment practices and levels of observation are consistently delivered to patients who present with defined risk levels. For example, a patient who is assessed as being at high for suicide risk will most likely be placed on a 1 to 1 observation, where the patient who presents as a low risk for suicide might be placed on the Q15 minute observation. The stratification will also be important in determining if a patient needs to be situated in a ligature-safe environment or room (18).

The psychiatric triage nurse should also use an evidence-based tool to measure a patient's potential for violence. Standardized tools such as the Broset Violence Checklist, the "Staring and eye contact, Tone and volume of voice, Anxiety, Mumbling, Pacing" or STAMP tool, or danger assessment tool, are examples of acceptable instruments (19,20). When evaluating a patient's risk for violence, it is important not to make assumptions that just because the patient is experiencing psychiatric emergency or has a history of mental illness, it is not an automatic indicator that a patient will become violent (21). The psychiatric triage nurse should attempt to remain nonjudgmental through the process of assessing this area of risk, and rather than deferring to an emotional response, substitute the appropriate tools to assess the patients' potential for violent behavior. A common mistake that is made by assessing a patient's potential for violence is assuming that that potential indicates likelihood or certainty and an overreaction results. For example, just because a patient has been violent in a past visit, it does not mean that they need to be placed in restraints upon arrival to ensure that they do not become violent during the current visit.

An effective triage and intake process allows the nurse to integrate the findings from the suicide and violence screens, along with pretriage and nonverbal information, to synthesize a clear clinical picture that can be used to mitigate patients' clinical risks and direct their immediate care.

Post Triage

Post triage, the patient will continue to a full nursing intake assessment by the triage nurse or has a warm handoff to the assessment nurse who will complete this comprehensive psychiatric nursing assessment. Thorough and clearly communicated documentation, along with good clinical evaluation and judgment, is a key aspect. The psychiatric nurse conducting the comprehensive assessment should be able to collect information that fills in the gaps from the triage documentation, such as psychosocial indicators of what may be contributing to the patient's current condition, psychiatric history, nonverbal assessment, and when possible, the existence of crisis plans and/or factors that might decrease or increase the patient's acuity. Mental status triage evaluation should include any elements of the appearance, behavior, activity, attitude, speech quality and rate, mood, affect, perception, thoughts, cognition, judgment, attention span, and psychotic symptoms relevant to the presenting complaint. It is important that the psychiatric nurse synthesizes and analyzes the information and writes a narrative note that creates a well-defined clear picture of the patient.

"Mitigating factors" can also be important to add to the assessment in determining overall level of concern (22). Does a patient appear to be in good control and trustworthy? Are they discussing spiritual or family concerns that would prevent them from acting upon risk factors? Do they clearly appear to want help, or do they appear to be an elopement risk?

It is also critical that the psychiatric nurse use descriptive words that provided substance to narrative of the documentation (23). For example, the statement "patient is delusional" gives far less information or evidence than "patient believes that they are the past president of the United States" which clearly indicates that the patient has a delusional belief that is not validated by reality. This type of documentation is very important for the psychiatric nurse's triage to be of value to the rest of the clinical team.

CONCLUSION

A strong psychiatric nursing triage process sets foundation and tone for how the patient and clinicians experience the overall emergency encounter, while also establishing connection and trust. When handing the patient off to the next practitioner, the psychiatric triage nurse should introduce the patient and explain what will happen next. A good psychiatric triage process facilitates safety, a collaborative workflow, and a positive patient experience.

REFERENCES

1. Clarke, D. E., et al. (2005). Psychiatric emergency nurses in the emergency department: The success of the Winnipeg, Canada experience. *Journal of Emergency Nursing, 31*(4), 351–356.
2. Morphet, J., et al. (2012). Managing people with mental health presentations in emergency departments—A service exploration of the issues surrounding responsiveness from a mental health care consumer and carer perspective. *Australasian Emergency Nursing Journal, 15*(3), 148–155.
3. AHRQ. (2018). *Emergency Severity Index (ESI): A triage tool for emergency departments.* Agency for Healthcare Research & Quality. Retrieved December 30, 2018, from https://www.ahrq.gov/professionals/systems/hospital/esi/index.html.
4. Broadbent, M., Moxham, L., & Dwyer, T. (2007). The development and use of mental health triage scales in Australia. *International Journal of Mental Health Nursing, 16*, 413–421. doi:10.1111/j.1447-0349.2007.00496.x.
5. Downey, L. V., Zun, L. S., & Burke, T. (2015). Comparison of Canadian triage acuity scale to Australian Emergency Mental Health Scale triage system for psychiatric patients. *International Emergency Nursing, 23*(2), 138–143.

6. Zun, L. (2016). Care of psychiatric patients: The challenge to emergency physicians. *The Western Journal of Emergency Medicine, 17*(2), 173–176. doi:10.5811/westjem.2016.1.29648.

7. Zhou, W. H., Hu, J. B., Hu, S. H., Wei, N., Huang, M. L., & Xu, Y. (2008). Application of the triage assessment system for a rapid assessment of mental health of the referral wounded and their family members in Wenchuan earthquake. *Chinese Journal of Preventive Medicine, 42*(11), 798–801. Retrieved from https://www.ncbi.nlm.nih.gov/pubmed/19176137.

8. The Joint Commission. (2018). *EP 3 & 4: Validated/evidence based suicide risk assessment tools*. Retrieved December 30, 2018, from https://www.jointcommission.org/assets/1/18/Suicide_Prevention_Resources_EP3_4_NPSG150101.pdf.

9. ENA. (2018). *Care of the psychiatric patient in the emergency department*. Retrieved December 30, 2018, from https://www.ena.org/docs/default-source/resource-library/practice-resources/white-papers/care-of-psychiatric-patient-in-the-ed.pdf?sfvrsn=3fc76cda_4.

10. The Joint Commission. (2015, December 7). *Standards BoosterPak for suicide risk (NSPG. 15.01.01)*. Retrieved December 30, 2018, from https://www.jointcommission.org/search/?keywords=suicide+risk+score&f=sitename&sitename=Joint%20Commission.

11. Patient Safety Advisory Group. (2016, February 24). Detecting and treating suicide ideation in all settings. *Sentinel Event Alert*, (56), 1–7. Retrieved from https://www.jointcommission.org/assets/1/18/SEA_56_Suicide.pdf.

12. Biro, D. (2010). Is there such a thing as psychological pain? And why it matters. *Culture, Medicine and Psychiatry, 34*(4), 658–667.

13. Nordstrom, K., Zun, L. S., Wilson, M. P., Md, V. S., Ng, A. T., Bregman, B., & Anderson, E. L. (2012). Medical evaluation and triage of the agitated patient: Consensus statement of the American Association for Emergency Psychiatry Project BETA Medical Evaluation Workgroup. *The Western Journal of Emergency Medicine, 13*(1), 3–10.

14. Holloman, G. H., & Zeller, S. L. (2012). Overview of project BETA: Best practices in evaluation and treatment of agitation. *The Western Journal of Emergency Medicine, 13*(1), 1–2.

15. Stowell, K. R., Florence, P., Harman, H. J., & Glick, R. L. (2012). Psychiatric evaluation of the agitated patient: Consensus statement of the American Association for Emergency Psychiatry Project BETA Psychiatric Evaluation Workgroup. *The Western Journal of Emergency Medicine, 13*(1), 11–16.

16. Baker, S. N. (2012). Management of acute agitation in the emergency department. *Advanced Emergency Nursing Journal, 34*(4), 306–318.

17. University of Notre Dame. (2018). *Assessing the risk of suicide*. University Counseling Center. Retrieved December 30, 2018, from https://ucc.nd.edu/self-help/depression-suicide/helping-someone-in-a-suicidal-crisis/assessing-the-risk-of-suicide/.

18. Beebe, C. E. (2018, November 9). *Separating fact from fiction in ligature risk. Health Facilities Management*. Retrieved April 8, 2019, from https://www.hfmmagazine.com/articles/3515-separating-fact-from-fiction-in-ligature-risk.

19. ACEP. (2015, November). *Risk assessment and tools for identifying patients at high risk for violence and self-harm in the ED*. Retrieved December 30, 2018, from https://www.acep.org/globalassets/sites/acep/media/public-health/risk-assessment-violence_selfharm.pdf.

20. CDC. (2013, August 12). *NIOSH-WPVHC-violence risk assessment tools*. Retrieved December 30, 2018, from https://wwwn.cdc.gov/wpvhc/Course.aspx/Slide/Unit6_8.

21. Large, M., & Nielssen, O. (2017). The limitations and future of violence risk assessment. *World Psychiatry, 16*(1), 25–26.

22. Cole-King, A., & Lepping, P. (2010). Suicide mitigation: Time for a more realistic approach. *The British Journal of General Practice, 60*(570), e1–e3. doi:10.3399/bjgp10X482022.

23. Mohr, W. K., & Noone, M. J. (1997). Deconstructing progress notes in psychiatric settings. *Archives of Psychiatric Nursing, 11*(6), 325–331.

8

Safety and Security in Psychiatric Emergency Services and Emergency Departments

Victor G. Stiebel

The emergency department (ED) of today must be open and available for all who come, but concurrently, the safety of everyone present must be assured. This complex balance is increasingly hard to maintain as violence has escalated in our society. The first edition of this textbook focused specifically on the psychiatric emergency service (PES). In these last 10 years, much has happened and far more mental health care is provided in the general medical ED. This chapter will focus on developments since the first edition and explore issues that affect safety and the opportunities for improvement that can occur.

Safety in the healthcare setting is ambiguous at best and even more confused in the ED. One can have high security or open access, but it is difficult to have both. The ED must offer round-the-clock access to all comers while at the same time ensuring the safety of all those present. Into this add the ill, the traumatized, the potentially violent, and the mentally ill. Family may be fearful for their loved ones and often do not understand a very complex system. The presence of police and security can be unsettling to many. Mental health patients, although a small percentage of those treated in the ED, may be agitated or suicidal and necessitate a disproportionate amount of staff time. In combination with ubiquitous waiting times and ever present staff shortages, a potentially volatile mix is created.

EPIDEMIOLOGY

The Occupational Safety and Health Administration (OSHA) defines workplace violence as "any act or threat of physical violence, harassment, intimidation or other threatening disruptive behavior that occurs at the work site." Their 2015 report noted that healthcare workers suffer serious workplace violence at a rate four times that of private industry (1). The risk starts prehospital with 80% of emergency medical service (EMS) suffering some form of assault, though not even half were treated or even filed reports of the incidents (2).

A prospective survey of violent acts against ED physicians in 2012 found that 78% reported at least one incident of verbal or physical aggression in the previous 12 months (3). Phillips reported in 2016 that violent acts by a patient or an authorized visitor (family, customer, or employee) accounted for 93% of all assaults against hospital workers (4). These numbers have not improved in the last 10 years. A 2018 survey of emergency physicians found that the percent of respondents reporting any form of violence remained level at 72% in the previous 10 years. The percent reporting actual physical assault however rose to 38% from 24% (5). The immediate impact of violent acts includes the actual physical injury and time off, acute stress reactions, and workplace fears leading to loss of productivity. The long-term sequelae include posttraumatic stress disorder (PTSD) and depression, cognitive effects of head injuries, physical debility preventing return to work, and general burnout. The public often believe that mentally ill patients are at higher risk for violence then the rest of the population and this may be influenced by media coverage of mass shootings and publicized suicides. However, Choe (6) and Elbogen (7) showed that while there is a slightly elevated risk, when patients with substance abuse are excluded, not only were the mentally ill less likely to be violent, they were more likely to be victimized themselves. In 2017, The Joint Commission updated their determination that healthcare violence was a sentinel event (8). They reported that problems in policies and procedures were a factor in 62% of cases of violence. Human resource–related factors were a factor in 60%. Problems in assessment and observation were in third place at 58%. Inadequate communication, both among staff and with patients or families, was 53%. Last, physical plant was cited in 36% of the cases.

ADMINISTRATION

In these last 10 years, much has changed in emergency medicine, but the prevalence of violence directed to staff has not, vexing administrators. Traditional predictors of violence risk were based on a relatively stable inpatient model and included things such as patient census, percentage of patients with a history of violence, the number of female staff, and the level of overall mental health training in staff (9). In contrast to the relative stability of inpatient units, the ED is likely more unpredictable. Average daily census figures can fluctuate widely, with less ill patients often being diverted to non-ED settings, resulting in a higher-acuity mix. An average number of staff can safely care for their average number of patients, but that average can often be exceeded. Patients with a history of violence, aggression, or impulsivity are now brought to the ED by police for evaluation and disposition prior to legal processing. The number of guns being carried by non-law-enforcement individuals has only grown, yet aggressive screening for weapons at entry points may convey a public relations message that is not ideal (10). In the last 10 years, traditionally defined roles in medicine have evolved, and currently 50% of medical students are women. The number of men employed in traditional nursing fields has also grown to 10% (11). This has resulted in a new dynamic, which has not been studied, where it is not unusual to have an ED staffed with a majority of nurses being men and all physicians being women. Training opportunities for ED staff and security are more widely available and have become more standardized (12) as computer-based learning has become ubiquitous, although this is still a costly endeavor that requires yearly training to be effective. The perennial problem of capturing the revenues that

the ED brings into the hospital has not changed. Effective leadership can ensure that these resources are allocated back to the ED to address these issues; however, finances are not always the only answer. The Emergency Nurses Association (ENA) surveillance survey (13) showed that EDs with violence reporting policies and an administration committed to minimizing workplace violence were less likely to experience violence.

STAFF CHARACTERISTICS

The unique staffing models and needs in the ED are often not reflective of the general hospital. The camaraderie in a well-functioning department is unusually tight. However, many disciplines are often thrown together for the first time, during a critical situation, each with their own training and experience. Adding to the confusion is that when critical staffing levels are reached, shortfalls can be more easily covered pulling staff from other departments or using outside agencies. These staff may not be familiar with the general nuances of the ED. Specifically, this can have significant implications for the psychiatrically unstable patient, as many of these "part-timers" lack experience with these patients. Students, residents, and other trainees are often used to fill out staff functions and are often the first to see a patient, even though they are the least experienced. The triage nurse can be especially vulnerable, meeting an unknown patient for the first time, alone, in the setting of a relatively isolated triage or examination room. It is the rare ED that is staffed with full-time psychiatrists, although the expanding use of telepsychiatry is providing a solution.

RESIDENT CHARACTERISTICS

Residents fill a critical staffing role in the ED. Because of their lack of experience, they may miss subtle nuances of a patient's mental status that could presage violence or decompensation. Not being aware of transference issues could lead to a patient feeling disrespected or misunderstood. Countertransference can result in anger or feelings of helplessness toward a difficult or agitated patient. Nuanced speech patterns by both the resident and the patient could be perceived as provocative. Lack of situational awareness such as allowing for adequate interpersonal space or location of escape routes and alarm buttons can contribute to unfavorable outcomes. Many of the medications used in mental health will be unfamiliar and can contribute to errors. Additional resident factors include the ubiquitous lack of sleep, service obligations mandating ED coverage, and reluctance to come to attending staff with clinical concerns. Behnem in 2011 (14) found that residents early in training were more likely to be verbally threatened, but senior residents were more likely to be physically assaulted. It may be that a patient's initial anger may be directed at a trainee early in the ED process. A more experienced resident may not get involved until a patient becomes more agitated or has been in the ED process for an extended period of time and is thus more likely to act out violently. Interestingly, attending staff reported verbal or physical violence much less frequently, suggesting that experience matters.

NURSING CHARACTERISTICS

In 2011 the National Crime Victimization Survey, the US Department of Justice (15) found nurses accounting for 4% of workplace violence. Law enforcement was the only field with higher rates. The survey noted that there has been no decline in workplace incidents in these last 10 years. Half of nurses reported experiencing verbal abuse and 12% had suffered from physical violence in the previous week. Over 80% of the episodes occurred in patient rooms when the nurse was most likely to be alone. This becomes a critical factor as younger nurses with less experience are more likely to be filling these roles. Nurses in general spend more time with patients than the rest of the healthcare team placing them at greater overall risk. They are more likely than other staff to be at the front line when restraining patients and therefore more likely to be injured. While nurses are a source of comfort for patients providing for their multiple needs, they are also the ones responsible for painful procedures. Education clearly plays a role with graduate level nurses being less likely to be threatened than those with a 2- or 4-year degree (3).

PATIENT CHARACTERISTICS

Staff are at greatest risk when the potential risk of a patient's actions is not recognized in advance. A preexisting diagnosis can be a warning sign of possible acting out. A patient with changes in mental status due to an underlying medical issue, a risk factor for violence, is unlikely to be missed. A delirious or demented patient may also have their striking out excused. In both cases however, staff injuries suffered while caring for the patient will remain. Studies of violence can be informative for our work in the ED. A meta-analysis of 24,000 inpatients in 35 studies done in 2015 concluded one in five psychiatric inpatients may commit an act of violence. The characteristics associated with violence were male sex, involuntary status, diagnosis of schizophrenia, and patients with alcohol use disorder.

It is noteworthy that while the current trend toward open-door policies encourages visitors and family members to remain with the patient, visitors can be the perpetrators of staff-directed violence. Gang-related issues or family feuds can find their way into the hospital and into the laps of unsuspecting staff. Basic underlying personality structure can also be important to note. Antisocial, histrionic personalities may present with violence directed toward others while a patient with borderline features may be more at risk for self-injury. However, psychiatric illness is not responsible for the majority of today's violence (16,17). Patients with mental illness who do act violently are more likely to harm themselves than anyone else. In total, violent acts related to the mental illness constitute less than 5% of all violent acts committed in this country. However, this clearly does not apply when drugs or alcohol enter the picture.

Intoxication due to any substance is a major risk factor for violence, and this has only worsened in these last 10 years. A 2013 British National Health Service survey noted that 30% of violent episodes were related to intoxication (18). Substance abuse in any form, even if not associated with the current presenting problem, increases the risk of violence. Traditional stimulants such as cocaine have been replaced by methamphetamine and various hallucinogens. Nontraditional CNS stimulants, such over-the-counter dextromethorphan, are becoming more popular. Narcotics have branched out to the more toxic synthetic opioids such as subfentanyl. Many of these substances are not detectable by routine drug screens, so ED staff must be on alert to recognize patients who may be using. In addition to substance use and intoxication increasing the risk of violence, acute withdrawal can be associated with agitation and violent acting out.

Patients arriving from jails, detention settings, or those who are gang members, have accounted for 29% of shootings in EDs. As we will discuss shortly, 11% of these shootings occurred during an escape attempt, and these patients typically did not come to the ED with their own weapons (19). Staff must be vigilant about the environment and assure that knives and other sharps, sprays, and items that can be used as nontraditional weapons are not available to patients. Gang membership may provide access to guns or weapons, and the related culture may normalize violent behaviors. Youth are more at risk for violent acting out due to multiple factors including immaturity, lack of socialization, and strength. Those in jail may feel as if they have nothing more to lose.

ASSESSMENT TOOLS

The ideal risk assessment tool for the prediction of violence has remained elusive. A violent act is a state of being, not a Diagnostic and Statistical Manual of Mental Disorders (DSM) diagnosis. It can be verbal, sexual, or physical, or a combination. It may be a proactive or reactive. It can be perpetrated by the old or the young, in the inpatient or outpatient setting, or just on the street. This ambiguity and ubiquity mean that no one tool will fit every need and the ED setting brings this all into focus. Into this uncertainty, various tools have been developed to make risk assessment determinations in various settings including inpatient utilization review; civil and criminal court proceedings; and level of care determinations. This is very different than the psychiatric risk assessment of the past which was used clinically following a prolonged inpatient hospitalization for a patient who was very well known to their providers. This last point highlights that the end result of any tool is only as good as the historical information entered into it.

Singh (20) reviewed 68 studies for predictive accuracy. They noted over 120 different risk assessment tools that were available as of 2011. These had been developed in multiple settings including inpatient and outpatient clinical settings, civil and criminal court systems, in the United States and abroad. Their conclusion was that substantial differences were found in the tools surveyed and that accuracy was related to the population for which it was originally validated. Generally, the best predictive rates were for older predominantly white populations, which likely does not accurately reflect current clinical reality. The American Psychiatric Association in 2012 issued a paper on psychiatric risk assessment. They reviewed various instruments and found that structured approaches to risk assessment performed better than unstructured (21). They found that the overall accuracy of prediction tools has increased from 1970 to 2000. However, in the end, a test cannot substitute for clinical judgment in interpreting that test result. A broad understanding of multiple risk factors and social issues is critical.

One of the biggest problems with any form of standardized risk assessment tool is that ultimately, clinical judgment comes to the fore. If it is felt that violence risk is high, a moral and ethical obligation to act ensues, regardless of what a test might conclude. Using the "number needed to treat" concept from medication trials is informative. When assessing violence, one needs to think about the number needed to detain (NND). If a baseline level of violence could be set at 10%, then 10 people would need to be detained to prevent one violent act. However, as the base rate declines the NND would rise. The Epidemiologic Catchment Area study found a baseline rate of violence of 17% which would result in the NND of 3.5 people. The NIMH CATIE study found that prevalence of assault was 3.6% and so the NND would rise to 15 (at the same levels of sensitivity and specificity). This has significant ethical ramifications for clinicians who must balance competing clinical interests of patient autonomy and the safety of others (21,22).

CRITICAL COMMUNICATIONS

Communication flow between hospital staff and outside agencies and effective transfer of information is one of the biggest considerations in mitigating risk of violence in the ED setting. Poor communication can lead to catastrophic results. The 2017 Joint Commission Sentinel Event

Advisory noted that failures in communication comprised almost 60% of the human-related factors that were associated with ED violence (23). In 2015, communication failures accounted for 30% of malpractice actions.

It is given that critical information is often lost during change of shift. This has been discussed extensively, but has gained even more support recently. The "patient handoff" sequence for the ED actually starts in the field with police and/or EMS receiving a call for agitation or violence. These units gather critical data about the setting and circumstances, where the patient is found, evidence of alcohol or drugs, and other collateral information. If staff do not aggressively reach out for this information, it may be lost for all practical purposes: The police may not arrive when the patient does; medics may be called away before staff can question them; the completed trip reports may only arrive in batch form at some later time. Hospital security may be present but not briefed about their role in the crisis situation. Further, nursing staff, social workers, and other nonmedical ED staff may be reluctant to ask key questions due to concerns about overstepping boundaries, perceived weakness for asking questions, or even uncertainty about what to do with the information. Residents may not want to share their lack of knowledge, and staff physicians may be called only after a situation develops.

Despite all these issues, good communication is possible and has recently been studied (24-26). A well-organized team helps to ensure that information flows seamlessly from prehospital to security personnel to staff and nurses and finally to physicians. Use of a standard "handoff template" ensures consistency in data transmission, limits duplication, and enhances timeliness. In these last 10 years, this is becoming a standard of care. More recently, electronically based handoff systems have gained acceptance. Whatever format is used, an adherence to standardized workflow will clearly improve quality of care and staff-patient satisfaction.

A discussion of communication would not be complete without a brief summary of de-escalation techniques and the importance of training and yearly reviews for all staff. There is no one correct definition for the term de-escalation. It is more effective to consider this a sound-bite for a range of nonphysical verbal and environmental interventions whose goal is redirection of the agitated patient to a calmer state of mind. In an emergency, these are critical skills akin to the advanced cardiac life support (ACLS) protocols and all staff should be trained. The Project BETA from 2012 has been the most widely cited overview on this topic (27). Berring in 2016 used a meta-analysis to break this process into its various parts (28). The formal basics however date back to 1991 (29) and today would likely be called situational awareness and include: Knowing yourself; knowing the patient; knowing the situation; and knowing how to communicate. Verbally engaging the patient with empathy and clearly letting them know they will be cared for go a long way. Offering food, drink, or other comfort measures can often be helpful to establish collaboration. Humor, when effectively administered, and calmness, always, can often turn a potentially dangerous situation around. However, ensuring the safety of everyone is always paramount. Current thinking remains that avoiding restraints and other coercive steps is critical.

PHYSICAL ENVIRONMENT AND SECURITY

The actual physical layout of the ED is the final piece creating the perfect storm in which violent acts can occur. Identification of factors that might contribute to violence and the development of solutions to these factors is key, although no two settings will likely come to the same conclusions or plans. A recent review (30) noted that physical conditions commonly associated with EDs that contribute to violence include high acuity, crowded areas, noise, and the presence of substitute personnel. Additional issues identified include long waiting times, lack of information being passed to patients and families, and the presence of loud or agitated patients or visitors (31). With the understanding that none of these factors are going to be easily resolved in our current medical system, awareness remains the key to mitigating risk.

As mentioned above, security and access are generally mutually exclusive domains. An open-model ED allows rapid patient movement and staff efficiency and promotes a feeling of community to the department. Monitoring of all this movement is problematic. Metal detectors, security cameras, increased security presence, and multiple controlled access doors have been shown to be highly effective security measures. They also contribute to a "lockdown" feeling that can be alienating for a community-based hospital (10). In the last 10 years, however, there has been more acceptance of the need for security. More EDs are using things like disposable colored wristbands placed on the patient at triage to provide critical information about the patient. The requirement that all visitors to wear identification badges has become ubiquitous and acceptable.

An ENA study (8) noted the greatest risk for violence occurred in patient rooms, corridors, halls, stairwells, and elevators. These are all highly difficult areas to monitor closely for multiple reasons. Privacy issues place further limitations to patient rooms and public bathrooms or changing areas. In some cases, there may have no better option than having staff carry personal alarms or "panic buttons" when needed, though systems must be in place for rapid response when they are activated. All areas should be well lit and blind spots or hiding places should be minimized.

Security cameras can further assist in monitoring less accessible areas, but they are a mixed blessing and can lead to a false sense of security. Watching a camera feed can induce a low level of stupor which can be experienced by anyone who spends even a few minutes in their security office. It has been shown that individual attention span when monitoring a bank of monitors begins to drop after just 20 minutes (32). Increasing the number of monitors is directly correlated with decreased accuracy of detection. A single person watching one monitor can maintain accuracy of 85% for up to 2 hours; however, this drops to 53% with nine monitors, and it is not uncommon to have far more than this in a security office. With attention to these limitations, video monitoring will likely remain at the center of a comprehensive security plan.

The stated goal of ensuring that weapons do not enter the hospital is for the very reasonable purpose of protecting staff and patients. However, today it is also a potential political Pandora's box that public facilities may not want to open. Specifically, metal detectors, handheld

or walk-through, elicit visceral responses both for and against their use. Use of metal detectors requires continuous security personnel and also ongoing training which becomes a budgetary consideration, and it is not clear that they reduce violent acts in the ED setting. One 1999 study showed that after a metal detector system was put in place, the number of weapons confiscated increased but there was no drop in violent episodes (33). A 2003 survey found that 41% of weapons were confiscated from patients who arrived by ambulance and had bypassed security (34). In 2015, Malka et al. confirmed an earlier study in finding that metal detectors were effective at finding weapons. In contrast to a 2003 finding where guns made up less than 1% of confiscated items, they found the number of guns found had risen to 4.5%. Knives were the most common weapon confiscated, but chemical sprays made up 9% and other weapons including brass knuckles, stun guns, and box cutters made up 5%. This knowledge should inform the day-to-day practice of hospital security.

Security personnel have become a generally accepted reality of life in the violence-prone setting of the emergency service. Hospital security staff come from many backgrounds and their past training varies widely such that not all fit easily into the hospital environment. A young physically fit off-duty police officer will respond quite differently than an elderly deconditioned retired government employee. Furthermore, some hospitals arm security with guns, some with Taser-type devices, and some with a simple uniform. Few have ever had formal training with mental health patients and the unique aspects associated with seclusion and restraint. Their presence however does seem to be associated with decreased violent episodes (35). A 2014 survey showed that the number of hospitals authorizing handguns and Tasers doubled between 2010 and 2014. Fisher (19) reported that as of 2016, 52% of hospitals had personnel with guns and 47% with Tasers. The first survey found that allowing Tasers to be carried had a 41% lower risk of physical assault, controlling for other factors. An unanswered question is if it is the presence of security personnel that lowers aggressive acts or the presence of weapons. Unfortunately, weapons can have a mixed risk/benefit effect. In the last 10 years, incidents of patients being killed or injured by hospital security personnel have been reported (36). Between 2000 and 2011, the National Crime Victimization Survey noted 154 shootings on American hospital campuses with 41% occurring within the general hospital. Fully one-third occurred in the ED. In 20% of the cases, the perpetrator did not bring their own firearm (implying that someone else brought it for them). In 8% of the cases, the perpetrator took the gun from the police or security officer on scene (37).

CONCLUSIONS

Every patient under our care, every worker, and everyone who enters our hospital environment has the right to mental and physical safety. How each emergency service designs their safety program will depend on their unique philosophy, physical setting, and financial resources. There has been significant progress in our understanding violence and safety in these last 10 years. However, medical staff, and in particular nurses, continue to lead national statistics in physical injuries and resulting disability. There is still no "ideal" solution to this problem, and every ED and community will need to find their own balance. Safety begins with strong proactive leaders and extends to a tight team of professionals who practice effective communication and have ongoing training. Continuous risk mitigation strategies that are literature based can be broadly implemented to make emergency services as safe as possible.

REFERENCES

1. OSHA. Guidelines for *preventing workplace violence for healthcare and social service workers*. Retrieved May, 2018, from www.osha.gov/dsg/hospitals/workplace_violence.html.
2. Furin, M., Eliseo, L. J., et al. (2015). Self-reported provider safety in an urban emergency medical system. *The Western Journal of Emergency Medicine*, 16(3), 459–464. Retrieved from https://westjem.com/originalresearch/self-reported-providersafety-in-an-urban-emergencymedical-system.html.
3. Kowalenko, T., Cunningham, R., Sachs, C. J., et al. (2012). Workplace violence in emergency medicine: Current knowledge and future directions. *The Journal of Emergency Medicine, 43*(3), 523–531.
4. Phillips, J. P. (2016). Workplace violence against health care workers in the United States. *The New England Journal of Medicine, 374*(17), 1661–1669.
5. Omar, H., Yue, R., Amen, A. A., Kowalenko, T., & Walters, B. L. (2018). Reassessment of violence against emergency physicians. *Annals of Emergency Medicine*, 72(48), S144.
6. Choe, J. Y., Teplin, L. A., & Abram, K. M. (2008). Perpetration of violence, violent victimization, and severe mental illness: Balancing public health concerns. *Psychiatric Services, 59*, 153–164.
7. Elbogen, E. B., & Johnson, S. C. (2009). The intricate link between violence and mental disorder: Results from the National Epidemiologic Survey on Alcohol and Related Conditions. *Archives of General Psychiatry, 66*(2), 152–161.
8. The Joint Commission. (2010, June). Preventing violence in the health care setting. *Sentinel Event Alert*, (45). Retrieved from https://www.joint-commission.org/assets/1/18/SEA_45add.pdf.
9. Owen, C., Tarantello, C., Jones, M., et al. (1998). Violence and aggression in psychiatric units. *Psychiatric Services, 49*(11), 1452–1457.
10. L.A. County removing metal detectors from some hospital facilities. *Los Angeles Times*. (2013, February 3). Retrieved July, 2018, from https://www.latimes.com/health/la-xpm-2013-feb-03-la-me-metal-detectors-20130203-story.html.
11. US Census Bureau. (2018, March 19). *Table B24020, Sex by occupation for the full-time, year-round civilian employed population 16 years and over*. Retrieved July, 2018, from https://www.census.gov/newsroom/stories/2018/nurses.html.
12. Holloman, G. H., & Zeller, S. L. (2012). Overview of project beta: Best practices in evaluation and treatment of agitation. *Western Journal of Emergency Medicine: Integrating Emergency Care with Population Health, 13*(1). doi:10.5811/westjem.2011.9.6865.
13. Emergency Nurses Association. (2011, November). *Emergency department violence surveillance study*. Retrieved from https://www.ena.org/practice-research/research/Documents/ENAEDVSRcportNovember2011.pdf.
14. Behnam, M., Tillotson, R. D., Davis, S. M., & Hobbs, G. R. (2011). Violence in the emergency department: A national survey of emergency residents and attending physicians. *The Journal of Emergency Medicine, 40*(5), 565–579.
15. Harrell, E. (2011, March). *Workplace violence, 1993–2009*. US Department of Justice. Retrieved from https://www.bjs.gov/content/pub/pdf/wv09.pdf.

16. Pinals, D. A., Anacker, L., et al. (2016). Mental illness and firearms: Legal context and clinical approaches. *Psychiatric Clinics of North America, 39*, 611–621.

17. Pinals, D. A., Appelbaum, P. S., et al. (2015). Resource document on access to firearms by people with mental disorders. *Behavioral Sciences & the Law, 33*, 186–194.

18. Knowles, D., Mason, S. M., & Moriarty, F. (2013). I'm going to learn how to run quick: Exploring violence directed towards staff in the emergency department. *Emergency Medicine Journal, 30*, 926–931.

19. Kelen, G. D., Catlett, C. L., et al. (2012). Hospital based shootings in the United States: 2000–2011. *Annals of Emergency Medicine, 60*(6), 790–798.

20. Singh, J. P., Grann, M., & Fazel, S. (2011). A comparative study of violence risk assessment tools: A systematic review and metaregression analysis of 68 studies involving 25,980 participants. *Clinical Psychology Review, 31*, 499–513.

21. Buchanan, A., Binder, R., Norko, M., & Swartz, M. (2012). Resource document on psychiatric violence risk assessment. *The American Journal of Psychiatry, 169*, 3, data supplement.

22. Swanson, J., Swartz, M., Van Dorn, R., Elbogen, E., Wagner, R., Rosenheck, R., ... Lieberman, J. (2006). A national study of violent behavior in persons with schizophrenia. *Archives of General Psychiatry, 63*, 490–499.

23. The Joint Commission. (2017, September 12). *Preventing violence in the health care setting.* Retrieved from http://jointcommission.newmedia-release.com/2017_hand_off_communication.

24. Debelle, A., Dashwood, M., Bird, L., Rao, R., & Reilly, T. (2017). Improving handover between triage and locality wards in a large mental health trust. *BMJ Open Quality, 6*(2), e000023.

25. Tobiano, G., Bucknall, T., Sladdin, I., Whitty, J. A., & Chaboyer, W. (2018). Patient participation in nursing bedside handover: A systematic mixed-methods review. *International Journal of Nursing Studies, 77*, 243–258.

26. Sonis, J. D., Lucier, D. J., Raja, A. S., Strauss, J. L., & White, B. A. (2018). Improving emergency department to hospital medicine transfer of care through electronic pass-off. *The American Journal of Emergency Medicine, 36*(11), 2122–2124.

27. Richmond, J. S., Berlin, J. S., Fishkind, A. B., et al. (2012). Verbal de-escalation of the agitated patient: Consensus statement of the American Association for Emergency Psychiatry Project BETA De-escalation Workgroup. *Western Journal of Emergency Medicine, 13*(1), 17–25.

28. Berring, L. L., Pedersen, L., & Buus, N. (2016). Coping with violence in mental health care settings: Patient and staff member perspectives on de-escalation practices. *Archives of Psychiatric Nursing, 30*, 499–507.

29. Stevenson, S. (1991). Heading off violence with verbal de-escalation. *Journal of Psychosocial Nursing and Mental Health Services, 29*(9), 6–10.

30. Fisher, K. (2016). Inpatient violence. *Psychiatric Clinics of North America, 39*, 567–577.

31. Tadros, A., & Kiefer, C. (2017). Violence in the emergency department: A global problem. *Psychiatric Clinics of North America, 40*, 575–584.

32. Einsbruch, J., Breiner, A., & Gorman, E. (2016, March 23). *Security system monitoring in health care facilities.* International Association for Healthcare Security and Safety Foundation.

33. Rankins, R. C., & Hendey, G. W. (1999). Effect of a security system on violent incidents and hidden weapons in the emergency department. *Annals of Emergency Medicine, 33*(6), 676–679.

34. Simon, H. K., Khan, N. S., & Delgado, C. A. (2003). Weapons detection at two urban hospitals. *Pediatric Emergency Care, 19*, 248–251.

35. Schoenfisch, A., & Pompeii, L. (2014). *Weapons use among hospital security personnel.* International Healthcare Security and Safety Foundation.

36. Rosenthal, E. (2016, February 12). When the hospital fires the bullet. *The New York Times.*

37. Harnum, J. (2014). Hospital gun discharge events 2011–2013. *Journal of Healthcare Protection Management, 30*(2), 36–46.

9

Medical Evaluation of the Psychiatric Emergency Patient

Katrina A. Bozada, Leslie Zun

Patients with psychiatric emergencies may be seen in a variety of settings including emergency departments (EDs), psychiatric emergency services (PESs) or other emergency care settings. It is important that the psychiatric provider at these facilities, either in concert with a medical provider or alone, fully evaluate the patient to determine treatment needs and appropriate disposition. This assessment should include a thoughtful medical evaluation driven by the history, mental status examination (MSE), physical examination (PE), and any necessary testing to determine if an underlying medical etiology is either responsible for or exacerbating the patient's presentation. It is also important to identify any medical conditions needing treatment in an ED or medical inpatient setting, requiring continued care or special accommodations in the psychiatric inpatient setting, or needing follow-up in the outpatient setting (ie, by a primary care physician).

The medical evaluation of patients presenting with psychiatric complaints is an essential component of the assessment as studies have shown the incidence of underlying medical problems resembling psychiatric illness range from 15% to 90% (1-13). Missing a serious medical problem in an apparent psychiatric presentation can lead to significant morbidity and mortality. For example, the mortality rate in the elderly population with delirium is 25% (14). Common medical conditions presenting with psychiatric symptoms include dementia, delirium, medication issues, drug and alcohol intoxication and withdrawal, infections, central nervous system disease, metabolic and endocrine conditions, and cardiopulmonary disease (14), among others (see Table 9.1). If a serious medical condition is found, one may consider treatment either in the ED

prior to disposition or a medical inpatient admission with concomitant treatment of psychiatric symptoms as necessary.

The components of the medical evaluation of the patient presenting with psychiatric symptoms include a full history and PE, an MSE, and additional testing as indicated. While performing this evaluation, remain cognizant of potential "red flags" that may indicate a medical etiology for the patient's presentation including age greater than 40 without a psychiatric history, abnormal vital signs, recent memory loss, and clouded consciousness (15), among others (see Table 9.2). When working with the pediatric population, age less than 12 would also indicate a possible "red flag" (16), as psychiatric illness rarely presents before age 12. During this process, keep in mind possible medical conditions that can be deadly if misdiagnosed as a psychiatric illness (see Table 9.3).

HISTORY

A detailed history of the symptoms and timeline of events leading up to presentation is an essential component of any evaluation. If the patient is unable to communicate or guarded regarding details, information should be sought from collateral informants including family, friends, bystanders, paramedics, or peace officers, as well as prior inpatient and outpatient visits. Occasionally, the patient may need medications, such as an antipsychotic or an anxiolytic, prior to being able to participate in the assessment.

The history includes obtaining information regarding past psychiatric illness (including details regarding patient's past presentations during crisis), past and current medical conditions, past surgeries/trauma, and a review of systems. It is important to review current medications

TABLE 9.1 Common Medical Disorders that May Present With Acute Behavioral or Psychiatric Symptoms

Medication/Toxic Effects	Infections	CNS	Metabolic/ Endocrine	Cardiopulmonary	Miscellaneous
Alcohol and drug abuse Drugs of abuse • Cocaine • Marijuana • PCP • Amphetamines Prescription medications (common causes) • Digitalis • Tricyclic antidepressants • Steroids • Anticonvulsants	Pneumonia Urinary tract infection Sepsis Syphilis	Subdural hematoma Tumor Subarachnoid hemorrhage Hypertensive encephalopathy Meningitis Normal pressure hydrocephalus Seizure Complex migraine	Thyroid disease Adrenal disease Diabetic ketoacidosis Hypoglycemia Hepatic encephalopathy Electrolyte disturbances	Dysrhythmias Myocardial infarction Congestive heart failure COPD/asthma Hypoxia	Vasculitis Anemia Lupus Sarcoidosis

CNS, central nervous system; PCP, phencyclidine.

TABLE 9.2 Clues to Differentiation of Medical Versus Psychiatric Cause for Behavioral Symptoms[a]

	Medical	Psychiatric
Age	<12 or >40 y	12–40 y
Onset	Sudden	Gradual
Consciousness	Decreased	Normal
Hallucinations	Visual	Auditory
Course	Fluctuates	Continuous
Orientation	Disoriented	Scattered thoughts
Vital signs	Abnormal	Normal
Prior psychiatric history	No	Yes

[a]These are general clues and may not always differentiate. A full assessment is still needed to make the diagnosis.

including the use of over-the-counter medications and supplements (17). Review of substance use history including use of alcohol, illegal drugs, or misuse/abuse of prescription drugs is an important component keeping in mind that clinical intoxication may necessitate delay of the interview until the patient is able to effectively communicate. The history is also the time to identify any medical conditions or issues needing stabilization prior to disposition such as uncontrolled diabetes or problems resulting from self-injurious behavior (eg, laceration from cutting or a fracture from punching a wall). It is also important to recognize issues that may affect placement as not all psychiatric facilities may be able to accommodate the patient's needs (eg, need for nightly tube feeds, morbid obesity requiring a higher weight limit bed, need for a fall risk prevention).

TABLE 9.3 Potentially Fatal Medical Conditions That Can Present With Psychiatric Symptoms

Serotonin syndrome
Neuroleptic malignant syndrome (NMS)
Thyroid storm
Malignant catatonia
Anticholinergic poisoning
Hypoglycemia
Post ictal state
Medication overdoses (eg, tricyclic antidepressant, monoamine oxidase inhibitors).

PHYSICAL EXAMINATION

The PE provides another checkpoint in the evaluation to identify possible medical causes for the patient's presentation. Ideally, the patient needs an unclothed examination in a gown to allow for a full assessment although not all psychiatric crisis centers are set up to offer appropriate privacy for this type of examination. In these settings, providers should do the most thorough examination possible. Vital signs should be obtained on all patients although occasionally these may need to be delayed until the patient is cooperative. Abnormal vital signs need to be investigated further as they may indicate a "red flag" for an underlying medical condition and can be associated with many deadly conditions if missed (eg, neuroleptic malignant syndrome [NMS], serotonin syndrome, etc.).

A head-to-toe examination is the standard of care for proper evaluation. In cases of patient agitation, the PE may need to be delayed for patient and staff safety until the patient is better able to cooperate. The overall hygiene and appearance of the patient give clues to the patient's condition. Pulmonary, cardiac, abdominal, and neurologic examinations may point to need for further workup and testing if abnormalities are found. An examination of the patient's neck may indicate meningeal signs or thyroid disease. Loss of bowel/bladder or other focal neurologic signs may suggest the presence of concerning lesions requiring further imaging. Abnormal findings on PE would lead to further workup including indicated testing.

MENTAL STATUS EXAMINATION

For all providers, the MSE is an unwavering part of the psychiatric assessment. Most of this information is gathered as one is conducting other portions of the overall evaluation. When attempting to rule out medical etiologies of the patient's psychiatric presentation, it can be helpful to focus on the patient's level of consciousness, orientation, attention, concentration, and memory. It can be impractical to perform longer assessments in a crisis situation, but in select patients, it can be useful to use shorter assessment tools. The Montreal Cognitive Assessment or Mini-Mental Status Examination are both useful tools (18,19). Another shorter assessment tool is the Brief Mental Status Examination which consists of six questions and has been researched in the ED setting (20). If attempting to more formally assess the patient's cognition, it is important to use a formal assessment tool and not simply piecemeal portions of the different tests together as these pieces are not validated and cannot be used to follow the patient's progress over time needed in the future.

TESTING

The need for testing during the evaluation of psychiatric patients has evolved over time and often appears to be dependent on the culture of the locale and institutions involved. Disagreement often exists between ED medical providers and psychiatric providers as to how extensive testing should be. In efforts to bridge this gap, many groups and organizations have come together to form recommendations and consensus statements regarding testing needs. Additionally, many states in the United States have taken it upon themselves to create protocols in attempts to standardize this process in a way that is agreeable to both ED physicians and psychiatrists.

In 2014, the American College of Emergency Physicians (ACEP) released a consensus statement created by the ACEP Emergency Medicine Practice Committee regarding the care of psychiatric patients in the ED that further solidified their initial guidelines released in 2006 (21). Based on review of the literature and expert consensus, the committee made three recommendations on the medical clearance of patients in the ED. First, diagnostic testing should be directed by the history and PE and routine laboratory testing should not be performed on all patients. Second, routine urine toxicology screenings do not affect management in the ED, thus, if obtained only because they are required by receiving psychiatric facility, the screenings should not delay evaluation or transfer. Third, the timing of the assessment of patients intoxicated by alcohol should not be based on the specific alcohol level but instead on the patient's cognitive abilities.

In 2017, the American Association of Emergency Psychiatry (AAEP) released a two-part consensus statement created by a task force consisting of both emergency medicine physicians and psychiatrists regarding the medical evaluation of adult psychiatric patients (22,23). The task force made two conclusion statements regarding patients they deemed low and high risk. Low-risk patients are "young, present to the ED with an isolated psychiatric complaint, have a past history of psychiatric disease, are not using illicit substances, have normal vitals, and have a history and physical exam that does not suggest medical illness." High-risk patients may have the following: "older age, abnormal vitals and/or disorientation, no previous history of psychiatric disease, or a history and/or physical exam that suggests medical illness." Per the task force, the latter group of patients needs a thorough medical evaluation, whereas the former may have testing deferred.

PEDIATRIC POPULATION

Most recommendations regarding the issue of medical clearance have been made with a focus on the adult population; however, more recent studies in the pediatric population confirm that routine laboratory testing is largely unnecessary as it rarely changes disposition, increases cost, and increases length of stay in the ED (24–29). The American Academy of Pediatrics wrote a clinical report in 2016 in coordination with the ACEP in which the literature was reviewed and recommendations were made regarding the medical clearance of pediatric psychiatric patients (30). Overall, this report advocated for the thoughtful use of laboratory testing that is driven by the history and PE, not routine in nature, and in collaboration with the mental health provider when further testing is thought necessary.

Although the most controversial part of the medical evaluation is need for testing (ie, laboratory, imaging, etc.) as ED physicians and psychiatrists can often disagree regarding how comprehensive testing should be, the research to date as described above suggests testing is often unnecessary as well as costly. However, concern that something medical may be missed and a patient may be in a psychiatric facility without medical capabilities continues to drive many psychiatrists and psychiatric facilities to require testing beyond what is clinically indicated. It will take time to shift this perspective and encourage collaboration between psychiatrists and their medical colleagues. When psychiatric providers feel more testing is required in a given case, a discussion with the ED or PES provider about the patient's presentation and risk factors for medical issues is the best way to resolve the conflict.

DISPOSITION

The medical evaluation helps to determine if the patient is in need of inpatient medical admission, inpatient psychiatric admission, or discharge with outpatient follow-up (either medical, psychiatric, or both). Sometimes the patient's symptoms and their etiology are unclear, and inpatient medical hospitalization with psychiatric consultation may be necessary to further clarify the clinical picture. In such cases, the psychiatric consult team can help to determine if subsequent inpatient psychiatric hospitalization is necessary. The medical evaluation process also allows for the identification of medical conditions that may need treatment in a medical ED prior to transfer to an inpatient psychiatric hospital or discharge, those that may need concurrent treatment on an inpatient psychiatric unit or those simply needing outpatient medical follow-up. This is why the authors choose not to use the term medical clearance. Patients with psychiatric emergencies need evaluation and management of medical issues, not a statement they are clear for hospitalization.

When a patient is transferred to another facility, the Emergency Medical Treatment and Labor Act (EMTALA) requires that the patient is stabilized prior to transfer, that the patient's medical records are forwarded, and that there has been acceptance by a physician at the receiving facility (31). Patients need to be psychiatrically and medically stabilized within the capabilities of the transferring institution prior to transfer, and, to do this properly, a medical evaluation has to have taken place.

CONCLUSION

In a psychiatric emergency, the medical evaluation is an important component of the overall assessment in patients with a psychiatric presentation so as not to miss an underlying medical condition, which if missed could have serious or deadly consequences. It is also the time to identify other medical conditions that need treatment in an ED, need continued treatment while the patient is admitted to a psychiatric hospital and/or follow-up in the outpatient setting. The combined use of the history, PE, MSE, and testing (driven by the preceding components) will aid the provider in diagnosis and disposition decisions.

REFERENCES

1. Roca, R. P., Breakey, W. R., & Fisher, P. J. (1987). Medical care of psychiatric outpatients. *Hospital & Community Psychiatry, 38*, 741–745.
2. Hall, R. C., Popkin, M. K., Devaul, R. A., Faillace, L. A., & Stickney, S. K. (1978). Physical illness presenting as psychiatric disease. *Archives of General Psychiatry, 35*, 1315–1320.
3. Bunce, D. F., Jones, L. R., Badger, L. W., & Jones, S. E. (1982). Medical illness in psychiatric patients: Barriers to diagnosis and treatment. *Southern Medical Journal, 75*, 941–944.
4. Hall, R. C., Beresford, T. P., Gardner, E. R., & Popkin, M. K. (1982). The medical care of psychiatric patients. *Hospital & Community Psychiatry, 3*, 25–34.
5. Ferguson, B., & Dudleston, K. (1986). Detection of physical disorder in newly admitted psychiatric patients. *Acta Psychiatrica Scandinavica, 74*, 485–489.
6. Hall, R. C., Gardner, E. R., Stickney, S. K., LeCann, A. F., & Popkin, M. K. (1980). Physical illness manifesting as psychiatric disease. *Archives of General Psychiatry, 37*, 989–995.
7. Osborn, H. (1978). Medical clearance of the patient with psychiatric symptoms. *Archives of General Psychiatry, 35*, 357–371.
8. Koran, L., Sox, H. C., Marton, K. I., et al. (1989). Medical evaluation of psychiatric patients: Lawsuits in a state mental health system. *Archives of General Psychiatry, 46*, 733–740.
9. Koranyi, E. K. (1979). Morbidity and rate of undiagnosed physical illnesses in a psychiatric clinic population. *Archives of General Psychiatry, 36*, 414–419.
10. Hoffman, R. S. (1982). Diagnostic errors in the evaluation of behavioral disorders. *JAMA, 248*, 964–967.
11. Summers, W. K., Munoz, R. A., Read, M. R., & Marsh, G. M. (1981). The psychiatric physical examination – Part II: Finding in 75 unselected psychiatric patients. *The Journal of Clinical Psychiatry, 42*, 99–102.
12. Hall, R. C., Gardner, E. R., Popkin, M. K., Lecann, A. F., & Stickney, S. K. (1981). Unrecognized physical illness prompting psychiatric admission: A prospective study. *American Journal of Psychiatry, 138*, 629–635.
13. Beresford, T. P., Hall, R. C., Wilson, F. C., & Blow, F. B. (1985). Clinical laboratory data in psychiatric outpatients. *Psychosomatics, 26*, 731–741.
14. Williams, E. R., & Shepherd, S. M. (2000). Medical clearance of psychiatric patients. *Emergency Medicine Clinics of North America, 18*(2), 185–198.
15. Dubin, W. R., Weiss, K. J., & Zecccardi, J. A. (1983). Organic brain syndrome: The psychiatric impostor. *JAMA, 249*, 60–62.
16. Nwaobiora, C. J. (2017). The SMART medical clearance protocol as a standardize clearance protocol for psychiatric patients in the emergency department. *International Journal of Current Research, 9*(9), 57140–57147.
17. Medical Letter. (2002). Drugs that may cause psychiatric symptoms. *Medical Letter, 44*, 59–62.

18. Nasreddine, Z. S., Phillips, N. A., Bedirian, V., Charbonneau, S., Whitehead, V., Collin, I., ... Chertkow, H. (2005). The Montreal Cognitive Assessment, MoCA: A brief screening tool for mild cognitive impairment. *Journal of the American Geriatrics Society, 53*(4), 695–699.

19. Folstein, M. E., Folstein, S. E., & McHugh, P. R. (1975). "Mini-mental state": A practical method for grading the cognitive state of patients for the clinician. *Journal of Psychiatric Research, 12,* 189–198.

20. Kaufman, D. M., & Zun, L. S. (1995). A quantifiable, brief mental status exam for emergency patients. *American Journal of Emergency Medicine, 13*(4), 449–456.

21. ACEP Emergency Medicine Practice Committee. (2014). *Care of the psychiatric patient in the emergency department   A review of the literature.* American College of Emergency Physicians.

22. Anderson, E. L., Nordstrom, K., Wilson, M. P., et al. (2017). American Association for Emergency Psychiatry Task Force on medical clearance of adults. Part I: Introduction, review and evidence-based guidelines. *The Western Journal of Emergency Medicine, 18*(2), 235–242.

23. Wilson, M. P., Nordstrom, K., Anderson, E. L., et al. (2017). American Association for Emergency Psychiatry Task Force on medical clearance of adult psychiatric patients. Part II: Controversies over medical assessment, and consensus recommendations. *The Western Journal of Emergency Medicine, 18*(4), 640–646.

24. Shihabuddin, B. S., Hack, C. M., & Sivitz, A. B. (2013). Role of urine drug screening in the medical clearance of pediatric psychiatric patients: Is there one? *Pediatric Emergency Care, 29*(8), 903–906.

25. Donofrio, J. J., Santillanes, G., McCammack, B. D., et al. (2014). Clinical utility of screening laboratory tests in pediatric psychiatric patients presenting to the emergency department for medical clearance. *Annals of Emergency Medicine, 63*(6), 666–675.

26. Donofrio, J. J., et al. (2015). Most routine laboratory testing of pediatric psychiatric patients in the emergency department is not medically necessary. *Health Affairs, 34*(5), 812–818.

27. Conigliaro, A., et al. (2018). Protocolized laboratory screening for the medical clearance of psychiatric patients in the emergency department: A systematic review. *Academic Emergency Medicine, 25*(5), 566–576.

28. Riccoboni, S. T., & Darracq, M. A. (2018). Does the U stand for useless? The urine drug screen and emergency department psychiatric patients. *The Journal of Emergency Medicine, 54*(4), 500–506.

29. Santillanes, G., Donofrio, J. J., Lam, C. N., & Claudius, I. (2014). Is medical clearance necessary for pediatric psychiatric patients? *The Journal of Emergency Medicine, 46*(6), 800–807.

30. Chun, T. H., Mace, S. E., Katz, E. R., AAP FACEP. (2016). Evaluation and management of children and adolescents with acute mental health or behavioral problems. Part I: Common clinical challenges of patients with mental health and/or behavioral emergencies. *Pediatrics, 138*(3), e20161570.

31. Moy, M. M. (2000). *EMTALA and psychiatry in the EMTALA answer book* (2nd ed.). Gaithersburg, MD: Aspen.

10

Types of Initial Psychiatric Interviews in Emergency Settings

Jon S. Berlin

The difficulty and complexity of the initial psychiatric interview in the emergency setting can range considerably, from relatively straightforward and candid conversations to more complicated interactions with people determined to present an exaggerated or minimized picture of their condition to very challenging communications with individuals with grossly altered mental states. In all three groups, modification of the standard psychiatric interview is the rule: in the first group, selective abbreviation in the interest of time and efficiency is common practice in emergency departments (EDs) and psychiatric emergency services (PESs); in the second group, the evaluator must navigate a highly charged and high stakes disagreement with the patient; and in the third group, even a fragment of intelligible or meaningful dialogue is considered a success.

In the first edition of this textbook, my chapter on interviewing (also Chapter 11, this volume) emphasized assessment (1). Elements of engagement and treatment emerged but only as beneficial byproducts of an examination that succeeded in accessing underlying issues. As the title of the chapter suggested, "Interviewing for Acuity and the Acute Precipitant," the emphasis of the material was on elucidating the underlying crisis and crisis state of mind that led to the emergency visit, in order to accurately stratify the clinical acuity. This particular slant was due to my influence, not my coauthor's; I felt the emergency psychiatry audience at the time needed a reintroduction to the practical benefits of psychodynamic interviewing, and I thought the most compelling way to make the case would be to show its impact on the risk formulation. Since then, however, I have been increasingly impressed with the importance of having an engaging and therapeutic mindset that is integrated with the diagnostic mindset. As will be discussed, these are synergistic and intertwined, not separate.

In the present chapter, the focus shifts to the ways in which interviews might achieve both enhanced self-disclosure of material pertinent to risk *and* noticeable degrees of engagement and crisis reduction. The interview has a therapeutic component as well as an evaluative one. I consider how the therapeutic impact might become evident in the course of one initial interview, in a series of initial interviews during one episode of care, or in the course of multiple visits to an emergency service. Finally, I describe the case of a gentleman with severe and persistent alcoholism and suicidality who decided, one day, to transcend an extended phase of his life as an inveterate and virtually "uninterviewable" PES visitor.

This chapter summarizes, and in some cases extends, parts of this topic that I have explored elsewhere (1-5). It also presents ideas for interviewing the third, most difficult group of emergency patients. Unifying concepts throughout include engagement, resistance, safety, iterative process, interviews that unfold, treatment versus triage (6), motivational interviewing, and the turning of an acute patient into an outpatient. At the heart is an abiding impulse to connect with the part of the person that feels congruent, coherent, and authentic. Winnicott is among the first to articulate this as a goal of psychoanalysis (7), yet clinicians in the emergency setting can have an instinct for it, too.

SELECTIVE ABBREVIATION

The standard psychiatric interview includes a list of well-known categories: Identification, referral, chief complaint, history of present illness, past psychiatric history, substance abuse history, family psychiatric history, medical history, social history, developmental history, school and work history, military history, legal history, abuse and trauma history, mental status examination, patient strengths, differential diagnosis, assessment and formulation, prognosis, and treatment plan (8).

Given adequate time, a methodical emergency practitioner may choose to cover it all. If the patient is being admitted and the PES note will also be serving as the inpatient admit note, the practitioner will need to include much of it. However, busy working conditions usually require us to be much more selective, even when the patient is open to a full examination. One learns to say things like, "You know, this is a very important subject, and I'd like to hear about it, but given our limited time I think we'd better focus on…." When a patient has a known illness and is already receiving care, the PES visit is handled more as a follow-up visit or a consult, not as a workup for a new onset of illness. Most experienced practitioners focus the interview on what the patient wants, what he needs today, and why he is presenting now. The interview covers the chief complaint, history of present illness, acute precipitant, mental status examination, diagnosis, assessment, and plan. If treatment is provided, whether medication or therapy, we also note the response to intervention, which is in essence a brief reevaluation. The other categories of data are usually explored only if they are relevant to the reason for the current visit (9).

Consider a common example: a man comes into a PES asking for a fluphenazine injection, which he takes for his schizophrenia. For the most part, the real question is not his diagnosis or his general treatment, but why he is coming to this PES at this particular time asking for something he should be getting as part of his regular outpatient care. Is he late for his depot injection and feeling symptomatic and if so, how symptomatic? What is his risk assessment and does he need some additional oral fluphenazine or other acute care? Or is the gentleman avoiding his clinic for some reason? Have the staff there been using the injection appointments as an opportunity to talk to him about personal hygiene or drug use? These are the kinds of questions that help the story and the presentation fall into place.

MINIMIZING AND EXAGGERATING

When we talk about the second group of individuals, the ones that under- or overestimate the presence of a psychiatric emergency condition, we are referring mainly to three types of clinical situations: superficially composed people who minimize underlying suicidal or homicidal conditions; people with overt psychotic agitation and dangerousness to others but very little insight into their need for help; and individuals often well known to EDs who are exaggerating or feigning psychiatric symptoms in order to gain restricted medication or hospitalization.

Table 10.1 puts these interviews and the straightforward interviews in the first group into perspective. It is obviously oversimplified, but

TABLE 10.1 Emergency Interview Through The Lens of Acuity and Engagement

Emergency Interview	Needs PES	Does not Need PES
Wants PES	1 Doctor-patient agreement	4 Doctor-patient disagreement
Does not want PES	3 Doctor-patient disagreement	2 Doctor-patient agreement

Numbering of quadrants corresponds to the increasing degrees of difficulty of the interview.
PES, psychiatric emergency services.

it helps to orient trainees and other newcomers. The *x*-axis indicates whether or not the patient has an acute condition and *needs* PES. The *y*-axis indicates whether or not the patient *wants* PES.

In quadrants #1 and 2, the patients understand the severity of their condition and we have clinician-client agreement. For example, in quadrant 1, a person with a bipolar disorder who has become severely depressed might present to an ED with suicidal risk and a request for hospitalization. He both wants and needs care. Quadrant 2–type interviews usually occur when a patient with a nonacute condition has been pressured by someone to come in for acute care services. For example, parents want their adolescent son hospitalized for a handwashing compulsion because he keeps using up all the hot water. Family concern may be genuine but misguided. The interview with the patient is uncomplicated, while the real work involves assisting the family member(s) or others to see there is no need for emergency care and possibly collaborating more closely with an outpatient provider.

In quadrant #3, the patient does have an acute condition, either suicidality or dangerousness, but is typically on a mental health hold and arrives in the custody of law enforcement. He may be superficially composed or have psychotic agitation but in either case is refusing services. In quadrant #4, the patient is exaggerating or feigning symptoms of an acute condition in order to obtain emergency services. In both types of cases, the doctor and patient have a serious disagreement about the appropriate level of care. Patients with poor impulse control may turn aggressive, and staff without a good handle on their countertransference feelings may become cold or sarcastic. Trainees have been observed to become indecisive out of self-doubt, whereas experienced practitioners are prone to reach premature closure, opting for simple triage rather than real treatment.

This graphic can also be used to illustrate the theme of therapeutic movement within the interview. For example, when patients in quadrant 3 start to become engaged in treatment, they move into quadrant 1, and when they overcome their crisis, they move into quadrant 2. When patients in quadrant 4 engage in treatment, they move into quadrant 2. Conversely, when a case goes poorly,

for iatrogenic or other reasons, movement can go in the reverse direction.

Gudeman and I described actual cases of minimizing and exaggerating that had an optimal outcome in one interview (1). To review briefly, the interviewer often had a sense that the patient's presenting mental status examination was superficial and not representative of the reason for the visit. It did not feel entirely authentic or believable, and it was not congruent with the history or presentation. Typically, the history of present illness in particular felt incomplete and was missing an acute precipitant.

Our recommendation was to get below the surface to the underlying issues. However, the first step had to be to appreciate the patient's resistance to our investigation. We viewed the exploration as part of a normal examination but the patient experienced it as probing. Similarly, what we viewed as defensiveness, the patient experienced as necessary guardedness. From the analytic perspective, we explained how we had to appreciate that the patient might have all kinds of reasons, conscious and unconscious, not to trust us with intimate details of his inner life or a true picture of his acuity. He also might not trust his own ability to bring difficult thoughts and feelings into fuller awareness.

In less-difficult scenarios, the interviewer invites the individual to speak freely, and the person more or less welcomes the chance to share his troubles with a sympathetic listener. However, almost by definition, people who need to come to an emergency service involuntarily are individuals who do not welcome talking and who handle a crisis by resorting to very extreme types of coping: acting out behaviors, threatening statements, heavy drug use, breaks from reality, et cetera. Rationally talking out their problems is not something that comes naturally to them. Therefore, we cannot expect them to have an easy time with the interview when they sit down with us. In particular, experienced interviewers note the difficulty with obtaining a coherent history of present illness or mental status that feels real. Shea talks about the skill required to get in touch the patient's "nitty-gritty" state of mind (10).

From a dynamic standpoint, the symptomatic behavior that triggered the emergency visit, for example an overdose, may be a patient's archaic attempt to cope with the disturbing state of mind instigated by the acute precipitant, for example a romantic breakup. If the patient were capable of talking about it, and talking it out, he would have sought the counsel of a friend or therapist or confidante. He might still have a crisis to some degree, but not an emergency, which becomes life or death as he acts impulsively. In other words, the overdose is an attempt at self-cure of the real problem, which is an intolerable feeling state.

Even these individuals have a need to be understood but only if their defenses are treated with the utmost respect. Our trying to understand both sides of them helps tip the balance in favor of greater self-disclosure. Then, we can continue with attempting to reconstruct the history of present illness, searching out in particular the acute precipitant, or what is sometimes referred to as the "Why now?" question.

In the cases we described, unearthing the signal event led to a reconstruction of the original crisis state of mind, now relived in the interview. This might be called the preconscious mental status examination, which we find to be more congruent with the history. It also feels more authentic to us, and not incidentally, we also feel the beginnings of a genuine connection with the person we are speaking with, the birth of a doctor-patient relationship, as it changes from adversarial in nature to engaged, affective, and collaborative.

The collaboration means that the patient helps with both assessment and treatment. First, regarding risk assessment and risk stratification in particular, our task is simplified considerably. Rather than approaching the patient as an object of study (11), and having to rely solely on the actuarial guesswork of weighing risk factors against protective factors, the patient *tells us* how dangerous he really is, and it is believable, or at least it rings true. Moreover, the emerging realness and connectedness between the doctor and patient is itself an important protective factor (12). Incidentally, this approach was demonstrated with a patient who exaggerated her symptoms as well as with a patient who minimized his.

Second, from a treatment perspective, what we find with this type of interview is not only engagement but also some catharsis and crisis resolution. Patients start to feel better for having talked about the acute precipitant and painful emotions surrounding it. They begin to see how their symptomatic behavior, such as an overdose, was an understandable but desperate and maladaptive way of coping with a difficult situation. They see the need to have someone who can help them think and talk like this again. If medicine is indicated, they become more receptive to the idea. They become motivated to be in therapy, and the interview has supported the overarching goal of emergency care: to turn an acute patient into an outpatient (13). Again, a similar therapeutic outcome may be seen with persons initially exaggerating their risk.

Despite some good results, we are powerfully reminded of how unreliable in general self-reports of suicidal ideation are. In an excellent recent paper, Berman reported on 157 patients who died by suicide (14). Two-thirds of them denied having suicidal ideation when last asked within the last 30 days of their life and "one-half of these patients were dead by suicide within 2 days." However, experienced clinicians and instructors know that it takes years to learn how to ask about suicide with any finesse or evaluate the nuances of answers we receive. Berman's article is both a sobering reminder of the challenge of suicide assessment and a stimulus to keep working on interviewing skills.

VERBAL DE-ESCALATION AS AN INTERVIEW TECHNIQUE

In looking at the interviews of people in the emergency setting who minimize their condition, the other major group to consider is individuals with psychotic agitation who are refusing help. Typically, they are violent or threatening, and they are forcibly transported to an ED or PES on a mental health hold. Very often, too, these individuals are unknown to us, yet the standard psychiatric interview is usually so premature that descriptions in our literature of the right kind of initial verbal interaction have coalesced around the term "verbal de-escalation" (15). Yet it may be useful to conceptualize verbal de-escalation itself as a specialized kind of initial interview in its own right, where the emphasis is addressing the problem of the alliance and being helpful and gathering a very specific kind of information.

In the classic case of psychotic agitation, we encounter an individual who does not think his condition is serious, at least not consciously, or knows it is serious but is unwilling to acknowledge it or to engage with us. Traditional history-taking usually deteriorates rapidly—no matter how reasonable the questions might seem to us—and the evaluator ends up reverting first to coercive stabilization with restraint and medication, followed by medical screening, and then triage, which in most cases would mean psychiatric hospitalization. But a better understanding of de-escalation teaches us to shift gears quickly. The patient is overwhelmed; he is drowning. We should put our agenda on hold and move directly to questions he cares about: What can I do for you? What do you need? What do you want? What's wrong?

We fix our attention on the missing ingredient in this patient's presentation, which is rapport—rapport which will hopefully be followed by trust, openness, and a willingness to engage in a doctor-patient relationship. We must remind ourselves that management of psychotic agitation is much less difficult when the patient *is* requesting our help. Therefore, engagement, if possible, is key. This is the goal. Everything else is secondary.

The patient has an emergency condition, a dysphoric state of inner tension and behavioral dyscontrol, which is only made worse by the infringement of freedom. He says he does not want our help, but he clearly needs it. Therefore, we make the assumption that on some level, he probably does want it. If only he knew our ability and our good intentions. His distrust may be the product of paranoia or trauma or negative transference. But we do not let that cloud our focus: we see someone flailing and we reach out. Paranoid glares and accusations are to be met with constant reassurance that we have only one goal in mind: to be helpful.

This key element of verbal de-escalation, the focus on engagement, might be considered somewhat new. Yet in another respect, it is not new at all. Gill, Newman, and Redlich analyzed the initial psychiatric interview in the 1950s, both by reviewing the literature and studying audio recordings of initial assessments (16). They identified two different approaches to the interview that still persist to this day: one that focuses on gathering data and one that focuses first on forming an alliance and letting data flow secondary to that. They concluded that the latter approach was far superior. Of course, they were not looking at initial interviews in the ED or PES, yet if anything, their approach is even more applicable to an emergency setting.

In a de-escalation interview, the evaluator keeps a safe distance and obtains staff backup. He introduces himself and makes it clear that he has something to offer, that he wants to be useful. He makes every attempt to find out something the patient wants that makes sense in some way and that can be granted in some way. Even if the patient says something seemingly nonsensical, that he wants to be in outer space, for example, the interviewer might ask if he wants some private time and offer a quiet room or area away from the crowd.

Fishkind explicated this principle in 2002 (17). If the patient makes some overtly threatening statements or behaviors, the interviewer must of course set limits but, more importantly, wonders what the person is angry about. The evaluator might say "I didn't know we had a problem. Have I offended you in some way, or have any of us here offended you?" Or perhaps the patient is feeling threatened and needs us to emphasize safety. "Let me reassure you, Mr. Smith, all of us here are committed to nonviolence. We don't want anyone to get hurt. Not you or anyone else. We'll do whatever we can to solve this problem without getting physical." Or make the invitation explicit: "Work with us. We stretch ourselves to avoid resorting to violence. Let us help you do the same."

Most commonly, what the agitated person wants is to be left alone, released immediately from the confines of our establishment, expressed in the bluntest of terms. The interviewer aligns himself with the positive part of this: "Great. That's my job, to jumpstart the process of your getting out of here. It just has to be safe for you to go. Let's work on showing everyone that--that it's safe for you to go."

Note the motivational interviewing, the invitation to immediate behavioral change (18). We have identified what the person wants yet also the discrepancy and alluded to his looking stressed and dangerous. If the patient slams his fist into the desk and says, "I am safe to go!" we say, "Stop.

I can't use that." We might add, "What works for you when you're feeling like this?" If the patient challenges the interviewer and asks, "What d'you mean? Feeling like what!?" the interviewer can say, "I'm not sure what you'd call it. But it doesn't look like you're feeling good. What works for you when you're not feeling good like this?"

Often, patients with serious mental illness have avoided taking their medication and feel that others in their life nag them about it. By trying not to be the one to mention medication first and asking patients instead more generally what works for them, the interviewer tries to restore the patient's personal agency and can sometimes avoid a coercive intervention. Experienced patients may know that something else works better. Or they might request medication. Hostile patients have even been known to ask for an intramuscular injection when it was their idea and it was presented to them as a way to feel better more quickly. The patient with a new onset of illness may not know what he needs, but after acknowledging how poorly he feels may be open to the clinician's suggestions.

Some of the most challenging de-escalation cases we encounter are those when the only thing the individual wants is for us to leave him alone *now*. His paranoid view of us seems fixed, and he leaves no opening to find common ground or even to talk for a minute. In this fleeting moment, our only hope may be to point out the futility of rejecting us and the possible benefit of giving us a chance. For example, after being told by a patient to "get out of my face now," it may work to respond with, "That's what I'm trying to do, to get me, and people like me, out of your face. But if I go, someone else will come. Give me a try, why don't you? I really want to help get people like me out of your face for good."

Agitated patients may require involuntary measures. But even in these cases, the interviewer should resume his interviewing and engagement as soon as possible. This is sometimes referred to as debriefing. The interviewer may say: "I wish that had gone better. How are you doing?" and "What was that like for you?" Also, "Hopefully, you don't run into that degree of difficulty again, but if you do, any idea how we could all handle it better in the future?" Comments such as these demonstrate a continuing desire to work *with* the

individual, not on him. This is all part of the initial interview, and hopefully a de-escalating interview will go better the next time.

Once de-escalation is achieved, the interviewer is ready to conduct a second phase of the initial interview, which will be a second round of data gathering, data synthesis, and treatment planning. This will fill in many of the blanks of a standard psychiatric evaluation, to fine-tune the assessment and treatment plan. Naturally, obtaining collateral history from key informants and the medical record is also a key part of the data gathering. But engaging with the patient first and trying to establish a therapeutic alliance keeps him from feeling like we are only talking to others or going behind his back.

Verbal de-escalation is a specialized form of initial interview with evaluative and therapeutic components. It also highlights the value of initially focusing on rapport and engagement.

EXTREME MENTAL STATES

It is not uncommon to hear practitioners say that extremely psychotic or intoxicated individuals cannot be interviewed: that the mind is gone, buried alive under an impaired brain. But if we ask ourselves the question, "why is this person here, in this condition, at this particular time?" we must consider the possibility that it may be, on some level, intentional on the patient's part. Presenting to the emergency service represents the combination of two opposite needs, conscious or unconscious: the overt need to avoid any meaningful interaction with an evaluator, but also, by virtue of the fact of his being here with us today, an embryonic need to make some human contact. Of course, this is a psychodynamic formulation, and it is purely conjectural. Regardless, practitioners of different theoretical persuasions know empirically that these patients often can repeat verbatim what was said and done in the first interview, and it lays a foundation for subsequent interviews, of which some of these patients will have many. Therefore, the interviewer is well-advised to take the long view, understanding that whatever verbal and nonverbal interaction takes place between the two participants *is* the interview, namely, the *initial* interview (Case Examples 10.1 and 10.2).

CASE EXAMPLE 10.1

Ms. Z, a single, unemployed refugee from the Middle East was brought to see a psychiatrist at a walk-in clinic connected to a PES. Since losing her job as a chemical engineer in the United States a year earlier, she had become increasingly mute and begun staring bizarrely at her young nieces and nephews. She had no known history of mental illness or violence and did not possess weapons, but her family had understandably become very uncomfortable around her, even frightened. They took her to an ED, but she denied harmful ideation, declined hospitalization, and was released. Another time, the county crisis mobile team was summoned and went to her apartment, but she refused to let them in, and her case was put on hold. A community agency that worked with immigrants then became involved and assigned a therapist to work with her, who discovered that Ms. Z's goal was to leave America and return to her native country. Ms. Z was obviously psychotic but would not consider any kind of mental health evaluation and treatment. The case was at an impasse and no one knew how to proceed. The therapist eventually persuaded Ms. Z that seeing a psychiatrist was the first step to going home.

The psychiatrist's first impression of Ms. Z was in the waiting room: she was standing in the middle of the room almost immobile and hesitated a long time before coming into his office. She presented as a thin, hypervigilant woman in her mid-30s wearing black trousers, a navy-blue windbreaker, and dark sunglasses. Her head was shaved on both sides and had a shock of blue hair on top. Once seated, she mumbled, and only minimally, in a regional Arabic dialect. The therapist, who accompanied her in the interview, explained that Ms. Z, who spoke no English, refused to converse using a formal translation service but had agreed to talk by means of a bilingual ex-coworker in England who was standing by to be called long-distance. The interview was conducted via a cell phone speaker.

The psychiatrist told Ms. Z it was nice to meet her and thanked her for coming in. He explained that he was not connected to the immigration service and had no knowledge of what she needed to do to return to her native country, but perhaps he could help her to feel better and talk to the right people in immigration services more successfully. Her verbalizations were muffled and indistinct, as was the phone translation at times, but from her brief comments he learned that the Central Intelligence Agency (CIA) had changed the chemicals in her brain to control her thoughts. It was also doing something terrible to her neck and her back, making them hurt constantly. Ms. Z was focused on the somatic symptoms and reiterated her refusal to consider any kind of mental health evaluation or treatment. Her level of psychological distress seemed moderate, but her engagement with psychological help was virtually nonexistent. She never removed her sunglasses or looked in his direction, and she quickly ran out of things to say.

He sensed her impatience with the interview and felt the need to evaluate emergency psychiatric conditions before his time with her ran out. The ED had already ruled out emergency medical conditions. He said he could not think of a reason why the CIA would mistreat her, but knew it seemed very real to her, and he asked what it was like living with this feeling of persecution on a daily basis. He had to rephrase this question in a couple of different ways, but when she finally understood it she said it made her very angry. He asked if she ever wanted to do anything about it, and she said yes, but the CIA was all-powerful and faceless, and there was no one to confront. She reconfirmed the family's history that she had never been violent, and she said she did not plan on becoming so.

He then asked if she ever became discouraged or hopeless living a life like this. She suddenly turned very serious and still. With a little probing, he determined that she was depressed and had suicidal thoughts, but that her commitment to her family, especially her nieces and nephews, prevented her from acting on these thoughts. There was no history of suicidal behavior, and her self-report sounded believable. The psychiatrist said he thought she was dealing with a lot, and he was glad she had such good family support. He added that mental health treatment might also be very helpful, but perhaps she wanted to think about it. She said absolutely not, there was nothing to think about. The therapist added that Ms. Z had not agreed to counseling with her; she was only coming in for what amounted to case management.

CASE EXAMPLE 10.1 *(continued)*

At this point, Ms. Z stood up and left the room, ending the interview, and the psychiatrist and therapist discussed the case. They both had the feeling they had only scratched the surface, but all things considered, the visit might have been a positive step. It sounded like she was staring at the nieces and nephews with love and care, not animus. That was reassuring. He wanted to review the evaluation Ms. Z had in the ED and order any additional studies necessary to rule out medical causes of psychosis. Ms. Z might agree to them if they also helped to locate the source of her pain, or better yet, helped her to get some relief from her pain. Of course, the clinical history and presentation were more suggestive of a primary mental illness. The psychiatrist and the therapist discussed the differential diagnosis. Trauma needed to be considered. They also discussed Ms. Z's risks for harm to self and others. Both were clearly elevated, but not yet enough to meet the standard for commitment in the county where she was living. To get her more definitive evaluation and treatment, their only option was to continue trying to engage her or waiting till her level of risk increased. They would also support and educate the family, make sure that weapons, alcohol, and drugs were kept out of the picture, and be ready to call in reinforcements if the clinical picture deteriorated. The psychiatrist also realized he had not explored with Ms. Z her reasons for wishing to return home. Given her modern appearance, he had assumed it that made more sense for her to be living in a more modern society and that the wish was symptomatic of psychosis. But perhaps not. This was something for the therapist to ask about. For her part, she finally felt she had an ally and a coherent assessment and game plan.

This was a nearly impossible interview conducted under suboptimal conditions, though in emergency psychiatry it is all in a day's work. That it may have accomplished anything at all seemed to stem from two or three factors: a nascent wish on Ms. Z's part for a professional to know her psychiatric distress, the psychiatrist's attempt to think and feel his way into her experience, and the possible therapeutic effect of his having been a good listener and offering to help without being intrusive. Their having had an interaction that attained some emotional resonance was a sign that engagement might be achieved in time. The meeting was like an audition, with an equally uncertain outcome. In locales with more liberal commitment law, perhaps a mandated referral of someone like Ms. Z to a higher level of care, such as an Assertive Community Treatment program, could speed up the process. But it also goes without saying that, with cases like this, in today's practice environment, as hospitalization becomes less and less accessible, an initial interview that focuses on engagement and therapeutic action becomes increasingly important.

 ## CASE EXAMPLE 10.2

Mr. A was a middle-aged, homeless man who was repeatedly brought to a PES on a police mental health hold for being highly intoxicated and suicidal. He was always too drunk to be interviewed except to say that he drank to the point of blacking out and he had suicidal ideation. The routine disposition was a locked detoxification center, where he was always held for a few days, then released with follow-up, which he never had attended. He cycled over and over through the PES with the same diagnoses of alcohol dependence and depression, not otherwise specified. Initial interviews became brief and mechanical. On occasion, he was in the PES long enough to sober up, and one of the attending physicians or nurses would sometimes try talking to him, but he was not a conversationalist, and nothing ever came of it.

This went on for several years. However, one day, one of the psychiatrists sat down with him during rounds the morning after Mr. A came in,

CASE EXAMPLE 10.2 (continued)

while he was waiting for the transport service to take him to detox. As they met, the attending noticed a little more eye contact than usual, and he told Mr. A that he really ought to consider outpatient follow-up. He knew Mr. A did not want to go to Alcoholics Anonymous, but how about some counseling? To his surprise, Mr. A said, "Well, I'd see you." The attending did have a part-time practice and agreed to see him. To his greater surprise, Mr. A kept his appointment, and the next appointment, and the one after that. Almost overnight, Mr. A's drinking and visits to the PES stopped. The duration and frequency of their appointments quickly stabilized at 20 minutes every 2 weeks.

Mr. A was never comfortable meeting for longer sessions, but a standard psychiatric interview conducted over several weeks' time revealed a clinical depression, persistent suicidality, and a posttraumatic stress disorder with chronic nightmares. Pharmacologic treatment and supportive psychotherapy provided partial relief of the depressive and traumatic symptoms. There were still suicidal crises but never to the point of high risk. Mr. A had his psychiatrist's telephone number but never called it. He never became a talkative person and never felt comfortable elaborating on his painful past history, including any specifics of his past traumas, but for years never missed a session or returned to PES.

Like with severe psychosis, a case of extreme intoxication that presents in a PES or ED can be viewed, among other things, as an instance of extreme psychological guarding combined with an underlying wish to connect. It was far from obvious at the time, but with hindsight Mr. A might have been using alcohol partly to self-medicate his trauma and depression and his fear of engagement. Nor was it likely that Mr. A's various evaluators were consciously aware that he was responding to, or remembering, how they treated him. But they must have treated him with enough respect collectively that, even in his multiple drunken states, he developed a positive attachment to their PES. At a minimum, staff must have processed their countertransference feelings of hopelessness sufficiently to help Mr. A with his. We also have to wonder if the therapeutic strand of his serial initial interviews had a cumulative effect of building trust and motivation over a period of years. The suddenness of Mr. A's engagement in treatment was unexpected. Yet it is not unusual for patients to hide their progress until they are reassured that a therapist will continue working with them in their improved, but not fully improved, state.

ITERATIVE PROCESS

Conceptually, the clinical discipline of psychiatry is a repeating process of gathering data, interpreting and synthesizing the data, and intervening.

The three elements are systematic and sequential, but they are also integrated and simultaneous. In an emergency, practitioners must spring into action (19), followed by more definitive diagnosis and treatment. In less-urgent cases, triage is followed by treatment. In emergency psychiatry, practitioners are doing more of the second rounds of diagnosis and treatment themselves, rather than referring patients to an inpatient setting. We have also reviewed an example of how repeated rounds of seemingly superficial triage might add up to something more substantive, apparently because of, at least in part, an occult therapeutic thread in the patient's experience of his PES visits.

As with engagement in the initial interview, treatment from the start is not a new idea either. Gabbard (20) presents a succinct history of the hypothesis that, in the psychodynamic interview, "any distinction between diagnosis and treatment would be artificial." He articulates the therapeutic effect of active listening and "validating that the patient's life has meaning and value." He quotes Menninger that, "In a sense, treatment always precedes diagnosis" (21). Although this may be a novel concept for some, it suggests an approach to the initial interview that can produce greater trust, greater self-revelation, better risk assessment, and more meaningful clinical engagement and crisis resolution.

CONCLUSION

The drama of the initial emergency encounter and assessment—sometimes successful, sometimes Sisyphean—remains our most basic competency. Whether an emergency patient is seen once or dozens of times, the interview is our only opportunity to engage the real self. Setting the bar so high may seem mystifying or idealistic, yet its worth is borne out by initial interviews that are by turns focused, restrained, therapeutic, and searching, as well as by an approach to recovery that takes the long view and attempts to coordinate crisis work with the work that the patient is, or some day will be, doing in other settings, such as inpatient and outpatient.

REFERENCES

1. Berlin, J. S., & Gudeman, J. (2008). Interviewing for acuity and the acute precipitant. In Glick, R. L., Berlin, J. S., Fishkind, A. B., & Zeller, S. L. (Eds.), *Emergency psychiatry: Principles & practice* (1st ed.). Philadelphia, PA: Lippincott Williams & Wilkins.
2. Berlin, J. S. (2013). Advanced interviewing techniques for psychiatric patients in the emergency department. In Zun, L. S., Chepenik, L. G., & Mallory, M. N. S. (Eds.), *Behavioral emergencies for the emergency physician* (1st ed.). Cambridge: Cambridge University Press.
3. Berlin, J. S. (in press) The modern emergency psychiatry interview. In L. S. Zun, et al, (Eds.), *Behavioral emergencies for the emergency physician* (2nd ed.). Cambridge: Cambridge University Press.
4. Berlin, J. S. (2017). Collaborative de-escalation, In Zeller, S. L., Nordstrom, K. D., Wilson, M. P. (Eds.), *The diagnosis and management of agitation*. Cambridge: Cambridge University Press.
5. Berlin, J. S. (2007). The Joker and the Thief: Persistent Malingering as a Specific Type of Therapeutic Impasse. Psychiatric Issues in Emergency Care Settings. *Cliggott Publishing Group*. 6(2). Retrieved from http://www.psychiatrictimes.com/joker-and-thief-persistent-malingering-specific-type-therapeutic-impasse. Accessed September 15, 2018.
6. Allen, M. H. (1996). Definitive treatment in the psychiatric emergency service. *Psychiatric Quarterly, 67*, 247–262.
7. Winnicott, D. W. (1976). The aims of psychoanalytic treatment (1962). In *The maturational processes and the facilitating environment*. London: Hogarth.
8. Waldinger, R. J. (1990). The clinical interview: Fundamentals of technique. In *Psychiatry for medical students* (2nd ed.). Washington, DC: American Psychiatric Press, Inc.
9. Riba, M. B., & Ravindranath, D. (2010). *Clinical manual of emergency psychiatry* (pp. 12–15). Arlington, VA: American Psychiatric Press, Inc.
10. Shea, S. C. (1999). *The practical art of suicide assessment*. New York: John Wiley & Sons.
11. MacKinnon, R. A., & Michels, R. (1971). *The psychiatric interview in clinical practice* (pp. 6–7). Philadelphia: W. B. Saunders Co.
12. Benglesdorf, H., Levy, L. E., Emerson, R. L., & Barile, F. A. (1984). A crisis triage rating scale. Brief dispositional assessment of patients at risk for hospitalization. *Journal of Nervous and Mental Disease, 172*(7), 424–430.
13. Sederer, L. I. (1991). *Inpatient psychiatry: Diagnosis and treatment* (3rd Sub ed.). Baltimore: Lippincott Williams & Wilkins.
14. Berman, A. L. (2018). Risk factors proximate to suicide and suicide assessment in the context of denied suicidal ideation. *Suicide and Life-Threatening Behavior, 48*(3), 340–352.
15. Richmond, J. S., Berlin, J. S., Fishkind, A. B., et al. (February 2012). Verbal de-escalation of the agitated patient: Consensus statement of the American association for emergency psychiatry project BETA workgroup. *The Western Journal of Emergency Medicine, XIII*(1), 17–25.
16. Gill, M., Newman, R., & Redlich, F. (1954). *The initial interview in psychiatric practice*. New York: International Universities Press, Inc.
17. Fishkind, A. B. (2002). Calming agitation with words, not drugs: 10 commandments for safety. *Current Psychiatry, 1*(4), 32–39.
18. Miller, W. R., & Rollnick, S. (2013) *Motivational interviewing: Helping people change* (3rd ed.). New York: Guilford Press.
19. Petit, J. R. (2004). *Handbook of emergency psychiatry* (p. 1). Philadelphia: Lippincott Williams & Wilkins.
20. Gabbard, G. O. (2005). *Psychodynamic psychiatry in clinical practice* (4th ed., pp. 70–71). Washington, DC: American Psychiatric Publishing, Inc.
21. Menninger, K. A., Mayman, M., & Pruyser, P. W. (1962). *A manual for psychiatric case study* (2nd ed.). New York: Grune & Stratton.

11

Interviewing for Acuity and the Acute Precipitant

Jon S. Berlin, Jon E. Gudeman

Significant strides have been made in recent years in the assessment of psychiatric acuity, particularly with respect to appreciating the role that empirically validated risk factors play in determining an individual's potential for harming self or others (1). However, as the importance of compiling and weighing the various conditions, characteristics, and behaviors that increase the likelihood of a bad outcome has increased, the place of the clinical assessment in determining acuity has become an enigma: Studies have not demonstrated its independent value for estimating degrees of dangerousness, yet no one is willing to dispense with it.

Undoubtedly, this unwillingness stems partly from the multitude of other diagnostic and therapeutic purposes that a clinical assessment interview serves and partly from the understanding that the concept of acuity includes incapacity and subjective distress and is a much broader domain than that of risk alone. However, in our view, another reason is the awareness that the clinical dialogue, conducted skillfully, does seem to produce reliable subjective and objective findings to use in the assessment of acuity and risk. We, along with many others, believe that the science and art of clinical interviewing are worth preserving and may be essential (2-4).

This chapter discusses the role of the initial interview in assessing acuity in the emergency setting. The guiding principle is the value of drawing out the patient to elucidate the underlying acute precipitant for the current visit, sometimes referred to as asking the "Why now and how come?" questions (5). Using multiple case vignettes, we illustrate how, if one appreciates the protective roles of resistance and defense, a sensitive probing interview produces a clearer chief complaint, more valid mental status findings, more pertinent history of the present illness,

and ultimately a more accurate diagnostic formulation and treatment plan. In helping to estimate acuity, a good interview therefore holds the promise of reducing false positives (ie, unnecessary admissions) and false negatives (inappropriate discharges). This approach to interviewing may help mitigate the adversarial aspect of some patient-clinician interactions that are endemic in the emergency setting, thereby increasing patient satisfaction and adherence. It may also set the stage for crisis resolution (6), thereby potentially reducing both risk and return visits to the emergency service for a problem that was not adequately addressed the first time.

When the presenting acuity is obvious and vivid, as it is, for example, with cases of psychotic agitation, rage, mania, intense despair, or acute catatonia, actively pursuing the acute precipitant should be deferred until emergency measures have been implemented. Later, however, clinical assessment helps to ascertain the underlying nature of the problem, to engage the patient, and thus to resolve the problem more rapidly at the most therapeutic level of care (7). This can sometimes mean handling the problem in the crisis situation instead of utilizing scarce hospital resources.

Acute presentations demonstrate the importance of preliminary stabilization and securing the foundation or "frame" before attempting to delve into the underlying problem. We address the important contraindications of an uncovering approach, as in acute traumatic stress conditions. In all cases, regardless of presenting acuity, the importance of appreciating the type and current state of an individual's defense mechanisms remains unaltered.

Our discussion also assumes that the individual has been carefully assessed medically for delirium, dementia, substance-induced disorders, mental disorders secondary to medical conditions (organic disorders), and emergency medical conditions in general. To the extent possible, these states must be ruled out or stabilized before undertaking the type of examination described.

ACUITY AND CHIEF COMPLAINT

The emergency practitioner places emphasis on two tasks: (a) determining and managing acuity, and (b) determining and addressing the real chief complaint. Both are integral to good practice. One can be wrong, for example, about whether an individual being discharged from a psychiatric emergency service (PES) has a bipolar manic psychosis versus a schizoaffective disorder–bipolar type, but one really does not want to be wrong about his or her suicide risk or appropriateness for outpatient follow-up. We also do not want to misunderstand the patient's view of the problem and his or her specific treatment request.

We concur with Allen's articulation (8) of the difference between the *triage model* and the *treatment model* in emergency psychiatric practice and his advocacy for a treatment model based on more concerted efforts to definitively diagnose and treat psychopathology. The number of patients in the community with incompletely characterized, "not otherwise specified" diagnoses receiving nonspecific treatment is a real concern. Unfortunately, ever-increasing volume surges are forcing the triage model in many emergency centers to become the default mode, leaving the nuances of psychopathologic axes I and II diagnosis to other settings. But nuances of acuity cannot be ignored. In *DSM-IV* terms, it might be said that the approach we are describing is the focus of our attention on not only axis I but also on the defenses of axis II (9), the acute precipitants of axis IV, and the acuity of axis V.

TIME

The time element in an emergency setting is crucial. Working conditions sometimes require clinicians to see two to three patients per hour. Does an interview focused on the acute precipitant take too long? In our experience, it either shortens the interview or the overall time that the person spends in the emergency department (ED) or PES. Sometimes this more in-depth approach does lead to a longer stay in the crisis service but less time in the hospital. Of course, sometimes one barely has enough time to identify medical emergencies, keep everyone safe, and rapidly triage to a variety of settings. But if the patient goes to the observation area of the PES or ED, or if no beds are available and the patient ends up remaining in the waiting room, one may pursue the acute precipitant at a slightly later time but still prior to a final disposition.

Time is also crucial in relation to how long a patient waits to be seen. People seeking mental health services want relief of suffering. The sooner they are seen, the more willing and able they are to open up. After a certain point, they start to wonder if their concerns are of any interest or importance to the ED staff, and they start to shut down or act up.

REVIEW OF THE LITERATURE

The tasks of any initial psychiatric interview include a sequence of establishing rapport, inquiring how the person sees his or her problem, gathering subjective and objective data, collating these data with information from other sources, formulating a biopsychosocial assessment, and collaborating on a biopsychosocial treatment plan. The main adaptations of this schema described in the emergency literature are triage and the necessity at times to act decisively with incomplete information (3,5,10-12). The clinician evaluates and treats simultaneously. Although this idea is not new or limited to emergencies (2,13-15), its usefulness in this situation is unmistakable. For example, faced with an acutely agitated, unknown patient without identification who is brought in by police, the emergency clinician quickly works through the above sequence of interview tasks not once, but in repetitive cycles, each time with greater precision and depth.

In their chapter "The Emergency Patient," MacKinnon, Michels, and Buckley (3) identify overwhelming anxiety and urgency as a predominant feature. They emphasize both the importance of authoritativeness and self-assuredness on the clinician's part and of helping to instill or restore a personal sense of initiative and effectiveness on the patient's part. Interestingly, these are both important techniques in the intervention currently referred to as psychological first aid (16).

The ultimate goal with any patient is to have a real conversation. In classic chapters on validity techniques and on eliciting suicidal ideation, Shea (4) stresses the importance of the depressed patient inviting the clinician "into the nitty-gritty details" of his or her inner world. Shea explicates how histories and mental status examinations become increasingly valid with improving interview technique. He also recognizes the need for interviews to be time-efficient.

In a related vein, Gabbard (2) highlights the need to go beyond the descriptive diagnoses of axes I and II and to consider the psychodynamic importance of the precipitants on axis IV. He also talks about axis V as a summation of a person's level of functioning, although from an emergency perspective the acuity component of axis V has more immediate relevance. Gabbard and Shea both stress the importance of understanding one's own feelings that are activated in the assessment process, not only to keep them from interfering but also to use them as potentially useful clues about the patient.

Psychoanalysts, including Langs (17) and Gill (18), have demonstrated that a contemporary psychodynamic approach—far from being passive, slow, or focused on the deep unconscious—capitalizes on the preconscious derivatives of a person's relevant underlying issues that have made their way in decipherable form into the here-and-now interaction. Langs (19) also emphasizes doing what one can to establish an appropriate "frame" for the clinical interview, including those undertaken in the ED. He recommends establishing as much privacy and confidentiality as is practical and safe. He points out the negative effects that seeking out unnecessary collateral history can have on the alliance.

In a 1995 critical appraisal of axis IV, Forman et al. (20) sum up its clinical utility as "at once self-evident and uncertain." They allude to "the significant literature on the effects of stressful life events in psychiatric and general medical conditions," and they cite the major emphasis of the brief, focused therapies on current problems. On the other hand, they acknowledge that the underlying biology of a mental illness appears to be the dominant etiologic factor at times, and for acute episodes of these conditions, caution the clinician not to give psychosocial factors "a false, preeminent position."

PSYCHODYNAMIC PERSPECTIVE

Psychiatric crises and clinical presentations may be viewed as an amalgam of an acute precipitant; a preexisting biologic, psychological, or interpersonal vulnerability; an unbearable, painful mental state; and a maladaptive response of conduct, thinking, and/or subjective distress. These four elements make up a *precipitant complex*. Descriptively speaking, the maladaptive response (eg, a suicide threat) is viewed as the presenting problem, whereas in reality the suicide threat is really the individual's own misguided attempt to cope with a painful mental state. This state is the result of an acute precipitant that has set off or stimulated a preexisting diathesis.

The individual has a hard time talking about, or even being aware of, the acute precipitant, out of fear that the painful affect connected with it will be intolerable, forcing the clinician to pick up various clues. Quite frequently, there is an associated fear that a helping professional will not understand or react appropriately. Under more normal circumstances, a person who has experienced a painful event, such as a loss or failure, will be able to process it in his or her own way or be able to talk about it with friends, family, or a trusted confidant of some type. When in need, this person is more likely to be seen in an outpatient setting, if at all. Conversely, people who end up needing emergency services often lack the necessary internal and external resources to cope on their own.

Resistance and Defense Mechanisms

From this perspective, a clinician attempting to get at the acute precipitant should expect to be met with some degree of resistance (2,3), for he or she is asking the individual to abandon his or her usual coping skills of guardedness, denial, minimization, repression, and so on. The clinician will encounter individuals who may expect him or her to be unsympathetic, self-serving, incompetent, or disinterested (21,22). The interviewer must counter these expectations with genuine interest and expertise: the desire to help, the ability to listen, knowledge, and professional self-confidence. His or her handling of patients' defenses against the attempt to get to know them is key: The evaluator must understand that the presenting problem is the person's attempt at self-cure and must respect his or her difficulty talking about the issues underlying it. The clinician must also remain determined and not give up prematurely. He or she should expect that the same defensive maneuvers and coping skills that lie behind the presenting problem will pervade the person's interaction with the evaluator. It will come as no surprise, for example, when a woman minimizing and rationalizing a suicide attempt says she really will become suicidal if the evaluator decides not to discharge her home and instead says she requires hospitalization.

Patients seen in emergency settings often use primary defense mechanisms to protect themselves. These are denial, distortion, projection, avoidance, acting up (sometimes referred to as "acting out"), and minimization. All of them can be used by both neurotic and psychotic patients, but in psychosis they are used more tenaciously and with a loss of reality testing (23). Denial is an active process of refusing to acknowledge reality. It is a conscious or unconscious warding off of pain. With distortion, the ego fools itself into believing its self-flattering ideas to gratify unobtainable wishes. This defense also serves the purpose of keeping people at a distance. Projection transfers blame to outside people or things: "It is not I who controls the situation; it is others who are controlling me." Avoidance is the act of looking elsewhere and getting away from where it hurts.

In borderline conditions, somewhat higher-level defenses such as splitting, projective identification, identification with the aggressor, and acting up are often seen. As with neurotic defenses, there is no loss of contact with reality, although there may be significant difficulties imagining, or "mentalizing," what the evaluator is realistically thinking and feeling. One should also look for brief periods of lost reality testing in borderline individuals, lasting minutes to hours. People who act up when they are stressed are

particularly likely to behave in ways that result in referral to PESs. They use actions instead of words to handle their problems and have an especially hard time discussing them at all. Neurotic defenses are, among other things, an attempt to gain support. By and large, individuals use reaction formation, rationalization, doing and undoing, and intellectualization in obsessive-compulsive personality conditions. In hysterical conditions, repression, dissociation, and depersonalization are seen.

Simultaneous with an appreciation for the different anxieties and fears these various defenses keep at bay, the clinician must be on the lookout for the area of greatest psychological tenderness. He or she is well served to operate on the assumption that what may be most diagnostic and therapeutic for patients is to help them to acknowledge their painful feelings, to bear them, and to put them into some kind of perspective (24).

We begin our discussion of diagnosing acuity with three cases in which the clinician's idea and the patient's idea of acuity are not in accordance with one another, as when the patient appears to be minimizing or exaggerating his or her clinical distress.

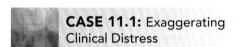

CASE 11.1: Exaggerating Clinical Distress

Ms. A, a 42-year-old woman, presents to a PES one evening complaining of hearing voices telling her to kill herself. She had scratched her arm and called the police. In the interview, she says her depression and suicidality increased out of frustration that her psychiatrist in her intensive community support program has variously referred to her condition as bipolar, schizoaffective, and borderline. She asserts that hospitalization is necessary now to ensure her safety and clear up nagging questions about her diagnosis.

Ms. A does not look hopeless or suicidal. In fact, her presentation is quite similar to all the other documented times she has gone to the PES recently, which could be described as mildly to moderately discontented. The evaluator determines that she has been frustrated with her psychiatrist about her diagnosis for 2 years and that she last saw him 10 days ago. Next, he inquires about how her daily life is going and how her day went today. Ms. A becomes irritated and resists this line of questioning. He asks if she is angry with him for not immediately acceding to her request for hospitalization. She says, "Yes, you have to admit me. I'm on a hold. I'm suicidal." The psychiatrist says he knows she has a serious psychiatric illness and that ongoing suicide risk is an important aspect of it, but he wants to understand her current situation better. She replies, "You're not listening to me. No one ever listens to me. . . . No one cares. . . . I don't know why you should be different than anyone else in my life. I wish I was dead." She gazes at the scratches on her arm.

Pursuing this affect, the psychiatrist says it sounds like not being listened to really bothers her and asks if anyone else had not listened to her today. Ms. A looks down for several moments and stops talking, and then, giving up her defense of denial, relates that one of the 800-number crisis lines she calls across the country every day had told her she had already used up her five calls for the day and hung up on her. She explains she keeps careful track of her calls and was certain that that one was her fifth. Recalling the experience of being rejected and disbelieved makes her tearful. She goes on to talk about her loneliness in life and her lack of friends. As the clinician pays close attention to her hurt feelings, her mood brightens. She then starts to talk about the many abuses she had experienced in her life. He handles this by acknowledging that there are a great many things she has yet to work through, but that she had worked on some important issues tonight.

Ms. A smiles and says she feels she could go home now. Her suicidal urges had not entirely disappeared, but they had subsided. He agrees. As they stand up, she says she hoped to get a job working in this PES as a peer support specialist next year. The psychiatrist remarks that working hard in therapy does help people become good therapists. He also asks for her permission to relay some information about this visit to her psychiatrist. Total time spent on case: 15 minutes.

Precipitant Complex

In attempting to delineate the components of the precipitant complex, the interviewer was met with a variety of defensive maneuvers that nonetheless allowed him to fill in a number of blanks about the patient. One should gather this information while at the same time recognize its defensive function. With Ms. A, a detailed discussion of the diagnoses in axis I and II would have been a diversion. The goal for the evaluator was not to be thrown off course but to continue the search for the real reason for her visit. Despite her playing up her stated symptoms, he uncovered actual painful feelings and the precipitating event associated with her real chief complaint, which had to do with loneliness and rejection, feelings that seemed too painful to acknowledge or bear. He also judged it might have been too reinforcing of the victim role to dwell on the childhood or historical antecedents of her vulnerability, as well as undermining of her efforts to become independent and to recognize her own tendency to put upon others.

Preconscious Mental Status

In the course of this evaluation, the mental status examination became more congruent and more reliable. By focusing on the recent events and getting the person to tell her story, there was an increase in believable affect, a decrease in reported suicidal ideation, and a decrease in apparent symptom embellishment for secondary gain. This may be conceptualized as a deepening of the mental status by bringing some of the preconscious mental contents into the conscious mind. Parenthetically, in a brief interview, a patient may demonstrate good reality testing, orientation, intact memory, and most of the categories associated with a formal mental status. In general, the mental status regarding suicidality, although important in suicide assessment, is widely regarded as quite unreliable. This interview approach appears to increase its validity and value.

Crisis Resolution

Identifying the acute precipitant in this case allowed an opportunity to begin addressing the crisis. As it turned out, it was something that could be handled in the assessment interview. Ms. A's ability to talk it through was indicative of previous work in therapy, and talking it through that night was another little piece of treatment. As is often true in cases such as these, her fears of being unable to handle feelings were unjustified.

Therapeutic Alliance

Another common feature of this type of interview is the transformation of the clinician-patient relationship. Initially, the evaluator warily perceives Ms. A to be trying to obtain a hospitalization that would risk only promoting her dependency, and she perceives him as someone she must convince of her need for hospitalization, in order to get what she has decided on her own that she needs and suspects will not be forthcoming. She probably felt at risk for feeling humiliated if the full extent of her clinging dependency was made known. But by the end of the interview, the clinician has brought forth her more positive attributes and been useful to her. For her part, she feels a bit more understood and somewhat accepted—at least enough to assuage the hurt from earlier in the day—and this adds a thread of strength to the therapeutic alliance.

This woman has also once again briefly made the connection between her long-standing sensitivity to rejection from early experiences (real or imagined) and current events. The interviewer recognized her sensitivity and chose to keep the discussion in the here and now. However, Ms. A has seen that talking helps and that some people can be trusted to be interested in her plight. She has gone from being an emergency patient to being someone appropriate for ambulatory follow-up. This will not be her last visit to the crisis service, but she has been steered in the direction of using it more appropriately. Her idea of working in the crisis service in a year's time is probably unrealistic, yet the idea of doing it at all helps give her some purpose in life and indicates a positive identification with the evaluator.

Exaggeration of the Chief Complaint and Acute Precipitant

Ms. A's dependence on crisis services is a frequently seen type of problem. It is common anywhere that deinstitutionalization has not been coupled with adequate development of non–hospital-based services such as housing, day programming, socialization, work programs, and case coordination. It is also common in persons with character pathology who routinely draw people into playing out victim-victimizer types of scripts.

Elements of malingering are a common comorbidity with psychiatric illness in the crisis population (25). One key to its assessment and management is to follow the agenda of searching out the acute precipitant. One must assume that one does exist. There must be reasons why a person comes one day and not another. The precipitant may not be serious enough to explain the stated complaint, but it may still be an issue with which the person is having some trouble. Identifying it and working with it will help the story and the clinical picture to come into better accordance.

Risk Management

Finally, the evaluator does not ask Ms. A to "contract for safety" at the end of the interview. They do not have a long-standing treatment relationship wherein such a commitment to him would actually mean something. But this type of interview does give one much to document on the rationale for discharge: that there is a history of overstated suicide threats, that the severity of the acute precipitant is not great, that as she became more open and honest her mental status findings became more congruent and reliable, that there was some resolution of the immediate crisis, that the good response to the interview suggested that outpatient therapy was a viable option, and that in hoping to work in the PES one day, Ms. A indicated she was looking to the future.

CASE 11.2: Minimization of Chief Complaint and Denial of Acute Precipitant

In contrast to the preceding scenario, another common emergency presentation is when a patient is seen following a suicide attempt and says that he or she is "fine." Either a cursory search for an acute precipitant is noncontributory or evaluators do not even undertake it because superficially the patient does seem fine to them and they can document many different reasons why the person is not high risk. Despite a clear impression of minimization in the interview, one sees so many of these cases that one can become inured to them and sign off on them without thinking. The rate of successful suicide is low, even in populations with an elevated risk, so statistically most of the discharges will survive (26). But the danger and liability of a false negative do exist, and they at least warrant an attempt to search out any hidden acuity.

Mr. D is a 45-year-old accountant who had an emergency consultation after spending the night in a general hospital for treatment of an overdose of 20 Tylenol taken while intoxicated. He was on a police mental health hold but felt much better later and was ready to go. He presented as sober, nondepressed, and politely pleading to be released. An admitted recovering alcoholic, he said his drinking the day before was a one-day relapse. There was no reason for the overdose other than that he was drinking, and he was committed to sobriety again. He had a job and a family to get home to. He also had an outpatient psychiatrist, who was contacted and confirmed the history that Mr. D had not been under any new stresses lately, that he was being treated for major depression, and that he had not attempted suicide for several years. The psychiatrist was comfortable seeing him for follow-up in the office.

The evaluator, a female psychiatry resident, gleaned this information from the chart in a few minutes. She started her interview asking Mr. D for more information about his life situation. He admitted he did not like his marriage or his job that well. He complained that all that his psychiatrist ever wanted to talk about were medications. He had thoughts of making many changes in his life but had not done anything about it yet. Things were going along okay and he had them under control. The resident asked him about the circumstances surrounding his overdose. His wife and children were away visiting her mother. He was glad to have the day to himself. He had simply made the mistake of taking a drink, and then could not stop. The next

thing he knew it was afternoon, and he had overdosed and was calling for an ambulance. It was all just a strange aberration, and he was fine. He acknowledged he did not attempt suicide every time he drank too much, but nothing had triggered the event in particular.

The resident asked Dr. D to take her through that day, starting with when he awoke. He proceeded to describe the events up until early afternoon, then faltered and had trouble continuing. The expression on his face changed. She gently persisted. Speaking more haltingly, he said he had called his AA sponsor to tell her about his relapse. He also told her about his being free for the day. He asked her to rekindle the romance and sexual relationship they had had 1 year ago. She said no. He pleaded with her. She rebuked him. He said he was starting to feel suicidal and accused her of being unfeeling and selfish. She suddenly turned on him then, saying she never had romantic feelings for him and never wished to see him again. It was at this point that he turned upon himself and overdosed. He had called for help right away, but for a moment he really wanted to die.

As Mr. D related this part of the story, his eyes moistened. This woman had been his best friend over the past year—actually, his only friend. She was the bright spot in his life. His sobriety had been tied up with his strong attraction and fantasies about her. He turned to the psychiatry resident and said he did not know what to do. He did not know if he could handle going home yet or not. What did she think? He also asked if he could see her for therapy. A bit surprised, she said that these were really good questions. They needed to think about them. She would also be staffing the case with his attending psychiatrist.

She asked Mr. D what his thoughts were about his problems and his treatment. He told her about his disillusionment with AA, the difficulty he had had finding a sponsor, and his beginning awareness of what good therapy really was. Eventually, when it was clear that with help he could handle this situation, it was decided he would return home, entering more intense therapy the next day with the psychiatry resident, who could see him in the outpatient setting. Duration of the interview: 20 minutes.

The patient Mr. D in case 2 illustrates the danger of simply cataloging risk factors to determine suicide risk. Examining the patient produced essential information. Shea (4) refers to the technique of reviewing the day as "behavioral incident." As in the previous case, the search for the acute precipitant helped to bring out preconscious elements of the mental status examination, allowing the evaluator to examine the crisis state of mind that resulted in the suicide attempt, namely, profound feelings of loss and failure. This enabled her to assess her patient's ability to bear these painful feelings and his response to a potentially therapeutic interaction. The positive response strongly suggested the reasonableness of beginning treatment in an intensive outpatient treatment setting. Mr. D might have been discharged in either case—with or without recovery of the acute precipitant—but the resident's sensitive persistence transformed a polite but evasive man trying to sell his own version of his self-assessment and avoid involuntary hospitalization into a real patient who was aware of and sharing his vulnerability, asking for the doctor's recommendation, and motivated to continue this work collaboratively on an outpatient basis.

Countertransference

A variety of personal reactions to patients that have the potential to interfere with clinical work can instead enhance this work if one is aware of them. With the minimizing individual who tries extremely hard to put on a good front, one might expect to feel an inkling that something poignant lies beneath the surface. One might experience an urge to collude with the patient's avoidance and naive hope that all is well. The urge can become stronger if one senses the possibility of activating strong emotions toward the evaluator, as happened with the apparently complex feelings that Mr. D developed toward the female resident. Recognizing uncomfortable reactions in oneself with minimizing patients provides a clue that some important material is waiting to be unearthed. If these clues are missed, the clinician will risk overidentifying with the patient's forced cheerfulness and unknowingly acting out the role of a poorly attuned and ineffectual parent or guardian figure.

In contrast, the patient who seems to be exaggerating his or her symptoms can quickly generate negative emotions in practitioners. These include feelings of being manipulated and trapped, which in turn can give rise to distaste, avoidance, and even retaliatory impulses. The agenda of searching for the acute precipitant can easily get lost in the rush to end the interview as quickly as possible, a heightened risk in a setting without set interview times. One might be in danger of reenacting the behavior of past abusers. By becoming aware of these personal reactions, the interviewer quickly gets insight into the types of reactions that the patient may be getting from other people in his or her life. For example, in case 1, upon recognizing some negative feelings in himself about Ms. A playing the suicide card, the psychiatrist was on the lookout for recent instances where people were trying to get away from her. This helped him uncover the acute precipitant of her feeling rejected by the crisis line staff. In both types of cases, the false self that is constructed to escape examination (21) leaves the examiner with a familiar yet hard-to-describe sense of interpersonal "fog" that may be more easily appreciated in its absence. The clinician must respect the protective function of the patient's lack of authenticity while seeking to piece together a story or narrative that has some coherence.

Broadly speaking, fear of the unknown may restrict clinicians' curiosity about acute precipitants, but with experience and self-knowledge comes an awareness of this fear that frees them to be more venturesome. Good interviewers are explorers.

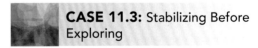

CASE 11.3: Stabilizing Before Exploring

Most practitioners intuitively grasp the importance of helping an acutely agitated or psychotic individual de-escalate before prematurely exploring the life circumstances that might underlie the presenting picture. There is a need first to engage the person, persuade him or her of one's professional interest, and attend to any real or perceived mistreatment by police, staff, or oneself leading up to the initial encounter. One must attempt to establish a clinician-patient relationship and address any iatrogenic precipitants. There are also medical issues and an array of interventions for reestablishing self-control and reality testing to consider. But even in a seemingly nonagitated person, it is important to appreciate fully how unsettling delving into underlying issues can be without securing a solid framework within which to work. Failing to do so can have serious consequences.

Mr. Z, a 47-year-old man, presented voluntarily to a PES with the request to be hospitalized and to restart his carbamazepine and olanzapine. Before moving to town, he had been seeing a psychiatrist regularly but had not found a new one yet. Things in his life had been going along all right; he just had not had any meds for several months and needed to get back on them. He was well groomed and polite and presented with only low-grade tension. There were no obvious symptoms or signs of depression, euphoria, or irritability. There was no evidence of impaired reality testing or cognition. He described a history of depressive and manic episodes and a suicide attempt in the distant past. He also had a history of substance abuse problems, primarily with cocaine. He had been in jail for disorderly conduct. Medical history was noncontributory. Urine drug screen was positive for marijuana, but he said he had not smoked recently.*

While considering a number of diagnostic possibilities, the evaluating psychiatrist asked to get a clearer idea about what had led him to decide to restart treatment at this particular point. Showing the slightest trace of annoyance, Mr. Z said there was not anything; he just thought it was a good idea. The psychiatrist agreed it was a good idea but reiterated that he wanted to get a clearer sense of what was going on in the patient's life that might be motivating him right now. The patient repeated there was nothing.

During a brief psychosocial review of systems, the psychiatrist learned that the patient was unemployed but came to town after having met his girlfriend on

the Internet. He looked after her house and kids while she worked. She gave him enough spending money, and their relationship was going fine. The psychiatrist asked how things were going with the kids. The patient said tersely, "Fine." Sensing some increased tension, the psychiatrist asked to hear a little bit more about that, but the patient said he did not want to go into it. After another unsuccessful appeal for more information, the evaluator said, "You don't have to if you don't want to. I respect that. It's just that the better I understand your situation, the better I can help you... You see, at this point, you're saying you need hospitalization, but I don't have enough information yet to justify that. I know some things can be very hard to talk about, but one of the things we do for people here is to listen to what is really bothering them most, and then help them to understand and handle their feelings better." Mr. Z's expression darkened. He said, "I can't..."

The evaluator paused for several seconds and then said carefully, "Let me ask it differently. What are you concerned would happen if you were to talk about it?" Mr. Z closed his eyes slightly. Suddenly, flashing with anger, he erupted into a loud tirade about his girlfriend's teenage children: They disobeyed him, they made fun of him, and they called him a loser. He then slammed his open hand onto the interview room table and jumped up, kicking his chair back against the wall, shouting, "I'm not going to take that shit anymore! I'm going to kill those little bastards! I'm going to wring their f— necks until their goddamn heads pop off!" He leaned forward and pounded his fist on the table, shouting, "I swear, I'll kill them; so help me God, I will!"

The psychiatrist sat very still. He glanced at the closed door, and then back at Mr. Z. "I see now why you need to be in the hospital. Can I get you some of your medication?" he asked. The patient glared at him and said, "Godammit! That's what I asked you for in the first place, isn't it?" The psychiatrist quietly acknowledged that he could have offered it sooner, then briefly discussed with him what would be the best dosages and excused himself from the room. Security stood by outside the door as Mr. Z took his medicine. His anger and escalation subsided, and he was admitted to the hospital without further incident. Clarification of the axes I and II diagnoses was deferred to the inpatient setting. Total interview time: 20 minutes.

The case of Mr. Z first appeared in slightly different form in an article by one of the authors Berlin, J. S. (2007), Managing malingering in the emergency setting. Psychiatric Issues in Emergency Care Settings, 5(2). It is reproduced here with permission of the publisher.

Reenactments

Although the pursuit of the "Why now?" question was ultimately essential in evaluating and managing Mr. Z's acuity, it was rather like doing surgery without an anesthetic. His affect tolerance, impulse control, and trust needed bolstering first. In retrospect, he may have experienced the examiner's very gentle prodding and deferral of his request for hospitalization as a reenactment of the goading and criticism he felt from his girlfriend's children. When encountering the increased tension and resistance, the psychiatrist might have thought back to Mr. Z's initial request (27), prescribed some medicine, given him some time, and then reconvened the interview in a more open area of the PES. Other stabilizing maneuvers might have included developing more of a rapport, moving less quickly, talking about his strengths, asking more about helpful past hospitalizations, inviting him to speak with a peer support specialist, offering food and drink, and so on. Unfortunately, today's practice environment often does not allow one to spend more time, so the interviewer pursued the underlying complaint. The interviewer as an explorer must be sensitive to the impact his or her venturing into unknown territory can have, but even then some unintended reenactments are inevitable.

False Negatives

False negatives are always a risk with individuals minimizing their symptoms. Mr. D, who was trying to avoid admission, is such an instance where pivotal information might easily have

been missed. But the case of Mr. Z illustrates the role that a thorough examination can play in preventing false negatives with individuals who are seeking admission. This point is not insignificant. Given the prevalence of hospital seeking for reasons other than medical necessity, emergency practitioners are often skeptical of such requests. However, it is a good idea to defer judgment until crucial history and preconscious elements of the mental status regarding acuity are apprehended.

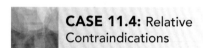

CASE 11.4: Relative Contraindications

Contraindications to an uncovering interview generally include organic mental states and acute or psychotic agitation, as discussed earlier. Another relative contraindication is acute trauma states. Discussed elsewhere in this text is the trend away from debriefing for these latter conditions in favor of what is now referred to as psychological first aid. A common complaint of people seen in emergency care settings who are already in office-based therapy for past trauma is that their therapist is moving too fast. When it is necessary in the emergency setting to discuss recent or past traumas, it is usually done for the purpose of putting old material back into the past.

Ms. T was a 35-year-old woman who presented to the emergency department voluntarily for intense anxiety symptoms related to intrusive memories of a rape she had experienced approximately 10 months ago. She thought she had put this experience behind her but inexplicably had been experiencing a resurgence of panic and other traumatic symptoms for the last 2 weeks. In the course of a brief interview, she recalled that her car had also been broken into 2 weeks ago. With a little bit of questioning, she realized this event had made her feel very violated and vulnerable, and it had reinflamed vestiges of the rape memory. Ms. T was helped to see that the break-in of her vehicle was very unfortunate but not of the magnitude of the prior violation. Upon making this connection, she quickly felt calmer and less out of control. She was easily referred for outpatient therapy. Total interview time: 15 minutes.

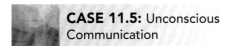

CASE 11.5: Unconscious Communication

A person's conflict between the desire to be understood and the fear of dealing with complicated emotions and events may result in a compromise formation that contains elements of content and defense. The individual communicates in symbolic, disguised ways. For the reasons discussed earlier—a tendency to resort to extreme defenses, distrust of helping professionals—people in the emergency setting often do not produce these indirect clues. However, when they do, interpreting or decoding them allows for a better evaluation and faster, more definitive treatment. This can even be done with individuals who are psychotic (23,24,28).

Ms. M, a 49-year-old woman, asked the police for a ride to PES and requested hospitalization on the day after Mother's Day. Her chief complaint was that she had been raped as a child, and her voices were telling her that invisible "military men" were putting their hands down her pants. Another mysterious force was turning her hair gray. She reported that the voices were worse than usual, and her level of distress seemed moderate, but she was not acutely agitated and had no thoughts of hurting herself or others. Except for signs of tardive dyskinesia, the rest of the triage findings and medical screening examination, including urine drug screen and urine pregnancy test, were noncontributory.

The triage nurse pulled the medical record and, with Ms. M's consent, called her treatment clinic for background information. Not a frequent visitor to the hospital, she was taking her medication for schizophrenia as prescribed, and her psychosis was known to be subacute at baseline. She was a somewhat dependent person. Her health was good. Her course of treatment over the past several years had been uneventful. She had some contact with family and lived alone on Social Security. There were no unusual stressors. She had never been a significant danger to herself or others.

The psychiatrist had this information when he sat down with Ms. M. Her thought processes were a bit tangential and idiosyncratic, but she essentially confirmed all of the information in the triage report, adding only that she had decided to come to PES that morning. She repeated her request for hospitalization. Something was clearly troubling her, but her presenting acuity did not seem to justify the use of such a limited resource.

This case is a familiar scenario. The emergency practitioner may not be sure what is causing this woman's disequilibrium, but he does have a fairly good idea of her diagnosis and acuity. Accustomed to making rapid decisions with incomplete information, he might offer her some as-needed medication and suggest either more frequent outpatient contacts or a short stay in an observation area or other intermediate care setting for further evaluation. These are reasonable choices.

But using the conceptual model we describe in this chapter, the clinician could remind himself of several things: (a) that an acute precipitant usually underlies a presenting problem; (b) the acute precipitant is associated with anxiety and other painful feelings that are difficult to bear; (c) awareness and discussion of the associated feelings are consciously and unconsciously defended against, often by denial, avoidance, projection, or distortion but potentially accessible in the initial interview; and (d) discovering the acute precipitant will result in a better picture of what the problem is and what needs to be done.

Complementing the "Why now?" line of questioning is active listening for indirect, unconsciously disguised references to the acute precipitant and its associated feelings. These references are found in stories, memories, dreams, slips of the tongue, and symptoms (17). Even when symptoms have a biologic basis, as they clearly do with psychosis, they often have symbolic or figurative meaning as well. In general, the more comfortable a person feels opening up to the evaluator, the more likely that the references will be able to be deciphered. The evaluator can increase an individual's comfort level by combining respect for her need to keep the precipitant to herself—or from herself—with an appreciation for her simultaneous wish to have her precipitant recognized and treated.

Returning to our case example: Overtly, Ms. M's conversation displayed a paucity of content, and her psychotic symptoms seemed devoid of any meaning. But then the psychiatrist allowed his mind to reflect on the specifics of her chief complaint. They involved themes of sex, rape, childhood, and aging. Perhaps the paranoid fears concealed a wish. Suddenly, it dawned on him that yesterday had been Mother's Day. He had not remembered until that moment.

He asked how the holiday had gone for her. Not good, she said. She had had a big argument with her mother last evening, big enough to make her leave her mother's house and return to her rooming house. Ms. M made real eye contact with the interviewer for the first time, and then smiled slightly. She looked relieved and seemed less distressed.

Wondering if it might be useful to explore this theme a little further, he asked if she had any children. No, she did not. Abruptly, she stood up and said she was ready to go. She felt fine. He asked if she had really covered everything she wanted to discuss and if she really felt safe to go. She said yes. The doctor then took the time to suggest that the recent disagreement with her mother would be worth talking over with her community support caseworker and her psychiatrist. He obtained her permission to let them know about their conversation. She was discharged uneventfully. Total time for the medical record review, the nursing triage assessment, and the psychiatric examination: 20 minutes.

Everything about Ms. M's clinical presentation suggested that full hospitalization was not indicated, but the deeper evaluation helped the clinician be more certain. It helped initiate a process of working through a stressor that this woman could continue on an outpatient basis, and it is an example of how an assessment in depth can be therapeutic. Her good response to evaluation and treatment in the PES suggested that she would be successful in continuing with treatment on an outpatient basis, and this was documented.

This PES intervention progressed from the triage model to the treatment model. It allowed treatment to take place right away, rather than postponing it and trying to pick it up later. This is better for the patient and avoids potential overuse of valuable inpatient or intermediate care resources. Ms. M's abrupt termination of the interview when the psychiatrist brought up the subject of children was a clear message that she would need to go very slowly with processing the various midlife issues she was facing. He might have expected this from her need to elaborate her feelings about motherhood and daughterhood into her psychotic symptoms, which were a complicated mix of paranoid projection, reaction formation, and condensation. Clearly, part of her sudden improvement was a flight into health, but for the moment she had apparently received the help that she needed.

WHEN NO ACUTE PRECIPITANT IS FOUND

It is hoped that presenting different types of cases has demonstrated that an acute precipitant can be occult but discoverable. Because defenses such as distortion, denial, and avoidance either carefully disguise the precipitant or block it from view, evaluators must start with the assumption that one does exist. Although success is never assured, it is almost certainly true that it will not be found if it is not looked for. It is a rare occasion indeed for an emergency department patient, resisting the pursuit of the acute precipitant and trying to be released from a mental health hold, to quickly do a sudden about-face, as one of ours did, and say with self-deprecating humor, "You want to know the straw that broke the camel's back, right?"

In reality, emergency patients such as the ones we have described here are not in the majority. The practitioner is therefore often left to decide what to do. A good rule of thumb is to let the unsolved mystery be the deciding factor in cases where one is debating which way to go. For example, in the case of Mr. D, his breakthrough about his AA sponsor suggested he could be referred for intensive outpatient therapy. Absent that insight, it would have been reasonable to prevail upon him to stay in a psychiatric facility until he knew what his trigger was, so that he could be properly prepared for it the next time. In a situation where a precipitant is not discovered but the individual still seems clearly safe enough for discharge, one might at least plant a seed and advise that he or she continue to think it over on an outpatient basis. Whether admitting or not, documenting "acute precipitant deferred" on axis IV calls attention to an interesting question that remains unanswered.

SUMMARY

These cases illustrate an approach that can help identify key underlying affective states and issues. With Ms. A, exploring her denial led to an appreciation of her acute feelings of rejection and loneliness. With Mr. D, understanding his avoidance led to the issue underlying his suicide attempt, which involved the lost romantic involvement of his AA sponsor. With Mr. Z, tuning into the issue of his girlfriend's children exposed his underlying rage that had been both denied and avoided. With Ms. T, it seemed she had distorted the recent trauma of the break-in and equated it with a rape from years past. And with Ms. M, who had a thought disorder with delusional projection and distortion, it was necessary to uncover the events of the prior evening when she argued with her mother.

Obtaining this kind of information allows the clinician to better choose the most appropriate and therapeutic level of care. Nonadmissions and shorter stays are more likely. By bringing the clinician's and patient's views of the acuity into better alignment, it also invigorates the assessment process and makes it the beginning of collaborative treatment. Biologic, psychological, and family interventions can all be brought to bear on the problems that are identified. One can imagine conjoint therapy being a useful adjunct in several of the cases we have described. Taken as a whole, clinicians find that this approach often proves to be very valuable for the patient.

We are at a juncture in our science where we recognize that clinical expertise produces very interesting and apparently useful data for the assessment of acuity, but not where it has the evidence base of empirically validated risk factors. In our opinion, evidence-based emergency psychiatry of this kind has not yet been demonstrated. In the future, one could imagine that postmortem review of medical records of completed suicides might perhaps reveal a disproportionate number of crisis cases in which the final acute precipitant was not identified. One could test the hypothesis prospectively by following two large cohorts of discharged patients longitudinally: one with the precipitant identified and one without. Studies over the last decade with functional brain imaging (29) raise the possibility of one day being able to objectify the moment when an individual dissolves a portion of his or her defensive facade and the clinician notices the emergence of an engaged and more real self. Until then, it would seem prudent for clinicians to continuously improve their interview technique for the reasons we have discussed.

REFERENCES

1. Jacobs, D. G. (Ed.). (1999). *The Harvard Medical School guide to suicide assessment and intervention*. San Francisco: Jossey-Bass.
2. Gabbard, G. O. (2005). *Psychodynamic psychiatry in clinical practice* (4th ed.). Washington, DC: American Psychiatric Publishing.
3. MacKinnon, R. A., Michels, R., & Buckley, P. J. (2006). *The psychiatric interview in clinical practice* (2nd ed.). Washington, DC: American Psychiatric Publishing.
4. Shea, S. C. (2002). *The practical art of suicide assessment*. Hoboken, NJ: John Wiley and Sons.
5. Hyman, S. E., & Tesar, G. E. (Eds.). (1994). *Manual of psychiatric emergencies* (3rd ed.). Boston: Little, Brown and Company.
6. Hoffman, D. L., & Remmel, M. L. (1975). *Uncovering the precipitant in crisis intervention* (pp. 259–267). New York: Social Casework.
7. Rosenberg, R. C., & Sulkowicz, K. J. (2002). Psychosocial interventions in the psychiatric emergency service. In Allen, M. H. (Ed.), *Emergency psychiatry*. Washington, DC: American Psychiatric Publishing.
8. Allen, M. H. (1996). Definitive treatment in the psychiatric emergency service. *Psychiatric Quarterly, 67*(3), 247–262.
9. *Diagnostic and statistical Manual of mental disorders: DSM-IV-TR* (4th ed., Vol. 28, pp. 807–813) text revision. Washington DC: American Psychiatric Association, 2000.
10. Lindenmayer, J. P., Crowner, M., & Cosgrove, B. A. (2002). Emergency treatment of agitation and aggression. In Allen, M. H. (Ed.). *Emergency psychiatry*. Washington, DC: American Psychiatric Publishing.
11. Petit, J. R. (2004). *Handbook of emergency psychiatry*. Philadelphia: Lippincott Williams & Wilkins.
12. Hillard, R., & Zitek, B. (2004). *Emergency psychiatry*. New York: McGraw-Hill.

13. Menninger, K. A., Mayman, M., & Pruyser, P. W. (1962). *A Manual for psychiatric case study.* (2nd ed.). New York: Grune & Stratton.

14. Stone, L. (1961). *The psychoanalytic situation.* Madison, WI: International Universities Press.

15. Winnicott, D. W. (1956). On transference. *The International Journal of Psychoanalysis, 37,* 369–376.

16. Raphael, B. (1986). *When disaster strikes: A Handbook for the caring professionals.* Boston: Unwin Hyman.

17. Langs, R. J. (1985). *Workbooks for psychotherapists.* Emerson, NJ: New Concept Press.

18. Gill, M. (1982). *Analysis of the transference: Vol I, theory and technique.* New York: International Universities Press.

19. Langs, R. J. (2000). Unconscious communication in the emergency room. *Emergency Psychiatry, 6*(4), 111–112.

20. Forman, L. M., Jones, C., & Frances, A. (1995). The multiaxial system in psychiatric treatment. In Gabbard, G. O. (Ed.), *Treatments of psychiatric disorders* (2nd ed., Vol. 2). Washington, DC: American Psychiatric Press.

21. Rinsley, D. B. (1983). *Treatment of the severely disturbed adolescent.* New York: Jason Aronson.

22. Adler, G. (1979). The myth of the alliance with borderline patients. *The American Journal of Psychiatry, 136*(5), 642–645.

23. Gudeman, J. E. (2000). Psychodynamic approaches to the person with psychosis in the emergency situation. *Emergency Psychiatry, 6*(4), 113–116.

24. Semrad, E. V. (1969). *Teaching psychotherapy of psychotic patients.* New York: Grune & Stratton.

25. Yates, B. D., Nordquist, C. R., & Schultz-Ross, R. A. (1996). Feigned psychiatric symptoms in the emergency room. *Psychiatric Services, 47,* 998–1000.

26. American Psychiatric Association. (2004). *Practice guideline for the assessment and treatment of patients with suicidal behaviors.* Washington, DC: American Psychiatric Publishing.

27. Diamond, R. J., & Scheifler, P. L. (2007). *Treatment collaboration.* New York: WW Norton.

28. Arieti, S. (1974). *Interpretation of schizophrenia.* New York: Basic Books.

29. Jung-Beeman, M., Bowden, E. M., Haberman, J., et al. (2004). Neural activity when people solve verbal problems with insight. *PLOS Biology, 2,* 500–510.

12

Advanced Interviewing Techniques

Ron C. Rosenberg

"A Stitch in Time Saves Nine"
"Haste makes waste"

PROLOGUE

Imagine this: You have arrived at your new assignment at an acute care center; perhaps, it is an emergency department (ED) or a walk-in clinic. A family arrives with a young man claiming that the "patient" broke furniture after visiting his ex-girlfriend's Facebook page. For days he had been sleeping and eating poorly, not attending classes, and his hygiene has been deteriorating. His family states to the triage staff that he has never been like this. He is demanding to leave.

Now:
1. What is the first issue to address? And to whom?
2. Do you let him leave? How do you decide that?
3. What treatments are appropriate now? Later?
4. How do you handle staff concerns? Safety concerns?

A critical tool for resolving these issues is one's skill as an interviewer. Patient and family disclosures are needed to provide data for an assessment and intervention. Understanding the patient's ability to manage his impulses and current needs and his capability to make and execute coherent and rational future acts must be understood to answer question 2 and 3. Your own training, experience, and skill will bear on question 4.

Now consider another question:
5. What literature, empirical research, and data are available to help you chose and master these tasks?

For a variety of reasons, research on the techniques of interview and intervention in an acute care setting itself is difficult to perform (1). Safety, capacity to consent, privacy concerns, mandated reporting, Health Insurance Portability and Accountability Act of 1996 (HIPAA), ethical issues, and limited resources contribute to barriers to performing needed evidence-based work. Are we simply following protocols? Should we consider the ED as a hopeless nontherapeutic environment as Gerson lamented (2)? In addition, the ED has increased its responsibilities toward assessment and management of risk: it is expected to provide elements of treatment (3). Can we provide the stitch that saves nine without undue haste?

Despite skepticism, interviewing in an acute care setting is simply a practical necessity and may provide an opportunity for change. So, what do we do when we get "stuck"? The purpose of this chapter is to give the reader hints, tools, and strategies for either avoiding impasses or for getting out of them. The focus is on pragmatism, not dogmatism. Theories are useful for generating solutions but detailed theoretical discussions are not possible within the limits of this chapter.

The term "technical eclecticism" has been used by Lazarus (4), and a transtheoretical therapy has been proposed by Prochaska (5) in which techniques are applied that are seen as the most appropriate to the patient's current state. The need to have a "toolkit of interventions" is another way of formulating this idea (6). Sometimes melding seemingly conflicting theories can make for even more useful tools in an acute care environment. For example, behavioral rewards can be combined with psychodynamically rich disclosures.

Three tools valuable for avoiding impasse are 1) establishing a working **alliance**, 2) providing real resources (**crisis** management), and 3) performing some element of a trial of **therapy** (7). When one melds these three components, the odds of a successful acute intervention improve. Work is optimized when it proceeds in a logical and disciplined order. In this model, establishing a working alliance usually precedes crisis work which often precedes therapy work (hence referred to as the **"ACT" paradigm**).

ESTABLISHING A WORKING ALLIANCE

The establishment of a working alliance has become mandated by the increasingly customer-oriented approach toward patient care. One would think that the severity of emergency patients would preclude issues of building an alliance, and classical psychoanalysts were initially doubtful about the possibility with anyone of a genuine working alliance uncontaminated by unconscious elements (8); however, there is abundant evidence that building an alliance improves treatment success (4,9). A review of the techniques advocated by a recent handbook for customer relations demonstrates surprising overlap of good customer relations methods with effective interviewing (10). In addition, these efforts overlap with emerging efforts to improve patient experience to yield better outcomes (11). Techniques advocated such as active listening, allowing venting (within limits), giving assurance, and empathic statements would be part of most therapy approaches. Despite the scripted and nonmedical orientation, these techniques do provide an approach to building an alliance in a stressful environment.

Staff: How can we help you? **
Patient: I need a rest.
Staff: Ok. Can you tell us what you think has made you so tired?
Patient: A lot of things. I just lost my job and now my girlfriend wants to leave me. Etc.

** All vignettes are similar to real cases but simplified for didactic purposes.

Recent research highlights the value of providing a safe environment, assessing and addressing immediate real needs, advocating for the patient, and demonstrating the potential of treatment (9). Good practices and good alliance building can involve addressing real physical concerns:

A middle-aged man cut his arms in a suicide attempt.

Staff: Does this hurt?
Patient: Not too much.
Staff: You must have been quite upset when you did this?
Patient: I don't even remember doing it. I guess I was "distracted."
Staff: Let's take care of this first, then we can talk about what was going on.
Patient: Thanks.
Some like to use a conversational tone:
Staff: [Noticing that the patient wears a baseball cap] Hello! Are you a Zooters fan?
Patient: Yeah, I went to the game yesterday.
Staff: Great catch by Simpson!
Patient: Yeah.
Staff: So what's going on?
Patient: I cut myself. … etc.
But take care with paranoid patients:
Staff: Hello! Are you a Zooters fan?
Patient: How do you know that?
Staff: Your hat?
Patient: What about my hat?!

Every step of the interview requires constant vigilance. Foreknowledge is highly desirable.

The provider of care must in the broadest sense engage the *reward system* of the patient/client. The patient/client should *want to* speak, disclose, and be ready to problem solve with the staff. One's theoretical orientation may call this being a positive reinforcement, establishing a positive transference, being a good object, etc. The manifest work is the same. But it usually requires some active work by the provider. Many years ago, the interviewer might have offered the patient a cigarette. Today, it is likely to be a nicotine patch or gum (12). It might also be juice, a sheet of paper, a quiet place to lie down, or a consoling positive thought. This leads us to crisis intervention.

CRISIS MANAGEMENT

The Crisis intervention prescribes replacing in some manner what has been lost from the patient's life and reestablishing equilibrium. Acute care frequently involves dealing with recent loss of persons, relationships, jobs, residences, etc. Giving patients specific advice and resources to replace these losses not only strengthens the alliance but may strengthen a sense of equilibrium that will foster self-reflection and self-direction in therapy. Since the tragedy of 9/11, there has been the evolution of the concept of psychological first aid (PFA) (13). The focus is on assessing and filling immediate needs rather than debriefing or retelling.

The application of the ACT paradigm can be seen:

Staff: Hello.
Patient: [No response]
Staff: What happened?
Patient: [After a pause …] I lost my mother. She might be dead.
Staff: This must be so upsetting. (Alliance building).
Patient: [Whimpers but no clear response]
Staff: When did you last see her?
Patient: This morning before the storm.
Staff: That *was* a terrible storm. Well we are all *safe* here. Please have a seat. Are you okay? (Support and alliance building before confronting the emotionally laden material. Note the importance of establishing safety)
Patient: I don't know.
Staff: Have you eaten anything today?
Patient: A little.
Staff: How about having something to eat first. Then you can help us find out about your mother. If you could, we would need you to fill out a small questionnaire. (Engaging support before challenge).
Patient: I don't know if I can handle that now. I'm *very* upset.
Staff: Have a little something. One of our staff can help you when you are ready.
Patient: I am not hungry…I am just a little thirsty.
Staff: I think when you feel a little stronger you'll be able to. Can I get you some juice?
Patient: Okay. [Takes a sip]
[Long pause]
Staff: Want to start now?
Patient: Okay.
Later that afternoon:
Patient: Any news?
Staff: Sorry. No reports so far.

Patient: I know it. She is dead. When I came back to the house and it was totally collapsed.
Staff: Have you seen any friends or family here?
Patient: I didn't really look.
Staff: We have some people in Room 4 from your neighborhood here. Perhaps you will find some friends there. There is staff there also. You might want to speak to them, and I'll still be here for a while too.

Using therapy techniques, the staff encourages self-support, network support, and coping behavior, and in a symbolic way staff becomes a kind of mother substitute. The point here is that therapy follows alliance building (empathic listening) and some crisis work filling tangible needs (food, drink, companionship), and this enables fulfilling other crisis needs (finding housing, missing relatives, etc.).

Note what is not recommended by PFA at the acute stage (13):

1. There is no encouragement to retell details of the trauma. For example, What happened? Where was your mother? Did you see people getting crushed in their houses? Did you smell something burning? Etc.

2. No premature and dismissive rationalizing of her experiences such as, "If she is dead, she is probably in Heaven so don't worry." (However, it is possible that much later on this may be a comforting thought appropriate to the patient's culture but only after the patient feels support and a sense of security.)

THERAPY IN ACUTE SITUATIONS

There are common elements of many therapies which can be enlisted when approaching an acute patient. Two particularly important features are the concept of **support** and **challenge**. Support involves statements, gestures, and actions that indicate empathic understanding of the pain and discomfort that the patient/client is experiencing. There may be common neurological mechanisms for this phenomenon (14). Indeed, there also may be common mechanisms for reflection and modification of affective material (15) which is part of challenge.

Defining challenge is more difficult. Challenge may raise the patient's anxiety. Patients are encouraged by questions, inflections, gestures, actions to reflect upon their own behavior, associations, thoughts, speech, and their effect upon others. Another form of challenge is trying to change, revise, or redirect thoughts and plans when a person becomes aware of emotionally laden sensations, associations, thoughts, etc. Enhancing these capacities for self-reflection and self-redirection is critical to the success of challenge. Many statements and efforts that are part of traditional interviewing protocols do not take this into consideration. (see example below).

Compare two interviews.

Interview as challenge without support:

Interviewer: So you were brought here by the police because you tried to hit someone with a baseball bat. Do you want to hurt anyone now?
Patient: I did not.
Interviewer: You did not want to hit someone?
Patient: No. Now can I leave?
Interviewer: We can talk about that later. Can you tell me about this?
Patient: These are all lies! I want to leave now!! You can't keep me! I will sue you and the hospital!

A central strategy for managing challenge is to manage support. Support should always precede challenge and, if possible, follow it. As previously stated, it should be rewarding to speak to the interviewer and one should be rewarded for having managed a challenge. Consider now how the previous interview could combine challenge and support:

Interviewer: Hello. Are you okay? (Support).
Patient: I shouldn't be here. (Protest. Unjust treatment)
Interviewer: That has to be difficult. (Support and empathy)
Patient: [Silence] (Processing statement)
Interviewer: Can you help me understand why you are here? (Slight challenge, but coupled with an empowering statement).
Patient: My sister called the police. (Patient is willing to make a disclosure).
Interviewer: That must have been upsetting to you. (Support; reward for having given some information)
Patient: Hmm.
Interviewer: "What is this stuff about a baseball bat?" (Challenge but avoids a direct confrontation)

Patient: I don't know. (No information yet).
Interviewer: Well it says here that you tried to hit someone. Can you tell me what was going on. (Challenge again, but avoiding blame)
Patient: I was defending myself. Someone stole from me. (More data given).
Interviewer: That's a shame that happened. (Again, support for having "survived" a challenge)

Some questions that are part of a routine mental status have the properties suggesting challenge: Do you hear voices? How much is 100-7? Do you want to hurt yourself? While others have properties suggesting support: Have you been sleeping well? How has your appetite been? How has your mood been lately?

It would be wise to use supportive questions earlier in the interview and be mindful of challenging questions. A suggested litmus test that can help inform the interviewer regarding the impact of a question is the following consideration: Would the question upset a colleague or a friend if posed in conversation.

Have you slept okay? (Not a challenge; likely a support).

Do you hear voices? (Clearly a challenge)

Before attempting therapy, one should always learn about previous therapies, what worked and what did not. This form of "debriefing" can help you avoid foreseeable situations that lead to an impasse.

Staff: What did you speak about with Dr. Smith?
Patient: Mostly about my job.
Staff: Did it help?
Patient: Sometimes. But he upset with me with his explanations when I just wanted advice. He always wanted me to talk about myself and not my job.

Interviews in the ED or an acute care environment get "stuck" for a variety of reasons.
1. Failure to consider how the working environment affects technique.
2. Failure to obtain information available from the patient and other sources that would allow one to choose an optimal approach.
3. Failure to take the time to establish a working alliance.
4. Failure to treat severe anxiety or psychosis that makes a working alliance impossible because of disorganization and distortions.

5. Failure to adequately address real stressors and real needs.
6. Failure to appreciate that the experience of the acute care environment can be traumatic to certain patients.

CHALLENGE ATTENUATION

Challenge attenuation is one way to avoid getting stuck when interviewing a patient. While the nature of ED crisis work requires asking questions that challenge the patient, the author has noticed that the challenge once recognized can be *attenuated* with *less emotional reactivity* from the patient. As important as medication and a supportive environment are to allow challenge, care about one's words is paramount. Three techniques to attenuate a challenge are (1) linguistic attenuation, (2) indirect reference, and (3) metaphorical techniques.

Linguistic methods involve modifying the words used when a challenge is posed.

Classic version: "Do you hear voices?" An attenuated version: "Have you been troubled by voices that bother you that aren't your actual thoughts?"

Classic: "Have you ever attempted suicide in the past?" Attenuated: "Have you ever had times when you felt so bad that you felt like harming yourself or others or actually tried to hurt yourself (or others)?"

Indirect reference asks the patient to consider a problem-solving approach.

Classic: "Have you ever tried to harm your mother?"

Attenuated: "So what do you do when your mother upsets you?" (Then go on to discuss possible violence).

Metaphoric approach. The use of metaphors in therapy is common (16). This technique has been helpful to break an impasse with a number of difficult-to-reach patients.

Sometimes the metaphor comes from the interviewer:

Direct: "You need (inpatient) treatment for your mania."

Metaphorical: "You have a lot of energy. Sort of like a sports car. But sometimes a Ferrari can be in a ditch. We need to help get you back on the road." (This approach is often well received by angry, manic patients.)

Sometimes the metaphor comes from the patient:

Classic: "You need (inpatient) treatment for your psychosis."

Metaphoric: Interviewer: "So how do you support yourself?"

Patient: "I used to teach piano."

Interviewer: "So what happened".

Patient: "The piano *stole* my fingerprints".

Interviewer: "I see. So sorry to hear. Maybe we can help you get your fingerprints back!"

Patient: "Can you do that?"

Interviewer: "Maybe; how about you stay with us for a few days and perhaps even take some medication?"

Patient: "I'll think about it."

ASSESSING AND REDUCING RISK

ED providers struggle to figure out which psychiatric patients need to be hospitalized. Approximately 10% of all adult ED patients, regardless of chief complaints, have recent suicidal ideation or behaviors but will often not mention this (17,18), and patients who are admitted because of concern for harm to self or others are sometimes noted to be fine once they are admitted. Overcoming emotional obstacles to disclosure of information needed to assess appropriateness for inpatient care is a significant burden on ED staff. Yet such assessment is now a universal requirement.

It has been shown that interventions in the ED can reduce risk of self and other harm (3). Examination of the tools that assist assessment (eg, CAMS-R) demonstrates opportunity for additional support (19). Elements of assessment of risk, such as reflecting on what makes life worthwhile, are a form of supportive work that is both revealing and an opportunity for assistance. Contrast the two interviews below:

1. **Interviewer:** "What do you do to relax and enjoy life?" **Patient:** "Nothing."
2. **Interviewer:** "What do you do to relax and enjoy life?" **Patient:** "I take walks. Sometimes I visit my sister."

Why not suggest a few items to the first patient in this example and monitor the patient's response?

Interviewer: "How about music, movies?"
Patient: "Yes I like reggae." versus: **Patient:** "Nah. I just do nothing."

An interactive approach that blends assessment and treatment can prove more productive and practical than a static approach (20). Management of violence potential has similar characteristics. For example, borrowing elements from dialectical behavior therapy (DBT), one can have patients reflect on their anger.

Interviewer: "What can you do when your roommate upsets you?"
Patient: "Walk away?"

The inquiry regarding suicidal or aggressive thoughts and acts requires skill. It is an opportunity to choose words carefully and attenuate the challenge. But take care when patients are brazen about aggression. Example: "If you don't give me …I will kill someone (or myself)!"

THE WORKING ENVIRONMENT

Interviewing technique focuses on the dyadic nature of the identified patient/client and the interviewer/therapist/examiner. Frequently ignored is the context of the interview, except as defined by an institutional label, eg, "Mental Health Clinic", "Emergency Department", etc. There is an increasing awareness that timing has an effect on institutional performance (21). As anyone who has labored long in acute care settings knows, the context can significantly alter individual performance, technique, and outcome. The availability of beds, staffing patterns, day of the week, time of the day, whether it is a holiday weekend, who is supervising or helping or on vacation or sick, etc. can have a profound effect on how an interview is approached.

Low staffing levels, many clients registered, no beds or appointment slots available can so tax the interviewer that there is not enough time to build a working alliance, and patients are challenged too early, supported too little, and rushed—often with unfortunate outcomes of an incomplete history, more use of medication, more use of restraint, caregiver burnout, etc.

Example: A patient is brought by ambulance Saturday night after a superficial cut of his wrists. There are eight patients waiting to be seen and a staff member is late.

Staff: "So why did you try to cut yourself?"
Patient: "I don't know."

The same patient appears on Sunday at noon. He is the first patient of that quiet morning.
Staff: "Hello."
Patient: "Hello."
Staff: "So tell me how are things going?"
Patient: "So so."
Staff: "Something bad happened?"
Patient: "Yeah, my girlfriend left me."

One can appreciate the mental energy needed to overcome institutional and time pressures. Sometimes, paradoxically, even when resources are abundant, less time is spent examining the patient, and patients are quickly admitted or referred. Not enough time is taken to understand the significant factors that led to a visit or to engage the patient and his support network. Arranging a disposition takes the place of finding a quality solution. Obtaining desired data must be balanced with the opportunity to make change.

Same patient as above (Sunday morning):

Staff: When your girlfriend left you, is that when you cut yourself?
Patient: I am not sure. I wasn't thinking.
Staff: Were you upset?
Patient: Maybe… maybe she would understand how upset I was.
Staff: Who could have helped you?
Patient: I don't know. My friends. My therapist maybe. [Pause] I don't really want to kill myself. [Pause] I just needed something… maybe to talk to someone.
Staff: Do you think it would help to be in a hospital?
Patient: I don't know. Maybe I should just go and see my old therapist.
Same patient (Saturday night):
Staff: Are you suicidal?
Patient: I don't know. Maybe.
Staff: You can sign yourself in as a voluntary patient.
Patient: Okay.

OBTAIN ENOUGH INFORMATION BEFORE THE INTERVIEW IS ATTEMPTED

Although some prefer to interview the patient "cold" and then consult the medical record or other sources, this approach is not recommended.

Rather one should learn as much as possible beforehand. Often this is a safety issue. One caveat is to avoid reacting too strongly to the first information you received, a phenomena known technically as "anchoring" (21) and engendering "confirmation bias" (22), the tendency to prove what you first believe. In a word, be cognizant of the "chief complaint," eg, "I want to kill myself" or "Brought by the police for throwing objects in the street." Be aware of the need to follow up on these issues, but do not be blinded or shackled by them. It is useful to consider a number of possibilities simultaneously. Note how in the example above the Sunday morning interviewer did a little exploration before addressing the chief complaint. The Saturday night interviewer felt pressed for time and "got down to business." The results were quite different.

Better care and better results come from an enlightened skepticism. When speaking to collateral sources try to be open-minded and see both sides of the situation. Paranoid patients, for example, can have (or acquire) real enemies (23). One can delay approaching the "chief complaint" until there is a working alliance (see below). Alternate explanations become possible. One might then appreciate that a suicide attempt was in fact an accidental overdose. Throwing an object might have been a defensive move. A hallucination might have really been tinnitus or a symptom of an infection.

TREATING PSYCHOSIS AND ANXIETY

Neuromodulatory dysfunction plays an important role in the severe anxiety, mood dysregulation, psychosis, or aggression that often triggers an ED or crisis visit. Disruptions in executive functioning can interfere with alliance building and processing of emotionally painful material. All too frequently, the outcome of the use of acute medication has been sedation rather than calming the patient. A consensus of experts seems to appreciate the increasing potential of newer atypical antipsychotic medications (24). Yet there is always staff pressure to make the patient quiet rather than informative. The goal should be a calm, awake patient who can give needed history. However, even an agitated patient must still be approached and interviewed to determine *if* medication is needed, which medication is optimal, and how it can be administered. The term "de-escalation" is used; but it is really a form of skilled interviewing.

Typical example:

A 44-year-old male with a previous psychiatric history was brought in an agitated state after pushing a woman on the bus.

Patient: Let me go! [Staring intensely in a strange way]

Staff: Can we talk about what happened?

Patient: No. get away! [Patient turns to avoid all eye contact]

Staff: Should we use something to calm you so we can talk?

Patient: [Still no eye contact] I don't want to be drugged!

Staff: We don't want you to fall asleep, just to be calm so we can talk.

Patient: What are you going to give me? [Begins to look at the interviewer]

Staff: A small amount of XX.

Patient: I am allergic to everything! [Looks at the interviewer]

Staff: What happens?

Patient: My throat tightens up.

Staff: The record shows you have had XX before. You seemed to have done okay with it in the past.

Patient: Oh, uh, yes, but don't use too much. How much are you going to give me?

Staff: A low dose, XX milligrams. Will you take it as a pill rather than as an injection?

Patient: A pill. [Looks away again]

The patient takes an oral dose; the interview resumes in 20 minutes.

Staff: What happened on the bus?

Patient: A woman was staring at me. She was putting thoughts in my head.

Note the use of alliance-building techniques, even prior to medication administration. The patient is empowered, given choices. Notice how the adjuvant use of medication facilitates the assessment as well as enables a therapeutic dialogue. Had medication been highly sedating, this assessment and treatment would have been delayed. Also note the importance of nonverbal cues to how the interview was received.

But sometimes initial attempts to build an alliance fail:

Patient: You are the devil! You are evil! Medication is the work of the devil!
Staff: We are trying to help you calm down so we can help you.
Patient: You just want to make money! I'll call my attorney!

Sometimes all one can do is use medication and be persistently supportive, even if it sounds like a broken record: "We are trying to help you. Let's talk when you are feeling a little calmer." Usually it is better for one person to speak calmly to the patient. This may not be the provider, but the physician in charge should not forget to try again to speak directly to the patient when the patient is calmer and more receptive to some questions that can be experienced as provocative.

Staff: "So how can we help you?"
Patient: "Call my mother."
Staff: "What shall we tell her?"
Patient: "To come here and get me out of here."

The patient provides the phone number and calms somewhat.

Direct confrontation can be problematic:

Interviewer: Do you hear voices?
Patient: "No. Do you? I am not crazy!"
Embedded support can help:
Staff: "Have you slept well?"
Patient: "No, I get up all the time."
Staff: "Do voices bother you at night."
Patient: "No".
Staff: "During the day?"
Patient: "Sometimes… I don't want to talk about it."

SELF-REFLECTION

Tools are not useful if they are not used. While institutional and workplace challenges play a role, it becomes increasingly useful to consider one's own emotional reactions as part of treatment and informing care. Consider your reaction to statements typical of patients in the ED.

1. If you don't admit me I will jump in front of a car!
2. I don't need to stay. I just said I would hurt myself to upset my wife.

3. Can I use my cell phone when I get admitted? (Many inpatient services forbid use.)
4. Why are you asking me all these questions? What is your name? Let me write this down. Give me a piece of paper!
5. Can I get a sandwich?

An important issue is not the interviewer's degree of empathy or antipathy but the impact of emotions on one's technique and approach. Does this decrease the resolve to build an alliance? To use supportive statements? To attenuate challenge? Often these are good opportunities for a valuable reflective response by the interviewer, eg, "How do you think that makes us feel?" or "It must be upsetting to talk about these things." Rehearsal, role playing, group discussion, and personal reflection and journaling can prove helpful to improve one's interviewing performance.

THE SHADOW OF STIGMA

Much has been written lately about the negative effects of stigma on mental disorders (25). When interviewing patients, be careful to avoid or not respond to words that are provocative or stigmatizing. Whereas mentioning common medical diagnoses are part of the medical interview, be sensitive to any mention of psychiatric disorders in the psychiatric interview. Recognize that there is an emotional cost to such disclosures and discussion.

Patient: I am schizophrenic.
Staff: What does that mean?
Patient: It means I am crazy.
Staff: I am not sure what you mean. Has someone said that to you?
Patient: Yeah, my girlfriend thinks I am "crazy."
Staff: Let's find another word. What is it your girlfriend doesn't like?
Patient: She says I call her too often.
Staff: Let's talk about that and figure out if there are ways for you to call her less often.

CONCLUSION

This chapter has outlined an approach to interviewing in the acute setting. It emphasizes the importance of rapport building as a crucial first step, even for the very acute patient. Then questioning (challenging) can take place. In summary, to avoid an impasse in acute interviews:

1. Do not pursue your evaluation and disposition until taking the time to build, or at least attempting to build, a fledgling alliance with the patient. If possible, delay pursuing the chief complaint until this begins to happen.

2. Do not confuse sedation with calmness. You should generally avoid sedation in acute situations; it can cause a delay in obtaining critical information.

3. You increase your effectiveness and do not diminish your authority by meeting real needs for patients in crisis.

4. Give the patient a choice whenever possible. If you must choose, eg, to medicate, tell patients about future choices. "When you are calm let's discuss what are the possibilities."

5. Avoid high-voltage words and phrases. Practice customer friendliness and when possible, attenuate challenge.

6. Be aware of, and learn from, your own and other staff's emotional reactions to patients. Be aware of institutional and workplace pressures.

REFERENCES

1. Litz, B. T., & Gibson, L. E. (2006). Conducting research in mental health interventions. In Elspeth, C. R., Watson, T. P. J., & Friedman, M. J. (Eds.), *Interventions following mass violence and disasters* (pp. 387–404). New York, NY: Guilford Press.

2. Gerson, B. (1980). Psychiatric emergencies: An overview. *American Journal of Psychiatry, 137,* 1–9.

3. Bridge, J. A., Horowitz, L. M., et al. (2017). ED-SAFE—Can suicide risk screening and brief intervention initiated in the ED save lives? *JAMA Psychiatry, 74,* 555–556.

4. Lazarus, A., & Wachtel, P. (2007). Integrative and eclectic therapies. In Prochaska, J. O., & Norcross, J. C. (Eds.), *Systems of psychotherapy* (6th ed., pp. 474–506). Belmont, CA: Thomson Brooks/Cole.

5. Prochaska, J. O., & Norcross, J. C. (2007). Comparative conclusions towards a transtheoretical therapy. In Prochaska, J. O., & Norcross, J. C. (Eds.), *Systems of psychotherapy* (6th ed., pp. 507–539). Belmont, CA: Thomson Brooks/Cole.

6. Rosenberg, R., & Sulkowicz, K. (2002). Psychosocial interventions in the psychiatric emergency service. In Allen, M. H. (Ed.), *Emergency psychiatry* (pp. 151–183). Washington, DC: American Psychiatric Press.

7. Crits-Christoph, P., Beth, M., & Hearon, B. (2006). Does the alliance cause good outcome? Recommendations for future research on the alliance. *Psychotherapy: Theory, Research, Practice, Training, 43,* 280–285.

8. Brenner, C. (1979). Working alliance, therapeutic alliance and transference. *Journal of the American Psychoanalytic Association, 27*(Suppl.), 137–157.

9. Rosenberg, R. (1994). The therapeutic alliance and the psychiatric emergency room crisis as opportunity. *Psychiatric Annals, 24,* 610–614.

10. Bacal, R. (2005). *Perfect phrases for customer service.* New York, NY: McGraw Hill.

11. Stewart, M. (1995). Effective physician-patient communication outcomes: A review. *Canadian Medical Association Journal, 152,* 1423–1433.

12. Allen, M., Debanne, M., et al. (2001). Effect of nicotine replacement therapy on agitation in smokers with a double-blind, randomized, controlled study. *American Journal of Psychiatry, 168*(4), 395–399.

13. Young, B. (2006). The immediate response to disaster: Guidelines for adult psychological first aid. In Elspeth, C. R., Watson, T. P. J., & Friedman, M. J. (Eds.), *Interventions following mass violence and disasters* (pp. 134–154). New York, NY: Guilford Press.

14. Singer, T., Seymour, B., O'Doherty, J., Kaube, R., & Dolan, J. (2004). Empathy for pain involves the affective but not sensory components of pain. *Science, 303,* 1157–1162.

15. Ochsner, K. N. (2007). How thinking controls feeling. In Harmon-Jones, E., & Winkielman, P. (Eds.), *Social neuroscience.* New York, NY: Guilford Press.

16. Berlin, R., Olsen, M. E., et al. (1991). Metaphor and psychotherapy. *American Journal of Psychotherapy, 45*(3), 359–367.

17. Ilgen, M. A., Walton, M. A., Cunningham, R. M., et al. (2009). Recent suicidal ideation among patients in an inner city emergency department. *Suicide and Life-Threatening Behavior, 39,* 508–517.

18. Claassen, C. A., & Larkin, G. L. (2005). Occult suicidality in an emergency department population. *British Journal of Psychiatry, 186,* 352–353.

19. Feldman, G., Hayes, A., et al. (2006). Mindfulness and emotional regulation: The development and initial validation of the cognitive and affective mindfulness scale-revised (CAMS-R). *Journal of Psychopathology and Behavioral Assessment, 29,* 177–190.

20. Stanley, B., Brown, G. K., et al. (2018). Comparison of the safety planning intervention with follow-up vs usual care of suicidal patient treated in the emergency department. *JAMA Psychiatry, 75*(9), 894–900.

21. Tversky, A., & Kahneman, D. (1974). Judgment under uncertainty: Heuristics and biases. *Science, 185,* 1124–1130.

22. Baron, J. (Ed.). (2000). Chapter 7: Hypothesis testing. *Thinking and deciding* (3rd ed., pp. 162–164). New York: Cambridge University Press.

23. Kantor, M. (2004). *Understanding paranoia: A guide for professionals, families, and sufferers*. Westport, CT: Praeger.

24. Allen, M. H., Currier, G. W., Hughes, D. H., et al. (2001). The expert consensus guideline series: Treatment of behavioral emergencies. *Postgraduate Medicine,* (Special no), 1–88.

25. Link, B., Struening, E. L., Asmussen, S., & Phelan, J. C. (2001). The consequences of stigma for the self-esteem of people with mental illnesses. *Psychiatric Services, 52*, 1621–1626.

13

Principles of Emergency Psychopharmacology

Herbert J. Harman, Scott L. Zeller

The guiding principles by which emergency psychiatrists perform their craft are best described by the American Psychiatric Association's Task Force on Psychiatric Emergency Services. The task force defines an emergency "as a set of circumstances in which 1) the behavior or condition of an individual is perceived by someone, often not the identified individual, as having the potential to rapidly eventuate in a catastrophic outcome and 2) the resources available to understand and deal with the situation are not available at the time and place of the occurrence. Thus emergencies frequently involve a mismatch of needs and resources for which the emergency service must compensate" (1).

Emergency psychiatrists must draw on all their experience and skills they have developed to conduct a rapid assessment and formulate an effective treatment plan in a limited amount of time (2). The stakes are much higher in the emergency settings. Patients are in acute crisis, putting them and others at risk for severe adverse events, so delays can be invitations to bad outcomes.

The lens through which the emergency psychiatrist views risk must account for many unknowns while evaluating acute agitation, psychosis, suicidality, intoxication, and a host of possibly deteriorating comorbid medical problems, and thus it is different than the lens used in a typical clinic during a scheduled visit. As a result, the emergency clinician's approach to prescribing medications is differentiated from other clinical scenarios. This chapter explores the general mind-set of emergency psychopharmacology.

SPECIFIC AIMS

When a person comes to the emergency setting in crisis, the role of the emergency psychiatrist is to intervene and initiate treatment as quickly as possible. The main focus is safety, and staff must be proactive to ensure the well-being of the patients and those who may come into contact with them. Decreasing distressing symptomatology and calming agitation are primary interventions toward this goal.

Historically, severely agitated patients would routinely be restrained and given intramuscular (IM) medications against their will. However, there has been a paradigm shift in the treatment of such patients in the last decade (3). Now, techniques such as verbal de-escalation, compassionate and collaborative interactions, ensuring comfort with calming spaces and food or drink, and offering medications to be taken voluntarily are the standard of care for emergency psychiatry even with the most difficult of patients.

Past practice with medications frequently was to heavily sedate, or "snow," the patient. However, the complications of oversedation are numerous, including interfering with the patient's ability to participate in treatment through actions such as answering questions, hydrating themselves, or undergoing medical examinations and procedures. Oversedation hampers not only the psychiatric interview but also the medical evaluation, which thus might mask medical comorbidities (4).

In 2012 the Project BETA Psychopharmacology Workgroup published consensus statements and included the following idea: *"If an agitated patient is medicated too aggressively or too early, it may hinder psychiatric evaluation. If the patient is medicated too late, it places the patient, staff, and others at increased risk for harm. In addition, the agitation may also become more pronounced, and greater doses or repeated medication administration may be required to abort the agitation (5)."*

Important factors in selecting a medication include the desire for an immediate effect on symptoms with the intent of reducing the odds for dangerous behaviors, the patient's history of response to the medication, patient preference of medication, limited risk of side effects, and ease of administration (eg, no need for lab tests and simple dosing requirements) (6). It is tempting for many clinicians to oversedate patients, with the idea being a sleeping person does not cause much disruption or violence. Yet the advantages of having a calm, awake, and conversant patient outweigh those of having a patient who is unresponsive for several hours, which can delay the medical clearance and evaluation of the patient for an appropriate disposition. An overly sedated patient is unable to explain their history or any social problems they might have and cannot describe recent events or symptoms that might offer clues to their diagnoses. The pressures of overcrowded emergency facilities, with space and resources at a premium, no longer allow for unnecessarily obtunded patients to be occupying beds.

TIMELINESS OF MEDICATION ADMINISTRATION IN EMERGENCIES

Patients with agitation, psychosis, and/or acute anxiety may require medication to treat symptoms, to alleviate the patient's suffering, while ensuring the safety of the patient and others. A proper screening assessment includes a brief medical evaluation and mental status examination, review of available medical records, and consideration for known medical problems, allergies, and possible toxic syndromes. There is commonly not enough time to complete a comprehensive psychiatric examination or seek routine consultation before deciding to use emergency medication.

After efforts to use calming techniques, environmental change, verbal de-escalation (7), and show of force have failed to resolve acute agitation, when possible, the patient should be involved in decision-making regarding the specific medication to be used. If the patient declines, or the condition is such that they lack the capacity for decision-making, and there is evident imminent danger to life or limb, then intramuscular medication may be necessary. Federal, state, and local laws should be considered as decisions are being made to ensure the patient's civil rights are protected. Every effort should be made to describe to the patient the risks, benefits, side effects, and treatment alternatives to the use of medication. The reasons for the involuntary administration of medication must be documented clearly in the medical record to justify these actions.

MEDICATION CHOICES IN THE EMERGENCY DEPARTMENT SETTING

Route of Administration

There is a clear need for the use of both oral and parenteral medications in the emergency setting (5). This can give patients a choice and allows them some control in their own treatment. During what may be perceived as a very scary situation for a person in crisis, the opportunity to make this choice can help a patient feel more in control, reduce the patient's anxiety, and help foster trust and cooperation with the treating physician.

Rate of Onset of Action

Oral and Voluntarily Accepted Medications

When giving an oral medication in the ED, the most common choices for those in crisis are formulations that deliver the medication and treatment response as quickly as possible. Medications such as extended-release formulations are usually not a reasonable first choice in emergencies because they do not have as rapid an onset of symptom relief as the regular formulation of the drug. Similarly, medications that take several days or weeks to take full effect, such as antidepressants, are usually not given in emergency situations unless needed to halt discontinuation syndrome, although they may be started in the acute care venue when planning for longer-term care or inpatient admission.

Rapid-dissolving formulations of the atypical antipsychotic medications are absorbed more quickly, and thus achieve effective plasma concentrations more promptly, than the regular tablets (8). Because the increased absorption rate leads to earlier initiation of medication effects, these agents are especially useful in crisis cases.

Newer medication delivery systems such as inhaled agents, intranasal agents, and sublingual agents appear to combine a more immediate onset of action along with a voluntary, cooperative administration involving a willing patient (9). Although these agents as of this writing have not achieved widespread use and can be difficult to initiate because of such factors as cost, potential side effects, and cumbersome mitigation strategy requirements, there is nonetheless optimism these could play an important role in clinicians' formularies in the future.

Parenteral Medications

Intramuscular medications have a brisk onset of action and can be administered involuntarily, if needed, to treat acute agitation and address imminent danger. They should only be used in emergency situations unless the patient requests an injection rather than an oral dose. Several atypical antipsychotics are available in the IM formulation that can bring about speedy behavioral control in the agitated, out-of-control patient. This has given emergency psychiatrists more choices than the traditional option: injectable, high-potency conventional antipsychotics, which have possible adverse reactions such as acute dystonia and severe drops in blood pressure. In addition, coadministration of either an anticholinergic or a benzodiazepine, or both, may not be needed in conjunction with these newer medications.

Side-Effect Profile and Drug Interactions

Although time is often of the essence, this should not preclude considerations of prospective drug-drug interactions, the patient's health status, possible substance abuse, and potential side effects in choosing a medication. For example, many antipsychotic medications can lower the seizure threshold (10), so caution must be used with these in patients with a history of epilepsy or those who might be in alcohol withdrawal. It is important to know as much as possible of a patient's medical history, present drug regimen, allergies, and current physical condition when making decisions on administration of medications. In cases of agitation due to stimulant intoxication or alcohol withdrawal, oral or intramuscular benzodiazepines may be preferred to antipsychotic medications.

Clinicians should proceed only after carefully weighing the potential risks and benefits of the treatment choice.

MEDICATION CHOICES

Consensus guidelines have suggested that first-generation antipsychotics, second-generation antipsychotics, and benzodiazepines are the three classes of drugs to most strongly consider in the case of a patient needing treatment for acute agitation or agitated psychosis (5).

First-Generation Antipsychotics

First-generation antipsychotics, once the primary option, remain in use to treat agitation. Medications such as chlorpromazine have risk for lowering blood pressure and are known to lower the seizure threshold, so they are now used less often. The most commonly used first-generation antipsychotic is haloperidol. Haloperidol has more risk for extrapyramidal side effects, dystonic reactions (including laryngospasm, oculogyric crisis, and torticollis), akathisia, dysphoria, and QTc prolongation (which could lead to severe cardiac conditions and even death) than some newer medications (11). Not every patient responds to newer medications, and a good interview or review of health history might uncover cases of patients preferring haloperidol. Haloperidol might be the best choice for agitation related to alcohol intoxication but not alcohol withdrawal. The use of droperidol, also a first-generation antipsychotic, has fallen out of favor since the medication was given a black box warning for QTc prolongation despite there being concerns for the same problem in other medications, including haloperidol, in this same class.

Second-Generation Antipsychotics

Second-generation antipsychotics (such as ziprasidone, olanzapine, aripiprazole, risperidone) are used in emergency settings for calming patients in acute agitation and have become the treatment of choice for agitation due to psychosis. Some studies have found the incidents of extrapyramidal symptoms to be much less with second-generation drugs when compared to medications such as haloperidol (12). Medications such as ziprasidone, olanzapine, and aripiprazole have both oral and intramuscular delivery options. In modest doses, use of these medications may increase the odds that a patient will have agitation successfully treated without putting the patient to sleep. Compared to a traditional approach of giving a patient high doses of haloperidol, diphenhydramine, and lorazepam; giving a patient a single dose of a second-generation antipsychotic alone maintains the goal of quelling agitation while helping the patient retain their ability to communicate about their symptoms, discuss their health history, and share with their treatment team their wishes regarding the next steps in their care. One study did find there was some risk for oversedation when intramuscular olanzapine was given with intramuscular lorazepam (13). Clinicians should take caution when giving multiple medications with sedating effects and extra carefulness when both are given intramuscularly simultaneously or with very little time between each injection. Some medications, including olanzapine, can be given in a rapidly dissolving oral form. Rapidly dissolving medications are preferred in scenarios when patients are agreeable to treatment and exhibiting psychotic symptoms that might make it challenging for them to follow through with swallowing a standard pill.

Benzodiazepines

Patients with agitation due to alcohol intoxication and alcohol withdrawal are often best treated with benzodiazepines, unless the patient is severely intoxicated. In the case of serious alcohol intoxication, the patient should not be oversedated to the point of lowering their respiratory drive. If the patient has symptoms of psychosis from intoxication, an antipsychotic is preferable to a sedative. Other drugs of intoxication may respond to benzodiazepines as well. Patients with stimulant intoxication, from methamphetamines for instance, will respond best to treatment with benzodiazepines, allowing them an opportunity for sleep and time for detoxification, which often is all that is needed for resolution of transient symptoms.

NONEMERGENT MEDICATIONS

It is often the case that patients boarding in emergency departments will miss doses of medications while an evaluation is taking place, a treatment plan is being formulated, or the patient is waiting for transfer, discharge, or admission to an inpatient setting. Prescribing standing doses of home medications for regular administration during the boarding period can avoid a worsening of symptoms. Missing doses of the selective serotonin reuptake inhibitor (SSRI) and selective norepinephrine reuptake inhibitor (SNRI) class of drug can result in discontinuation syndrome. Medications with relatively short half-lives (paroxetine and venlafaxine for instance) can be more likely than others to lead to these problems. On the other hand, missing a dose of fluoxetine, which has an active metabolite with a half-life of 5 to 7 days, is not likely to create problems for the patient in the ED—but nonetheless, remaining on regular outpatient medication regimens can reassure patients that their regular daily medication practices are recognized and being met appropriately. Careful attention should be given to mood stabilizer and antiepileptic medication as patients will have better mood regulation if their medication is kept at a steady state.

It should be remembered that blood levels of medications such as valproate and carbamazepine will most likely not be trough values when drawn in the emergency department, and thus the physician should be observant for toxic levels as verified by clinical examination in congruence with serum levels. Additionally, nondetectable levels can offer clarity regarding compliance and further guide decision-making. Lithium, in particular, is sensitive to changes in hydration and electrolyte intake and output which are often in flux during a psychiatric disturbance. For patients known or suspected to be on lithium for mood stabilization, serum levels should be measured for patients in psychiatric crisis. The mood stabilizer lamotrigine should be continued for patients known to be consistently taking the medication, but caution should be exercised for patients who may have stopped taking lamotrigine, since a rapid change in serum levels of lamotrigine correlates with an increased risk for Stevens-Johnson syndrome (14).

TREATING ACUTE PSYCHOSIS

It is common for clinicians to suggest that acute psychosis is best treated with drugs known to cause sedation, or even worse, using medication as a "chemical restraint" (defined as "a drug or medication, or a combination, when it is used as a restriction to manage the patient's behavior, restrict the patient's freedom of movement, or to impair the patient's ability to appropriately interact with their surroundings – and is not standard treatment or dosage for the patient's condition.") (12). Despite the historic assumption that psychosis will definitely take many weeks to respond to antipsychotic medication, there are studies showing the benefits of directly treating the positive symptoms of psychosis (hallucinations, paranoid, disorganized thoughts) with antipsychotic medication in the emergency department itself. In fact, it is possible to see a reduction in these symptoms in as little as 2 hours in the emergency setting (13). When a patient's symptoms of psychosis are reduced, their capacity to engage in a meaningful interview may improve, and alternative disposition options such as crisis residential, partial hospitalization, or even a return to home with follow-up at their established outpatient provider can then be considered. A thoughtful emergency psychiatrist is carefully weighing the importance of treating psychosis and at the same time trying to avoid oversedation which might render the patient unable to participate in their own care through shared decision-making.

USING MEDICATIONS IN THE MEDICATION-NAIVE PATIENT

The emergency psychiatrist will often be faced with the challenge of treating patients who have no evident history of receiving psychiatric medications. It may be difficult to ascertain if a patient is truly "medication naïve," as a subset of chronic patients may deny previous experience with psychotropics, especially if they also report no past history of mental illness, hospitalizations, drug abuse, or suicide attempts. To clarify whether a patient has taken medications in the past may require gathering as extensive a collateral history as possible. Although this can be very time consuming and difficult, it is time well spent if a report from a reliable source can be obtained.

If a patient is truly naïve to psychiatric medications, then this factor must be taken into consideration—along with factors such as age and body habitus—before choosing a specific agent and its dosage. Though the general recommendation is to aggressively medicate patients in psychiatric emergencies, in the medication naïve, it is

prudent to start with lower doses when possible. Medication-naïve patients might respond to doses that patients with a long history of treatment might not, and cautious dosing reduces the risk of untoward side effects.

New-onset symptoms of psychosis or agitation may be from several causes, not just primary psychiatric illnesses such as schizophrenia. Because of this, in the initial evaluation period, it may be sensible to avoid antipsychotic medications with their potential for severe side effects, as they may end up being unnecessary if the symptoms resolve without neuroleptic administration. Mild and relatively safe, benzodiazepines can be a good first choice in these cases. If the symptoms of the psychosis were due to substance intoxication, postictal state, withdrawal phenomenon, or other organic conditions, a fast-acting benzodiazepine such as lorazepam may allow the patient rest and time to improve. If the patient does not improve after rest and promoting sleep, and the patient experiencing a reduction in anxiety and agitation from a benzodiazepine, then the case for psychosis from a primary psychiatric illness is stronger and antipsychotic medication should be considered.

Preventing unpleasant medication experiences can assist in developing a more positive therapeutic alliance for new-to-medication patients, which may result in better long-term outcomes and future treatment compliance (15).

BALANCING RISK: SIDE EFFECTS VERSUS THE NEED FOR IMMEDIATE TREATMENT

Whether in the acute or nonacute setting, psychiatrists must weigh the risks against the benefits of any potential treatment. This involves judging the usefulness of a particular medication, which can be broken down into three aspects: 1) efficacy, 2) tolerability and safety, and 3) adherence and persistence. Research has suggested that an urgent care strategy should be selected when the priority is immediate efficacy, whereas a sequential strategy should be selected when the priority is tolerability (5).

For the emergency psychiatrist, efficacy is the primary consideration when choosing a medication. Side effects which develop over a longer time course—such as weight gain or increases in glucose levels—are not a primary concern for the emergency psychiatrist. In treating patients in immediate need of behavioral symptom control, physicians should use their own clinical judgment and acumen in deciding which agent would be most efficacious.

Unfortunately, owing to overcrowding and limited resources, emergency psychiatrists may often treat a patient for up to several days before an inpatient bed can be procured (16). Once a patient is awaiting admission, the emergency psychiatrist should start a regular medication schedule with the long term in mind; often, the inpatient psychiatrist will continue this regimen if there was a good initial response. In these circumstances, the second criteria, tolerability and safety, becomes a concern along with efficacy. This is when the longer-term adverse effects such as metabolic concerns enter into the process of selecting an agent.

The third aspect of treatment effectiveness, persistence and adherence, is often why patients return to the emergency department—because of noncompliance with medications, leading to relapse of symptoms. There are several factors that can lead to noncompliance or discontinuation of treatment by patients. The CATIE study phases I (17) and II (18) investigated these phenomena and found that more patients discontinued their medications because of a lack of efficacy than to intolerability. Taking this into consideration, although side effects are very important to consider in selecting an agent, the primary concerns for emergency psychiatrists are efficacy and compliance—to help patients become well, encourage recovery, maintain stability, and thus hopefully prevent symptom relapse, which will reduce the chances of a return visit to the emergency department.

WORKING WITHIN A LIMITED FORMULARY

Limited formularies can be a challenging situation in any of the multiple treatment settings of psychiatry but is especially so in the emergency setting, where having all available agents in the armamentarium is very useful. As patients in emergency settings are frequently in urgent need of medications, having to substitute one medication for another can

involve risk. Although a patient may have done well in the past on a specific unavailable medicine, even the closest replacement might be ineffective or cause side effects.

When faced with formulary restrictions, the safest and most logical substitutions should be considered. For example, an unavailable atypical antipsychotic should be replaced with a different atypical rather than commencing a first-generation neuroleptic.

Economic reasons are usually at the root of limited formularies. If an agent is older and seldom needed, the cost of stocking the medication might not justify its availability for such infrequent use. On the other hand, widely used and effective newer medications might at the same time be quite expensive, which might make a pharmacy committee reluctant to add them. In the latter case, the emergency psychiatrist might wish to provide data to the formulary committee showing that a certain medication can be justified as cost-effective, due to favorable outcomes, and no comparable agent is currently on hand to substitute. Often formulary committees might be willing to conduct a limited trial of newer medications, during which time, the usefulness of the medication in emergency settings can be demonstrated.

Even if a particular medication is available in the hospital or clinic formulary, it might not be advisable to prescribe the agent if it is not on the patient's outpatient provider formulary. There is little to be gained by starting a patient on a medication which will be unobtainable—or obtainable only at steep cost—after discharge. Such financial issues could lead to patient nonadherence (19). It is thus practical for the emergency psychiatrist to have a working knowledge of the major outpatient provider formularies in their area.

TO PRESCRIBE AN OUTPATIENT SUPPLY OF MEDICATION OR NOT: THE EMERGENCY PSYCHIATRIST'S QUESTION

Owing to the shortage of access to psychiatrists in the United States, there can be a long wait between the time of discharge from an emergency setting and the first appointment with an outpatient psychiatrist. Wait times for appointments are often many weeks (12).

The period after discharge from a hospital or emergency department is a significantly high-risk phase for many patients. Whether they are returning to their own psychiatrist or hoping to start with a new one, care must be taken to do as much as possible to bridge the gap successfully. It is common for many psychiatrists to be reluctant to prescribe for a patient they may never see again, but prescribing at discharge may be the key to maintaining stability between emergency and outpatient care.

Medications at Discharge

Antidepressant medications are not commonly initiated in emergency settings. The beneficial effects of antidepressant medications can take weeks and sometimes months to be realized. Additionally, when starting treatment, patients are at increased risk for developing side effects from antidepressant medications, and it is best for patients with depression to have a physician in the community to offer continuity of care. Typically, patients are referred to their primary care doctor and to a psychiatrist when a patient should be considered for starting psychotropic medication long term.

Some medications used in the emergency setting to treat acute symptoms, such as benzodiazepines for anxiety and antipsychotics for agitation or psychosis, may be continued from the emergency department for a short period of time—after confirming that the patient has supports in the community and the possibility of close follow-up with a physician. Physicians should consider collaborating with social workers, clinical navigators, case managers, or similar professionals when securing follow-up.

Occasionally patients present to the emergency department seeking "refills" to ensure they do not run out of medication and have a relapse or recurrence of symptoms. The safety and utility of writing a prescription for refills should be considered on a case-by-case basis, and patients should be encouraged to obtain refills from their outpatient provider rather than inappropriately relying on the emergency department for this. Antidepressants, antipsychotics, and mood stabilizers with discontinuation syndromes can be prescribed to help patients avoid suffering and possibly worsening of depression, mood

instability, anxiety, or agitation. Although benzodiazepines can be drugs of abuse and are perceived as somewhat risky to prescribe from the emergency setting, a short supply of benzodiazepines may be necessary to help patients prevent withdrawal symptoms such as severe anxiety and seizures.

ADDITIONAL IMPORTANT ASPECTS OF EMERGENCY PSYCHOPHARMACOLOGY

Psychoeducation: The encounter in the emergency setting may be a patient's first introduction to the mental health system—but could also be the last, depending on the experience. The patient should be educated about their condition, the medication prescribed, the possible side effects of that medication, and treatment alternatives (including no medication) should be offered and discussed. If permission is given and time permits, the family, caregivers, and/or significant others should also be educated. This will help to increase the patient confidence in the treatment plan, by giving patients more support and understanding through important persons in their lives.

Patient reliability: This is assessed during the patient's evaluation and will help with the psychiatrist's decision-making process. Will the medication prescribed be taken appropriately and will the patient follow up with an outpatient psychiatrist, or instead return to the emergency department when the medications run out? It is easier to prescribe with confidence to a patient who appears reliable and involved in the care planning.

Aftercare: With the assistance of a social worker or a case manager, a good follow-up plan can be devised to improve the chances that the patient has enough support on the outside to help them receive the appropriate resources and prevent any adverse outcomes. When solid aftercare is in place, a clinician should also feel more assured about providing discharge prescriptions.

SUMMARY

The use of pharmacotherapy in the emergency setting is best understood as one important piece of the complete approach to managing acute symptoms, with effective communication and active listening being the first line of treatment. A rapid assessment to rule out emergency medical conditions other than psychiatric afflictions and an effort at understanding patients' current and past medical history are both indicated. Medication choices should be made with the goal of speedy improvement, but attempts should be made to minimize side effects and drug interactions. Understanding the realities of economic constraints and lack of access to timely care can also drive decision-making. The goal of the treatment plan should be to decrease the suffering of the patient, to preserve the patient's dignity, to resolve acute and severe symptoms, and to ensure the immediate safety of the patient, the staff, and the community in the process. Ultimately, emergency psychiatrists play pivotal roles in acute care but should always prescribe with an eye toward the long-term benefit of their patients.

REFERENCES

1. Allen, M., Forster, P., Zealberg, J., & Currier, G., for the APA Task Force on Psychiatric Emergency Services. (2002). *Report and recommendations regarding psychiatric emergency and crisis services*. Washington, DC: American Psychiatric Association.
2. Zeller, S. L. (2010). Treatment of psychiatric patients in emergency settings. *Primary Psychiatry, 17*, 35–41.
3. Holloman, G. H., Jr., & Zeller, S. L. (2012). Overview of project BETA: Best practices in evaluation and treatment of agitation. *The Western Journal of Emergency Medicine, 13*(1), 1–2.
4. Battaglia, J., Lindborg, S., Alaka, K., et al. (2003). Calming versus sedative effects of intramuscular olanzapine in agitated patients. *American Journal of Emergency Medicine, 21*(3), 192–198.
5. Wilson, M. P., Pepper, D., Currier, G. W., Holloman, G. H., Jr., & Feifel, D. (2012). The psychopharmacology of agitation: Consensus statement of the American Association for Emergency Psychiatry Project BETA Psychopharmacology Workgroup. *The Western Journal of Emergency Medicine, 13*(1), 26–34. Retrieved from https://www.ncbi.nlm.nih.gov/pmc/articles/PMC3298219/.
6. Allen, M. H., et al. (2005). The expert consensus guidelines series: Treatment of behavioral emergencies 2005. *Journal of Psychiatric Practice, 11*(Suppl. 1), 5–108.
7. Richmond, J. S., Berlin, J. S., Fishkind, A. B., Holloman, G. H., Jr., Zeller, S. L., Wilson, M. P., Rifai, M. A., Ng, A. T. (2012). Verbal de-escalation of the agitated patient: Consensus statement of the American Association for Emergency Psychiatry Project BETA De-escalation Workgroup. *The Western Journal of Emergency Medicine, 13*(1), 17–25. Retrieved from https://www.ncbi.nlm.nih.gov/pmc/articles/PMC3298202/.
8. Bartko, G. (2006). New formulations of olanzapine in the treatment of acute agitation. *Neuropsychopharmacologia Hungarica, 8*(4), 171–178.
9. Zeller, S. L., & Citrome, L. (2016). Managing agitation associated with schizophrenia and bipolar disorder in the emergency setting. *The Western Journal of Emergency Medicine, 17*(2), 165 172.
10. Alper, K., Schwartz, K. A., Kolts, R. L., et al. (2007). Seizure incidence in psychopharmacological clinical trials: An analysis of Food and Drug Administration (FDA) summary basis of approval reports. *Biological Psychiatry, 62*(4), 345–354.
11. US Food and Drug Administration. Information for healthcare professionals: Haloperidol (marketed as Haldol, Haldol Decanoate and Haldol Lactate). Retrieved September 28, 2019, from http://www.fda.gov/Drugs/DrugSafety/PostmarketDrugSafetyInformationforPatientsandProviders/DrugSafetyInformationforHeathcareProfessionals/ucm085203.htm.
12. Longtin, Y., Sax, H., Leape, L. L., Sheridan, S. E., Donaldson, L., & Pittet, D. (2010). Patient participation: Current knowledge and applicability to patient safety. *Mayo Clinic Proceedings, 85*, 53–62.
13. Kapur, S., Arenovich, T., Agid, O., Zipursky, R., Lindborg, S., & Jones, B. (2005). Evidence for onset of antipsychotic effects within the first 24 hours of treatment. *American Journal of Psychiatry, 162*(5), 939–946.
14. Parveen, S., & Javed, M. A. (2013). Stevens Johnson syndrome associated with Lamotrigine. *Pakistan Journal of Medical Sciences, 29*(6), 1450–1452.
15. Correll, C. U., & Schenk, E. M. (2008). Tardive dyskinesia and new antipsychotics. *Current Opinion in Psychiatry, 21*, 151–156.
16. Wilson, M. P., MacDonald, K., Vilke, G. M., et al. (2012). Potential complications of combining intramuscular olanzapine with benzodiazepines in agitated emergency department patients. *The Journal of Emergency Medicine, 43*(5), 889–896.

17. Lieberman, J. A., Stroup, T. S., McEvoy, J. P., et al., for the Clinical Antipsychotic Trials of Intervention Effectiveness (CATIE) Investigators. (2005). Effectiveness of antipsychotic drugs in patients with chronic schizophrenia. *The New England Journal of Medicine, 353,* 1209–1223.

18. McEvoy, J. P., Lieberman, J. A., Stroup, T. S., Davis, S. M., Meltzer, H. Y., Rosenheck, R. A., Swartz, M. S., Perkins, D. O., Keefe, R. S. E., Davis, C. E., Severe, J., Hsiao, J. K., for the CATIE Investigators. (2006). Effectiveness of clozapine versus olanzapine, quetiapine, and risperidone in patients with chronic schizophrenia who did not respond to prior atypical antipsychotic treatment. *The American Journal of Psychiatry, 163,* 600–610.

19. Dolder, C. R., Lacro, J. P., Dunn, L. B., & Jeste, D. V. (2002). Antipsychotic medication adherence: Is there a difference between typical and atypical agents? *The American Journal of Psychiatry, 159*(1), 103–108.

14

Engaging the Crisis Patient in Medication Decisions

Ronald J. Diamond

Most people in crisis feel chaotic and out of control. Often there is a complicated admixture of other feelings as well. Feeling anxious, frightened, or angry is common. Frustration, a sense of desperation, and embarrassment are part of the mix. The goal of crisis intervention is to help the person[1] reestablish control, cope more effectively with whatever is happening, and manage risk. The role of medication in a crisis situation is to support this reestablishment of control and support the person's own coping mechanism. Most people in crisis want to get back in control, feel better, and have a way to handle the overwhelming situation that led to the crisis. A person is likely to accept the use of medication if it is perceived as something that will help accomplish these goals. The use of medication will be fought if it is perceived as one more way of having control taken away. At times a person is so out of control that he or she needs to "be medicated." Even in this extreme situation and even when the circumstances of the crisis require that medication be forced, the goal is to move to a more collaborative approach to both the resolution of the crisis and the use of medication. This chapter is about engaging clients in a collaborative decision about the use of medication to help stabilize the crisis situation. Although this work has been strongly influenced by the growing literature on recovery and motivational interviewing, it is based on my own experience over the past 40 years (1).

---

[1]Both the term "patient" and "person" are used in this chapter. A person experiences a crisis and assumes the role of the patient as he or she comes into an emergency department seeking help. As professionals, we are in the role of helping patients, without ever forgetting that they are first of all people.

ENGAGING THE CRISIS PATIENT AROUND MEDICATION STARTS WITH THE ENGAGEMENT, NOT THE MEDICATION

Chapters on the use of medications in a crisis usually start with a discussion about when medication is needed, what medication to use, and how it can be used to decrease agitation (2,3). That is, the discussion typically starts from the professional view of both the problem and the range of possible solutions. The problem from the clinician's point of view is the patient's agitation and irrationality, and medication is a readily available solution to this problem. Engaging crisis patients around issues of medication requires that we start with a collaborative process of engagement rather than starting with the medication. Engagement requires that we start with the patient's own experience. Solutions, as much as possible, should relate back to that experience. Often the most useful question in the initial assessment and calming of an agitated patient is "how can we help you?" (4) Engagement is a two-sided process. It requires collaboration between the patient and the clinician. Engagement does not begin with the expectation that the patient will understand the clinician's point of view; it begins with the clinician's willingness to understand the patient's point of view (5).

Start From the Patient's Point of View

Think about the experience of most patients who are brought into emergency departments (EDs). How would you feel if you were brought to the hospital ED?

> Your parent, partner, friend, or a stranger has become upset by some part of your behavior and called the police. The police picked you

up even though you were not breaking any laws, and you have spent the last 2 hours in the hospital ED in handcuffs. You have not been allowed to smoke, or call anyone, or go to the bathroom by yourself, or given anything to eat. Your own clothes have been taken away and you are in a hospital gown. You have demanded to be able to call a lawyer, but everyone around explains that you are not being arrested and that no lawyer is needed.

A person in crisis is often feeling frightened, confused, angry, frustrated, and embarrassed. Nurses and doctors and social workers try to placate him or her, but it is obvious that no one is really listening, and certainly no one really believes the patient's account of what has happened. As time passes and no one believes what the patient "knows" to be the real situation, he or she may become increasingly desperate.

Think about how yosu would feel if your home had been ransacked by a burglar and a large amount of money had been stolen. When you called the police they came and looked around, but obviously did not believe your story, even though you knew it to be true. You point out evidence of the burglary; locks that had been broken or jewelry that you knew had been in the apartment but were now missing. The more you tried to explain this to the police, the more it seemed they did not believe you. You tried calling a friend or family member to explain what had happened, but they too seemed to just be placating you and refused to believe that anyone had broken in or that the money had been stolen. As you continued to try to convince the police (perhaps getting a bit frustrated and angry in the process), they suggest that perhaps you should let them take you to the hospital so that you could talk to a doctor about why you are so upset.

Of course it is not always this difficult. Not all patients are brought in by police against their will, not all patients are psychotic, and treatment staff may well believe the patient's experience. Often a patient will feel relieved that help is now available. Engagement is easy when there is agreement on the nature of the problem and agreement on the nature of possible solutions.

Engagement is much more difficult, and more important, when there are very different views of the problem and the possible solutions. Even when the patient is cooperative and rational, it is the clinicians who have the last word in defining the problem. Clinicians decide whether the problem is caused by the patient or by some outside stress. Clinicians decide whether the patient is seeing the world accurately or is misrepresenting the world in some major way. Clinicians decide whether the patient's view of the problem is, itself, the problem. It is the clinician who "decides" that the patient is psychotic or not. Even very rational, nonpsychotic patients are aware of the power that the clinicians have in labeling the nature of the presenting problem.

Not only do clinicians define the nature of the problem, clinicians also decide on the kind of solutions that are "most appropriate." For example, a patient may believe that the problem is that someone has broken into his apartment and stolen things, whereas the crisis staff may feel that this is a false belief that is part of a delusion. The patient wants the police to investigate, and the crisis worker feels that the patient should start taking antipsychotic medication. In most crisis situations, even with a cooperative patient, clinicians are the final arbiter of the nature of the problem and the nature of the appropriate solution. Patients' own views are considered, but it is the clinician's final belief that is held most accurate and definitive.

THERE IS A POTENTIAL CONFLICT BETWEEN THE NATURE OF CRISIS AND THE NATURE OF COLLABORATION

A crisis is often a very difficult time to develop a collaborative relationship. Time is short, there is pressure to act rapidly, anxiety is high, and the patient and clinicians typically have no previous relationship. Crisis clinicians are focused on ensuring the physical safety of both patients and staff. Crisis intervention and collaboration often seem to be in conflict with each other, and it is often difficult for crisis staff to know how to do both at the same time. Within this context, it is easy to see medication as the solution to reestablish control and to see engagement as a luxury that can be put off until later after the immediate crisis has stabilized. Medication is available as the "trump card" that clinicians can use as necessary if the relationship is not going well. Both clinicians and patients are aware that "medicating the patient" is always an available option. Both clinicians and patients are aware that in the final analysis, clinicians have the power to exert their will and their solutions on patients, and this asymmetry of power is an inherent part of the relationship between the crisis staff and the crisis patient.

Effective engagement requires collaboration. The term "crisis" comes from Greek krisis, literally, decision, from krinein *to decide*. Crisis, by definition, is chaotic, unstable, and requires rapid decision-making. It is inherently unpredictable. Needs, capacities, and goals are constantly changing.

Collaboration comes from the Latin *com-* + *laborare* to labor—to work jointly with others or together especially in an intellectual endeavor. A decision made in collaboration between patient and clinician working together may, initially at least, take more time than a decision made by just the clinician. It is sometimes felt that the time and trust requirements for effective collaboration are not readily compatible with the need to impose a structure to rapidly organize and resolve a chaos. Actually, collaboration can help crisis resolution (6). The conflict between crisis and collaboration is more often an issue of perception than of necessity. In most situations it is possible to carve out the time and structure for at least some level of collaboration to take place. In rare cases, this is not possible and the immediate need to ensure safety must take precedence over other issues. There is a dynamic tension between the need for safety, the time constraints of a crisis service, the need to impose order and structure, and the need to engage the patient and begin the process of collaboration. Engagement is critically important but so too is establishing safety and decreasing the sense of chaos. It is the process of balancing these issues that lies at the art of crisis intervention. Too often, the importance of collaboration and engagement is considered less important in the immediacy of the crisis situation.

GOALS FOR CRISIS INTERVENTION

There are three primary goals for crisis intervention:

I. The first goal must be to contain the risk of immediate harm (7). It is always possible to medicate a patient into submission, and in some cases rapid pharmacological control may be required. More often, risk containment requires working with the patient to help him or her calm down. Although medication can be helpful, having someone take you seriously and listen to your version of your own story can be extremely validating, as can the experience of having someone really on your side. Patients are often agitated because they are afraid, confused, overwhelmed, and alone. Patients will very often calm down if they feel some sense of hope, and a sense that they are not alone. This is not accomplished by talking "at" the patient; it is accomplished by listening with the patient. Patients often feel very out of control and usually would like to be more "in control." Medication can be something that is "done to" the patient or a tool that the patient can use to help reestablish control over him or herself. When medication is imposed, it can increase the patient's sense that he or she is out of control. Even when medication needs to be imposed over the patient's objection, it can be framed as something that will help the patient get back in control. Collaboration can be encouraged even when some part of the treatment may be involuntary.

It is also important to manage the postcrisis risk. It is not possible to eliminate all risk. Not all risk can be predicted. Not everyone who is angry or threatening or feeling somewhat suicidal can be or should be hospitalized, and although hospitalization may decrease the immediate risk, it can exacerbate long-term risk in some situations. Risk assessment requires that the patient be willing to share his or her thinking, and this requires some degree of trust and collaboration. How the initial phase of crisis intervention handled can significantly increase the quality of the postcrisis risk assessment.

II. The second goal is to help resolve the crisis. This typically involves helping to replace the chaos and loss of control of the crisis situation with a sense of order and direction. Crisis resolution requires some understanding of the cause of the crisis, putting the crisis into the larger context of the patient's life, and coming up with a plan for how the patient and staff can resolve the crisis. Crisis resolution is much more than just sedating or placating the patient. It is helping the person reestablish control over his or her own behavior. This is much more likely when the person in crisis can partner with the crisis clinician. It is more difficult if the patient feels he or she must reestablish this control alone, without any outside help. Help in this sense requires collaboration. Collaboration requires working together toward some common goals. It is difficult to imagine working together if there are no goals with at least areas of overlap.

III. The third goal is to use the crisis to support postcrisis recovery. The goal is not only to resolve the immediate situation but also to help avoid similar crisis events in the future. Even more may be possible. By definition, a crisis period is a period of flux and change that is both a time of opportunity as well as a time of risk. The period of crisis can often lead to permanent change. The goal is to use the crisis intervention to make this change positive rather than negative. Crisis staff and ED staff should understand that their intervention at the moment of crisis can make the patient's ongoing quality of life better or worse. Attending to the immediate crisis alone is not enough. The long-term consequences of the crisis treatment should always be considered.

Collaboration is required for all three of these goals. Trust and communication is required to partner with a person. Collaboration is required to conduct an optimal risk assessment. And collaboration is critical to increase the likelihood that the crisis period will lead to permanent improvement. Crisis resolution is not something that can be "done to" the patient; it is a process that must be done with the patient. Medication can help a person calm down, communicate more clearly, and feel better. Medication can help a person enter into a collaborative relationship with the clinician. Medication can also interfere with this collaboration.

A COLLABORATIVE APPROACH TO CRISIS RESOLUTION

Engaging patients around medication requires engaging patients in the entire process of crisis resolution. There are four parts of a collaborative approach to crisis resolution:
1. Plan for the crisis before the crisis occurs
2. Use the person's telling of the crisis story as a way to organize the chaos of the crisis
3. Look for small areas of collaboration, even in the midst of the crisis
4. Consider the long-term consequences of all parts of the crisis treatment

Plan for Crisis Before the Crisis

It is often thought that the crisis begins when the patient presents in the ED or psychiatric emergency service or begins the escalation that leads to the need for emergency treatment. The reality is that the vast majority of people who have a mental health crisis have had a similar crisis before and are at high risk for having one again. Most people now in crisis have a chronic or at least a relapsing illness. In the midst of the crisis, it may be very difficult to have a rational discussion about what led to the crisis and what the person thinks would work as a solution. Planning ahead is much more effective and is generally welcomed by people when they are not in crisis.

Involving a person in developing a written plan for the next crisis can help ward off the crisis before it ever begins, can help to empower the person, and can keep the person more involved if a crisis does ensue. The patient should have his or her own copy, and it can be filed in the chart of the crisis service or ED so it is available when needed. Knowing the person's own preferences and what the person thinks will work is likely to lead to much more effective solutions to the crisis. A number of structured approaches to crisis planning have been developed, most of them from a strong consumer-centric point of view. The best-known structured approach to collaborative crisis planning is the WRAP: Wellness Recovery Action Plan approach developed by Mary Ellen Copeland (8). This is manualized, practical, and very user-friendly for both the patient and clinician.

A WRAP plan, like other effective collaborative crisis planning tools, needs to be developed by, or at least with the strong input from, the person who will be using it. It is designed to keep the person in crisis in the active role and keeping his or her preferences in the forefront at a time when it may not be able to easily express those preferences. Ideally, it is a written "contract" that is signed by the person who may be in crisis in the future, along with the person's clinician and other members of the person's support system. It includes a "toolbox" that includes:

• Daily maintenance activities that maintain wellness and help avoid crisis
• Personal triggers the increase risk of crisis
• Early warning signs that a crisis is impending
• Signs that things have gotten worse, when you can still do something about it

A WRAP plan then goes on to plan how to cope with a crisis if one ensues. This is based on the person's preferences, but is much more effective if the ongoing clinician can agree and both "sign on." For example, a typical WRAP plans includes:

• Whom to involve in a crisis
• What medication helps, and what does not
• When should the hospital be used
• What other options should be considered during the crisis

A typical WRAP plan gets even more detailed than just this bare structure. WRAP plans often include "scripts" of how the clinician or family should approach the person in crisis, interventions that the person has agreed to accept, and other, negative interventions that the person has clearly specified as not helpful or not acceptable. Going to hospital A may be unacceptable, but hospital B may be much more acceptable if needed, and staff have agreed in the event of a crisis to try and arrange to use hospital B. Going to stay with parents may be unacceptable, but spending a few days with a sibling in the event of a difficult time might be seen as a good option as a way to head off a crisis before things get out of control.

Another part of a WRAP plan includes specifying, ahead of time, what helps, and what does not. Writing in a journal may help; being alone in one's own apartment may make things worse. Watching TV with someone else may help, being touched may not. Patient, family, friends, and clinician can all decide who is willing to do what, what helps, and what does not. This often leads to much better solutions than would be the case at 3 o'clock in the morning in the midst of a crisis that makes problem solving difficult.

The use of medication becomes one part of a WRAP plan. A person may agree that he or she hates medication but acknowledge that it helps. As part of a WRAP plan, the person may agree to take an extra dose of a medication for a few days or a few weeks or agree to use one medication but not another. Although there is no legal way to enforce such an agreement, having worked it out with the person's own agreement makes it much more likely to be accepted when needed. A WRAP plan is most likely to be effective when medication is not the only kind of help offered and not the only issue that staff is willing to discuss.

Not all crisis contracts need to be as elaborate as a WRAP plan:

Seth is a man with a history of four manic episodes. In his first episode, he accidently set a fire and came very close to going to jail. In his most recent episode, he borrowed more than $10,000 from various credit cards to capitalize a new business idea. The idea was a good one and could possibly have worked, but as he became more grandiose, the initial business plan became too large, grandiose, and expensive to be viable. By the end of the episode, he was left with significant debt. His mood is now stable, but he is very concerned that he keeps having to start his life over every time he has an episode.

He has drawn up a written contract that specified that for a 4-week period he will accept an increase of both his antipsychotic and mood-stabilizing medication if both his psychiatrist and his mother agree that this is necessary. The contract states that he will go along with this, even if at the time he feels it is unnecessary and even if he feels it would be counterproductive. He, his mother, and his psychiatrist have all signed it as well, and each has a copy.

He, his mother, and his psychiatrist all realize that there is no legal standing to such a contract, but it can hold enough moral sway to help ensure that medication is a useful tool right when it is needed the most.

Use the Person's Telling of the Crisis Story as a Way to Organize the Chaos of the Crisis

Crisis, by definition, is a place of chaos and uncertainty. There is concern about physical risk. The unpredictability of crisis means that there is a risk that something bad could happen at any time. Staff are legitimately concerned about what the patient could do, and the person in turn is often very concerned about what the staff will do. Will the patient hit someone, storm off, pull out a weapon? Will the staff tie the person down, force him into the hospital, call police, or force him to take medication that will cause him to lose control of what is happening? The chaos and anxiety affect both sides of this interface. There is sometimes the sense that the immediate use of medication is needed to ensure safety and reestablish order.

Medication is rarely an effective way to establish immediate control of a situation when the person is physically out of control. If someone is assaultive or throws things around in the ED, the first priority must be to establish physical control. Even injectable medication will not work fast enough to provide immediate physical safety for a person physically out of control. In this kind of extreme situation, physical restraint may be required. Once there is physical containment, the immediate risk is over. The person may continue to yell or be agitated, but once the person is in restraints, there is no longer any immediate physical risk. This period of safety allows for at least a brief pause while the clinician can try to empathize with and validate the feelings of the crisis patient before immediately imposing medication. Trying to tell an angry, agitated person what he or she needs to do is unlikely to be helpful. For example, telling a patient "you need to calm down and stop yelling" is likely to provoke more of the same. What is more likely to help is to validate the person's feeling and actively listen to the person's story. For example, an invitation such as "It must

feel terrible to be dragged into this place by the police. What happened?" is much more likely to start a conversation.

If physical control is not lost, then verbal de-escalation can help the person calm down. Encouraging the person to tell his or her own story along a chronological timeline helps provide a sense of order, decrease anxiety, and increase a sense of personal control (9). Even a person who is angry and uncooperative, even a patient in restraints, will often be willing to tell his or her own story if allowed to do it his or her own way. What does the person think about the crisis? Who does the person think is involved? How does the person think the crisis developed? Try to establish a behaviorally specific description of events. How did it begin, and then what happened next, and what after that? Look for gaps and assumptions.

Collecting this organized history helps to organize the chaos of the crisis. It also provides information about what the person wants, and what the person in crisis is most afraid of. It provides a sense of how the person sees the problem that has led to the crisis. Too often medication is something that is "done to" the patient, to force the person to be calm. At times this may be necessary, but medication is more likely to be useful, both in the short term of the crisis resolution periods and longer term during follow-up care, if medication is thought of as a tool that the person can use to reestablish control over him or herself. This means not rushing into the use of medication as the way to start the dialogue and force calmness but rather to find specific problems that the person agrees might be helped by the use of medication.

There are, of course, some crisis situations where a person is so upset or out of control that it is difficult to have any kind of verbal dialogue until some sedation is in place. Even when medication seems needed, the purpose is to help the upset person have enough control so that dialogue can take place. Crisis resolution is not just sedating a person into submission. Effective crisis resolution involves finding ways to help the person reorganize and cope with the events that led to the crisis in some different and more effective way. Medication may have a role as a tool to this process, but it is not itself the solution to the crisis.

Look for Small Areas of Collaboration, Even in the Midst of the Crisis

The goal for crisis resolution is to help the patient reestablish control of him or her. There is a need to minimize risk of harm while the person is still out of control and some coercion may at times be needed. The goal is NOT to "win." The goal is not to get the patient to do it "our way" or just accept our treatment. The goal is to do as much as possible the patient's way (10).

What does the person want? Everyone in crisis wants something. He wants to go home, or get a smoke, or have something to eat, or call his girlfriend. He wants the world to calm down and for you to stop asking him dumb questions. There is always something that the patient wants.

Of all of the things that the person wants, what can you help him or her obtain? It may not be possible to let the person leave the ED, but it may be possible to get him some food or something to drink or make a phone call. Focus on what you can help with and acknowledge those things you cannot help with.

Start first, and then invite the person in crisis to follow. Too often, we start by requiring the patient to change first, to calm down, or become rational, before we are willing to change. What can we do/give/say to demonstrate good faith?

A young woman was brought into the ED by police after having been found wandering outside not making any sense. When police tried to talk with her, she became increasingly agitated, and by the time of her admission, she was in handcuffs and then placed in four-point restraint because of her incessant attempts to grab or punch anyone within range. When I saw her, she was furious and refused to answer any questions even her name. I empathized with her predicament and shared how frustrating, embarrassing, and defenseless it must be to be strapped down the way she was. She demanded to be let out of restraints, which was her first clear verbal communication.

I indicated that I would like to be able to do this, but that the police had had a ruckus bringing her in, and she and I would need to convince them that she could stay in control if she were not strapped down. At that point, I
got the police to unstrap one hand and let her know that she and I now had the job of convincing the cops that it would be safe to let her out of the rest of restraints. She then demanded a cigarette, and I responded that I would need her help in making this happen, as no one was allowed to smoke in the ED and no one was going to be comfortable just letting her walk away. At each step, I sided with her and her goals and encouraged her to join with me on further goals. As we talked, she calmed down, and at each step, I got the police to release another limb. By the time she and I went outside for her smoke, she had told me her story. She had a long-standing psychotic disorder but had been mostly stable. She and her boyfriend had gotten into a fight over another women, and she had left the apartment very upset. When the police tried to talk with her, she became very frightened, paranoid, and angry. When they grabbed her, she "lost it" and felt that she was fighting for her life.

At times, a patient demands something that you cannot deliver. "I want to just go home," or "I want you to stop asking me all of these dumb questions." We could respond rationally with explanations about why the demand is unreasonable or what the patient has to do first. This is all true and clear, but it also puts a barrier between us and the person we are trying to connect with. It is likely to be more effective if we clearly side with the person and indicate our desire to help. We can then go on to calmly talk about our limitations in the situation and how the patient can help us out so that we can try and help with his request. "I am not allowed to just let you go unless I can get enough information to explain why I am letting you go after the police were so upset." The job of the crisis clinician is to be in the role of helping the person and avoid being in the role of being the barrier between what the person wants and what is allowed to happen. The crisis clinician should try to avoid any kind of personal confrontation or a test of wills with the patient. Neither should the clinician be passive and allow the chaos to continue. The clinician needs to be clear, assertive, and impose an anxiety reducing organization on the situation but needs to do this to help the person get his or her story out and get his or her needs met.

It is easy to talk about how a patient is not cooperating. It takes two people to "not cooperate." The skill of the crisis clinician is to find ways to cooperate with patients with whom this is difficult (11). At times we can get provoked into being more rigid than even we would think reasonable, if only we were able to step back and put the situation into a broader context.

George came into the ED with the complaint that his long-standing voices were getting worse and "driving me crazy." He had a history of many previous hospitalizations but had been stable for several years. He first talked to the reception clerk who asked "a bunch of questions" and then asked him to wait. After an hour or so, he then talked to a nurse who asked another list of questions and found him "flagrantly psychotic." He then waited for another hour before talking to a medical physician who asked more questions and who then called the crisis team. When the mental health crisis team arrived, he refused to talk with them or answer any more questions until he was allowed to smoke. He was told he was not allowed to smoke until the assessment was completed and that he needed to answer some questions first. His behavior began to escalate and security was called. Medication was offered but was refused.

George was a voluntary patient who at no point expressed a threat to himself or anyone else. He was agitated, pacing, and upset, but not more. As soon as the crisis worker offered to join George for a walk outside of the ED so he could have his smoke, he calmed down and was willing both to continue the conversation about what may have caused the voices to become worse and to take the same medication that had been refused a short time before.

A key ingredient in helping someone calm down is empathy. People, whether they are patients, friends, or lovers, calm down when they feel heard and when they feel someone is on their side. People who are very upset rarely calm down when told about the irrationality of their own behavior.

How to Respond to Someone Who is Angry

Think about what you want when you are angry. As a "thought experiment," think of how you would feel if you were having a terrible, very bad day. Your supervisor just criticized you, two clients told you that you were incompetent, your car had a flat tire, and then on the way home you got a speeding ticket. You walk into the house and you spew out your frustration and anguish to your loving partner, who then responds by suggesting that at least some part of the supervisor's comments may have merit and reminding you that you should not have been speeding anyway.

Most of us can immediately recognize that this is not a helpful response. When we are angry, we do not want our support person to be rational, we want the person to empathize with how terrible the world is, we want the person to take our side, and to be there with us. Later there is a time and place to help us rationally look at our participation in the events of the day, but in the first throes of anger, few of us would find this useful.

Yet this initial assumption of being rational is exactly what we give to our angry patients, and we are then often surprised that they get more angry rather than less. Someone who is angry wants to feel heard, supported, and have his or her feelings validated. Later he or she can join a dialogue about what happened and what else could have been done. Angry people can rarely tolerate unsolicited advice. Problem solving too early will prolong the anger and dyscontrol. Validation can lead to a joining and partnering that can support later problem solving.

This does not mean pretending to agree with an idea or belief that one really disagrees with. It is not about supporting a delusion or pretending support that is not really there. It is about finding some belief or issue that one can really agree with. It also means not always feeling the need to correct every belief that one disagrees with (12).

John was brought into the ED after neighbors called the police after he pounded on their door and threatened to hurt them if they did not stop what they were doing. Police reported that when they tried to talk with him he was angry and uncooperative and did not appear to be making sense. John was angry that neighbors kept "playing tricks" on him. He believed they would sneak into his apartment and steal things, eat his food, spill things on his rug, and generally cause mischief. He felt they were malicious and trying to drive him crazy, probably because they wanted him to move.

He began to calm down when he was given the chance to tell his story without being challenged. He calmed down even more when the crisis therapist empathized with how bad it felt for the police to grab him and force him into the police car in front of his neighbors, and how bad it felt to have bad things happen and not even be believed. As the crisis interview proceeded and after he felt heard, John began to agree that he had probably overreacted to the police who were, after all, not at fault. By the end, he agreed that his story "sounded crazy," even though he continued to maintain that it was really true. He agreed to take some medication to help himself calm down as he did not want to get so upset that police would again be called. He ended up going home with a friend and agreed to come into the mental health center a few days later to continue the conversation.

Consider the Long-Term Consequences of all Parts of the Crisis Treatment

The crisis clinician must focus on the immediate crisis at hand but also be aware that whatever occurs during the crisis period will impact how the patient feels about follow-up treatment. If the person feels treated with respect, listened to, validated, then he or she is more likely to be willing to avail himself of follow-up treatment. If the person feels that medication was imposed and led to further loss of control, he or she will be likely to associate medication with this loss of control in the future. If, on the other hand, the person felt that medication was a useful tool that helped in a way that he or she felt was useful, then this too influences follow-up treatment. This means that long-term consequences must be allowed to influence what the clinician does during the crisis period. This may mean taking a bit more time and working to ensure that the patient feels listened to. In particular, it means trying to find problems or at least part of a problem that both the clinician and patient feel that medication could possibly help. Whenever medication is used as part of the crisis treatment, the clinicians should ask themselves about long-term consequences. "How will the use of this medication at this time help the person's quality of life a year from now?" "Is this experience with medication likely to encourage the patient to use medication in the future?"

Most patients in crisis have an ongoing, persistent illness. At times, the only contact they have with the treatment system is recurrent visits to the emergency service. Every contact with the emergency clinician will help promote a more effective engagement or will discourage that connection.

THE USE OF MEDICATION AS PART OF THE ENGAGEMENT PROCESS

Medication can support the process of engagement (13). Medication can also interfere with engagement. When used to support engagement, mutual goals are established that both the patient and clinician feel might be helped by medication. The medication might help the agitated person calm down, feel less frightened, feel in more control, help him to express himself in a more organized fashion, or allow him to feel that something is being started that might help. This engagement is part of a process of collaboration in which both the patient and clinician agree on common goals and on the use of medication as one way of helping to achieve these goals. It also requires that both the patient and clinician collaborate in assessing how well the medication is actually working (14). This may sound like an impossible goal, but it is actually much more possible, even during a crisis, than many clinicians think. It does require some time to talk with the patient, skills in how to connect with the patient, and an attitude that this is important.

At times, even with time, skill and the desire to engage in this way, the crisis situation is too volatile or the person in crisis is too traumatized or too stuck to find areas of collaboration, in the use of medication or much of anything else. There are situations in which medication is imposed over the patient's objection and without any sense of collaboration goals for what the medication might accomplish. Even in this situation, the clinician can try, as much as possible, to stay in communication with the patient and put the medication into a context that is most likely to be acceptable to the patient. This requires thinking about the situation from the patient's point of view, even if the patient is not a willing participant in the collaboration.

I know that you are angry about being here, and angry that we are forcing you to take medication. I am hoping that the medication will help you calm down and get in enough control that we can talk about what happened to get you here.

I know that you are very afraid that people are trying to kill you. I am also aware that you are very afraid that any medication we give you might be poison, and that you would like to just go home and see if you can figure this out on your own. The police brought you in because they got worried after you threatened your neighbors. At this point, I cannot just let you go home. I can promise you that the medication is not poison and that you will be safe here. I know that you do not completely believe me, but I hope that if the medication is useful in helping you calm down and be less frightened, we can talk some more and figure out what can happen next.

The process starts by empathizing with the patients' view of the world and then framing what will happen next as an invitation that at some time in the near future, the medication will help some kind of collaboration to take place. Giving medication is not the end of the discussion or the resolution of the interaction. The goal is not to "get the patient to take the medication" but rather to use medication so that joint planning is easier.

Even when medication is imposed over the patient's will, it is often possible to engage the person in some element of the decision. For example, a person who is being forced to take medication can be given the choice of some liquid in juice or an injection. If the person cannot participate at all, then little is lost by giving him or her the choice. If he or she chooses the oral medication, then he or she is partially participating in the decision and this begins the process of negotiating about his or her own treatment. The very slight extra time required to obtain an effective serum level of oral medication over injection may be a good tradeoff over having the person feel completely uninvolved in the treatment decision. Similarly, a person may refuse one medication but be willing to take another. He or she may be unwilling to take 30 mg of a medication but be willing to take

15 or 20. Often there is no good scientific data that demonstrate that one medication is significantly better than another or that one dose is necessarily better than another. What is clear is that patient involvement and engagement will probably lead to better resolution of the crisis and more likely follow up with ongoing care.

John had been very aggressive in the ED and ended up in four-point restraints. Since he was in restraints, neither he nor staff was in immediate danger and taking a few minutes to try and engage him did not increase risk, although his level of agitation was such that some medication seemed clearly needed. He was told that he had frightened a number of the staff, seemed very much out of control, and was going to have to take some medication to help him calm down. He was told that he was going to be given some intramuscular haloperidol. He responded, angry and upset but cogently, that he hated Haldol and wanted something else, anything else but Haldol. He then bargained for some Xanax instead. Staff responded with a choice of ziprasidone or risperidone. He asked about the side effects, while continuing to argue that he did not need any medication and should not be forced to take it. Given a forced choice, he finally agreed on getting an injection of ziprasidone, which he had not had before. By this point, he was at least talking with staff, expressing a preference, and beginning to tell his story of what had happened to get him to the ED.

SUMMARY

Medication is a tool, not a goal. The goal of crisis intervention should not be to get a patient to take medication. The goal should be to help a person in crisis to reestablish control, be less frightened, and be better able to cope with the world. Patients and clinicians often have very different views of both the problem and the solution. It is easy to point out where the person is irrational or in error or just not making much sense. The focus should not be on these areas of disagreement, but on finding legitimate and real areas of agreement. This starts with empathizing with the person's view of the world, validating the person's feeling, and listening to the person's understanding of the problem. Patients are unlikely to listen to us if we are not willing to listen to them first.

Medication is a tool that can help this process of collaboration. Medication can help a person be more in control of his or her own life. Medication is not the end of the crisis intervention but only one part of the resolution process. Too much of a focus on the medication can get in the way of focusing on the patient and the relationship.

At times, patients and clinicians will disagree. Even when there is little area of agreement, clinicians can invite engagement by demonstrating an understanding of the patient's view of the problem, validating the patient's feeling, and laying out the nature of the disagreement that respects both the patient's and the clinician's point of view. At all times, clinicians need to keep in mind that the goal is to develop the collaboration and relationship between the patient and clinician and to help the patient reestablish control. Medication can be an important tool that can support this process.

REFERENCES

1. Diamond, R. J. (2006, August). Recovery from mental illness: A psychiatrist's point of view. *New Directions in Schizophrenia*, A Post-Graduate Medicine Special Report, 54–62.
2. Tan, D. T. (2007). Medications for psychiatric emergencies. In Khouzam, H. R., Tan, D. T., & Gil, T. S. (Eds.), *Handbook of emergency psychiatry* (pp. 22–31). St. Louis, MO: Mosby.
3. Allen, M. H., Currier, G. W., Carpenter, D., Ross, R. W., & Docherty, J. P.; & Expert Consensus Panel for Behavioral Emergencies 2005. (2005, November). The expert consensus guideline series. Treatment of behavioral emergencies 2005. *Journal of Psychiatric Practice, 11*(Suppl. 1), 5–108.
4. Berlin, J. (2017). Collaborative de-escalation. In Zeller, S., Nordstrom, K., & Wilson, M. (Eds.), *The diagnosis and management of agitation* (pp. 144–155). Cambridge, UK: Cambridge University Press.
5. Lipp, M. R. (1986). Psychiatric emergencies. In *Respectful treatment: A practical handbook of patient care* (pp. 51–70). New York, NY: Elsevier.
6. Scharfetter, J. (2017). The psychiatric evaluation of patients with agitation. In Zeller, S., Nordstrom, K., & Wilson, M. (Eds.), *The diagnosis and management of agitation*. (pp. 88–103). Cambridge, UK: Cambridge University Press.
7. Havens, L. (1986). *Making contact*. Cambridge, MA: Harvard University Press.
8. Copeland, M. E. (2002). *Wellness recovery action plan*. West Dummerston, VT: Peach Press.
9. Factor, R. M., & Diamond, R. J. (1996). Emergency psychiatry and crisis resolution in community psychiatry. In Vacarro, J. V., & Clark, G. H. (Eds.), *Practicing psychiatry in the community: A manual*. Washington, DC: APA Press.
10. Meichenbaum, D., & Turk, D. C. (1987). Enhancing the relationship between the patient and the health care provider. In *Facilitating treatment adherence* (pp. 71–109). New York, NY: Plenum.
11. Miller, W. R., & Rolnick, S. (2013). *Motivational interviewing: Helping people to change* (3rd ed.). New York, NY: Guilford.
12. Shea, S. C. (1998). The art of moving with resistance. In *Psychiatric interviewing: The art of understanding* (2nd ed., pp. 575–621). Philadelphia, PA: W.B. Saunders.
13. Diamond, R. J., & Scheifler, P. L. (2007). *Treatment collaboration in mental health: Improving the therapist, prescriber, client relationship*. New York, NY: WW Norton & Co.
14. Ellison, J. M. (2000). Enhancing adherence in the pharmacology treatment relationship. In Tasman, A., Riba, M. B., & Silk, K. R. (Eds.), *The doctor-patient relationship in pharmacotherapy* (pp. 71–94). New York, NY: Guilford.

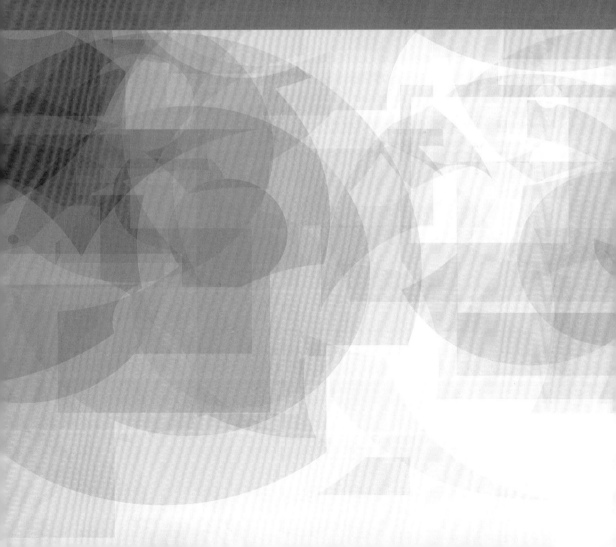

PART III

Staffing and Support

Section Editor: Divy Ravindranath

15

Staffing: Models, Knowledge, and Skills

Tony Thrasher

It has been well publicized that the incidence of mental illness nationally is rising (1) whereas available services and funding are either decreasing or not escalating to meet the demand (2). Even more daunting is the fact this is happening in the setting of deinstitutionalization, lack of parity for mental health care, funding shortages, and continued stigma. Consequently, there are more patients with mental illness either finding themselves in crisis or seeking care from crisis services (3).

This chapter will cover the staffing requirements of such services as well as the training, skills, and knowledge crisis workers must have to function well. Different healthcare organizations choose to handle behavioral crisis care in different ways and staffing of these services can be quite variable. Some of this variability is based on state statutory requirements (4,5), so those who are developing new services need to be aware of the rules in their own jurisdiction. But other variables may be specific to each organization's history, style, and goals.

STAFF

In addition to the administrative and clerical support staff who are needed to run any clinical service (and who in the emergency behavioral health setting should at least be aware of the areas of knowledge, competencies, and skills that will be discussed in this chapter), clinicians working in crisis settings can come from several disciplines.

Licensed clinical social workers (LCSWs) commonly staff crisis services. Their breadth of training allows them to function well in a number of ways including but not limited to on mobile crisis teams, in clinics, as therapists

(depending on state certification/licensure), and/or as short-term or longitudinal crisis case managers. Some programs require these social workers to be masters trained as per state licensing or billing requirements. In some states, social work staff members (or even nursing staff as described below) are required to go through certification steps to be identified as a "crisis clinician" or other similar title.

Registered nurses (RNs) are also of great utility depending on the degree of medical interventions provided by a given crisis services group. One role could be that of a "clinic" or ambulatory care role where they provide medical care under their scope either in a primary fashion or that of assisting other medical professionals. It should also be noted that RNs can be useful in mobile outreach teams as they will often be able to assist their LCSW colleagues in identifying and assessing comorbid medical issues that are endemic in the chronic mentally ill (CMI) (6). RNs can also administer long-acting injectable medications, which are noted to be critical to maintaining the well-being of many patients and for mitigating future crises. A RN presence on the team can assist with making home health nursing visits as well. RNs may be assisted by LPNs, medical assistants, and other direct care workers as well.

Psychologists (PhD, PsyD, and in some states licensed master's level psychologists) can also lend a great deal of assistance to the crisis team, depending on the manner by which the state defines the scope of practice for psychologists in comparison to other mental health professionals. In some states, psychologists are considered equivalent to other nonprescribing mental health professionals whereas, in other states, specific actions, eg, placing patient on a mental health hold, are limited to only psychiatrists and psychologists. Regardless of their role, there are many clinical avenues of care where psychology can assist in diagnosis, treatment planning, risk assessment, and crisis management. Another item to consider when adding psychology to the team is what level of supervision they may be able to provide for the LCSW and Master of Social Work (MSW) roles as it pertains to cosigning and monitoring of supervision hour requirements.

Finally, there is always a need for strong psychiatric providers to be present on a crisis service team to not only handle medical assessment/leadership issues but also to provide physician assessments, certifications, detention proceedings, and to supervise the myriad of professionals described above. Psychiatrists serve as the subject matter experts in many of the items to be described under the training sections below (risk assessment, delirium, addiction, and de-escalation). Psychiatrists can also provide supervision for other prescribing professionals such as advance practice nurses and physician assistants, if these individuals are part of the team as physician extenders. If the system chooses to use a centralized psychiatric emergency service (PES), then the physician role is even more important as they often serve as a liaison to hospital administration and the emergency department (ED) leadership.

STAFFING MODELS

Many different staffing models are used to provide crisis services across many different venues/locales. All are similar in some ways, but more often than not, there are significant differences tied to funding (county vs state), public health versus private health system oversight, and statutory obligations noted in the civil commitment statutes.

Staffing can vary significantly depending on whether a service is in a centralized versus decentralized location. Centralized locations, such as a PES, especially one that is separate from an ED offer many advantages in terms of colocation of professionals who can provide risk assessment, immediate treatment including psychiatric medication, and the ability to handle increasing acuity of patients. But staffing of such a service is resource intensive. The volume of patients seen needs to be large enough to justify this level of resource commitment. This model of care is most often led by psychiatrists, who have higher market value salaries to support.

Alternative options include decentralization of services into drop-in facilities such as peer run centers, observational units, ambulatory care centers, mobile crisis units, and linkage sites providing a bevy of services. These allow for patients to arrive directly from the community which not only assists in patient care but also allows for ease of transport from external stakeholders (such as case managers and law enforcement). An additional advantage to this model can be that patients may feel like they are not going to a hospital as much as a community center. These centers may be run by social workers and other behavioral health clinicians, with or without psychiatric input depending on services provided. Although these staff may be less expensive to hire, a rate limiting factor for the more decentralized options include the need for more funding/staffing to account for varied geographic sites.

CRITICAL KNOWLEDGE AND SKILLS

By virtue of their training and certification or by virtue of experience on the job, mental health professionals involved in emergency mental health work will become experts in many of the following areas. Depending on the scope of practice, a given professional may be (or become) more proficient in one category, eg, suicide safety planning, than in another, eg, distinguishing between delirium, dementia, and depression. This textbook offers a number of critical categories for providers in this arena and Table 15.1 offers a partial list to consider.

Categories of Major Mental Illnesses

Although understanding the illnesses they will deal with may seem obvious for clinicians, it is beneficial to make sure that all major categories are covered in orientation. Table 15.2 lists categories that should be covered. Although this knowledge is important for patient care, crisis service staff are often in the public eye and speak with concerned stakeholders so it is important that the definitions, wording, and information be evidence based and professional at all times. Staff who are armed with correct information/phrasing can

TABLE 15.1 Critical Knowledge and Skills for Emergency Psychiatry Clinicians and Staff

- Psychiatric diagnosis/categories of mental illness
- Assessment for general medical comorbidities and for nonpsychiatric behavioral emergencies (recognition of delirium)
- Brief psychotherapeutic interventions
- Management of substance intoxication and withdrawal
- De-escalation of agitated behavior
- Risk assessment and mitigation
- Coordination of care with general medical providers and community partners
- Basic understanding of psychopharmacology (types of medications/common side effects)

help combat myths surrounding mental illness and help minimize stigma that can be accentuated by incorrect languages and definitions.

Delirium

Regardless of whether a crisis staff member is medically trained (MD/DO, PA, or RN/NP) or nonmedically trained (LCSW, MSW, PhD), it is vital that they understand and can recognize delirium. In addition to noting the waxing and waning nature of this illness, all staff must understand that this change in mental status is not indicative of a psychiatric illness and that the patient with delirium needs immediate medical assessment and care. This is especially important because of the high levels of morbidity and mortality associated with delirium (7).

Substance Use Disorders

Substance use disorders are among the most debilitating and destructive of the mental illnesses. These illnesses can present as the main disorder from which the patient is suffering or exist as a comorbidity for almost all other psychiatric conditions. Addiction is often misperceived as being "separate" from other mental illnesses or not being a true illness (8), which contributes to stigma. Knowledge about substance use disorders and addiction will lead to better outcomes and decreased stigma for these marginalized patients.

Intoxication is quite common in suicide attempts, so knowing about addiction is key in risk assessment. Also, the addition of intoxicants is one of the few things known to raise the violence risk in those with mental illness beyond that of the general population (9). Although most addiction has similar neurobiological roots, the social, legal, and medical consequences of each particular substance vary greatly. Consequently, it is suggested that education specifically addresses all substances listed in Table 15.3.

Legalization, usage, and long-term outcomes of cannabis use in patients is a current hot-topic. At a minimum, staff should know about the effect of cannabis in first-episode psychosis (FEP) patients, the usage of cannabis recreationally by those with no preexisting mental illness, and the

TABLE 15.2 Categories of Mental Illness Staff Must Understand

- Psychotic Illnesses including schizophrenia and prodromal variants
- Mood illnesses of the depressive subtype
- Mood illnesses of the bipolar subtype
- Anxiety illnesses
- Trauma-based illnesses
- Obsessive-based illnesses
- Substance use illnesses
- Personality/characterological illnesses
- Adjustment reactions

TABLE 15.3 Substances/Classes of Substances Staff Should Have Knowledge of

Alcohol	Hallucinogens
Amphetamines	Nicotine
Caffeine	Sedative/hypnotics
Cannabis	Opiates
Cocaine	Synthetic Cannabis (K2, Spice)
Inhalants	Synthetic stimulants (bath salts, Flakka)
Phencyclidine	Salvia
Dextromethorphan products	Kratom
Codeine/cough syrup products	Synthetic opiates (fentanyl, carfentanil)
Piperazines	

therapeutic investigations of cannabidiol (CBD) versus that of the intoxicant component of tetrahydrocannabinol (THC).

Risk Assessment, Management, and Mitigation

Many patients seen in crisis services have suicidal thoughts or behaviors, and suicide risk assessment is a key skill. This is particularly germane because of the ever increasing incidence of suicide nationally (10).

Assessing risk is not only important clinically, it is also addressed in accreditation requirements. As The Joint Commission noted in its 2016 newsletter focusing on National Patient Safety Goals (NPSGs 15A), the incidence of suicide has now surpassed that of homicides and motor vehicle accidents in certain populations. Additionally, there is no clear designation of a "typical" suicide victim. Many individuals with numerous risk factors never attempt suicide. Hence, risk assessments are more than a simple review of risk factors that have been determined in research (11). They require specific clinical skills.

In addition to well-described "traditional" risk factors for suicide (that likely were part of the initial training in team members' professional scopes), there are many other items to focus on that should be part of a biopsychosocial approach and subsequent education. These include but are not limited to sleep difficulties (12), major physical health conditions (13), recent medication changes, anxiety (14), and acute substance use (15).

Crisis services team members will need risk assessment training not only for their daily assessments of those in crisis but also for patients who are post crisis, as many crisis teams are providing care status post crisis or status post hospitalization due to the evidence supporting these contacts as items of mitigation for future episodes (16). Additionally, the education surrounding risk assessment should be focused not only on "time zero" assessments but also how this supports proper handoff and continuity of care with the receiving provider/institution/agency if so applicable (17).

When seeing patients who are status post self-harming behaviors, it is important for staff to focus upon not just plan/method but also the importance of expectations, future orientation, motivations, possibility of rescue, and presence of hopelessness and helplessness. Combining these with medical information can provide a better understanding of the medical significance and psychological significance of these behaviors.

Crisis workers will often be seeing patients with not only suicide risk but also risks pertaining to more externalized violence (assault, abuse, and/or homicide). Hence, discussion of harm to others is important not only for the safety of the patient but also that of the individual team member. When dealing with violence risk, it is also valuable to keep in mind those with mental illness are more often victims of violence as opposed to being perpetrators (18). It is also notable to emphasize that the same factors driving violent behavior in the mentally ill are akin to those driving violent behavior in the non–mentally ill, such as anger, intoxication, and access to firearms (19).

Regardless of the source of the risk, it is in the staff member's best interest to fully document the presence/absence of risk factors, protective factors, items that are able to be mitigated versus those that are not, and concluding statements based upon a synthesis of the above.

De-escalation Processes

Although many crisis episodes do not require de-escalation, there will be instances where the first step in engagement will be to use this skill set. Crisis service team members need to be experts at de-escalation for the good of the patient and the others who may be present.

There are many reasons why an individual may present to a medical ED, community drop-in center, or other crisis receiving venue with agitation as either a primary or secondary complaint (20). Regardless of the etiology of agitation, verbal de-escalation is the first-line intervention to handle these situations (21).

The primary teaching point behind all verbal de-escalations is respect. This cannot be overemphasized. All patients, regardless of illness and/or legal status, should be treated with respect. Simply taking extra efforts to not stigmatize, withhold care, or marginalize a person's suffering can lead to immediate de-escalation (22). In addition to verbal de-escalation, pharmacological interventions should also be taught to those whose scope of practice and certification includes prescribing.

CRITICAL TENETS OF CRISIS CARE

Trauma-Informed Care

Based on the fact that approximately 50% of patients presenting to safety net facilities (such as EDs and crisis centers) have previously experienced trauma in their lives (23), it is important that staff know how to handle those who have suffered traumas. Thus, Trauma-Informed Care (TIC) is a critical attitude to cultivate in staff who attend to psychiatric emergencies.

TIC specifically focuses on a trauma-informed approach that supports patient autonomy and avoids coercive measures. It speaks to the fact that patient's actions (including fearful,

paranoid, or otherwise dangerous behavior) are often being driven by past traumas; hence, it is in the best interest of the crisis services staff member to approach in a calm manner, avoiding any behaviors or language that may trigger (or exacerbate) any traumatic memories or feelings.

The patient's trauma may in fact be with the system of care itself. There are many complications in accessing care when in crisis, and many historical methods are not as patient centered as the current state. Hence, it is important to note that the patient's trauma may be tied to past emergency visits, contact with law enforcement, or court-ordered interventions. This is of immense importance to the crisis team working with these patients so this history can be acknowledged, accounted for, and hopefully mitigated in the present situation.

In contrast to the many patients presenting to crisis services with histories of trauma (either recent or historical), it should also be noted that for other patients, this may be their only time of crisis. Hence, the very nature of having to use such services or engage emergency care can be traumatizing in of itself. Noting the above is very important not only for good patient outcomes but also for the longitudinal well-being of the crisis services staff. More of this will be covered in the section later focusing on burnout and support, but it should be noted here that repeated exposure to traumatization and its victims is its own form of secondary trauma. Hence, supervisors and other leadership should be using the ideas of TIC with their staff and not just teaching it for the purpose of patient care.

Psychological First Aid

Psychological First Aid (PFA) has replaced the process of "debriefing" (or CISD/CISM: critical incident stress debriefing or management) in disaster situations (24). Although PFA is often discussed in disaster response and/or mass casualty events, it is a tenet of care that is of use in ALL crisis services interactions. PFA notes that the best thing for the patient is what the patient actually needs in the moment. These immediate needs (safety, food, shelter, kindness, and contact with supportive loved ones) are often different than what healthcare workers see as immediate treatment (labs, meds, diagnostic tests, and answers to questions). Nonetheless, tending to what the patient needs is the most important thing in disaster situations and other crises and doing so can de-escalate potentially explosive situations. PFA is not the same as having to follow all patient requests at all times, as it includes therapeutic limits and engaging in constructive alternatives as mechanisms to use to resolve the crisis.

By focusing on what the patient needs at the time, the clinical team can better plan for an efficient response. Additionally, addressing urgent needs can lead to a quicker rapport, less anxiety from the patient, and a more valuable interaction between all parties. By moving the interaction away from an autocratic approach (as one might see with the legal system or law enforcement) and toward a partnership, the information gathering, crisis planning, and patient engagement all markedly improve.

It is recommended that all staff have TIC and PFA training as part of their initial orientation followed by annual updates as arranged by individual systems. Additionally, elements of TIC and PFA can also be shared with Crisis Intervention Training (CIT) partners in law enforcement or National Alliance on Mental Illness (NAMI) education for advocates. The tenets of TIC and PFA are of paramount importance in engaging with patients during a psychiatric crisis.

OTHER TOPICS CRISIS SERVICE STAFF SHOULD KNOW ABOUT

Abuse and Neglect

A strong understanding of abuse and neglect and the ability to recognize presentations that suggest the possibility of these issues is markedly important for a crisis services team member. This is often thought as being due to the mandatory reporting rules that are often covered in basic orientation; however, as alluded to in previous sections on PFA and TIC, a strong knowledge base in this area will benefit rapport, engagement, and longitudinal relationship building with patients.

A crisis service will, undoubtedly, have a high prevalence of those suffering from abuse and neglect than other settings because of many inherent factors. Victims of abuse often seek out medical settings rather than law enforcement, and there is correlation between increased victimization and

certain socioeconomic areas served by large-scale PESs (25). Also, exacerbations and symptoms of certain mental illnesses may make patients more prone to abuse and neglect; hence, they will often utilize safety net services such as these.

Staff members should not only be aware of the mandatory reporting laws in their jurisdiction but also be competent in assisting victims in engaging with the local network of services. This, in of itself, can be complicated as the support services may differ depending on whether the case is categorized as physical abuse, sexual abuse, neglect, involvement of minors, elder abuse, chronic domestic violence, and/or illicit sex trade avenues.

Regardless of the classification above, it is important to not only utilize prior training in PFA/TIC as previously mentioned but also to maintain interest in engagement over time. Many such cases are of a chronic nature and require frequent reassurances/supports for the individual to engage in change. A good parallel for staff to ponder would be the stages of change as noted by Prochaska/DiClemente (26).

Legal Responsibilities (Civil Commitment and Detention Statutes)

It is quite common for crisis services to deal with state commitment and detention statutes. Although laws differ state to state, every state has some process available to provide involuntary treatment. Although there are United States Supreme Court cases that speak to the overall framework (O'Connor v. Donaldson, Addington v. Texas, Cameron v. Lake), states are left with their own authority on how they choose to handle said commitments. As such, it would be very germane for staff members to be familiar with relevant statutes effecting local practice.

Crisis Plans

Being able to help a patient develop and write a crisis/safety plan is also a needed skill.

There is good research to note that the preparation and discussion of crisis plans are not only productive ways to mitigate suicide, but they are also a more preferred/accepted method of intervention by patients (27).

The specifics of a service's crisis plans will likely depend on the team's electronic health record and other interagency items. That being said, there are several components that are integral for safety planning: steps for safety, warning signs, internal coping mechanisms, people/places for distraction, and supports/people to call or contact when distressed, and staff should be well-versed at asking about these.

Cross Cultural Aspects of Care

It is important for front-line providers to remember that many of the current diagnoses and discussion of major mental illnesses are biased toward western medicine and western culture (28). The patient's cultural background and family history can greatly affect not only how they present in crisis but also how amenable they will be to accepting care.

The United States is becoming increasingly diverse, and it is paramount for mental healthcare workers to avoid a myopic view of how a specific group of people may respond to a patient's suffering from psychiatric illness. There should be discussions on different definitions and applications of the terms ethnicity, race, and culture included in the cross-cultural education. Additionally, there is benefit in considering a formulation touching on cultural identity, cultural explanations, cultural factors, and cultural assessment in how it affects the relationship between the patient and assessor (29).

Psychiatric Patient Boarding

It is well noted in the literature that there are more and more patients with mental illness either coming to EDs or being boarded in EDs because of lack of access to other services. More specifically, while the overall ED visits are increasing by 8% from 1992 to 2001, the number of mental health visits in that same period saw a rise of 38% (30).

As patients with mental illness are more likely to be "boarded" in EDs, psychiatric crisis services staff are often called upon to help. Additionally, regardless of statutory obligation, the crisis services team can serve a very valuable role in making sure that the ED employees are well versed in skills to ease the suffering of the patients being boarded.

Many of these skills have already been described above, but crisis services teams can often best help the patient by educating the ED staff about de-escalation, engagement, comorbid medical conditions, respite care, observation status, debriefing status post restraint episodes, and collaboration with law enforcement.

Harm Reduction

Members of crisis service teams are often involved in public health matters because of their subject matter expertise as well as frequently seeing the issues surrounding primary versus secondary prevention. The topic of harm reduction is well known in healthcare and social services realms; however, it is an item in which crisis services line staff and leadership should be fluent. The most notable examples of current harm reduction methods in crisis services work include needle exchange projects, FEP intervention programs, "wet" housing for patients suffering from addictions, and education surrounding birth control. An additional component that is highly linked to suicide prevention is access to firearms and safe storage of weapons (31).

Service Recovery

Patients in the ED will be undergoing some of the most difficult moments of their life. In accordance with this, ED staff can be the recipients of a great deal of displaced emotion, catharsis, and customer dissatisfaction even if they did nothing to cause said feelings. Hence, it is markedly important to eventually discuss the topic of service recovery.

Service recovery is defined as "a company's resolution of a problem from a dissatisfied customer, converting them into a loyal customer" (32). In fact, there is a related concept in business known as the "service recovery paradox" which defines the notice that a customer actually values a service more highly when they "fix" a situation that went poorly as opposed to as if the service existed without complications initially.

This can be of great assistance to a crisis service group both at the level of supervisors and line staff. In particular, this topic allows staff to objectively address someone expressing a grievance and maintain rapport and engagement for future crisis presentations. Concurrently, it can also be noted that engaging in effective service recovery allows for patients and external stakeholders (such as family or case workers) to receive what is perceived as "bad" news in a thoughtful, processed manner.

RETENTION/SUPPORT OF STAFF

As noted in previous sections, qualified mental healthcare staff are in short supply. Hence, it is important to think of long-term retention. Many programs tend to focus on recruitment; however, lost in this rush to obtain new employees is the fact that an employee is not fully considered part of the team by others until they have been there multiple years (33).

As will be described in the section below, crisis service employees face many issues that can contribute to burnout and dissatisfaction with one's role and job description. It is noted in historical employment literature that employees are more likely to leave a job because of "fit" and job duties rather than compensation or benefits (34).

Hence, it is incredibly important that crisis services leadership investigates the best ways to retain and educate talented staff. Much of this chapter is focused on the training aspects of line staff, but it is just as important to identify future leaders for the program. Once identified, these individuals can then be given separate trainings or opportunities to allow for growth in the fields of leadership, group management, and motivational dynamics.

This team member may then either be included in leadership succession to take up a current role or to begin new roles tied to program expansion. Ensuring succession plans among healthcare leadership is something that can set the program apart by ensuring sustainability and the ability to focus on more patient care items and not just staffing complexities.

Burnout

As mentioned above, support of team members is integral to future success as well as how the team is perceived in the community over time. This chapter has covered many of the stressful issues that the team may be exposed to because of their work with crisis situations. In particular, it is important to refer secondary trauma that has been noted by first-line responders in both a subacute and chronic nature (35) that is also present in crisis work.

To complement the education and support already being given, it is important to have awareness and knowledge pertaining to burnout and how this can affect a sustainable work force.

It is key to maintain vigilance for the three main warning signs of employee burnout: 1) emotional exhaustion, 2) depersonalization/lack of connection with others, and 3) losing sense of meaning within one's work. Keeping an eye out for these signs will allow the supervisor to keep their employees healthy, and it is well known that individual well-being is tied to better systemic outputs (36).

In addition to basic burnout education, there are related topics that can be covered in advanced didactics that can help empower employees in this area. Two of the most pertinent to crisis services would be fictive schedule (being assigned more patients to care for then physically possible) and cognitive scarcity (constantly needing to do more with less) (37). Employees should be empowered to look for these problems and report them if they develop.

By addressing all of this in a systematic fashion, one can maintain employees who manifest vitality, engagement, and self-efficacy, all of which combat burnout and improve performance with subsequent excellent patient care outcomes.

REFERENCES

1. Curtin, S. C., Warner, M., & Hedegaard, H. (2016). *Increase in suicide in the United States, 1999–2014*. NCHS data brief, no 241. Hyattsville, MD: National Center for Health Statistics.
2. McGinty, E., Pescosolido, B., Kennedy-Hendricks, A., & Barry, C. L. (2017). Communication strategies to combat stigma and improve mental health access. *Psychiatric Services, 69*(2), 136–146.
3. Zeller, S. (2010). Treatment of psychiatric patients in emergency settings. *Primary Psychiatry, 17*(6), 35–41.
4. Slobogin, C., Rai, A., & Reisner, R. (2009). *Law and the mental health system: Civil and criminal aspects* (pp. 74–75). St. Paul, MN: West Academic Publishing.
5. LeBlond, C. (2008). *A review of adult mental health mobile crisis programs*. Maine DHHS Report.
6. DeHert, M., Correll, C. U., et al. (2011). Physical illness in patients with severe mental disorders: Prevalence, impact of medications and disparities in health care. *World Psychiatry, 10*(1), 52–77.
7. Sadock, B. J., Kaplan, H. I., & Sadock, V. A. (2007). *Synopsis of psychiatry* (10th ed., pp. 322–327). New York: Lippincott Williams and Wilkens.
8. National Institutes of Health (NIH). (2007, Spring). The science of addiction: Drugs, brains, and behavior. *2*(2), 14–17.
9. Torrey, E., et al. (2008, February). The MacArthur Violence Risk Assessment Study revisited: Two views ten years after its initial publication. *Psychiatric Services, 59*(2), 147–152.

10. Klonsky, E. D., & May, A. (2015, June). The three step theory: A new theory for suicidal action. *International Journal of Cognitive Therapy, 8*, 114. doi:10.1521/ijct.2015.8.2.114.

11. *NPSG #15A: Crafting a suicide risk assessment policy.* (2016). Joint Commission National Patient Safety Goals: Update.

12. Bernert, R. A., Hom, M. A., Iwata, N. G., & Joiner, T. E. (2017). Objectively assessed sleep variability as an acute warning sign of suicidal ideation in a longitudinal evaluation of young adults at high suicide risk. *The Journal of Clinical Psychiatry, 78*(6), e678–e687.

13. Ahmedani, B. K., Peterson, E. L., & Hu, Y. (2017). Major physical health conditions and risk of suicide. *American Journal of Preventive Medicine, 53*(3), 308–315.

14. Lineberry, T. W. (2012, June). Seven clinical pearls for suicide risk assessment. *The Carlat Report, 10*(6), 1–2.

15. Bagge, C. L., & Borgas, G. (2017). Acute substance use as a warning sign for suicide attempts: A case-crossover examination of the 48 hours prior to a recent suicide attempt. *Journal of Clinical Psychiatry, 78*(6), 691–696.

16. Chung, D. T., Ryan, C. J., & Pavlovic, D. (2017). Suicide rates after discharge from psychiatric facilities. *JAMA Psychiatry, 74*(7), 694–702.

17. Murray, D. (2016, January). Is it time to abandon suicide risk assessment? *BJPsych Open, 2*(1), e1–e2.

18. Metzl, J. M., & MacLeish, K. T. (2015, February). Mental illness, mass shootings, and the politics of American firearms. *American Journal of Public Health, 105*(2), 240–249.

19. Skeem, J., Kennealy, P., Monahan, J., et al. (June 2015). Psychosis uncommonly and inconsistently precedes violence among high-risk individuals. *Clinical Psychological Science, 4*, 40–49.

20. Citrome, L. (2002). Atypical antipsychotics for acute agitation. *Postgraduate Medicine, 112*(6), 85–96.

21. Dawson, N. L., et al. (2018, March). Violent behavior by emergency department patients with an involuntary hold status. *The American Journal of Emergency Medicine, 36*(3), 392–395.

22. Richmond, J. (2013). Use of verbal de-escalation techniques in the emergency department. In Zun, L. S. (Ed.), *Behavioral emergencies for the emergency physician* (pp. 155–163). New York: Cambridge University Press.

23. Fallot, R. D., & Harris, M. (2009). Creating cultures of trauma informed care (CCTIC): A self assessment and planning protocol. *Community Connections, 2*(1), 1–17.

24. APA Presidential Task Force on Evidence Based Practice. (2006). Evidence based practice in psychology. *American Psychologist, 61*(4), 271–285.

25. Avdija, A. S., & Giever, D. M. (2012). The impact of prior victimization and socio-economic status on people's crime-reporting behavior. *International Journal of Applied Psychology, 2*(4), 59–70.

26. Velicer, W. F., et al. (1998). Smoking cessation and stress management: Applications of the trans theoretical model of behavior change. *Homeostasis, 38*, 216–233.

27. Richards, J. E., Whiteside, U., Ludman, E. J., et al. (2018). Understanding why patients may not report suicidal ideation at a health care visit prior to a suicide attempt: A qualitative study. *Psychiatric Services, 70*(1), 40–45.

28. Ton, H., & Lim, R. (2006). The assessment of culturally diverse individuals. In Lim, R. (Ed.), *Clinical manual of cultural psychiatry* (pp. 3–9). Washington, DC: American Psychiatric Publishing, Inc.

29. American Psychiatric Association (APA). (2013). Cultural formulation. In *Diagnostic and statistical manual of mental disorders* (5th ed., pp. 749–759). Washington, DC: American Psychiatric Publishing, Inc.

30. Larkin, G. L., & Beautrais, A. L. (2013). Magnitude of the problem of psychiatric illness presenting in the emergency department. In Zun, L. S., Chepenik, L. G., & Mallory, M. N. S. (Eds.), *Behavioral emergencies for the emergency physician* (pp. 1–10). New York, NY: Cambridge University Press.

31. Miller, M., et al. (2009, June). Recent psychopathology, suicidal thoughts and suicide attempts in households with and without firearms: Findings from the National Comorbidity Study Replication. *Injury Prevention, 15*(3), 183–187.

32. Hart, C. W., Heskett, J. L., & Earl Sasser, W. (1990). The profitable art of service recovery. *Harvard Business Review, 68*(4), 148–156.

33. George, G. (2011, September). 8 untraditional ways to retain the best and brightest in healthcare. *Becker's Hospital Review*, 1–2 (online).

34. Flowers, V. S., & Hughes, C. L. (1973, July). Why employees stay. *Harvard Business Review*, 1–12.

35. Pietrantoni, L., & Prati, G. (2008). Resilience among first responders. *African Health Sciences, 8*(Suppl. 1), S14–S20.

36. Nielsen, K., et al. (2017). Workplace resources to improve both employee well-being and performance: A systematic review and meta-analysis. *Work and Stress, 31*(2), 101–120.

37. Shanafelt, T. D., & Noseworthy, J. H. (2017). Executive leadership and physician well-being: Nine organizational strategies to promote engagement and reduce burnout. *Mayo Clinic Proceedings, 92*(1), 129–146.

16

Peer and Consumer Involvement in the Psychiatric Emergency Service

Howard D. Trachtman, Ken Duckworth

Emergency department (ED) caregivers, particularly when coping with psychiatric emergencies, face numerous challenges in the delivery of comprehensive and respectful care. These include challenging interactions with consumers (or survivors or ex-patients—there is a vibrant debate among people living with mental illness about the labels that should be used to refer to them) and family members, lengthy waits for inpatient beds, frequent understaffing, the risk of staff injury during a behavioral emergency, and other unpredictably difficult circumstances and risks. Further complicating the situation, coverage may be provided by an infrequent staffer who is not integrated into the clinical team. Despite these pressures, given the fragmentation and underfunding of mental health services (1), EDs will continue to be an essential element of psychiatric care.

Similarly, the consumer and family component of the service equation is fraught with challenges. The individual who arrives seeking services, or who is brought involuntarily, is likely to be experiencing fear, anxiety, desperation, rage, and shame (Case 16.1). Arriving in an involuntary manner compounds the intake process. In addition, the consumer may be delusional, manic, intoxicated, suicidal, abused, impoverished, or assaultive. Family members may be allies or in conflict with the individual seeking psychiatric services.

These two halves of this service equation can add up to difficult interfaces. In a 2006 Internet survey conducted by the National Alliance on Mental Illness (NAMI) of 465 consumer members and 254 family members or friends who accompanied the consumer to ED services following a suicide attempt, many troubling experiences were reported. Fewer than 40% of consumers felt that the ED staff listened to them, described the nature of treatments to them, or took their suicide attempt seriously. Additionally, more than half of the consumers and more than a third of family members felt directly rebuked or stigmatized by staff. Consumers and family members also reported negative experiences involving a perception of unprofessional staff behavior and long wait times (2).

A BRIEF HISTORY OF THE CONSUMER MOVEMENT

During the past decade, "recovery" has been the mantra bringing about massive change in the models that offer to explain mental health and inform mental health services. For example, the President's New Freedom Commission for Mental Health in 2002 endorsed a "recovery-based model of community services." Prior to this point, consumers had to reconnoiter a mental health system that considered serious psychiatric disorders harbingers of doom (3). Despite the longitudinal body of evidence by Harding et al. (4,5) demonstrating long-term improvements for many, people with serious mental illness were frequently told to accept that a "normal" life was impossible, independence unattainable, and institutionalization unavoidable.

As the voices of both family members and consumers have grown, some professionals have begun to change their views about the capabilities and aspirations of people living with mental illness.

CASE 16.1: First Person Experience 1: How EDs and I Have Evolved

EDs are a key gateway to hospitalization and levels of care. I have been hospitalized many times over the years. Sometimes I presented voluntarily, other times I was escorted by law enforcement. Over time I have noticed improvements in the procedures and I have also learned more about the process. I have also learned more about ways to identify crises and better manage my condition, so this may make EDs look better to me.

My very first time being brought to an ED was when my bizarre behavior at an airport led to police escorting me to a crisis center. I recall waiting to see the doctor. He asked me if I heard voices. Hearing voices is not one of my symptoms. When I said "yes" because I could hear people talking, I was put into restraints and injected with antipsychotic medication. Fortunately, they contacted my parents who flew in the next morning. While I was floridly psychotic, they discharged me to the care of my parents.

We flew back to Buffalo and within 10 minutes I was outside barefoot looking for a bible. My parents tried to get me hospitalized. They were reluctant to do so until they told the hospital I thought I was the Messiah. That was good enough for hospitalization in 1983, it may not be so any longer.

After returning to Boston, I soon became homeless and lost my temp job. I had another manic episode after being up all night. I now recognized more symptoms of mania. At another time, I told the admitting doctor that I was suicidal. She asked me if I had any prior attempts and I told her no. She let me go. I then went to a convenience store to buy sleeping pills and got in trouble with the store owner. Then I went to a friend's apartment and swallowed a whole bottle of medication and washed it down alcohol. In the morning, I presented in an ED, had my stomach pumped, spent a few days in medical unit then transferred to psychiatric hospital.

Later, I met the peer recovery movement and started taking a psychiatric medication that worked for me. I then went 5 years without a hospitalization until I experimented with going off that medication. Soon I was hospitalized. I spent a lot of my time isolated and living in "quiet rooms." Back on the medication I went 8 years without a hospitalization.

More recently I had two episodes where I could see the warning signs of breaking down. Each time I called a different good friend— both peers—people with lived experience of mental health treatment of their own. This time my experience was different. We called ahead to a crisis center in Boston that knew me. The first time we went directly to a CCS, a community crisis stabilization unit was an unlocked alternative to a hospital. The crisis team evaluated me there and had me admitted to the CCS. I stayed a weekend and felt better so I was allowed to go home. I stayed at another CCS this one longer but was grateful 1 day they gave me a pass to go to some doctors' appointments and a work meeting. This would not be allowed in a conventional hospital unit.

Finding alternatives to EDs such as mobile crisis assessment and CCS units is an important way to help people in crisis with a more consumer-oriented perspective.

One noteworthy example of this culture change is that the President's New Freedom Commission called for a "system driven by families and consumers" (6). Policy makers and professionals have started to include consumers as partners in the design and delivery of services (7,8). In describing a framework for the role of consumers as providers of psychiatric rehabilitation, Mowbray and Moxley (9) suggest that one rationale for peer-run programs is that "consumers have the ability to form creative, non-traditional, and more beneficial alternatives… to formal mental health services… [S]ince the consumer-controlled program is developed and delivered by consumers, it has the potential of contributing something that is very different in rehabilitation and community support than what individuals with professional training can do within existing structures."

Two forces converged over the past century to bolster peer-run support programs as they exist today for people with psychiatric diagnoses (10): the growth of self-help groups that address

CASE 16.2: First Person Experience 2: Unnecessary Restraint Left me Degraded and Powerless

Once I arrived at the ED, I was very compliant with the staff and after what I thought was an evaluation, I voluntarily agreed to be admitted, and I was not at all aggressive to the staff and did not pose as a safety risk either to myself or anyone else. Shortly after I was admitted to the ED, I was transferred from a wheelchair onto a sheet and placed in restraints with the upper half of my body in an upright position. I was restricted of movement on both my hands and feet and placed in a confined room.

As the staff was forcibly placing me in restraints against my will, I became very resistant and I started struggling and pleading to the staff to release me but to no avail. There was no evidence or proof other than struggling from restraints that I was exhibiting aggressive behavior. I felt terrified and powerless. I had no control over decisions that were concerning me by the staff regarding what methods besides physical restraint were to be used. There was no consent from me for the treatment I received, I wasn't offered any strategies to help calm me down and de-escalate the situation. I was not given a choice regarding the type of restraint and positioning, the gender of the staff restraining me, or any option to decide in which way I would like to be calmed.

While I was in restraints and the confined room, I was abandoned and ignored. After repeated attempts pleading staff to release me, I became more agitated and started to struggle and plead for more medication to calm me down. When I was finally acknowledged and asked to be released from the restraints, the staff alleged that I was a safety risk to myself and others and therefore denied my request. I pleaded with them to either release me from the restraints or to give me enough medication until I was sedated. The medication that was administered was ineffective and I increasingly became more agitated and restless.

I was then transferred against my will with restraints still on to another secluded room with no staff. At that point I completely broke down and started shouting and yelling to no avail. My pleas to access to the toileting facilites were ignored, and I had to resort to urinating in the bed.

I tried to release myself from one of the restraints and three male staff immediately came into the room and forced me down to the bed making the straps of the restraint so tight so that there was no movement on both my hands and the position of the restraint was so that it was physically painful.

Because I struggled against the unnecessary restraints, I was left with marks on my ankle where the restraints were and a bruise on my toe. This experience has left me feeling completely degraded and powerless.

I will be filing a complaint to the Department of Mental Health as a result of this experience.

CASE 16.3: First Person Experience 3: Remember How Hard It Can be for a Person to Get to the ED

For my ED evaluations, I was extremely depressed, had anxiety, and had an enormous amount of shame. When someone walks into an ED and says they have depression, they should be treated with a great deal of respect. People have been judging themselves for months if not years and it was very, very hard to walk in and ask for help. I was very in tune with how other people were perceiving me. I also did not have family members to help advocate for me either which made it harder to get the care I needed.

Although my memory isn't particularly great because of the nature of depression, I remember clearly how these experiences of ED assessments made me feel. They were not all bad and I did get care. I remember not feeling listened to, and sometimes the person didn't take my depression seriously.

I felt stigmatized by a lot of the staff I came across over the years. There were long wait times, but that negative experience paled in comparison to the way the staff was treating me. Maybe because in depression you have been judging yourself so negatively, you are more perceptive to any negative feeling coming off someone else. That is why staff needs to be sensitive to depressed people.

a broad range of medical conditions and disabilities, and the struggle of persons with mental illness to reenter community life following deinstitutionalization, along with the development of psychosocial rehabilitation programs to address their needs.

Peer support involves a wide range of services; almost all provide members with the opportunity to tell their stories of recovery to other members and to wider audiences. Through personal narrative, consumers combat societal stereotypes (11). One such program is NAMI's In Our Own Voice, a consumer recovery-based speakers' bureau for persons with serious psychiatric disorders who share their stories of coping mechanisms, recovery, and hope with a broad range of audiences, including hospital personnel (12). Because societal problems and injustices are commonly viewed as major contributors to individual problems, learning to speak for themselves encourages people with mental illness to act on their own behalf and to begin to advocate for the rights of others (13-15).

Some programs also formalize the role-modeling function of the consumer staff and assign peer mentors to individual participants. Peer mentors speak openly about their struggles and use their own experiences to provide encouragement and technical assistance to participants (16). One such program gathering momentum is Mary Ellen Copeland's Wellness Recovery Action Plan (WRAP), a structured system developed by each individual consumer, within the WRAP framework, with the assistance and support of peers, for monitoring uncomfortable and distressing symptoms and, through planned responses, reducing, modifying, or eliminating those symptoms. WRAP also includes a crisis plan "to identi[fy] those symptoms that indicate [a person] can no longer continue to make decisions, take care of [himself] and keep… safe. It is for use by supporters and health care professionals on… behalf [of the person] who developed the plan" (17).

Another sign of consumer strength in programming is the burgeoning growth of recovery learning centers, consumer-governed and consumer-staffed centers working to build a community that offers natural supports and a growth plan for people with mental health and addiction recovery needs. Recovery learning centers offer opportunities to learn about recovery, practical leadership skills that encourage growth and wellness, and the role of peer specialists or peer mentors in mental health services, as well as the impact of peer-operated services and the importance of advocating for positive changes in the mental health system. Examples in Massachusetts include Metro Boston Recovery Learning Community and the Southeast Recovery Learning Community (18).

The role of consumers as supports and advocates in emergency settings is relatively uncharted territory. There is a growing in the role of mental health peer supports which of course could be deployed in ED settings. Studies of decision-making in psychiatric emergency settings have indicated that "hospitalization could have been avoided if there had been a more supportive and protective milieu" (19). Warmlines staffed by people who offer support and who have lived experience also represent a growing resource (20).

CONSUMER VOICE IN CRISIS PLANNING

Frequently, individuals who present to EDs are experiencing flare-ups of long-standing symptoms, illnesses, or inadequate strategies to manage their distress. This challenge also presents an opportunity. When people can work to devise crisis plans that identify early warning symptoms, the best people to talk to, and methods to help reduce symptoms, ED visits can be reduced or even eliminated for an individual. In a field often lacking a preventive mind-set, crisis planning can literally be lifesaving and can reduce ED service use. Although these strategies can take structured forms, as in WRAP, they can also be more informally developed between service providers and consumers. Yet one vital key in a fragmented system is that the information must be available when the crisis occurs, because information not used is information wasted. There is recent evidence that a thoughtful and structured approach to assessing suicide risk in ED with telephonic follow-up reduces suicidal behavior and promotes outpatient follow-up (21).

The system of care that has more choices for disposition than simply inpatient or discharge is likely to be able to match individual needs better.

For example, respite/stabilization beds can be the appropriate level of care for some people. If these services are peer run and directed, the "culture mismatch" often experienced between consumer and professionally run programs can be reduced. Warmlines are phone support services, staffed by consumers, that can be used by peers to support one another, thus easing the feeling of being alone with their concerns, and possibly also reducing ED service usage (22).

In a more formal way, psychiatric advance directives (PADs) can formalize crisis planning. PADs empower consumers to plan for the type of interventions they would like in case they become incapacitated and unable to make decisions. Examples of such decisions could include choice of medication under what circumstances, to which hospitals the person prefers or refuses to be admitted, and who they want to help make decisions for them should they be unable to do so. States vary in their application of this concept and laws that make the agreements binding. The website of the National Resource Center on Psychiatric Advance Directives (www.nrc-pad.org) is an excellent source for state-by-state summaries of the status of psychiatric advance directives.

ATTENTION TO THE ENVIRONMENT OF CARE

Emergency services convey many messages in the design of their physical environment. A warm and humane environment that offers attention to safety, respect for privacy, and integrated access to medical assessment is essential. Given the modern crisis in ED boarding and access to psychiatric services that result in long wait times, the environment of care becomes even more salient.

Adequate staffing is also essential to afford individual attention during extended wait times. For example, adequate and well-trained staff may reduce the use of restraint and seclusion in ED settings. At one large ED in Boston in the 1990s, it was routine for individuals seeking psychiatric services to be restrained to a gurney. The thinking in this misguided practice was to ensure no one would harm themselves. After human rights concerns were raised to the leadership, additional staffing was deployed, which eliminated this alienating practice.

Minimal restraint use and sensitivity to trauma are good indicators of the commitment of staff to provide a humane environment of care. Restraints are now conceptualized as treatment failures, and a preventive approach is being promoted nationwide (Case 16.2). The national culture change to employ preventive de-escalation strategies to dramatically reduce restraint use is altering many aspects of inpatient care. In 1999 the National Association of State Mental Health Program Directors (NASMHPD) issued a seminal paper on the topic, and the recommendations of its National Technical Assistance Center (NTAC) for State Mental Health Planning have transformed this practice (23). The use of preventive safety and crisis plans has been effective in inpatient settings to substantially reduce restraint use, and leaders in the emergency psychiatry field also advocate verbal de-escalation as an approach to minimize and eliminate use of restraints (see Chapter 18).

There is evidence in ED settings that the use of restraint reduces the likelihood of follow-up with outpatient services. The authors in a novel study concluded that while physical restraint may sometimes be necessary to manage aggression and agitation in the emergency department, being restrained appears to be associated with decreased likelihood of attending prescribed outpatient follow-up mental health treatment. Avoiding physical restraints whenever possible may help minimize impact on treatment compliance after discharge from the emergency department (24).

Similarly, sensitivity to the likelihood that the consumer has a history of trauma must be incorporated into the clinical consciousness of a compassionate ED setting. For people who are dealing with difficult internal stimuli and who have a trauma history of physical violence, routine application of restraints to a gurney can be devastating. Similarly, mandatory clothes removal may inadvertently trigger severe reactions in a person with a history of sexual trauma. Policies and training that reflect the high incidence of psychological trauma in the psychiatric population reduce the risk of exacerbating a painful situation for the person seeking assistance.

EXAMPLES OF PEER SUPPORT

There are few examples of peer-run or active peer support programs in emergency settings, but this is an area that is likely to grow over time. An example of programs that incorporate the peer-driven principles are the People USA Programs in New York featuring Rose House.

As an alternative to hospitalization, People USA's Rose Houses offer temporary residential/respite care, for one to seven nights, in a house run by peers. In this setting, individuals learn tools for recovery and averting crises, with the goal of avoiding future hospitalization in a psychiatric facility. The program is peer-, support-, and skills-oriented. It offers 24-hour peer support, self-advocacy education, self-help training, and mutual understanding. People USA also offers in-home peer companionship if that is a better fit for a person in need. If an individual requires an assessment at a hospital ED, People USA has peer advocates who work directly with the ED staff to assist the consumer in navigating the challenges of that experience (Case 16.3). Support for this innovative program is funded by the county (25). More information on peer run respite programs and a directory of programs can be found at https://power2u.org/crisis alternatives/.

At a macrolevel, the state of Georgia has demonstrated tremendous leadership in the area of peer support. It has developed a certification program for peer specialists; by the end of 2005, 285 graduates had completed the training. The services are Medicaid reimbursable. The state's focus is now on the peer role in assertive community treatment teams and community support work. Georgia has shown pioneering leadership in what promises to be an important "growth stock" for the field of mental health—using peers to improve the quality of services for the people who use them (26). The peer specialist movement continues to grow and there are certification programs in 45 states as well as an international organization to support these efforts (27).

CONCLUSION

Emergency services remain one setting in which the failure to adequately fund a service system becomes evident daily. Consumer participation in service planning, environmental design, crisis planning, and dispositional outcome, wherever possible, will make a difference. With these efforts, the system of care can begin to move the culture of emergency services for those with psychiatric problems closer to the goal envisioned by the President's Freedom Commission—a consumer- and family-driven system.

REFERENCES

1. National Alliance on Mental Illness. (2006). *Grading the states: A report on America's health care system for serious mental illness, 2006.* Arlington, VA: National Alliance on Mental Illness.
2. Cerel, L., Currier, G. W., & Conwell, Y. (2006). Consumer and family experiences in the emergency department following a suicide attempt. *Journal of Psychiatric Practice, 12*(6), 341–347.
3. Ralph, R. O., & Corrigan, P. W. (2005). Introduction. In Ralph, R. O., & Corrigan, P. W. (Eds.), *Recovery in mental illness: Broadening our understanding of wellness* (pp. 3–4). Washington, DC: American Psychological Association.
4. Harding, C. M., Brooks, G. W., Takamaru, A., et al. (1987). The Vermont longitudinal study of persons with severe mental illness, I: Methodology, study sample, and overall status 32 years later. *The American Journal of Psychiatry, 144*, 718–726.
5. Harding, C. M., Brooks, G. W., Takamaru, A., et al. (1987). The Vermont longitudinal study of persons with severe mental illness, II: Long-term outcome of subjects who retrospectively met DSM-III criteria for schizophrenia. *The American Journal of Psychiatry, 144*, 727–735.
6. New Freedom Commission on Mental Health. (2003). *Achieving the promise: Transforming mental health care in America.* Final report. Publication No. SMA-03-3832. Rockville, MD: US Department of Health and Human Services.
7. Campbell, J. (1996). Toward collaborative mental health outcome systems. *New Directions for Mental Health Services, 71*, 68–69.
8. Campbell, J. (1997). How consumer/survivors are evaluating the quality of psychiatric care. *Evaluation Review, 21*(3), 357–363.
9. Mowbray, C., & Moxley, D. (1997). A framework for organizing consumer roles as providers of psychiatric rehabilitation. In Mowbray, C., Moxley, D., Jasper, C., & Howell, L. (Eds.), *Consumers as providers in psychiatric rehabilitation* (pp. 35–44). Columbia, MD: International Association of Psychosocial Rehabilitation Services.

10. Campbell, J. (2005). The historical and philosophical development of peer-run support programs. In Clay, S., Schnell, B., Corrigan, P., & Ralph, R. (Eds.), *On our own, together: Peer programs for people with mental illness* (pp. 18–19). Nashville, TN: Vanderbilt University Press.

11. Mead, S., Hilton, D., & Curtis, L. (2001). Peer support: A theoretical perspective. *Psychiatric Rehabilitation Journal, 25*, 136.

12. For information on this NAMI outreach program, go to http://www.nami.org/template.cfm?section=In_Our_Own_Voice. The brochure, In Our Own Voice: Living with Mental Illness—Learn about Mental Illness from People Who Have Been There, can be downloaded.

13. Zinman, S. (1986). Self-help: The wave of the future. *Hospital & Community Psychiatry, 37*, 213.

14. Zinman, S. (1987). Definition of self-help groups. In Ainman, S., Harp, H., & Budd, S. (Eds.), *Reaching across: Mental health clients helping each other* (pp. 7–15). Riverside, CA: California Network of Mental Health Clients.

15. Chamberlin, J. (1988). *On our own: Patient-controlled alternatives to the mental health system.* Manchester: Mind Publications.

16. Saltzer, M., & Liptzin-Shear, S. (2002). Identifying consumer-provider benefits in evaluation of consumer-delivered services. *Psychiatric Rehabilitation Journal, 25*, 281.

17. Copeland, M. E. (2000). *Wellness recovery action plan* (Rev. ed., p. 4). West Dummerston, VT: Peach Press.

18. For more information about the Massachusetts recovery learning centers see www.mbrlc.org and www.southeastrlc.org.

19. Marson, D., McGovern, M., & Pomp, H. (1988). Psychiatric decision-making in the emergency room: A research overview. *American Journal of Psychiatry, 145*, 918–925.

20. Warmline.org is an online resource guide for peer run supports by state.

21. Stanley, B., Brown, G. K., Brenner, L. A., et al. (2018). Comparison of the safety planning intervention with follow-up vs usual care of suicidal patients treated in the emergency department. *JAMA Psychiatry, 75*(9), 894–900.

22. Fisher, D. (2006). *Warm Lines: An alternative to hospitalization.* National Empowerment Center. Retrieved from http://www.power2u.org/articles/selfhelp/warm_lines.html. For perhaps the first published reference to the term warm line, see Adkins, P. G., & Ainsa, T. D. (1978). A primary prevention service. *Research Communications in Psychology, Psychiatry and Behavior, 3*, 173–176.

23. National Association of State Mental Health Program Directors. (July 13, 1999). *Position statement on seclusion and restraint.* Retrieved from http://www.nasmhpd.org. See also http://www.nasmhpd.org/ntac.cfm for NTAC's *Six Core Strategies to Reduce the Use of Seclusion and Restraint Planning Tool* and other prevention-based training curricula.

24. Currier, G. W., Walsh, P., & Lawrence, D. (2011). Physical restraints in the emergency department and attendance at subsequent outpatient psychiatric treatment. *Journal of Psychiatric Practice, 17*(6), 387–393.

25. See https://people-usa.org, the website of this innovative consumer-operated agency.

26. Sabin, J. E., & Daniels, N. (2003). Strengthening the consumer voice in managed care, VII: The Georgia peer specialist program. *Psychiatric Services, 54*, 497–498. See also the website of the Georgia Division of Mental Health, Developmental Disabilities and Addictive Disorders, http://mhddad.dhr.georgia.gov/portal/site/DHR-MHDDAD/.

27. https://www.inaops.org/.

17

The Family in Psychiatric Emergencies: An Across the Lifespan Approach

Sarah A. Nguyen, Alison M. Heru, Lee Combrinck-Graham

Families are an important resource for understanding and responding to the individual in distress. The family/home environment is also the patient's primary social milieu, so it is especially important to assess the family context when creating a comprehensive treatment plan (1). In this chapter, we review the evidence and rationale for family inclusion and outline how to work with families in psychiatric emergencies across the lifespan, using case examples to illustrate the best practice approach to family involvement.

THE RATIONALE FOR FAMILY INCLUSION

Families are a significant resource. In many situations, families report the emergency, accompany the patient to the hospital, and assume responsibility to care for the patient throughout the course of the illness. Family members provide important information about the patient and circumstances leading to the crisis, particularly if the patient is cognitively impaired, agitated, or psychotic or has difficulty communicating a clear history (2). The provider's message to family members should be, "You are my eyes and ears. We will work together to make sure your family member does the best they can." If families are not present initially, they should be invited to join in as soon as possible.

Outcomes improve when families are involved in patient care (3). In a Denver-based crisis intervention project, patients whose condition was deemed serious enough to warrant hospitalization were randomized to hospital treatment or discharge home from the emergency department

with a home-based family treatment intervention. Those in the family intervention group had a speedier recovery, shorter time away from daily activities, and decreased relapse rate compared with patients who were hospitalized (4).

Involving families in assessment and treatment substantially reduces risk for the patient and also for the provider (5). Good documentation and good rapport with family members provide a protective function against adverse provider outcomes such as lawsuits (5). Families may provide information that increases the likelihood of an accurate diagnosis or early detection of harmful behaviors such as substance misuse, self-injurious behavior, or even functional decline. Involving the family in decision-making about treatment and disposition is key to good patient compliance and will lead to more successful outcomes (6--8). Family members usually want to be helpful and appreciate guidance to lessen the likelihood of harm to their loved ones. Listening to the family, taking their fears and concerns seriously, and teaching them how to help keep their loved one safe are important first steps in providing optimal family-oriented patient care.

Furthermore, when a family is overwhelmed and can no longer care for a patient with behavioral issues, they may bring the patient to an emergency department. A family member may not be able to continue with caregiving any longer and may need a therapeutic space to talk through what is happening and be connected to available resources. Families may be beginning to face the impact of change in the relationship, their expectations, and their assumptions about recovery. Families may need guidance to reorganize

TABLE 17.1 How to Invite the Family Into the Conversation

- Sit and listen to family members, noting the roles that each person plays.
- Recognize that all stories are different and may provide clues about what is going on.
- Respond to the family's anxiety, reassuring them that their questions will be answered and they will be involved in the treatment plan.
- Display an attitude of interest, warmth, and appreciation of the multiple points of view of all family members.
- Understand the concerns of each family member.
- Appreciate the impact of illness across generations, recognizing that effects can be felt by the parents, spouse, and children of the identified patient.

the family functioning. This can be as simple as helping families coordinate schedules, organizing where family members are, deciding who should be involved, and determining their level of involvement and responsibilities. The provider can help set the best tone, begin to delineate the best path, and recognize how best to utilize and incorporate the specific family strengths. Compassionate emergency intervention can be the greatest gift to the family.

Given all of the reasons for family to be involved, why has family involvement not become the standard of care for psychiatric emergencies? Sometimes, families are not readily available or are unwilling to become involved with the patient. However, the main reasons are related to provider training and provider comfort level. Emergency providers are usually not trained to meet with families in a brief, directive but supportive manner. Providers may also view families as "toxic," meaning that families are somehow responsible for, or can worsen, the patient's distress and are avoided altogether.

Including families in a psychiatric emergency, however, does not require specific training, and when family distress is understood and acknowledged, more options for disposition from the emergency setting may emerge. In the following sections, patient vignettes will illustrate how an empathic and collaborative approach can engage families in a more constructive way. In a crisis situation, families are often upset or angry, and if the provider responds to the anger or misunderstanding with compassion, the initially "toxic" family member can become an ally and the course of the crisis changes for the better.

FAMILY ENGAGEMENT IN PSYCHIATRIC EMERGENCIES

Invite the Family into Conversation

Beginning to work with families means including family members in the assessment and treatment planning process. With family inclusion, no specific family intervention is provided: the family is simply present. Regardless of the diagnosis, when the family is included with the patient in the assessment, decision-making, and treatment planning, patients' adherence and outcomes to treatment improve (9-11). Family inclusion does not require any specific training and can occur as part of routine care. Table 17.1 summarizes how to invite the family into the discussion.

Two overall perspectives on families and family function may help the provider individualize their interventions to a particular family. First is the identification of family strengths, which can support recovery. For example, a family that lives in or is part of a supportive community can be encouraged to ask the community to help out in some small and specific ways. A family member who has a car can be asked to help with transport while other family members contribute by performing basic practical tasks such as cleaning or cooking. A family that enjoys spending time together can be reminded that setting time to celebrate good times can still be part of their lives, despite adversity.

A second helpful perspective is the developmental stage of the family and identification of any specific life cycle transitions. Families tend to be vulnerable at times of transitions such as changes in status and role functions when people come into the family (birth or adoption, marriage, assuming care of aging parents) or leave the family (adolescent

TABLE 17-2 Example Questions for the Initial Assessment

- What are the concerns of each person present?
- When did the family notice the problem and what attempts were made to solve it so far?
- How was it decided that they should seek professional help?
- Can a family member tell you what happened from their perspective?
- If someone refers to an important person who is not present, follow up with "Can we call your mother to get her point of view?"

leaving home, divorce, death of family member, or any other transition related to loss of independence or autonomy). Identifying these normative events and normalizing the family's distress may be sufficiently reassuring to alleviate a crisis (12).

What to Ask

The assessment should initially focus on the immediate crisis, with the priority being an assessment of safety. Upon being assured that the patient, family members, and provider are immediately safe, the provider can begin. Good structure and firm limit setting are keys to a successful family meeting (13).

In beginning the meeting, each family member needs to be introduced and invited to express their opinions and concerns. This might happen with a question, "Who can tell me what is going on?" Someone will identify themselves as a spokesperson at this juncture, and then the others can be asked. Remember, even young children have opinions and feelings, and it is OK to ask them. In fact, children who have parents with serious mental illness have expressed desire to be acknowledged and included in treatment planning (14). If an important person is not present, consider having them join by phone or ask if other family members can say what that person might think or say? Table 17.2 lists some useful questions for an initial family assessment.

Listen and Observe the Family

Observe the demeanor and attitudes of the patient and family members toward each other. Family members can be present voluntarily or grudgingly. Look for close and supportive relationships or distant, hostile, or even intimidating behavior. A good understanding of the family's perspective allows the provider to develop empathy and put themselves in the family's shoes. This information

can help manage the family meeting and inform the discharge plan. The following points can guide you:

- Validate everyone's efforts to manage the situation and their decision to search further for help. "I hear what you are all saying and that everyone has a different view of what happened. The good thing is that you all agreed that this was an emergency and brought John to the emergency room."
- Maintain good control of the meeting at all times, gently redirecting distressed family members and firmly setting limits. "We have a limited time to meet; it is important that everyone gets to express their concerns, and I will need to keep things moving in order to allow that to happen. Is that OK?"
- Appreciate different family members' perspectives. If tensions become too unmanageable, the family meeting may need to end. Some family members may be asked to wait outside or the patient may need to be seen by themselves. Keep in mind that even a brief engagement with the family may expose relevant conflicts and strengths of the family that will be useful for ongoing treatment after the emergency is settled.

Shared Decision-Making Between Professional, Patient, and Family

At the end of the meeting, it is important to summarize the information learned in the family meeting and synthesize an understanding of the problem from a family perspective as well as from a medical perspective. By giving the family the opportunity to be heard, they are more likely to listen and follow through with the treatment plan. As mentioned before, try to validate and provide emotional support and discuss options and resources, such as referral to a community support group, as you work with the family to develop a treatment plan.

THE FAMILY IN EMERGENCIES INVOLVING CHILDREN AND ADOLESCENTS

The American Academy of Child and Adolescent Psychiatry issued a "Facts for Families," on "What is a Psychiatric Emergency," that is based on three alarms—threats or actions to die; threats or actions to harm someone else; or not making sense/losing touch with reality. The recommendation for families is to bring the child or adolescent to the emergency department (ED) (15-17). However, in work with children and adolescents in the context of their families, the experience of emergencies is somewhat broader and more complex, as we will explore in Cases 17.1-17.3.

 CASE 17.1

A 7-year-old "freaks out" in school. Jimmy, the younger of two boys of divorced parents, becomes upset in his second-grade class. It is not clear what precipitated the episode of screaming, yelling, and shouted foul language at the teacher, followed by running around in the school, and then attempting to run out of the building. The ambulance is called, and he is brought to the ED. As often happens in such a case, by the time Jimmy gets to the ED, the outburst has diminished, he is exhausted, frightened, and overwhelmed. Both of his parents arrive in the ED shortly after he does. At first, because of their antagonistic relationship, his parents blame each other for Jimmy's outburst. The father, who favors a diagnosis of some form of mental illness, accuses the mother of being neglectful; and the mother observes that Jimmy is always fine when he is with her. However, she notes that whenever Jimmy talks to his father, she always has to calm him down afterward.

Inviting the family to the conversation. Hearing his parents argue in the ED, upsets Jimmy. He begins to scream, saying he wants to die. Sitting with the parents and Jimmy, the ED provider asks the parents how they might help comfort Jimmy and settle him down right now. After a brief argument because dad wants to give him medication whereas mom wants to comfort him with words, saying, "Jimmy, it's OK, we're going to take care of you," they both realize that what he needs right then is comfort, not an arbitration about who is right. Dad takes Jimmy tenderly onto his lap, while mom strokes his hair; Jimmy calms to sobbing, then breathing softly before he falls asleep.

Shared decision-making between professional, patient, and family. Because it is mom's time to have the children, Jimmy goes home with her that night, but it is agreed that the follow-up has to include the parents coming together to comfort both of their boys. For the moment, Jimmy's diagnosis is downgraded from dad's preference of bipolar disorder and attention-deficit hyperactivity disorder (ADHD) to adjustment disorder with anxiety.

 CASE 17.2

A child hallucinates. Clarissa, an 11-year-old girl, is awkward and uncomfortable in her school and reports hearing voices telling her to hurt herself and others. The school principal calls 911 and has her transported to the ED. Her mother is called. Her father is not available. The mother arrives in the ED and says she is "managing" Clarissa and two young sons, ages 4 and 3, and she is upset and angry about having to disrupt her day to go to the ED.

This is not Clarissa's first time hearing the voices, and, in the past, visits to the ED with this complaint have resulted in her being hospitalized, diagnosed with schizophrenia (because of hallucinations), and placed on medication that makes her hungry so that she has gained weight and feels even more awkward and uncomfortable with her peers. In a previous episode, her mother has become so exasperated that she has shouted, "I'm calling child protective services, and they can take you. I can't deal with you anymore."

Inviting the family to the conversation: When Clarissa's mother arrives in the ED, she

CASE 17.2 *(continued)*

is once again exasperated with her daughter and begins to yell at her. Clarissa responds by getting more upset and says she does not care and just wants to die. The ED staff sits down with the mother and Clarissa. Speaking to the mother, the professional says "Can you find out from your daughter what happened?" The mother starts to give her own explanation beginning with, "Oh she always wants her own way...." The professional persists, saying, "Ask her what happened, that she didn't get her own way." Her mother again resists and the professional persists. Finally, the mother addresses Clarissa in such a way that sobbing Clarissa replies that her classmates have called her fat and stupid. "And I just feel no good and nothing will be good," she said. "Do you think she's no good and fat and stupid?" the professional asks the mother. "Oh, no, I think she's beautiful and smart and good," said the mother, tearing up and turning to hug her daughter. "But it just scares me when she says all these things about hurting herself, and it makes me angry, because I don't know what to do."

Shared decision-making between provider, patient, and family. Clarissa's sobbing decreases and she says she thinks she can go home. The ED staff, Clarissa, and her mother develop a safety plan that all are comfortable with and it is recommended that the family pursue outpatient therapy. The family continues in therapy, with the mother working specifically on identifying when Clarissa feels ignored, awkward, or shunned by her peers and being sensitive about her hurt. Her mother makes more special time to spend with her, doing "girlie things" together, sometimes leaving the boys with their grandmother. Over time, Clarissa begins to identify the "voices" as thoughts and begins to recognize the situations in which these thoughts come up, what generated them, and what to do about them—that is, talk to a teacher, if at school, or her mother, when at home. In this context, her psychotropic medication is decreased, and she becomes less "hungry" and more active.

CASE 17.3

An adolescent threatens suicide. Liana, a 16-year-old high school junior, lives with her parents who immigrated from India. Her parents are observant Hindus and expect their children (Liana, her older sister, and younger brother) to participate in their religious practices. They are also traditional in their expectations of conduct, dress, and social behavior. Under the guise of doing extra schoolwork and having study meetings with her classmates, Liana has actually been smoking pot and drinking. In addition to flouting her family rules and expectations, she has been lying and living in a false relationship with her parents. On one occasion, she became overwhelmed and said she wanted to die. She told this to the school counselor who took her to the ED. Her parents were called and were extremely distraught. Liana was afraid that her parents would find out about her lies and begs the providers not to tell them. Because she was an adolescent, the providers had "maintained

her confidentiality." Liana was referred to the hospital for inpatient care, was diagnosed with depression, and was placed on a series of medications; sertraline "did not work," so she was also given aripiprazole. The tension continued, and Liana's "depression," which seemed to be a form of despair and desperation, got worse. She makes another suicide threat and is sent to the ED a second time, and this time, the ED providers meet with Liana and her family.

Inviting the family to the conversation. "Let's talk about what is happening," says the ED provider. The mother weeps and the father is very sad, and both say they feel excluded from what is happening with their daughter, and very helpless; however, they love her and want her better. Eventually, reluctantly, and ashamedly, Liana tells them what she has been doing and the lie that she has been living. They all weep. The parents are upset about what she has been doing, but with the encouragement of the ED

CASE 17.3 *(continued)*

provider, they move toward more understanding and remind her they will always love her.
Shared decision-making between professional, patient, and family. After the family meeting, the parents feel that Liana will be safe

to go home that night. Her mother sleeps with her, holding her tight. They have a follow-up family meeting during which she tells her siblings what has been going on, and the parents warn her siblings, "Don't get any ideas!"

Danger and Opportunity

A psychiatric emergency in a child or adolescent presents both a danger and an opportunity. The danger is that there will be a rift between the child and parent(s) that leads to a greater disruption to family functioning. Disruption occurs for several reasons:

- Parents are overwhelmed and helpless and do not know how to help their child or adolescent
- Parents are angry or embarrassed and blame the child
- Professionals step in as experts and either explicitly or implicitly take over from parents or are seen as being "better" than the parents in the child's eyes
- Children are rejecting, seeing their parents as not helpful or comforting

On the other hand, the crisis of an emergency presents an opportunity for the family to become a more reliable context for the child's comfort and safety by professionals respecting parents' familiarity and experience with their child through:

- Consulting parents about their understanding of what their child might be going through: the upset, the fear, the despair, the fury, or the outrage
- Encouraging parents to comfort their child using the skills they already have
- Asking parents to talk to their child to find out what the child thinks might be helpful
- Inviting the family members to soothe their children, perhaps hold them, stroke their cheeks, speak softly to them, or reassure them.

There is an opportunity to increase the family members' competence in managing the child's mood and behaviors when the provider invites the family to talk about what happened, how the child is feeling, and how the parent feels about the child. When children and adolescents have psychiatric emergencies, they are either inconsolable or uncontrollable or both. It is important to remember that these children usually live with

families who are responsible for their care and also for consoling and controlling them.

There is some debate about whether and when the parents should be seen with or without the child (15-17). Clearly, we believe that families should be involved as soon as possible, and that decisions about safety and subsequent care of the acutely disturbed child are best made through assessment and consultation with family and other resources. The presence of family members can provide the most immediately useful "collateral" information, including relevant history, but most importantly the display of family strengths and resources (or liabilities, if that is what appears). We always begin with the whole family, including siblings, aunts, uncles, and grandparents, if they happen to be present.

The following points can guide you:

- What happened? And who is going to tell the story?
- If something happened to the child away from the family, the parents can ask the child to tell them what happened. The professional is a witness to this interaction.
- If the parents are not understanding or even angry with the child, the provider might say something like, "You sound angry; let's hear more about what happened and see."
- If the child is reluctant to speak with parents present, the provider might ask the parents' permission to speak to the child alone with the understanding that then the child will then be able to say something about what happened so they can all work together.

If the parent seems to be annoyed with child because they have been inconvenienced or embarrassed by the child's behavior, the first step is to share concern with the parent—that is, "we are just as concerned as you are," or "we are not angry with your child, we are just concerned that he/she can calm down and be safe."

Safety and comfort are the objective outcomes for an upset child, so the question becomes who is capable of providing it, and how can they best do it? Usually the parents or adult family members are the ones responsible for keeping their children safe and comfortable. The professional intervention in an emergency is to assess both the capacity of the family to provide safety and comfort and to assist them in feeling confident and competent to do so.

When the emergency interventions focus only on the child, the child's distress, and the provisional diagnosis, a decision about care can result in further, often unnecessary distress. A child-focused intervention may separate the child from his/her family and be more upsetting if the child goes to an unfamiliar setting while the family is left feeling frightened and incapable. When hospitalization is the best disposition, this should be decided with the family, and hopefully a family member can be with the child in the hospital.

With adolescents, the danger of disruption of the family, particularly the parent-child relationship, is often even greater than with younger children. Unfortunately, the general societal interpretation of adolescent development is that we, as adults and especially parents, should not interfere or hinder the teen's individuation. This may be an extreme way of expressing this, but the common message to parents is "stay out of my/his/her business." With this message, the adolescent may feel that either they have the right to no parent interference, or for some reason they "should not" ask for help and should work things out for themselves or with their inexperienced peers. It is not uncommon to discover that an adolescent emergency occurs when the adolescent is disconnected from his/her family/parents. In addition to the reasons described above, this may also be driven by ongoing family conflicts where the adolescent is already feeling isolated and withdrawn.

These three vignettes illustrate the benefit of emergency interventions when parents and children are seen together. Without family involvement, there is the danger that parent(s) and child will move even further apart emotionally making the stresses even worse and further pathologizing the child's feelings and behaviors. In these vignettes, the crises provide an opportunity to restore respect and comfort in family relationships, leading to a better outcome for the child and family.

THE FAMILY IN EMERGENCIES INVOLVING ADULTS

In the adult emergency department, it is much easier to assess an adult when family members, police, or other concerned friends or colleagues accompany them. Healthcare providers are used to asking for "collateral"; that is information that can clarify their diagnostic reasoning, however, there are other reasons to include family or friends. These additional reasons include the needing to fully assess the environment, looking for risk and protective factors in the family, and most importantly, enlisting family and friends in a plan for treatment and recovery.

It is not immediately obvious that family meetings are helpful when the patient is very psychotic, cognitively impaired, or intoxicated. As Case 17.4 illustrates an initially clear picture can become complicated, a not infrequent occurrence in emergency settings. Complicated presentations can be difficult to disentangle for the emergency department providers, family, and friends. For successful care, family and friends may need detailed education about how to help with treatment, both in the short and the long term.

CASE 17.4

A patient whose physical and mental illnesses are complicated by substance abuse. Ms. Evans, a 37-year-old married white woman, presents to the ED, with a chief complaint of "not feeling good" Ms. Evans is anxious and tearful, reporting, "I got a letter and it says that I'm going to go to jail. The cops are watching all the time." She reports not taking any of her home medications for the past 3 to 4 months. Her ability to give an accurate history is impaired. She cannot say where she is living. She states her husband just left her. She is unable to identify any social support. Urine toxicology screen is positive for methamphetamines, Thyroid Stimulating Hormone (TSH) is 256.57 and T4 is 0.19. On examination, she is paranoid and disorganized. Her Montreal Cognitive Assessment (MoCA) score is 20/30 with deficits in executive functioning.

Inviting family into conversation. The provider calls the patient's mother, who is identified in the chart as her family contact. The mother is glad to hear her daughter is safe because she has not heard from her for a few days. She confirms that her daughter uses methamphetamine and does not go to her medical appointments. She also confirms that the patient's husband has left her but states that they have an "on-and-off-again" relationship. She believes that the patient's three children are with her daughter's in-laws. The provider asks the patient's mother if she would come to the hospital to meet with her daughter and the team and she agreed to do so.

The provider next asks the patient's permission to call her husband. The patient is initially reluctant to do so but with the support of her mother, she agrees. He also agrees to attend the meeting.

When the patient's husband arrives, the patient is more coherent, and she is able to take part in the discussion. The mother is calm and somewhat detached. The husband greets his mother-in-law with a resigned smile. At this point, it appears that they share the burden of caring for Ms. Evans and have an unwanted alliance, from which the patient is excluded.

The provider limits expectations for the meeting to "gathering information and deciding on a safe plan." The provider states that "at this point, no decisions have been made," and that what happens will depend on the outcome of the meeting. The mother is firm that her daughter cannot come home with her. The provider recognizes it is absolutely necessary to have the patient participate as fully as possible and not allow the husband and mother to take charge or gang up against her. This will allow the patient to "own" any decision she makes, rather than feel that it is her mother or her husband's decision.

The provider wants to hear each person's story but also gently reminds them that she might interrupt because of limited time. After each person shares their perspective, they are all educated about the role of her thyroid disease and the possible link to Ms. Evan's mental status and use of substances.

Shared decision-making between provider, patient, and family. The mother and husband both agreed on what needs to happen and are clear that they are both burnt out. The mother wants her daughter to be hospitalized: "She has a psychiatric problem; why can't you admit her and fix it?" The patient responds, "I want help but not as an inpatient." The husband intercedes impatiently, "Then get the help. I don't care if you go in-patient or sail around the world. But we have three little children who don't have a mother. And I'm not going to let you see them until you clean yourself up!" The patient begins to sob and her speech becomes incoherent. The husband turns away in frustration. The mother says she will take no more responsibility for her daughter, stating she has been burned many times and that her daughter should go to rehab. The patient begins to yell at her mother.

The provider asks the patient to quiet down so that any decision made can include the patient and not be made for her, stating, "If you can be calm and clear you can make decisions about what will happen next." Then the husband again asks the patient, "So, what is your plan? This is not about whether you do what your mother or I want; it is about you getting clean and staying clean so your mother can enjoy her life without worrying about you all the time, and so your children can have a mother."

The psychiatrist notes that the family is angry and understands their point of view. She redirects the family, bringing the focus back to the present. "We all need to decide on a safe plan for today." She asks about potential follow-up options as the patient does not want admission, such as a community mental health center or walk-in clinic where the patient can go when she has difficulty. The patient and her mother agree that the walk-in clinic down the street is the best option to take care of her thyroid disease. Her husband agrees and wonders if there is any way he can help to remind her or go with her the medical clinic. The patient also agrees to enroll in an outpatient co-occurring program and is given an appointment for the following week. She also agrees that if she should fail outpatient care, then she will consider inpatient rehab.

CASE 17.4 *(continued)*

The patient decides on a goal of having contact with her children as a longer-term objective, which her husband fully supports and he reassures her that the children are safe and that she can see them regularly when she is drug free.

Working to get someone into treatment can begin in the emergency situation, and this may be an opportunity to work toward an optimal outcome. After the immediate patient care needs are established, the provider can look for supporting community resources. Regarding substance use programs, Judith Landau's ARISE (Addiction Recovery in Supportive Environment) Family Interventions have shown efficacy in getting patients into treatment (18). This is a family approach that engages reluctant substance dependent individuals into treatment using families. It is an evidence-based intervention that empowers the family and attempts to break the isolation and "private struggle" of both the addicted individual and family.

THE FAMILY IN EMERGENCIES INVOLVING GERIATRIC PATIENTS

As people get older, they become increasingly vulnerable to disease and mortality. They are often lonely because friends die; they are less mobile and cannot get out to mingle and visit others as easily; they lose mental faculties and become disoriented and frightened; they are more prone to a variety of medical problems ranging from wear and tear on their systems to accidents and injuries; and they become more dependent. As they become increasingly dependent, the first caregivers are other family members, including partners, often aging themselves, or children, usually grown and with other responsibilities. Sometimes, they have committed caretakers—either a relative or someone hired for this job. All of these conditions of normal aging contribute to a sense of frailty and unfamiliarity in an emergency situation. Deterioration and changes in physical and mental status require review, reeducation, and possible redesign of living situation, treatment processes, and goals. In this context, everyone can easily become discouraged and exhausted, making it is especially important to involve family members and other caregivers (eg, relative/caregivers, other relatives, staff in a memory unit, home health aides) in evaluating what is happening and what needs to be done.

Details about the care of the geriatric patient are covered in Chapter 35, but often the most important part of treatment planning is figuring out who is going to help implement and carry out the plan. This is why family involvement (as illustrated in Case 17.5) is key when treating psychiatric emergencies in older adults. Although all questions about who will care for the patient in an ongoing way may not be answered in the emergency situation, they must be considered so that the acute emergency interventions include appropriate actions to minimize and avoid repeated emergencies. For older adults, family members and/or caretakers play a critical role particularly in an emergency situation. These supportive people should be involved as soon as possible to avoid the worst of possible outcomes, their abandoning the patient or becoming so overburdened that they can no longer provide care adequately.

CASE 17.5

The overwhelmed caregiver. *Mr. Kwok is a 69-year-old lawyer with a history of bipolar disorder, a traumatic brain injury (TBI) incurred in a fall 4 years ago, and vascular dementia with behavioral disturbances. He has become very agitated and exhibits sexually inappropriate behavior beyond what the staff in his nursing home can tolerate, so he is brought by an ambulance to the emergency department. He was hospitalized a few months ago for pneumonia, urinary tract infection (UTI), and associated delirium that appeared to be resolving*

CASE 17.5 (continued)

at the time of discharge. He presented to the emergency department 2 weeks ago for worsening behavior: not sleeping at night, throwing things around his room, and requiring 24/7 assistance because of wandering and falling. His wife of 22 years is his conservator of estate and person, and she is demanding hospital admission.

Inviting family into conversation. Usually, Mrs. Kwok accompanies her husband to the ED, but since he was sent from the nursing home, she arrives a little after he did. The ED staff began talking with the patient to get to know him but are grateful for his wife's arrival, greeting her warmly and assuring her that they are keeping her husband safe and comfortable. The evaluating provider sits with her to get background information: the patient's history, his level of function at baseline, and an account of the recent changes and deterioration. The provider also inquires about children and other family or caregivers involved in his care. Mrs. Kwok explains their children live out of state and says she does not want to bother them. The provider wonders if the children might have additional useful information, but more importantly, if they might offer more support to their mother—the primary caregiver—in this difficult situation.

Shared decision-making between professional, patient, and family. Although Mrs. Kwok insists that she does not want to bother her children, the provider persists, providing psychoeducation on caregiver burden and explaining and validating how much responsibility and stress she is enduring to manage things by herself. The provider suggests that even though her children may not be able to come in, they could certainly offer emotional support and even assistance with a range of things, including finances, legal concerns, and possibilities for securing support for more services at home or in a facility. Mr. Kwok finally agrees to call her 43-year-old daughter, a nurse, who is grateful to be included. After the provider outlines the situation and discusses the treatment plan with the patient's wife and daughter, the daughter agrees to take a more active role in helping her mother care for her father. The daughter also provides some additional information about

her father, confirming that he had been a brilliant trial lawyer who suffered several episodes of severe depression and had received two rounds of electroconvulsive therapy (ECT) when he was in his 50s. It seems that he has been deteriorating since then, and she thinks a lot of his deterioration is from depression about not being able to work.

The patient's daughter asks a number of questions and wonders why her father is suddenly getting worse expressing concern about whether his medications might be making things worse or whether he might have had a stroke. Mrs. Kwok said she had similar questions and asked, "Is this something that can be treated so he can get better?" The psychiatric provider, based on her examination and the history, thinks that a new acute process is unlikely and that his worsening symptoms are likely a part of the natural course of his progressing dementia. She provides more information about dementia, particularly about the neuropsychiatric and behavioral changes that can occur, which is all new information to Mrs. Kwok who is then referred to a caregiver support group and connected with a social worker to help her plan the next step for her husband's care.

Although acute inpatient hospitalizations are usually not the appropriate setting for dementia patients with behavioral disturbances, information from Mrs. Kwok reveals that this is a significant worsening from her husband's behavioral baseline. Mrs. Kwok says she wants her husband to be in the hospital saying, "This just keeps happening over and over, and we have to keep him safe. Even though he's in the nursing home, they keep calling me. I can't sleep because I'm worrying about him." Both the provider and her daughter understood Mrs. Kwok's desperation, and the provider agrees to admit Mr. Kwok, primarily to see if any interventions can help modify his behavior but also to give Mrs. Kwok respite and do some more thoughtful planning about the kind of living situation and supportive services that will make Mr. Kwok most comfortable.

Feeling somewhat better, Mrs. Kwok goes to sit with her husband, kissing his forehead,

CASE 17.5 *(continued)*

stroking his hand, and talking softly to him as he smiles back. This episode in the ED is different than the previous ones, because the provider had reached out to the family. The additional information and engagement of the daughter, even if long-distance, allows for a more positive intervention that was beneficial for everyone and will hopefully minimize the occurrence and severity of future crises.

While the outcome from this visit is good, this is unlikely to be Mr. Kwok's last visit to the ED for similar complaints. Crisis situations often

allow ED providers to begin the difficult conversation about goals of care with families of elderly loved ones with progressive physical and/or cognitive decline. Ultimately, a patient may require more than what a family can provide or support, and working to help the family make these challenging decisions can begin in the emergency situation. If Mr. Kwok is to be discharged back to his conservator or other caretaking persons, their ability to care for him and their understanding of his needs must be addressed.

When a patient can no longer return home, and nursing home or other placement is being considered, families are crucial in the decision-making process. Common reasons given for why placement is needed include, "my loved one needed more advanced or skilled care than I could provide," "my health would not permit me to continue caregiving," and "my loved one's behavior became too difficult to handle." Movement to a nursing home is a major life event for both the patient and caregiver, and informed guidance to the family can increase the chances for appropriate and timely nursing home placement and reduce caregiver guilt (19). Discussion about placement in the emergency setting is just a first step and should offer psychoeducation, teach problem-solving techniques, and mobilize existing family networks and the primary caregiver in order to improve emotional outcomes for the primary caregiver and other loved ones.

CONCLUSION

The family in crisis experiences fear, anxiety, frustration, and uncertainty. Emergencies are disturbances in ongoing life, both for the individual and for the family, and involve all in the family system. To resolve a crisis, it is important to learn what has been going in the family that may have upset the usual order of things, including transitions at all life stages. The provider can intervene to calm and engage the family, thus reducing anxiety and gaining a better understanding of the emergency. All family members can be welcomed and those

who cannot be present may be reached by phone. Although dealing with families in the context psychiatric emergencies can be time-consuming, including the family in the assessment and acute resolution of the crisis enhances the likelihood of a good outcome. As illustrated in the vignettes above, including families in a psychiatric emergency does not require any formal training but simply an attitude of interest, warmth, and appreciation for the multiple points of view of all family members.

A family's narrative about an illness is a window into the family's sense of confidence and efficacy in managing chronic illness (20). The presence of a coherent story that has an illness plan of management indicates a family at lower risk, whereas high-risk families appear to be disorganized and/or traumatized and do not have a coherent illness management plan. Observing the way in which family members interact during a routine interview not only helps identify family strengths but also helps determine family needs. If the family shows significant discord, overt disagreement about how to manage the illness, or admits to long-standing family conflicts present before the illness, referral to family therapy can be considered (21). In the case of older adults, referral to adult protective services should be considered if there is concern for abuse or neglect by family or caregivers. When a family participates in the process of managing an emergency, they may be able to plan ways to respond more quickly and appropriately to future conflicts before they become emergencies.

Meeting with the family, getting to know their stories about the emergency and the patient, identifying family strengths, and utilizing resources to manage and reduce the crisis are important for shared decision-making between the provider, patient, and family. However, the most valuable outcome in a psychiatric emergency is the family's grasp of the difficulties they are experiencing and the usefulness of continuing to work on these problems, whether they are family conflicts or serious illnesses. The family's ability to reflect on these problems occurs in a therapeutic space where the family members are able to express themselves and receive professional feedback on the illness, stages of the illness, and acknowledgment of how this affects the family and each individual's life stages (22).

In this chapter, we have provided the evidence and rationale for family inclusion and outlined how to work with families in a psychiatric emergency, using case examples across the lifespan. Flexibility is needed when managing the diverse population encountered in emergency situations. Providers who have flexibility can more easily manage the provider-family interaction (23). We do not recommend any specific model of family interaction; rather, we recommend that the provider bring a flexible attitude that allows the use of common factors found in all models: communication, empathy, and the ability to provide a rationale for the intervention (24).

Families are our allies in the care of the patient. Talk with the family members as if they are members of the team, as they will likely have a major influence on how the patient will manage after leaving the emergency department. One of the hallmarks of a successful encounter in the emergency department is whether the patient follows up with recommended care, and family is the best guarantee this will happen. It is therefore worthwhile spending time with the family, listening to their concerns, answering their questions, and providing psychoeducation.

REFERENCES

1. Lee, T. S., Renaud, E. F., & Hills, O. F. (2003). Emergency psychiatry: An emergency treatment hub-and-spoke model for psychiatric emergency services. *Psychiatric Services, 54*(12), 1590–1591, 1594.

2. APA. (2016). *Practice guidelines for psychiatric evaluation of adults* (3rd ed., p. 20). Arlington, VA: APA.

3. Doherty, W. J. (1995). Boundaries between patient and family education and family therapy. *Family Relations, 44*, 353–358.

4. Langsley, D. G., Kaplan, D. M., & Pittman, F. S. (1968). *The treatment of families in crisis*. New York, NY: Grune & Stratton.

5. Recupero, P. (2007). Risk management in the family. In Heru, A. M., & Drury, L. M. (Eds.), *Working with families of psychiatric inpatients: A guide for clinicians* (pp. 139–148). Baltimore, MD: Johns Hopkins University Press.

6. Baird, M. A., & Doherty, W. J. (1990). Risks and benefits of a family systems approach to medical care. *Family Relations, 22*, 396–403.

7. McDaniel, S. H., Campbell, T. L., & Seaburn, D. B. (1990). *Family oriented primary care: A manual for medical providers*. New York, NY: Springer-Verlag.

8. Lang, F., Marvel, K., Sanders, D., et al. (2002). Interviewing when family members are present. *American Family Physician, 65*(7), 1351–1354.

9. DiMatteo, M. (2004). Social support and patient adherence to medical treatment: A meta-analysis. *Journal of Health Psychology, 23*, 207–218.

10. Wolff, J. L., Clayman, M. L., Rabins, P., et al. (2015). An exploration of patient and family engagement in routine primary care visits. *Health Expectations, 18*, 188–198.

11. Scheurer, D., Choudhry, N., Swanton, K. A., et al. (2012). Association between different types of social support and medication adherence. *The American Journal of Managed Care, 18*, e461–e467.

12. Combrinck-Graham, L. (1985). A developmental model for family systems. *Family Process, 24*, 139–150.

13. Heru, A. M., & Drury, L. (2007). *Working with families of psychiatric inpatients: A guide for clinicians*. Baltimore, MD: Johns Hopkins University Press.

14. Cooklin, A. https://www.youtube.com/watch?v=uk9nHrlYF5U.

15. AACAP. (2018, July). What is a psychiatric emergency? *Facts for Families* #126.

16. Carandang, C., Gray, C., Marval-Ospino, H., & MacPhee, S. (2012). Child and adolescent psychiatric emergencies. In Rey, J. M. (Ed.), *IACAPAP e-textbook of child and adolescent mental health*. Geneva: International Association for Child and Adolescent Psychiatry and Allied Professions.

17. Gerson, R., & Havens, J. (2015). The child and adolescent psychiatric emergency: A public health challenge. *Psychiatric Times, 32*(11). Retrieved from http://www.psychiatrictimes.com/special-reports/child-and-adolescent-psychiatric-emergency-public-health-challenge.

18. Landau, J., Stanton, M. D., Brinkman-Sull, D., Ikle, D., McCormick, D., Garrett, J., Baciewicz, G., Shea, R. R., Browning, A., & Wamboldt, F. (2004). Outcomes with the ARISE approach to engaging reluctant drug- and alcohol-dependent individuals in treatment. *The American Journal of Drug and Alcohol Abuse, 30*(4), 711–748.

19. Buhr, G. T., Kuchibhatla, M., & Clipp, E. C. (2006). Caregivers' reasons for nursing home placement: Clues for improving discussions with families prior to the transition. *Gerontologist, 46*(1), 52–61.

20. Wamboldt, F. S., & Wamboldt, M. Z. (2013). Family factors in promoting health: The case of childhood asthma. In Heru, A. M. (Ed.), *Working with families in the medical setting* (pp. 23–40). New York, NY: Routledge.

21. Heru, A. M. (2015). Family-centered care in the outpatient general psychiatry clinic. *Journal of Psychiatric Practice, 21*(5), 381–388.

22. Rolland, J. S. (2018). *Helping couples and families navigate illness and disability. An integrated approach*. New York, NY: Guilford Press.

23. Perlmutter, R. A., & Jones, J. E. (1985). Assessment of families in psychiatric emergencies. *American Journal of Orthopsychiatry, 55*(1), 130–139.

24. Frank, J. D., & Frank, J. (1991). *Persuasion and healing: A comparative study of psychotherapy* (3rd ed.). Baltimore, MD: Johns Hopkins University Press.

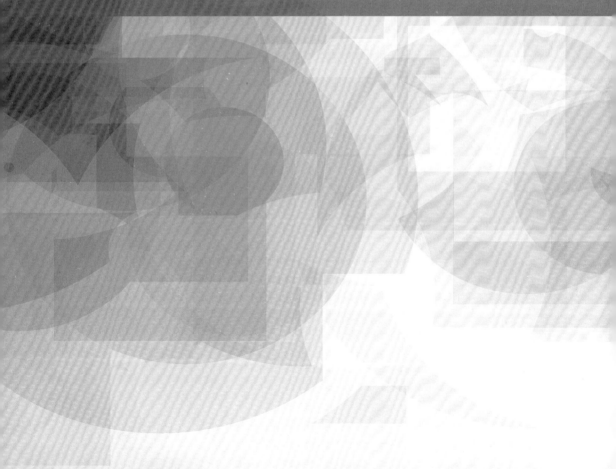

PART IV

Common Presenting Problems

Section Editors: Cheryl McCullumsmith and Scott A. Simpson

18

Agitation: De-escalation

Scott A. Simpson, Lucas Andrew Salg

INTRODUCTION

Agitation is a state of restlessness and motor hyperactivity. When present, agitation is an emergency that heralds medical or psychiatric deterioration (1). In this chapter, we discuss the importance of recognizing agitation in the emergency department (ED) setting and describe techniques for providing the first-line treatment for agitation, verbal de-escalation.

Agitation is common in EDs and important to recognize. Around 3% of ED patients exhibit agitation (2). The prevalence of agitation exceeds 10% of patients in specialty emergency psychiatric services (3). The myriad etiologies of agitation are discussed elsewhere in Chapter 19, Agitation: Evaluation and Management. At worst, agitation may herald a life-threatening condition such as delirium (4). At least, the presence of agitation complicates care through delays in treatment of comorbid conditions, the application of restraint or seclusion, and administration of involuntary medications.

Rapid and competent management of agitation is also an issue of occupational safety. All ED workers are exposed to physical and verbal violence (5,6). These experiences reflect a workplace in which patients are very ill, incapacitated, intoxicated, and maintained in an uncomfortable environment sometimes under circumstances of duress and uncertainty. Yet staff's sense of safety is less reflective of the actual incidence of workplace violence then with their own competence in addressing agitation (6,7). Thus, ED staff deserve training in effective, evidence-based treatments for agitation.

As difficult as agitation may be to manage, there is agreement as to the initial clinical approach to this syndrome. This approach comprises preventing agitation, identifying agitation and its causes early, and offering verbal de-escalation (8–11).

THE PHILOSOPHY OF TREATING AGITATION

Implementing specific techniques to identify or treat agitation requires that the clinician internalize several tenets that underlie the contemporary approach to treating agitated patients:

- Agitation is a symptom, not a disease (1).
- Verbal de-escalation is the first line of treatment for all agitation, regardless of etiology (9).
- The goal of verbal de-escalation is to help the patient regain control of their symptoms. No patient enjoys feeling agitated.
- De-escalation seeks to avoid restraint, seclusion, and coercive interventions.
- Medications are a helpful and sometimes necessary adjunct to treating agitation, and the patient should participate in the decision to take medications.

These principles reflect an approach to patient care that respects patients' preferences in clinical decision-making (12,13), incorporates our scientific understandings of agitation as a transnosologic syndrome and the benefit of medication treatment (1,14), and prioritizes patient and clinician safety by avoiding dangerous restraint episodes (3). Accepting these principles empowers more effective action in the treatment of agitation, whether one is a service leader implementing new processes or a clinician de-escalating an agitated patient.

IDENTIFICATION AND PREVENTION OF AGITATION IN THE EMERGENCY DEPARTMENT

EDs and crisis centers must be deliberative in creating environments that reduce the incidence of agitation as well as its dangers should it occur (15,16). These efforts require anticipatory investments in both physical plant and clinician education (17).

The physical space of the ED cannot approximate the sterility and safety of an inpatient psychiatry unit. EDs must accommodate a range of medical illnesses, are designed for short patient stays, and operate 24 hours a day. In service of these demands, ED rooms have beds with guardrails, wall monitors, sinks, and various objects that may pose a ligature risk, be thrown, or be damaged by an acutely agitated patient. Hallways are constantly lit, there are no windows, and the milieu is noisy and chaotic. Patient rooms are clustered for more efficient care. Staff change frequently, and the course of care is often unpredictable. For psychiatric patients at risk of behavioral instability, the ED is hardly calming.

There are regulatory expectations for EDs' physical space in regard to minimizing suicide risk; these regulations also aid in realizing a physical space that reduces risk to patient and staff should agitation occur (18). In the United States, regulations require that suicidal patients in the ED be treated in ligature-free environments if possible. When not possible, patients should be maintained under continuous observation and out of arm's reach from dangerous objects insofar as medical status allows. Staff observing patient should have ready access to assistance if necessary—the readily available presence of security staff and universal patient screening also appears to reduce the risk of violence (19,20). Environmental modifications should be attempted when necessary to address the underlying etiology of agitation. For example, patients presenting with hallucinogen intoxication should be treated in a low-stimulation environment with low lights and ambient noise.

Staff and clinicians themselves play a pivotal role in reducing the risk of agitation. Staff should be trained in the use of a standardized agitation scale. Examples of scales commonly used in EDs include the Richmond Agitation-Sedation Scale (RASS) (21) and the Behavioural Activity Rating Scale (BARS) (22). These tools require only seconds to administer and are reliable with minimal training. Routine administration of these scales enables staff to properly diagnose conditions associated with agitation (eg, delirium) and quickly communicate to colleagues that agitation is present. For example, a BARS score of 5 suggests the patient is hyperactive but verbally redirectable and requires immediate intervention to avert further escalation (7). Signs of developing agitation may include the rapid onset of irritability, confusion, pacing, fidgeting, or disorganized behaviors. The presence of acute clinical symptoms is a stronger correlate of restraint or seclusion than patient demography, diagnosis, or history (3).

Clinical leaders contribute to the prevention of agitation through supporting staff training in verbal de-escalation, personal safety and escape skills, and trauma informed care (TIC). TIC is a care model that recognizes the impact of trauma in patients' lives (23). TIC proposes that patient autonomy is served by clinicians' efforts to mitigate averse, trauma-related reexperiencing in the medical environment. These efforts include offering patients choices as often as possible, anticipating personally invasive procedures including the physician examination and recognizing that affective instability including irritation, is a common symptom of posttraumatic anxiety. Leaders should promulgate an expectation of decreased or no restraint in favor of even repeated efforts to verbally de-escalate agitated patients (11,24).

INITIATION OF VERBAL DE-ESCALATION

As with most interventions in medicine, verbal de-escalation comprises a core set of technical skills that become more effective with the clinician's artful practice. The core skills of de-escalation are centered around a stepped process described by the acronym RESOLVE:
- **R**eadying to engage,
- **E**ngaging the patient,
- **S**olving problems and **O**ffering choices,
- **L**imit-setting when necessary,
- **V**alidating the patient's perspective, and
- **E**nding the escalation event.

These steps are roughly chronological, although elements of these steps may happen in any order and may need even to be repeated during the patient encounter. Table 18.1 summarizes the steps of verbal de-escalation and their components.

Readying to Engage

As a clinician, it is impossible to effectively de-escalate a patient if you feel unsafe yourself. Upon recognizing agitation in a patient, the clinician prioritizes environmental safety. Staff should maintain a distance of about 2 arms' length away;

TABLE 18.1 The RESOLVE Model of Verbal De-escalation

Step	Component Parts	Example Phrases
Readying to engage	• Environmental preparations • Staff training • Use of standardized scales to assess agitation	
Engaging the patient	• Enter the patient's narrowed range of attention • Identify the patient's needs through active listening	"My name is Dr. Smith, I am the physician in charge of the service. How can I help you?"
Solving problems and offering choices	• Try to solve problems • Offer choices	"Let us help you make a phone call." "Would you like some food or water?"
Limit-setting when necessary	• Set clear limits and boundaries on behaviors • Use time limits	"You cannot leave the hospital right now." "I will not order opioid medications."
Validating the patient's perspective	• Affirm the legitimacy of the patient's concerns	"You are really upset right now." "This is a frustrating situation." "I would be angry if I were in this situation, too."
Ending the escalation event	• Debrief with the patient • Debrief with the staff • Note resolution in objective agitation score	With patient: "What can we do to help you if you are feeling out of control again?" "In the future, How can we tell if you are not doing well"? With staff: "Was anybody hurt?" "What went well during that episode?" "What could have gone better?"

this distance maintains physical safety and avoids the appearance of any threatening intentions. The area should be quickly scanned for objects that might be dangerous if thrown or broken. Wheeled furniture may be flipped or moved precipitously. When possible, dangerous objects should be removed from the patient's reach. Both the patient and clinician should have access to an exit. Staff should be provided with personal alarms or communication devices to quickly and easily summon help (25). If the clinician feels safe doing so, the process of verbal de-escalation begins.

Many ED de-escalation events involve a team of clinicians approaching the patient. If time and circumstance allow, the team should huddle to anticipate some basic aspects of the pending de-escalation intervention. Important considerations include which individual will be speaking to the patient, whether certain medications should be prepared for the patient, and what particular

limits need to be set. Parameters for the involvement of nonclinical security personnel should be established, and a backup plan for physical intervention should be made in the event that verbal de-escalation is inadequate for the patient's safety. The team's leader—most often a physician— should give the team as much guidance as possible to the range of outcomes for the patient, in particular whether the patient should be physically prevented from leaving the ED.

Engaging the Patient

Agitated patients have a narrow range of attention and have difficulty attending to multiple simultaneous stimuli (26). This narrowing of attention occurs regardless of the etiology of the agitation. It is vital for the de-escalating clinician to be within this narrowed range of attention when speaking with the patient. Only one clinician should be speaking at a time, and this person should use brief, concise phrases that

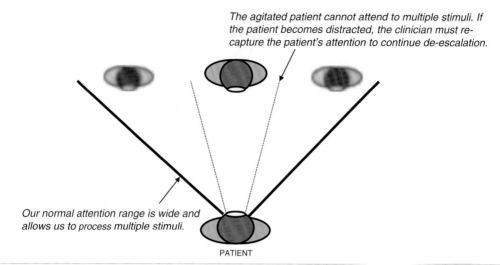

The agitated patient cannot attend to multiple stimuli. If the patient becomes distracted, the clinician must re-capture the patient's attention to continue de-escalation.

Our normal attention range is wide and allows us to process multiple stimuli.

PATIENT

FIGURE 18.1 • Narrowing of attention in agitation.

respect the agitated patient's difficulty attending to convoluted or ambiguous statements. Should the patient become distracted, the clinician must reengage the patient's attention, perhaps with a brief reiteration of the patient's name. Figure 18.1 illustrates this practice. This initial engagement sets the tone for engaging the patient. Common pitfalls include the clinician responding to the yelling patient with more yelling or orders, for example, "Sit down!" or "Be quiet!" A firm tone of voice is helpful, but the clinician must maintain self-control and recall that the patient does not want to be agitated, either. Agitated patients need collaboration not coercion. A more helpful initial approach might be a brief introduction and inquiry as to what the patient needs: "My name is Dr. Smith, I am the physician in charge of the service. How can I help you?"

In this early stage of de-escalation, the clinician seeks to identify the patient's needs. These needs may range from simply being heard to receiving material comfort (eg, food) to receiving an explanation of the treatment plan. Importantly, actively listening while allowing the patient time to speak uninterrupted is crucial to both identify their needs and to let them know they are being heard. The most common needs cited by patients for helping with psychiatric crisis include having enough time with a clinician and having the clinician listen to their story and perspective (12). Active listening is a way for the clinician not only to validate the patient's dignity and autonomy but also to

more quickly identify the patient's goals for the encounter. The active listener uses nonverbal cues including eye contact, nodding, and facial expressions to demonstrate engagement in what the patient is saying.

As the patient's needs are identified, the clinician should verbalize agreement with the patient as to their validity. Repeated validation builds rapport between the clinician and patient. The clinician can validate the patient's emotional state—perhaps frustration, anxiety, or anxiety—or the current circumstances ("It's not fun to be in the ED.")

One can neither listen nor validate the patient too much when providing verbal de-escalation. When the patient rambles or becomes difficult to direct, a brief validating statement provides the clinician leeway to reenter the conversation and move on to the next stage of de-escalation.

Solving Problems and Offering Choices

This step is the beginning of the resolution of the escalation event. Agitation can often result from a patient's subjective feeling that they have no control over their situation. Having recognized some of the patient's needs and validated their feelings, the clinician begins offering solutions and choices. In some instances, these needs are readily apparent: perhaps food, water, access to a telephone, or an explanation of events. Offering choices can help patients regain some sense of control. Other times, validation is sufficient for resolving the acute episode.

TABLE 18.2 Examples of Validating Statements

Statement	Level of Validation
"You seem really upset right now."	Validates the patient's emotional state
"You are stuck in the hospital right now."	Validates the facts of the situation
"I would be frustrated if I could not leave the hospital when I wanted."	Normalizes the patient's response and validates the likelihood of their reaction
"I understand that if you have been treated poorly in the hospital before, you would be right to worry about that again."	Validates the patient's response based on their prior experiences

Sometimes the clinician must be creative in offering choices based on the patient's request or history, but generally the patient should be offered the opportunity to show ownership over the escalation event and supported in making choices that will resolve the agitation episode. What has worked for them in the past? An anxious patient might benefit from a brief list of coping skills that can be practiced in the ED; a patient in withdrawal might require medications for detoxification. In helping reestablish a sense of dignity and control, soliciting the patient's participation in making choices is thus an important therapeutic intervention by the clinician.

Offering medications is a valuable component of de-escalation. The selection of medications can be based in part on patient preference but must also consider suspected etiology among other medical considerations. Many patients cite the opportunity to have a say in choosing medication as an important element of de-escalation their crisis state (12).

Limit-Setting when Necessary

Clinicians must be prepared to set clearly stated limits around behavior for patients' and others' safety. For instance, the clinician should feel confident in telling a demanding patient that they will not receive contraindicated medications. Ambiguously stated limits only further frustrate the agitated patient who will become confused over what is expected of them or fail to intuit the boundaries of acceptable behavior on their own. Limits should be explicated firmly and concisely. "If/then" statements should be avoided—"If you don't calm down, then I will call security."—in favor of setting limits, offering choices, and again validating the patient's feelings about that choice.

When appropriate, introduce time boundaries on these limits: for example, the patient can have the phone after they have shown that they are in behavioral control for 10 minutes. Thus, limit-setting serves to maintain a safe environment while also reducing the risk of iatrogenic escalation.

Unfortunately, not all verbal de-escalation events end well. Active violence is an indication for involuntarily administered medications, restraint, or seclusion. Whenever possible, patients who receive these interventions should be allowed to participate in treatment planning including being given the option to take oral medications instead of an injection.

Validating the Patient's Perspective

The clinician cannot validate too frequently when de-escalating an agitated patient. Validation should be offered throughout the de-escalation episode and particularly when limits have been set or when the patient is engaging in positive, de-escalating behaviors. When the patient makes a good decision such as practicing a coping skill instead of yelling, it is entirely appropriate to applaud this position decision and the effort required to undertake it. Table 18.2 demonstrates different validating statements and the levels at which these statements are construed by the patient as supportive.

Many agitated patients express sentiments that are gross thought distortions ("Everybody hates me") or even psychotic (as with paranoid delusions). These statements should not be validated as accurate if they are not, and the clinician should not collude with or accommodate psychotic statements. In these situations, the clinician should seek to validate the patient's emotional reaction to this content or their goals for treatment. For example, the clinician might recognize that, "It must be frightening to experience that," or, "I know you really do not want to be here." The clinician's statements of validation must be authentic to be effective.

Ending the Escalation Event

Verbal de-escalation has succeeded when the patient is no longer agitated and feels in control again. The patient may accept one of the offered choices or be satisfied with the clinician's efforts to problem-solve. Or perhaps medications have had an opportunity to ameliorate problematic symptoms. Most often, the patient and clinician acknowledge resolution of the event; a more formal assessment might reveal a repeat BARS score of 4 or RASS score of 0.

Patients who have been agitated once are at risk for becoming agitated again. A debriefing is helpful for providing some conclusion to the acute episode and anticipating an approach that will help the patient in the future. Essential elements of a debriefing with the patient include a review of what happened, what helped the patient feel better, and how the de-escalation episode might go better in the future. Writing the patient's common triggers and main coping skills on an erasable wall board or sheet of paper in the patient's room keeps these lessons readily accessible for patients and staff. Debriefing is not optional in cases where the patient has experienced restraint, seclusion, or involuntary medication management. Debriefings may need to be signed out to the next shift in cases where the patient's clinical condition precludes an effective debriefing in the moment.

Staff should not neglect to debrief with friends, family, or other patients who may have witnessed the patient experience a coercive event. This debrief may include a description of what happened, why restraints or coercive measures were applied, a reassurance of safety, or simply an acknowledgment of how distressing the event may have been. Other patients frequently worry that a similar event may happen to them and even may imagine restraints to be a punitive action.

Debriefing is also invaluable for staff who were involved in the de-escalation (27). A team debrief should begin by ensuring that all staff are safe. Participants may then share what went well, what could go better, and any final thoughts about the event. Some suggestions arising from staff debriefs are very practical—Did the alarm button work? Was an opportunity to treat the patient sooner missed? Moreover, the debrief also allows recognition of the strong countertransference induced by agitated patients. Working with agitated patients may incite fear, helplessness, impatience, or even a sense of incompetence among staff. Clinicians deserve a supportive hearing from experienced colleagues who can normalize these reactions and, when appropriate, provide constructive feedback.

Debriefing should be provided regardless of whether the de-escalation ends positively or negatively; reserving debriefs for adverse episodes makes debriefing feel like corrective action. In fact, a good debriefing should emphasize positive interventions as frequently as correct negative ones.

CONCLUSION

Verbal de-escalation is the first treatment for any agitated patient. Although verbal de-escalation certainly requires trial-and-error, fast thinking, and patience by the clinician, appropriately treating the agitated patient is a matter of practiced effort more than luck or innate skill. The process of de-escalation precedes the patient's arrival through adequate staff training and environmental modifications that enhance safety and treatment delivery. When the patient arrives, trained clinicians must be prepared to identify incipient agitation, maintain environmental safety, and engage the patient appropriately in regaining control. Consistent debriefings empower both patients and staff to more effectively treat agitation in the future. These practices embody a philosophical approach to treating agitation that respects our best scientific and ethical appreciation of this common, challenging clinical situation.

REFERENCES

1. Lindenmayer, J. P. (2000). The pathophysiology of agitation. *Journal of Clinical Psychiatry, 61*(Suppl. 14), 5–10.
2. Miner, J. R., Klein, L. R., Cole, J. B., Driver, B. E., Moore, J. C., & Ho, J. D. (2018). The characteristics and prevalence of agitation in an urban county emergency department. *Annals of Emergency Medicine, 72*(4), 361–370.
3. Simpson, S. A., Joesch, J. M., West, I. I., & Pasic, J. (2014). Risk for physical restraint or seclusion in the psychiatric emergency service (PES). *General Hospital Psychiatry, 36*(1), 113–118.

4. Tamune, H., & Yasugi, D. (2017). How can we identify patients with delirium in the emergency department?: A review of available screening and diagnostic tools. *American Journal of Emergency Medicine, 35*(9), 1332–1334.

5. Gacki-Smith, J., Juarez, A. M., Boyett, L., Homeyer, C., Robinson, L., & MacLean, S. L. (2009). Violence against nurses working in US emergency departments. *The Journal of Nursing Administration, 39*(7–8), 340–349.

6. Khademloo, M., Moonesi, F. S., & Gholizade, H. (2013). Health care violence and abuse towards nurses in hospitals in north of Iran. *Global Journal of Health Science, 5*(4), 211–216.

7. Simpson, S. A., Pidgeon, M., & Nordstrom, K. (2016). Using the Behavioural Activity Rating Scale as a vital sign in the psychiatric emergency service. *Colorado Journal of Psychiatry and Psychology, 2*(2), 61–66.

8. Richmond, J. S., Berlin, J. S., Fishkind, A. B., et al. (2012). Verbal de-escalation of the agitated patient: Consensus statement of the American Association for Emergency Psychiatry Project BETA De-escalation Workgroup. *The Western Journal of Emergency Medicine, 13*(1), 17–25.

9. Garriga, M., Pacchiarotti, I., Kasper, S., et al. (2016). Assessment and management of agitation in psychiatry: Expert consensus. *The World Journal of Biological Psychiatry, 17*(2), 86–128.

10. Berlin, J. (2017). Collaborative de-escalation. In Zeller, S. L., Nordstrom, K., & Wilson, M. P. (Eds.), *The diagnosis and management of agitation* (pp. 144–155). Cambridge, UK: Cambridge University Press.

11. Knox, D. K., & Holloman, G. H., Jr. (2012). Use and avoidance of seclusion and restraint: Consensus statement of the American Association for Emergency Psychiatry Project BETA Seclusion and Restraint Workgroup. *The Western Journal of Emergency Medicine, 13*(1), 35–40.

12. Allen, M. H., Carpenter, D., Sheets, J. L., Miccio, S., & Ross, R. (2003). What do consumers say they want and need during a psychiatric emergency? *Journal of Psychiatric Practice, 9*(1), 39–58.

13. Allen, N. G., Khan, J. S., Alzahri, M. S., & Stolar, A. G. (2015). Ethical issues in emergency psychiatry. *Emergency Medicine Clinics of North America, 33*(4), 863–874.

14. Simpson, S. A. (2017). The biology of agitation. In Zeller, S. L., Nordstrom, K., & Wilson, M. P. (Eds.), *The diagnosis and management of agitation* (pp. 9–20). Cambridge, UK: Cambridge University Press.

15. Stowell, K. R., Hughes, N. P., & Rozel, J. S. (2016). Violence in the emergency department. *Psychiatric Clinics of North America, 39*(4), 557–566.

16. Pati, D., Pati, S., & Harvey, T. E., Jr. (2016). Security implications of physical design attributes in the emergency department. *HERD, 9*(4), 50–63.

17. Tadros, A., & Kiefer, C. (2017). Violence in the emergency department: A global problem. *Psychiatric Clinics of North America, 40*(3), 575–584.

18. Joint Commission Online. (2017). *Special report: Suicide prevention in health care settings. Quality and safety.* Retrieved October 30, 2018, from https://www.jointcommission.org/issues/article.aspx?Article=GtNpk0ErgGF%2B-7J9WOTTkXANZSEPXa1%2BKH0%2F4k-GHCiio%3D.

19. Malka, S. T., Chisholm, R., Doehring, M., & Chisholm, C. (2015). Weapons retrieved after the implementation of emergency department metal detection. *The Journal of Emergency Medicine, 49*(3), 355–358.

20. Rankins, R. C., & Hendey, G. W. (1999). Effect of a security system on violent incidents and hidden weapons in the emergency department. *Annals of Emergency Medicine, 33*(6), 676–679.

21. Balleine, B. W., Delgado, M. R., & Hikosaka, O. (2007). The role of the dorsal striatum in reward and decision-making. *The Journal of Neuroscience, 27*(31), 8161–8165.

22. Swift, R. H., Harrigan, E. P., Cappelleri, J. C., Kramer, D., & Chandler, L. P. (2002). Validation of the behavioural activity rating scale (BARS): A novel measure of activity in agitated patients. *Journal of Psychiatric Research, 36*(2), 87–95.

23. Muskett, C. (2014). Trauma-informed care in inpatient mental health settings: A review of the literature. *International Journal of Mental Health Nursing, 23*(1), 51–59.

24. Ashcraft, L., & Anthony, W. (2008). Eliminating seclusion and restraint in recovery-oriented crisis services. *Psychiatric Services, 59*(10), 1198–1202.

25. Joslin, J. D., Goldberger, D., Johnson, L., & Waltz, D. P. (2016). Use of the Vocera communications badge improves public safety response times. *Emergency Medicine International, 2016*, 7158268.

26. Easterbrook, J. A. (1959). The effect of emotion on cue utilization and the organization of behavior. *Psychological Review, 66*(3), 183–201.

27. Simpson, S. A., Rylander, M., Monroe, C., Albert, L., & Seefeldt, T. (2017). Advanced skills in de-escalation. *Verbal de-escalation of the agitated patient* [Online video]. Retrieved October 30, 2018, from https://youtu.be/wl7yIF5KpfQ.

19

Agitation: Evaluation and Management

Marina Garriga, Justo E. Pinzón, Eva Solé, Eduard Vieta

Psychomotor agitation is a frequent and significant clinical phenomenon, not only in psychiatry, but in other somatic emergency settings (1,2). Patients might become agitated for a variety of reasons, ranging from altered mental status caused by shock or metabolic derangements, intoxication with alcohol/substances, and neurologic abnormalities, to exacerbations of psychiatric diseases such as schizophrenia or bipolar disorder (2).

Historically, little information on the epidemiology of agitation has been available. Difficulties in conceptualizing agitation or differentiating it from mere aggressiveness or assault also make it challenging to quantify the extent of the problem. A recent observational study of agitated patients in a trauma center emergency department found that the prevalence of agitation was 2.6% of all presenting patients, out of which 83% was related to alcohol use and the remaining 17%, to a psychiatric cause (2). Older publications have reported prevalence rates ranging from 4.3% to 10% in psychiatric emergency services (3). Despite the fact that agitation events are frequent and costly, strategies to reduce the incidence and severity of hospital agitation episodes would actually be expected to reduce overall healthcare systems costs and alleviate patient suffering (4–6).

EVALUATION OF AGITATION IN EMERGENCY SETTINGS

Emergent agitation requires timely recognition, appropriate assessment, and optimum management to minimize patient anxiety and reduce the risk of escalation to aggression and violence, which might be directed toward themselves or others (1). When agitation is suspected, the recommended first step before the evaluation takes place is ensuring safety, through moving the agitated patient to a safe environment, where the risk to themselves or others is minimized, and a prompt evaluation of their current clinical state and the risk of symptom escalation can be undertaken (7).

Initial assessment, when possible, should be made by healthcare professionals with expertise in the evaluation and management of patients with agitation. This first assessment should be done to 1) exclude potential somatic causes, 2) achieve a rapid patient's stabilization, 3) avoid the use of coercive measures, 4) ensure the least restrictive form of management, 5) reach a therapeutic alliance with the patient, and 6) develop an appropriate care plan (8).

Early Signs and Risk Factors

Agitation is a dynamic phenomenon that may rapidly escalate from anxiety and restlessness to aggressive or violent behaviors (9). Therefore, it is important to consider not only causative factors but potential early warning signs and risk factors of escalating agitated behavior. Evaluation on risk factors for agitation will include a wide range of demographic, psychosocial, diagnostic, and clinical aspects (Table 19.1) (7,10-12).

Several rating scales have been primarily developed in psychiatric settings to estimate the future risk of agitation, aggression, and associated violence. These include the Broset Violence Checklist (BVC; [13]), the Historical, Clinical, Risk Management-20 (HCR-20; [14]), and the McNiel-Binder Violence Screening Checklist (VSC; [15]). However, the lack of proper training on their use and the required time to be invested, make them difficult to be used widely in emergency settings.

TABLE 19.1 Potential Early Signs and Risk Factors for Agitation of in Mental Ill Population

Demographic
• Young age • Male • Low educational level • Unmarried • Same gender between aggressor and victim • Agitation from substance intoxication or withdrawal
Psychosocial
• History of conflict with staff or other patients • Recent stressful life event
Diagnostic
• Alcohol intoxication • Schizophrenia • Bipolar disorder
Clinical
• History of previous agitation episodes • Greater number of previous admissions • Extended hospital stays • Nonvoluntary admission • History of self-harm • History of suicide attempts • History of substance abuse • Low adherence to treatment • Impulsiveness and/or hostility • Disturbing clinical symptoms • Provocative attitudes • Verbally demeaning or hostile behavior

Some scales have been developed to evaluate the symptom escalation and severity of agitation, not only for psychiatric causes, but also for those due to a somatic condition. However, for agitated patients, rapid clinical decision-making is a priority, and action often must be taken to protect the safety of patients and staff before administering any standardized scale. Some tools that are easy to apply in the emergency settings include the Clinical Global Impression Scale for Aggression (CGI-A; [16]), the Positive and Negative Syndrome Scale—Excited Component (PANSS-EC or PEC; [17]), and the Behavioral Activity Rating Scale (BARS; [18]).

The BARS is a simple 7-point scale ranging from "difficult to rouse" to "violent," serves as a quick, informative way to communicate levels of agitation between clinical staff, and has the advantage of being both easy to learn and apply, with a perfect interrater reliability of 1.0 (Swift et al., 2002). Also, it has been shown an effective way to monitor the responses to medications, de-escalation, and other interventions for treatment of agitation.

Etiology of Agitation

A definitive etiological diagnosis is not considered a primary goal to first manage agitation. On the contrary, ascertaining a differential diagnosis and implementing immediate actions for safety and developing an appropriate initial management should be the main goals of the assessment (19). Once the patient is calm, a more extensive assessment should be more possible and able to be completed.

Agitation can arise from a wide range of causes, which can be classified according to four etiological groups: a general somatic condition, substance intoxication/withdrawal, a primary psychiatric disorder, and undifferentiated agitation (20,21). See Table 19.2.

Clinical Assessment: Signs and Symptoms

Although a prompt assessment of the agitated patient is critical for successful management (19,22,23), historically there has been a lack of standardized protocols and clinical tools to assist healthcare professionals in achieving the best possible outcome. General signs and symptoms that may help in the identification of agitation are shown in Table 19.3.

Included in the immediate evaluation of the patient's current state, when possible, a medical, toxicological, psychiatric, and pharmacologic history should be reviewed. Events leading up to the current agitated presentation should also be considered to identify possible precipitating factors. For a thorough and complete assessment of the cause of agitation, when practical, a physical examination should be done, including vital signs and blood oxygen saturation, as well as a general workup including glucose levels, hepatic and renal function, and urine drug test. An electrocardiogram, chest X-ray, lumbar puncture, and a pregnancy test for females may also be considered (1).

TABLE 19.2 Probable Etiological Causes to Consider as Cause of Agitation

Agitation from General Medical Condition
• Head trauma
• Encephalitis, meningitis, or other infection
• Encephalopathy (particularly from liver or renal failure)
• Exposure to environmental toxins
• Metabolic derangement (ie, hyponatremia, hypocalcemia, hypoglycemia)
• Hypoxia
• Thyroid disease
• Seizure (postictal)
• Pharmacological intoxications
Agitation from substance intoxication or withdrawal
• Alcohol
• Other drugs (cocaine, opioids, ecstasy, ketamine, bath salts, inhalants, methamphetamines)
Agitation from psychiatric disorder
• Psychotic disorder
• Manic and mixed states
• Agitated depression
• Anxiety disorder
• Personality disorder
• Reactive or situational situation
• Autism spectrum disorder
Undifferentiated agitation
• Must be used less frequently as etiological presumption
• Must be presumed to be from a general medical condition until proven otherwise

Adapted from Nordstrom, K., Zun, L. S., Wilson, M. P., et al.(2012). Medical evaluation and triage of the agitated patient: Consensus statement of the American Association for Emergency Psychiatry Project BETA Medical Evaluation Workgroup. *The Western Journal of Emergency Medicine, 13*(1), 3–10. doi:10.5811/westjem.2011.9.6863. With permission.

Differential Diagnosis Process

Given the clinical relevance and the global impact of agitation in psychiatry, in the best case, a prompt evaluation of causative factors and immediate management would be essential. However, an agitated patient's uncooperativeness and/or the inability to give a relevant history often forces clinicians to make decisions based on very limited information.

In the initial assessment and as a rule in an individual with no previous history of any somatic or psychiatric illness, or when the patient's status does not allow differential diagnosis, the agitation should be attributed to a general somatic condition until proven otherwise (1). In emergency settings, it is not uncommon for a diagnosis of delirium to be overlooked during an initial screening. The patient may be mistakenly diagnosed as psychotic, as delirium's physical signs and symptoms may be subtle and easily go undetected (19). Agitation due to somatic causes typically presents with an acute/subacute onset, frequently in advanced age patients, without prior psychiatric history, and follows a fluctuating course. Such patients tend to exhibit an altered level of consciousness, temporal-spatial disorientation, and alteration in physical parameters (sweating, tachycardia, tachypnea, fever, etc.). Visual hallucinations and delusional ideation as well as cognitive impairment may also be apparent. Therefore, the presence of a confusional state, cognitive impairment, and intoxication/withdrawal syndrome from substances should be ruled out before considering a primary psychiatric disorder, especially in cases without relevant past psychiatric history.

TABLE 19.3 Clinical Features of Psychomotor Agitation

Changes in Behavior
• Combative attitude • Inappropriate behavior without clear purpose • Hyperreactivity to stimuli • Restlessness or inability to remain quiet • Exaggerated gesticulation • Facial tension and angry expression • Defiant and/or prolonged visual contact • Raised tone of voice, silence, or refusal to talk • Altered emotional state with appearance of anxiety, irritability, or hostility • Verbal and/or physical aggression against self or others or objects
Cognitive changes
• Fluctuations in level of consciousness • Time-place disorientation • Tendency to frustration • Difficulty in anticipating consequences • Delusional ideas • Hallucinations
Changes in physical parameters
• Fever • Tachycardia • Tachypnea • Diaphoresis • Tremor • Neurological signs (ie, unstable gait)

Adapted from Vieta, E., Garriga, M., Cardete, L., et al. (2017). Protocol for the management of psychiatric patients with psychomotor agitation. *BMC Psychiatry, 17*(1), 328. doi:10.1186/s12888-017-1490-0. Retrieved from https://creativecommons.org/licenses/by/4.0/. Copyright © 2017 The Author(s).

Once an acute somatic cause of agitation is excluded and in order to confirm a primary psychiatric etiology, an accurate psychiatric and mental status examination should be performed. Little to no testing may be needed to confirm this in a patient with a preexisting psychiatric disorder who presents with symptoms such as previous psychiatric relapses and with normal vital signs (20). Agitation due to primary psychiatric causes tends to have an acute/subacute onset and presents without alterations in the level of consciousness.

The initial psychiatric assessment should include a complete clinical interview with the patient and collection of collateral information (medical records, interview with families, friends, outpatient care providers) when possible. History of the present illness, past psychiatric history, past medical history, substance use history, social history, family history, and the mental status examination should also be covered. A mental status examination might be directed to find auditory hallucinations (rarely visual hallucinations), persecutory and/or paranoid delusions (eg, schizophrenia and related disorders), grandiosity (mania), inappropriate mood (elation or irritability), and loud, rapid, or pressured speech (24). Although acute agitation is commonly associated with schizophrenia, schizoaffective disorder, and bipolar disorder, several other psychiatric conditions should be considered (see Table 19.2).

For those known mentally ill patients who present with atypical features (eg, delirium, history of head trauma, overdose, fever, headache), additional diagnostic tests should be considered to rule out comorbid somatic conditions. These may include neuroimaging, lumbar puncture, serum chemistry panel, complete blood count, endocrine tests, and toxicological screens (1,19,22).

MANAGEMENT OF AGITATION IN EMERGENCY SETTINGS

When a patient arrives in a state of agitation to an emergency setting, an initial evaluation, the triage, and nonpharmacologic preventive interventions (eg, de-escalation) must occur concurrently as all part of the initial assessment. An effective management of the agitation should be driven to stabilize the patient quickly, avoid coercive measures, treat in the least restrictive manner, form a therapeutic alliance, and ensure an adequate plan for subsequent care (25).

Triage of an Agitated Patient

Agitation in a Community Program or Clinic Setting

When agitation presents in an outpatient clinic setting, the immediate task is to determine if the patient needs transfer to a higher level of care (such as a hospital emergency department) based on whether a somatic etiology is suspected, by history or overt signs and symptoms (see Table 19.3) and on the patient's level of agitation. For any patient with suggestive somatic signs or symptoms or a possibly delirious patient, immediate transfer to a medical emergency department is indicated. This transfer should be performed in the safest possible manner. In this case, worldwide common emergency telephone number (112, or 911 in the United States) will provide help in contacting with an emergency medical service and/ or ambulance. The emergency department where the patient is being transferred to should be notified before their arrival to ensure that the staff is ready and has as much collateral information and relevant medical and psychiatric history about the patient as possible.

Agitation in a Medical Emergency Setting

When triaging an agitated patient in a medical setting, a brief history and vital signs should be obtained if possible. If any sign/symptom indicating a medical or psychiatric emergency is suspected at initial intake triage, immediate evaluation by a clinician is indicated. First examinations should be directed at identifying factors that could indicate serious, life-threatening conditions such as disorientation, incoordination, loss of memory, severe headache, severe muscle stiffness/weakness, difficulty breathing, abnormal vital signs, overt trauma, slurred speech, seizures, paresis, or other conditions suggesting serious risk for morbidity (20).

The agitated patient may, at any point during triage, require increased behavioral support, medication, or (least desirable) seclusion/restraint because of symptom escalation. History-taking and physical examination may have to be interrupted to address the treatment of the patient's agitation and would need to be resumed after the patient is less agitated. Once some level of de-escalation is accomplished, an important triage decision is to determine if the patient should have a directed physical examination in a general medicine emergency department to rule out an acute medical and/or substance intoxication/withdrawal condition. If a nonpsychiatric medical emergency can be ruled out, psychiatric evaluation and management are indicated and transfer to a psychiatric emergency department should be done if it exists at the center. If it does not, the patient should be treated in the general medicine emergency department, with behavioral health professional consultation if possible.

Nonpharmacologic Approaches

Treating an episode of agitation during the earliest stages and minimizing a possible escalation of symptoms is the chief aim of nonpharmacologic interventions for agitation (1,26). To enable this, all emergency settings should endeavor to have regular staff training in the management of agitation/assaultive behavior and to be familiar with how to utilize environmental modifications and verbal de-escalation processes. Because education in this arena is of major importance for achieving an optimal outcome in preventing violence and managing agitation, an entire chapter of this book provides dedicated outlines involved in these techniques (see Chapter 20). In addition, Table 19.4 offers a quick guidance on nonpharmacologic approaches for emergency settings.

Pharmacologic Treatment

In agitated patients for whom nonpharmacologic treatments are insufficient alone, medication can be an effective treatment strategy (27). The primary goal of pharmacologic treatment is to rapidly calm the patient without oversedation. A plan for treatment should follow a stepwise paradigm (see Figure 19.1). Initial interventions should always be tried in the least restrictive manner, mainly alongside environmental modifications and verbal de-escalation. Then, depending on the severity of the psychomotor agitation, these techniques might be supplemented by more restrictive

TABLE 19.4 Nonpharmacological Approaches: Staff, Environmental, and Verbal De-escalation Considerations

Healthcare Professionals Concerns
• Optimal updated, basic and practical, multidisciplinary educational program on agitation
• Coordinated and collaborative teamwork
• Availability and training on proper culturally and policy-adapted protocol and guidelines
• Sufficient staff in number and good disposition (try not to see patients by yourself)
• Avoidance of unsafe situations, such as closed rooms or blocked emergency doors
• Disarm patients
• Remove conflicting partners
Environmental modifications
• Reduction of external stimuli: (ie, irritating factors such as light, noise, cold, or hot air currents) to achieve patients' comfort
• Use rooms with simple and nonremoveable furniture
• Remove objects that may double as potential weapons
• Prefer rooms with two exit doors
Verbal de-escalation process during assessment
• Maintenance of an optimal safe distance to respect the patient's personal space
• Avoid prolonged or intense direct eye contact
• Be mindful of body language that could be considered menacing or confrontational
• Minimize waiting time
• Communicate in a caring, respectful attitude

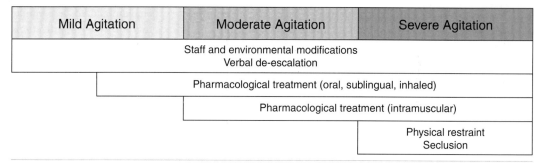

FIGURE 19.1 • Stepwise management for agitation.

options that may include injectable pharmacologic treatment and/or physical restraints, if needed.

When medication is indicated, noninvasive and nontraumatic routes of administration are preferred to preserve the physician-patient partnership. Where possible, medication should be given as monotherapy. A rapid onset of action is also a desirable feature of an ideal medication. All physicians should be familiar with the available pharmacologic options of their emergency departments, as well as well-trained on when and how to

use them. Despite worldwide differences, a small desirable list of optimal pharmacologic agents for psychomotor agitation is provided in Table 19.5.

Three classes of medications are traditionally used in the management of agitation: first-generation antipsychotics (FGAs), benzodiazepines (BZDs), and second-generation antipsychotics (SGAs) (23). During recent years, treatment options have grown with the development of new intramuscular (IM) SGA agents and different patient-friendly oral, sublingual,

TABLE 19.5 Minimal Desirable Medication Kit in an Emergency department

Types	Administration Route	Examples
First-generation antipsychotics (FGAs)	Oral	Haloperidol
	Inhaled	Loxapine
	IM	Haloperidol Levomepromazine Zuclopenthixol
Second-generation antipsychotics (SGAs)	Oral/sublingual	Aripiprazole Asenapine Olanzapine Quetiapine Risperidone Ziprasidone
	IM	Aripiprazole Olanzapine Ziprasidone
Benzodiazepines (BZDs)	Oral/sublingual	Clonazepam Diazepam Lorazepam
	IM	Diazepam Midazolam

IM, intramuscular.

and inhaled formulations (27-30). Presently, even though many algorithms for an appropriate treatment selection have been published, not all of them are adapted to local policy and culture of varied countries and regions, and specific agents may or may not be available in different locales. Therefore, this chapter provides an open, general first-line algorithm not containing active compound names but medication types and routes of administration (see Figure 19.2).

Specific considerations regarding this algorithm should first be clarified. The severity of the agitation, the cause of the agitation, and also the degree of patient cooperation are all key parts

for an optimal treatment choice decision-making process. In cases where a rapid onset is needed and the patient cooperates, consider an inhaled or oral/sublingual formulation. Oral medicines require time for absorption via the gastrointestinal tract, which tends to be slower in women, and after the presence of a large meal. Orally disintegrating tablets (ODTs, rapid-dissolving formulations) dissolve in saliva, but they also still require gastrointestinal absorption. Buccal, sublingual, and inhaled medications have a quicker onset than those going via the gastrointestinal tract. However, all these routes still require patient's cooperation.

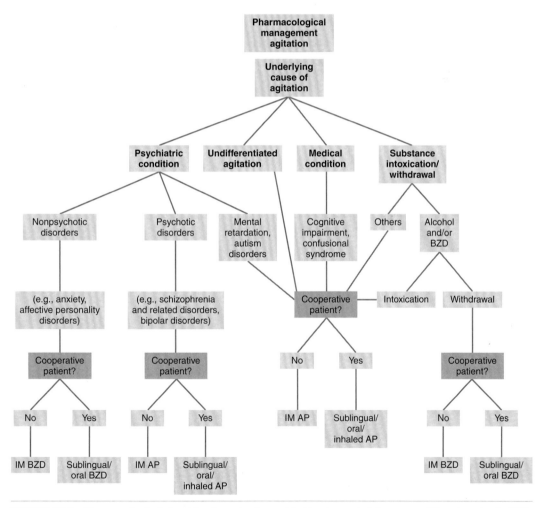

FIGURE 19.2 • Pharmacological algorithm for agitation guided by the underlying cause. AP, antipsychotic; BZD, benzodiazepine; IM, intramuscular. (Adapted from Vieta, E., Garriga, M., Cardete, L., et al. (2017). Protocol for the management of psychiatric patients with psychomotor agitation. *BMC Psychiatry, 17*(1), 328. doi:10.1186/s12888-017-1490-0. https://creativecommons.org/licenses/by/4.0/. Copyright © 2017 The Author(s).)

If patients are unwilling to comply, intramuscular (IM) injections are the next option, which being coercive and forcible are only for use when collaborative options are not possible. Injections ensure administration; however, its onset of action may not be significantly quicker than other routes (31). Although intravenous (IV) medications for agitation are another option and they do exhibit rapid efficacy, side-effect concerns (eg, oxygen desaturation, arrhythmias) should make them a consideration only in exceptional circumstances when other options have failed or cannot be attempted and when resuscitation facilities are available (32).

Special Circumstances
Agitation Associated With Delirium
When delirium presents with agitation, a prompt recognition of this type of agitation should drive determination of the underlying cause; an intervention aiming at correction of that cause is the best treatment.

If delirium is due to alcohol/BZD withdrawal, then treatment with a BZD is the agent of choice. If withdrawal from another substance is suspected, replacement with another substance with similar pharmacologic properties should be attempted if safe and appropriate. If the recent ingestion of a new agent (or an increased dose of a chronically ingested agent) is the suspected cause of delirium, then it will be self-limited, though the agitation may require temporary pharmacologic management (32).

If immediate pharmacologic control of agitation is required in a patient with delirium that is not due to alcohol/BZD withdrawal, SGAs are the preferred agents, with FGAs (eg, haloperidol) being also acceptable. BZDs should be then avoided because of the risk these might exacerbate the delirium. When delirium is presented in patients with Parkinson or Parkinsonlike disorder, FGAs should be avoided, and SGAs such as ziprasidone can be considered as an alternative. As an exception, for postictal agitated delirium, it may be advisable to use BZDs (1,7).

When an underlying somatic abnormality is the likely cause of delirium, the definitive treatment of the delirium and its associated agitation is correction of the underlying medical condition.

Substance Intoxication/Withdrawal
Alcohol, synthetic cannabinoids, gamma-hydroxybutyrates, and stimulants are most likely to be associated with acute agitation in substance users.

1. Substance use: In intoxications, especially due to stimulants, BZDs are generally considered first-line agents instead of antipsychotics, in order to decrease the potential risk of seizures (1,7,32). In those cases where the chronic use of stimulants has progressed into psychotic symptoms, an SGA may be useful in addition to a BZD. However, very often, the psychosis associated with a stimulant intoxication is correlated with lack of sleep, and giving the patient time to rest and detoxify with a BZD alone will commonly diminish the associated psychosis without the added risks of using antipsychotic medications.

2. Alcohol/BZD: Medication specifically to treat agitation symptoms associated with alcohol/BZD intoxication should be used carefully, if at all. If medication is required, BZDs should be avoided because of the potential risk of respiratory depression. Thus, antipsychotics are preferred. Among them, haloperidol has the longest track record of safety and efficacy with minimal effects on the central respiratory center. SGAs, such as risperidone, may be a reasonable alternative (33). When agitation is secondary to alcohol/BZD withdrawal, BZDs became necessary and preferred over antipsychotics to reduce the risk of seizures and *delirium tremens*. Agitation in a chronic alcohol/BZD user who exhibits features of *delirium* (eg, tachycardia, diaphoresis, tremors…) and a low alcohol blood level should be presumed to be due to withdrawal and treated accordingly with BZDs. Because *delirium tremens* can be life-threatening, its management might also include supportive care with intravenous fluids, nutritional supplementation, and frequent clinical reassessment. In these cases, where close monitoring is required, admission to an intensive care unit (ICU) should be attempted. In addition, administering B-vitamin treatment in these patients might also prevent serious complications in alcohol use patients (32).

Pregnancy

Commonly, psychiatric medicines would be avoided during pregnancy, but this is not always possible, in which case guidelines recommend treating the mother as per usual clinical algorithms (32,34), as the risks to the fetus from acts of agitation likely outweigh the risk of medications. Nevertheless, this population should be even more of a priority for the use of verbal and calming interventions from the earliest possible stages of agitation.

Changes in pregnancy affect drug management. Variations in clearance between trimesters, increased glomerular filtration rate, and expansion of plasma volume make necessary increase in dose for the same drug concentration but without knowing the effects of this in the fetus (35). Avoiding drugs that may accumulate in both maternal and fetal tissues is advisable, as well as selecting short half-life medication, such as lorazepam (32,34).

The risk balance of choosing one medicine over another, versus leaving the pregnant patient untreated, is difficult to assess. However, such concerns are more relevant in relation to ongoing medications, not single doses that are commonly used on agitation. Direct effects of single doses of medication on the fetus seem likely to be minimal, but the risks associated with the use of restraint and ongoing regular medications are more significant to the fetus. Further considerations, such as restraint positions (not prone or supine but semiseated), equipment (eg, use of beanbags), and suitable injection sites (gluteal or lateral thigh) have been suggested (32,34).

Seclusion and Restraint

There is worldwide controversy regarding the use of restraints and seclusion. However, under special circumstances and always as a last resort, the use of seclusion and/or physical restraint might be necessary to ensure the safety of the patient and the staff and to guarantee pharmacologic treatment is received. Unfortunately, the use of coercive measures generates an intensive depletion of health and nonhealth professional resources, because of the techniques themselves and subsequent required monitoring, so that reduction of their use could result in an economic savings and could also result in being able to allocate more resources to other types of measures (7).

Physical restraint is a procedure during which mechanical devices are used to limit the patient's physical mobility for the primary purpose of behavioral control (7,32). Seclusion has been defined as a supervised confinement of a patient in a locked room with the objective to contain severely disturbed behavior that is likely to cause harm to self or others.

When use of restraint (and seclusion) is unavoidable, healthcare professionals should be well-trained in advance how to implement these measures, and be knowledgeable about protocols and policies to decrease possible adverse events (both physical and psychological). From the beginning of the seclusion and/or restraint process, a single member of the staff should communicate with the patient and coordinate the restraint/seclusion team. From the very first moment, the patient must be informed about the reason for its indication and given a further opportunity to comply with alternative treatment options.

In most cases, medication should be administered to calm a patient who has been placed in restraints/seclusion. Choice of medication might contemplate both oral/sublingual/inhaled or IM medication, according to patient's cooperativeness (see Figure 19.2). The restrained patient should be clinically assessed at frequents periods with the goal of removing the restraints as soon as possible. Restraints should be removed gradually with a clear explanation of the behavior expected of the patient and with at least two healthcare professionals present. When restraints/seclusion has been removed and the agitation has been resolved, debriefing with patient and healthcare professionals is advisable to enhance therapeutic relationship and long-term outcomes.

Direct monitoring of restrained patients is necessary to assess medication response and adverse comorbidities due to the implementation of these techniques. This will also help lead to a prompter removal of forced seclusion/restraint. Physical adverse effects related with restraint and involuntary medication include extrapyramidal symptoms, sedation, respiratory depression, tachycardia, QTc prolongation, arrhythmia, postural hypotension, increased seizure potential, and neuroleptic malignant syndrome. Preexisting physical comorbidities, pregnancy, drugs/alcohol intoxication or withdrawal, and medication interactions confer further risks.

Physical health monitoring should include temperature, pulse, blood pressure, respiratory rate, oxygen saturation, and level of consciousness (32).

CONCLUSIONS

Agitation is a common clinical feature in emergency settings because of a wide range of causes (somatic and psychiatric). A prompt and early assessment and management, starting from the triage settings, will be key points for achieving the best possible outcome and avoiding the need for coercive measures.

Using a differential diagnosis algorithm for agitation will lead clinicians to the best intervention possible, although in seriously acute situations this might not be possible at first. Because of that, the first clinical question to be answered is whether the agitation is due to a medical/somatic condition. Once a medical/somatic condition has been excluded, psychiatric illnesses and substance abuse–related conditions are the most likely diagnoses that might present with psychomotor agitation.

Even if a clear cause of agitation is not clarified from the beginning, a stepwise management should be implemented as soon as a risk for agitation is detected, starting from nonpharmacologic interventions (eg, environmental modifications, verbal de-escalation) and evolving to medication management.

Appropriate treatment of agitation is of utmost importance. Regarding pharmacologic approaches, even though first-generation antipsychotics and benzodiazepines have been shown to be effective, because of the severe potential for side effects and oversedation in FGAs, the more recent guidelines and expert recommendations preferentially recommend the equally potent SGAs as first-line therapy.

REFERENCES

1. Garriga, M., Pacchiarotti, I., Kasper, S., Zeller, S. L., Allen, M. H., Vázquez, G., ... Vieta, E. (2016). Assessment and management of agitation in psychiatry: Expert consensus. *The World Journal of Biological Psychiatry, 17*(2), 86–128. doi:10.3109/15622975.2015.1132007.

2. Miner, J. R., Klein, L. R., Cole, J. B., Driver, B. E., Moore, J. C., & Ho, J. D. (2018). The characteristics and prevalence of agitation in an urban county emergency department. *Annals of Emergency Medicine, 72*(4), 361–370. doi:10.1016/j.annemergmed.2018.06.001.

3. Huf, G., Alexander, J., & Allen, M. H. (2005). Haloperidol plus promethazine for psychosis induced aggression. *The Cochrane Database of Systematic Reviews*, (1), CD005146. doi:10.1002/14651858.CD005146.

4. Peiró, S., Gómez, G., Navarro, M., Guadarrama, I., Rejas, J., Alvarez Díaz, A., ... Sorio, F. (2004). Length of stay and antipsychotic treatment costs of patients with acute psychosis admitted to hospital in Spain. Description and associated factors. The Psychosp study. *Social Psychiatry and Psychiatric Epidemiology, 39*(7), 507–513. doi:10.1007/s00127-004-0776-y.

5. Serrano-Blanco, A., Rubio-Valera, M., Aznar-Lou, I., Baladón Higuera, L., Gibert, K., Gracia Canales, A., ... Salvador-Carulla, L. (2017). In-patient costs of agitation and containment in a mental health catchment area. *BMC Psychiatry, 17*(1), 212. doi:10.1186/s12888-017-1373-4.

6. Warnke, I., Rössler, W., & Herwig, U. (2011). Does psychopathology at admission predict the length of inpatient stay in psychiatry? Implications for financing psychiatric services. *BMC Psychiatry, 11*, 120. doi:10.1186/1471-244X-11-120.

7. Vieta, E., Garriga, M., Cardete, L., Bernardo, M., Lombraña, M., Blanch, J., ... Martínez-Arán, A. (2017). Protocol for the management of psychiatric patients with psychomotor agitation. *BMC Psychiatry, 17*(1), 328. doi:10.1186/s12888-017-1490-0.

8. Zeller, S. L. (2010). Treatment of psychiatric patients in emergency settings. *Primary Psychiatry, 17*, 35–41.

9. Citrome, L., & Volavka, J. (2014). The psychopharmacology of violence: Making sensible decisions. *CNS Spectrums, 19*(5), 411–418. doi:10.1017/S1092852914000054.

10. Cornaggia, C. M., Beghi, M., Pavone, F., & Barale, F. (2011). Aggression in psychiatry wards: A systematic review. *Psychiatry Research, 189*(1), 10–20. doi:10.1016/j.psychres.2010.12.024.

11. Hankin, C., Bronstone, A., & Koran, L. (2011). Agitation in the inpatient psychiatric setting: A review of clinical presentation, burden, and treatment. *Journal of Psychiatric Practice, 17*(3), 170–185. doi:10.1097/01.pra.0000398410.21374.7d.

12. Kasper, S., Baranyi, A., Eisenburger, P., Erfurth, A., Ertl, M., Frey, R., … Winkler, D. (2013, November). Die Behandlung der Agitation beim psychiatrischen Notfall. Konsensus-Statement – State of the art 2013. *CliniCum neuropsy*. Sonderausgabe.

13. Almvik, R., & Woods, P. (1999). Predicting inpatient violence using the Brøset Violence Checklist (BVC). *The International Journal of Psychiatric Nursing Research, 4*(3), 498–505.

14. Webster, C., Douglas, K., Eaves, D., & Hart, S. (1997). *HCR-20: Assessing risk for violence* (Version 2). Vancouver, BC: MHLPI, Simon Fraser University.

15. McNiel, D. E., & Binder, R. L. (1994). The relationship between acute psychiatric symptoms, diagnosis, and short-term risk of violence. *Hospital & Community Psychiatry, 45*(2), 133–137.

16. Huber, C. G., Lambert, M., Naber, D., Schacht, A., Hundemer, H.-P., Wagner, T. T., & Schimmelmann, B. G. (2008). Validation of a clinical global impression scale for aggression (CGI-A) in a sample of 558 psychiatric patients. *Schizophrenia Research, 100*(1–3), 342–348. doi:10.1016/j.schres.2007.12.480.

17. Kay, S. R., Fiszbein, A., & Opler, L. A. (1987). The positive and negative syndrome scale (PANSS) for schizophrenia. *Schizophrenia Bulletin, 13*(2), 261–276.

18. Swift, R. H., Harrigan, E. P., Cappelleri, J. C., Kramer, D., & Chandler, L. P. (1998). Validation of the behavioural activity rating scale (BARS): A novel measure of activity in agitated patients. *Journal of Psychiatric Research, 36*(2), 87–95.

19. Stowell, K. R., Florence, P., Harman, H. J., & Glick, R. L. (2012). Psychiatric evaluation of the agitated patient: Consensus statement of the American Association for Emergency Psychiatry Project BETA Psychiatric Evaluation Workgroup. *The Western Journal of Emergency Medicine, 13*(1), 11–16. doi:10.5811/westjem.2011.9.6868.

20. Nordstrom, K., Zun, L. S., Wilson, M. P., Md, V. S., Ng, A. T., Bregman, B., & Anderson, E. L. (2012). Medical evaluation and triage of the agitated patient: Consensus statement of the American Association for Emergency Psychiatry Project BETA Medical Evaluation Workgroup. *The Western Journal of Emergency Medicine, 13*(1), 3–10. doi:10.5811/westjem.2011.9.6863.

21. Yildiz, A., Sachs, G. S., & Turgay, A. (2003). Pharmacologic management of agitation in emergency settings. *Emergency Medicine Journal, 20*(4), 339–346.

22. Allen, M. H., Currier, G. W., Carpenter, D., Ross, R. W., & Docherty, J. P. (2005). The expert consensus guideline series. Treatment of behavioral emergencies 2005. *Journal of Psychiatric Practice, 11*(Suppl. 1), 5–108; quiz 110-2.

23. Marder, S. R. (2006). A review of agitation in mental illness: Treatment guidelines and current therapies. *The Journal of Clinical Psychiatry, 67*(Suppl. 1), 13–21.

24. Hasan, A., Falkai, P., Wobrock, T., Lieberman, J., Glenthoj, B., Gattaz, W. F., … Möller, H.-J. (2012). World Federation of Societies of Biological Psychiatry (WFSBP) Guidelines for Biological Treatment of Schizophrenia, Part 1: Update 2012 on the acute treatment of schizophrenia and the management of treatment resistance. *World Journal of Biological Psychiatry, 13*, 318–378. doi: 10.3109/15622975.2012.696143.

25. Zeller, S. L., & Rhoades, R. W. (2010). Systematic reviews of assessment measures and pharmacologic treatments for agitation. *Clinical Therapeutics, 32*(3), 403–425. doi:10.1016/j.clinthera.2010.03.006.

26. Fishkind, A. (2002). Calming agitation with words, not drugs: 10 commandments for safety. *Current Psychiatry, 1*(4), 32–39.

27. Baker, S. N. (2012). Management of acute agitation in the emergency department. *Advanced Emergency Nursing Journal, 34*(4), 306–318. doi:10.1097/TME.0b013e31826f12d6.

28. Jarema, M. (Red.). (2015). Leczenie pacjentów pobudzonych. In Medica, V. (Ed.), *Standardy leczenia farmakologicznego niektórych zaburzeń psychicznych* (pp. 49–51). Gdańsk.

29. Popovic, D., Nuss, P., & Vieta, E. (2015). Revisiting loxapine: A systematic review. *Annals of General Psychiatry, 14*, 15. doi:10.1186/s12991-015-0053-3.

30. San, L., Estrada, G., Oudovenko, N., Montañés, F., Dobrovolskaya, N., Bukhanovskaya, O., … Vieta, E. (2018). PLACID study: A randomized trial comparing the efficacy and safety of inhaled loxapine versus intramuscular aripiprazole in acutely agitated patients with schizophrenia or bipolar disorder. *European Neuropsychopharmacology : The Journal of the European College of Neuropsychopharmacology, 28*(6), 710–718. doi:10.1016/j.euroneuro.2018.03.010.

31. San, L., Estrada, G., Oudovenko, N., & Vieta, E. (2017). Rationale and design of the PLACID study: A randomised trial comparing the efficacy and safety of inhaled loxapine versus IM aripiprazole in acutely agitated patients with schizophrenia or bipolar disorder. *BMC Psychiatry, 17*(1), 126. doi:10.1186/s12888-017-1291-5.

32. Patel, M. X., Sethi, F. N., With co-authors (in alphabetical order): Barnes, T. R., Dix, R., Dratcu, L., Fox, B., Garriga, M., Haste, J. C., Kahl, K. G., Lingford-Hughes, A., McAllister-Williams, H., O'Brien, A., Parker, C., Paterson, B., Paton, C., Posporelis, S., Taylor, D. M., Vieta, E., Völlm, B., Wilson-Jones, C., Woods, L. (2018). Joint BAP NAPICU evidence-based consensus guidelines for the clinical management of acute disturbance: De-escalation and rapid tranquillisation. *Journal of Psychopharmacology, 32*(6), 601–640. doi:10.1177/0269881118776738.

33. Pepa, P. A., Lee, K. C., Huynh, H. E., & Wilson, M. P. (2017). Safety of risperidone for acute agitation and alcohol intoxication in emergency department patients. *The Journal of Emergency Medicine, 53*(4), 530–535.

34. McAllister-Williams, R. H., Baldwin, D. S., Cantwell, R., Easter, A., Gilvarry, E., Glover, V., Green, L., Gregoire, A., Howard, L. M., Jones, I., Khalifeh, H., Lingford-Hughes, A., McDonald, E., Micali, N., Pariante, C. M., Peters, L., Roberts, A., Smith, N. C., Taylor, D., Wieck, A., Yates, L. M., Young, A. H., endorsed by the British Association for Psychopharmacology. (2017). British Association for Psychopharmacology consensus guidance on the use of psychotropic medication preconception, in pregnancy and postpartum 2017. *Journal of Psychopharmacology, 31*(5), 519–552. doi:10.1177/0269881117699361.

35. Wesseloo, R., Wierdsma, A. I., van Kamp, I. L., Munk-Olsen, T., Hoogendijk, W. J. G., Kushner, S. A., & Bergink, V. (2017). Lithium dosing strategies during pregnancy and the postpartum period. *The British Journal of Psychiatry, 211*(1), 31–36. doi:10.1192/bjp.bp.116.192799.

20

Psychosis

Joshua Niclas, Scott L. Zeller

Acute psychosis, although one of the most common presenting problems in emergency psychiatry, can be a very difficult diagnostic and therapeutic challenge (1). In addition to exacerbations of severe mental illnesses such as schizophrenia and bipolar disorder, medical and substance-induced conditions can present with symptoms of psychosis. Because many of the nonpsychiatric causes of psychosis can be life-threatening, the correct diagnosis of the origin of psychotic symptoms is one of the most important skills to develop for those practicing psychiatry in acute settings.

PRESENTING CLINICAL FEATURES

The predominant symptoms of acute psychoses include hallucinations, delusions and ideas of reference, and disorganized thought processes and behaviors. Other features of psychotic illnesses that might lead to an emergency presentation include catatonia and prominent negative symptoms.

Hallucinations

Patients with psychotic illnesses commonly complain of auditory hallucinations, sometimes referred to as "hearing voices." Often the auditory hallucination will be described as one person's voice or several different voices. Some patients describe the voices as an innocuous running commentary on daily activities, whereas other voices can be derogatory, threatening, or commanding. The latter are of the most concern in the emergency setting, because these hallucinations might induce dangerous behaviors toward self or others. A patient hearing a derogatory voice saying he is worthless might feel like killing himself. A patient hearing a hallucination telling her to strike a family member might act on the command.

Nonauditory hallucinations, such as tactile, olfactory, or visual, rarely occur in endogenous psychiatric disorders such as schizophrenia. The presence of these types of hallucinations should lead clinicians to investigate organic causes, especially toxic or withdrawal states.

Delusions and Ideas of Reference

Delusions, especially paranoid delusions, are frequently seen in psychotic illnesses. Many of the subtypes of delusions can lead to a presentation to emergency settings, sometimes with imminent danger. Paranoid delusions may lead patients to flee, hide, or strike out against the supposed persecutor. Ideas of reference include when patients believe that television programs or media stories are about them or are sending them secret messages, as well as the belief that surrounding objects and events are contrived only for the patient. Ideas of reference may lead patients to damage persons or property that they deem to be a threat.

For example, a person who believes that a television anchor's routine stories are really about the patient may destroy all the televisions in the house. Nihilistic delusions may result in a patient refusing to eat, because he or she is "already dead." Persons with somatic delusions may become very functionally impaired from a belief that their body is giving off a toxic odor or that they are infected with "bugs." Erotomanic delusions may lead to stalking behaviors and inability to obey restraining orders, leading to arrest.

A good history and collateral investigation are important in evaluating delusions. What might seem delusional at first glance may indeed be a true cause of concern. Many an emergency psychiatry veteran clinician can share experiences such as a patient, apparently delusional that the Secret Service was after him, who was shown to be otherwise minutes later—when a federal agent arrived seeking the patient for threats against the president.

Disorganized Thought Processes and Behaviors

Psychotic disorganization in a patient can lead to an emergency presentation when confusion becomes so prevalent that a person cannot adequately care for himself, or such behaviors endanger the patient. This might manifest itself in someone who wanders the streets, not knowing where home is; a person who turns on dangerous appliances or gas burners without realizing it; or a person who eats rotting food from garbage dumpsters or drinks drainage ditch water. Disorganization may be revealed in a person whose speech is rambling, confused, or circumstantial, leading to difficulty with conversations or making simple requests.

Catatonia

The term *catatonia* refers to a cluster of symptoms that can include mutism, negativism, grimacing, posturing, catalepsy, and apparent stupor. A patient in a catatonic state may display minimal spontaneous speech, lack of response to outside stimuli, purposeless resistance to commands, odd facial expressions or body positions, resistance to attempts by others to move the patient's limbs, or minimal spontaneous movement. A patient with catatonia may present to the emergency setting because of extremes of behavior, total lack of behavior, or violent activity associated with catatonia. The condition can rapidly evolve into a medical crisis because of inadequate oral intake and rhabdomyolysis induced by muscle contraction or increased psychomotor activity.

Negative and Cognitive Symptoms

Negative symptoms and cognitive symptoms are common in the psychotic illnesses. These include memory impairment, difficulty with decision-making, social isolation, lack of initiative, lack of social connectivity, and little or no spontaneous speech. Referrals to psychiatry will usually come from concerned family or friends, dismayed by the patient's change in affect and cognition. The acuity upon presentation from these symptoms alone rarely rises to the level of an emergency.

IMMEDIATE INTERVENTIONS FOR ACUTE PRESENTATIONS

The acutely psychotic patient needs to be immediately assessed for medical instability and should receive medical care promptly when indicated. Especially in the case of a highly paranoid or hallucinating individual, safety should be at the forefront; a calm, quiet observation room might be appropriate. For a patient who is highly agitated, clinicians may wish to use emergency antiagitation or anxiolytic medication to help calm the patient for the assessment.

ASSESSMENT

When a patient presents with a presumptive psychosis, the most important first step is an assessment of the individual, which should precede any interventions short of ensuring safety. This is because many organic, metabolic, and toxic etiologies—some of which are life-threatening—can mimic the symptoms of an acute psychosis.

A visual assessment, or "eyeball," of the patient should be the first step and can be done even when a patient is on a gurney or in the custody of police officers. Does the patient have markedly dilated pupils? Is the patient thrashing about, sweating profusely, or flushed? Readily observable signs such as these can be key indicators of the cause of current symptoms. If the patient can cooperate, a targeted review of systems should be completed. Medical and nursing personnel should look early on for easily recognized symptoms of delirium.

Next, it is essential to gather a quick and relevant initial history. Why is the patient here? What is the key presenting problem? Has there been any recent ingestion or substance abuse? While this is being ascertained, the taking of vital signs can commence. Fever, tachycardia, elevated blood pressure, and low oxygen saturation can all indicate a medical cause for the current symptoms. Acute conditions that warrant an immediate transfer from a psychiatric unit to an emergency medical unit or facility are listed in Table 20.1.

TABLE 20.1 Conditions Warranting Transfer to a Medical Emergency Department

Potential life-threatening illness or injury
Unconsciousness or unresponsiveness
Clear dizziness or signs of shock
Chest pain
Abdominal pain
Severe bleeding from trauma
Abrupt change in cognition in an elderly patient
Any evidence of an overdose of medication

Safety Interventions

Once obvious emergency medical conditions are ruled out, if a patient's psychosis is leading to the potential for self-harm or harm to others, ensuring safety is a fundamental next step. This will allow for further evaluation in an environment that minimizes risk.

De-escalation and calming techniques (see Section 4) should always be attempted and continued with agitated or hostile patients and can be done simultaneously during the evaluation or offering of medications. Additional safety options can include heightened supervision, one-to-one observation by staff, isolation in a quiet room with reduced stimuli, and, least desirably, coercive interventions such as seclusion, restraint, and forced medications.

EVALUATION

A thorough evaluation and history are essential for all presenting cases of acute psychosis. Even if a patient is familiar to emergency staff, it should not be assumed that the current presentation is a repeat of previous episodes. Even a recidivist patient with frequent past emergency visits because of exacerbations of psychosis might have the current presentation caused by a different etiology.

Nursing Evaluation

Nursing staff should do a proper triage evaluation, as described in Section 2. This should always include vital signs and a nursing physical history and examination where appropriate. If possible, pulse oximetry, breathalyzer, urine drug screens, and fingerstick glucose testing can be of great value.

Physician Evaluation

Medical staff should obtain as complete a history as possible, given the patient's current mental status. With an acutely psychotic individual, it is important for clinicians to be calm while being brief and direct with questions. Disturbing, challenging, or arguing with the psychotic patient should be avoided.

A careful mental status examination is a must prior to making any treatment decisions. At this point, a more careful assessment for delirium should be completed, with special attention being paid to the level of consciousness, orientation, and presence of waxing and waning features. Key to the mental status examination is inquiry about the symptoms of psychosis and whether the content and affect associated with the psychosis increase the potential for harmful behaviors.

A hands-on physical examination by the psychiatrist is usually not recommended unless there is clear evidence of an acute physical abnormality and no nonpsychiatric physician is present. Patients may have exacerbations of paranoia induced by the psychiatrist touching or invading their personal space. More delusional or sexually preoccupied patients might assign sexual intent to such an evaluation. Most physical determinations of the etiology of psychosis can be ascertained by visual clues or a thorough history.

Collateral Information

Obtaining as much collateral information about the patient as possible in the time available is essential. Significant others, roommates, board and care facility operators, case managers, and outpatient physicians are all good potential sources for collateral data. Any past medical or psychiatric records are helpful, especially in regard to the effectiveness and tolerability of previous medication. Clinicians should be aware that they must work quickly, regardless of the ability to obtain collateral information or medical records, and should not wait for either prior to beginning an assessment.

Laboratory Tests

If feasible, obtain a fingerstick glucose level, urine or serum toxicology, and pregnancy screen as soon as possible. Other key labs might be electrolytes (to check for metabolic abnormalities), complete blood count (CBC) and urinalysis (to rule out infectious states), and thyroid-stimulating hormone level (to rule out thyroid abnormalities). If there is an indication that the patient is on lithium, valproate, or other medications requiring monitoring, obtaining levels of these will help exclude toxic delirium states or noncompliance.

DIFFERENTIAL DIAGNOSIS

Nonpsychiatric Causes

A great many organic, toxic, and metabolic disorders may present with symptoms of acute psychosis (2). As many as 20% of episodes of psychosis presenting to a medical emergency department (ED) may be caused by medical reasons (3). The following syndromes, although constituting some of the most common nonpsychiatric causes, certainly do not represent all possibilities. It is very important for clinicians to always consider all of a patient's medical history and any ingested substances, including medication, food, and herbal supplements.

Substance-Induced

Amphetamines

Amphetamines stimulate dopaminergic pathways in the brain. Ingestion, inhalation, smoking, or intravenous injection of amphetamines

can lead to psychotic symptoms that mimic positive symptoms of schizophrenia. One study showed that methamphetamine abusers are 11 times more likely than the general population to experience symptoms of psychosis (4). These can include auditory hallucinations and paranoid delusions (eg, someone peeking at them through a window, making audio/video recordings of them, hacking their cell phone, following them, or trying to harm them). In addition, some patients intoxicated on amphetamines will have tactile hallucinations, often feeling they are covered with bugs (formication). This sensation will often lead to injurious self-picking behavior. Additional behaviors may include agitation, aggression, hyperkinesis, and repetitive, stereotyped body movements. Elevated blood pressure and tachycardia may be present. Amphetamine-induced psychosis usually resolves within 24 to 48 hours, especially with an opportunity for the patient to sleep and detoxify.

3,4-Methylenedioxymethamphetamine

3,4-Methylenedioxymethamphetamine (MDMA), also known as Ecstasy, is a popular substance of abuse at all-night dance parties and concerts. Although MDMA, like methamphetamine, stimulates dopaminergic pathways, it has much higher serotonergic effects, leading to its combination of stimulant and hallucinogenic properties. It can produce unpleasant psychotic phenomena, including paranoia, auditory and visual hallucinations, and delusions. In addition, depersonalization, derealization, and depression are common (5-7). Conversely, abusers of this drug often state that it induces feelings of love, empathy, and emotional closeness toward others.

Cocaine

Another dopaminergic agonist, cocaine, can be snorted, smoked, or injected. Studies of the effects of cocaine intoxication have found that 17% to 53% of patients under the influence of this drug experience psychotic symptoms (8-10). Patients abusing this substance can present with auditory hallucinations, tactile hallucinations including formication, and paranoid delusions. As with amphetamines, cocaine can also cause hyperkinetic, repetitive, and stereotyped behaviors as well as aggression and agitation. Elevated blood pressure and tachycardia may be present.

Cocaine-induced psychosis usually resolves within 24 hours, also responsive to sleep and detoxification time.

Synthetic Cathinones

Synthetic cathinones are stimulants related to the parent molecule cathinone which is found in the khat plant. The most commonly abused synthetic cathinones include mephedrone, methylone, and methylenedioxypyrovalerone (MDPV). They are structurally related to amphetamine and MDMA. Synthetic cathinones are commonly referred to as "bath salts" and are ingested, inhaled, or snorted. Use of high doses or chronic use can cause tachycardia, hyperthermia, delirium, paranoia, hallucinations, agitation, and violent behavior (11). As most currently available urine drug screens do not test for cathinones, intoxication with this category of substances should be considered in a patient presenting with this clinical picture and a negative urine drug screen.

Synthetic Cannabinoids

Although cannabis use can cause psychosis, there may be a much higher potential for synthetic cannabinoids, eg, "Spice," to do so as they are much more potent agonists of the cannabinoid receptors. In addition, synthetic cannabinoids do not contain cannabidiol which may protect against the psychotomimetic effects of delta-9-tetrahydrocannabinol (THC). A number of adverse effects have been documented in synthetic cannabinoid users including psychosis, mania, and suicidal ideation (11). As in the case of synthetic cathinones, currently available urine drug tests do not detect the presence of these designer cannabinoids.

Phencyclidine

The NMDA receptor antagonist phencyclidine (PCP) can cause symptoms that mimic both positive and negative symptoms of schizophrenia. This substance is usually smoked. Intoxicated patients have a high risk for experiencing hallucinations and paranoid delusions, in addition to displaying agitated, bizarre, or catatonic behavior. A study that examined clinical patterns of acute PCP intoxication found a state of toxic psychosis in 16.6% of its intoxicated subjects (12). Patients may exhibit hypertension, tachycardia, horizontal and vertical nystagmus,

ataxia, increased muscle tone, tremors, brisk deep tendon reflexes, diaphoresis, lacrimation, and increased salivary secretions. Decreased sensation may also be present and is sometimes associated with violent behavior regardless of self-induced injury.

Hallucinogens

Lysergic acid diethylamide (LSD), mescaline, and psilocybin cause perceptual disturbances that can include intensification of cognitive perceptions, depersonalization, derealization, illusions, hallucination, palinopsia, and synesthesias. Hallucinations are usually visual and not auditory or tactile.

Anticholinergics

Anticholinergic intoxication can result in delirium, agitation, and visual hallucinations. A physical examination may reveal dilated pupils; warm, dry skin; dry mouth; tachycardia; hypertension; and urinary retention. Constipation caused by anticholinergic medications may result in impaction with severe agitation and aggression in the elderly. Anticholinergic substances include both medications (eg, benztropine, atropine) and botanicals (eg, *Atropa belladonna* and *Datura stramonium*, or jimson weed).

Anabolic Steroids

Steroids may be abused by athletes and bodybuilders to enhance physical strength and muscle mass. It is not uncommon for amounts used to be one to two orders of magnitude greater than that needed to achieve therapeutic levels. Also, different anabolic steroids may be used simultaneously. A study of athletes and bodybuilders using anabolic steroids found that 12% displayed psychotic symptoms (13). Studies also suggest that abuse of these agents may lead to violent and homicidal behavior (14).

Other Sources

A great many substances have the potential for creating symptoms of psychosis when abused. Inhaling glues, paints, or fuels ("huffing"), especially in chronic abusers, can cause profound hallucinations, cognitive impairment, and paranoia (15). The seemingly innocuous spice nutmeg contains myristicin which is metabolized to MDMA and believed to be responsible for its hallucinogenic effects (16). Many legitimately prescribed and over-the-counter medications can induce psychosis when taken excessively or at therapeutic doses. Examples are digoxin, isoniazid, some vitamins, herbal remedies (17,18), and dextromethorphan (19). When doing a psychosis evaluation in the emergency setting, patients must be asked about every substance they have been consuming.

Withdrawal States

Alcohol Withdrawal

A patient with a history of alcohol dependence is at risk for alcohol withdrawal after cessation or reduction in consumption of alcohol. In addition to tremulousness, diaphoresis, hypertension, tachycardia, orthostatic hypotension, seizures, irritability, anxiety, depression, and insomnia, such a patient can also experience hallucinations. If the alcohol withdrawal is severe enough, the patient may suffer from delirium tremens. This syndrome usually begins 2 to 4 days after heavy drinking has stopped. In this case, the patient may experience auditory (eg, persecutory, threatening, derogatory), visual (eg, snakes, rodents), and tactile hallucinations, delusions, confusion, agitation, and autonomic instability (20). Alcohol withdrawal can be a life-threatening emergency, so monitoring of vital signs and regular reevaluation for worsening symptoms is essential (21).

Benzodiazepine Withdrawal

In similar fashion to alcohol withdrawal, patients with a history of chronic benzodiazepine use can undergo a withdrawal syndrome. The withdrawal syndrome can become severe enough that a life-threatening delirium occurs, characterized by auditory, visual, or tactile hallucinations. Additional symptoms include tachycardia, hypertension, nausea, vomiting, tremor, insomnia, anxiety, and agitation. There is a significant risk for seizures, particularly with short-acting benzodiazepines.

Opioid Withdrawal

Persons in acute opiate withdrawal frequently present to emergency settings. They may claim hallucinations or other psychotic symptoms, but these are unlikely in pure opiate withdrawal and should be viewed with skepticism. Drug-seeking behavior needs to be ruled out.

Metabolic Abnormalities

Hypoglycemia or Hyperglycemia

Low serum blood glucose levels can present with psychosis in the context of confusion, agitation, aggression, fatigue, headache, impaired cognitive functioning, seizures, and loss of consciousness (22,23). In addition, hyperglycemic patients in early diabetic ketoacidosis may present with psychosis and delirium.

Hypothyroidism or Hyperthyroidism

Hypofunction or hyperfunction of the thyroid can result in florid psychosis. In the hypothyroid state, both auditory hallucinations and paranoia (myxedema madness) can occur in the context of the physical symptoms related to metabolic slowing (24). In severe cases of hyperthyroidism (thyrotoxicosis), a patient may have psychotic symptoms such as hallucinations and paranoid delusions, as well as symptoms of depression or mania (25).

Hypocalcemia or Hypercalcemia and Parathyroid States

Hypocalcemia can present with mental status changes including psychosis, irritability, and depression. Carpopedal and laryngeal muscle spasms may be present, along with facial grimacing and convulsions. Hypercalcemia can lead to fatigue, depression, and mental confusion. Hypoparathyroidism, a cause of abnormally low serum calcium levels, causes psychiatric disturbances including psychosis (26,27). Primary hyperparathyroidism, a disorder that leads to hypercalcemic states, has been found to cause paranoid ideation and hallucinations (28). Psychosis in both hypocalcemic and hypercalcemic states usually resolves after normalization of serum calcium levels.

Hypercortisolemia

In patients presenting with mental status changes in the context of moon facies, buffalo hump, truncal obesity, fatigue, hypertension, and hirsutism, one must consider the hypercortisolemia of Cushing syndrome. The majority of patients with Cushing syndrome will display psychiatric symptoms. These can include florid psychosis, irritability, lability, depression, mania, and confusion (29-31). Such symptoms can also occur in patients taking prescription corticosteroids.

Hepatic Encephalopathy

Psychotic symptoms with alteration of consciousness and mood symptoms can occur in a patient with hepatic encephalopathy. This disorder can occur in acute and chronic liver failure, and patients will commonly display asterixis. It is believed that increased serum ammonia levels play a role in the altered mental status observed. The delirious state can last from a few days to weeks and can be fatal (32).

Infectious Diseases

Severe infectious states with high fevers have had associated psychosis or symptoms of delirium. A thorough medical evaluation should be done in any psychotic patient with an elevated temperature.

AIDS and Related Infections That Can Affect the Central Nervous System

Patients infected with the human immunodeficiency virus (HIV) are vulnerable to numerous central nervous system (CNS) diseases either because of actions of the virus or as a result of secondary infection by opportunistic organisms. These diseases include toxoplasmosis, cryptococcosis, progressive multifocal leukoencephalopathy, cytomegalovirus, syphilis, *Mycobacterium* tuberculosis, human T-cell lymphotropic virus 1 (HTLV-1) infection, aseptic meningitis, and HIV encephalopathy (AIDS-dementia complex). All these diseases can result in mental status changes, including the potential for psychotic symptoms. A study that examined patients infected with HIV found a prevalence of new-onset psychosis ranging from 0.23% to 15.2% (33). The types of psychotic symptoms that can occur include delusions as well as auditory and visual hallucinations (34).

Neurosyphilis

There are three types of neurosyphilis: meningeal, meningovascular, and parenchymatous. Meningeal syphilis may present with headache, nausea, vomiting, nuchal rigidity, cranial nerve palsies, seizures, and mental status changes. Meningovascular syphilis involves an inflammatory process that affects small vessels and usually presents with a stroke after a period that may include psychological changes. Parenchymatous syphilis is a condition with widespread degeneration of primarily cortical neurons. Patients in this stage of neurosyphilis exhibit delusions and hallucinations and significant cognitive abnormalities, as well as personality and mood changes (35).

Meningitis

Bacterial meningitis can present with altered mental status in the context of headache, fever, and nuchal rigidity. Nausea, vomiting, photophobia, and lethargy are common complaints. Seizures can also occur. Acute psychosis has been seen in patients with tuberculous meningitis (36,37). Both psychosis and mania have been documented in cases of cryptococcal meningitis (38,39). Sometimes patients being treated for meningitis can become psychotic from the treatment itself. Isoniazid, which is used to treat tuberculous meningitis, is known to cause psychotic symptoms (40,41). Patients with viral meningitis can also have a syndrome of signs and symptoms similar to that seen for bacterial meningitis, but the nuchal rigidity can be mild in some cases.

Neurologic Disorders

Stroke

An ischemic stroke must be considered in any patient who presents with acute onset of psychotic symptoms or altered mental status, or both, along with focal neurologic findings. In a review of poststroke patients with psychotic symptoms, the most common diagnosis was delusional disorder, along with schizophrenialike psychosis and mood disorder with psychotic features (42).

Central Nervous System Neoplasm

An intracranial mass must be considered in any patient who presents with psychotic symptoms or altered mental status, or both, along with focal neurologic findings. In the case of a CNS neoplasm, the symptoms may not have a history of acute onset. Delusions and hallucinations can be caused by tumors positioned in different regions of the brain (43-45).

Seizure Disorder

The possibility of a seizure event must be considered in a patient who is brought to an emergency treatment setting appearing confused, psychotic, and expressing a loss of memory for events prior to arrival. This could very well represent postictal disorientation. During the postictal phase, the patient may also complain of headache, fatigue, and muscle ache (46-48).

Hypoxic-Ischemic Encephalopathy

Hypoxic-ischemic encephalopathy is the result of a lack of adequate oxygen in the brain due to cardiac or respiratory failure. Events such as myocardial infarction, respiratory paralysis, shock, asphyxiation, and carbon monoxide poisoning can be causes. The degree of ischemic damage to the brain and resulting behavioral changes are dependent on the length of time of inadequate oxygenation. Carbon monoxide poisoning, for example, can cause symptoms of hysteria and psychosis at lower levels and encephalopathy or coma at more severe levels, along with more permanent neuropsychiatric sequelae (49).

Alzheimer Disease and Other Dementias

Patients with dementia frequently come to the attention of emergency settings either because the person was found aimlessly wandering the streets appearing confused or was demonstrating problematic behaviors at home. Psychotic symptoms appear after the development of progressive deficits in memory, language, and motor skills. In an analysis of studies published between 1990 and 2003, Ropacki and Jeste (50) found that 41% of patients with Alzheimer disease had psychotic symptoms, 36% with delusions, and 18% with hallucinations.

Multi-infarct dementia is associated with a history of one or more strokes, involves different regions of the brain, and has accompanying focal neurologic deficits and psychosis (51). Patients with frontotemporal dementia can be irritable, disinhibited, and socially inappropriate and then display mutism late in the course of the illness. A study attempting to identify behavioral clusters in frontotemporal dementia found that delusions, hallucinations, irritability, and agitation cluster together (52).

Pick disease (a subtype of frontotemporal dementia) can present with hyperoral behavior, language disturbance, irritability, disinhibition, and wandering. Cases have been reported of Pick disease first presenting with psychotic symptoms and even having been first diagnosed as schizophrenia (53,54). Diffuse Lewy body disease is characterized by parkinsonian features (rigidity, intention tremor) and fluctuations of cognitive function and behavior. Psychiatric symptoms include delusions, auditory hallucinations, prominent visual hallucinations, and depression (55,56).

Autoimmune Disorders

Systemic Lupus Erythematosus

Central nervous system involvement of systemic lupus erythematosus (SLE) has been clearly established to cause symptoms of psychosis (57,58). Additionally, psychotic symptoms caused as a side effect of the steroid medications often used to treat SLE should be ruled out before ascribing the symptoms to the CNS cause (59).

Autoimmune Encephalitis

Autoimmune encephalitis is characterized by brain inflammation and autoantibodies. Although relatively rare, psychiatrists need to be aware of this cause of psychosis. Anti-NMDA receptor encephalitis is the most common type. At least 80% of patients with this disorder initially presented with psychiatric symptoms (grandiose or paranoid delusions, auditory and visual hallucinations, bizarre behavior, agitation, and confusion) and had no past psychiatric history. It is important to determine if neurological features are currently or were recently present (seizures, dyskinesias, dysautonomia) (60). In the case of an acute presentation of psychosis in a patient with no such history, negative drug screen and presence of neurological signs, transfer to the medical ED for assessment including a neurology consult is essential.

Psychiatric Causes

The most prevalent cause for acute psychosis seen in the emergency setting is exacerbation of chronic schizophrenia (61). Psychotic symptoms might also be present in acute cases of bipolar mania, major depression, and delusional disorders. Some patients with personality disorders, such as borderline personality disorder, can develop psychosis when under pronounced stress (62). Although more rarely seen, atypical psychoses such as folie à deux—in which a more dominant, psychotic individual transfers delusional thinking to a susceptible other (63)—can at times present in emergency settings.

MANAGEMENT

Treatment Within the Emergency Setting

Patients who have been determined to have acute psychosis due to nonpsychiatric causes should be transferred to acute medical care. Patients at risk for new-onset, endogenous psychosis are detailed in a special section at the end of this chapter.

Patients whose psychosis has been determined to be from stimulant intoxication will likely see the psychosis diminish or disappear with sleep and time to detoxify. A reasonable approach for such patients is to use lorazepam 1 to 2 mg orally or intramuscularly every 30 to 60 minutes until the patient is asleep and then reevaluate after the patient has rested. If after several hours of sound sleep the patient awakens still floridly psychotic, an underlying psychotic disorder and not mere substance intoxication should be considered. Use of antipsychotic medications is likely unnecessary in pure substance-induced psychosis and should be avoided as they place patients at risk for the severe side effects these agents can cause.

For patients who appear to have an endogenous acute psychosis, it is prudent to commence antipsychotic therapy promptly. Although for many years it has been thought that true antipsychotic effects of neuroleptic medications might take several weeks, more recent research shows that antipsychotic effects are pronounced in less than a week (64), with noticeable effects even within the first 24 hours (65).

For patients with a well-established history of being on effective antipsychotic therapy, it is sensible to restart at least a full dose of their regular medication. Some clinicians will combine a full day's amount of medication into one initial dose.

Because the patient will be under supervision in the emergency facility, clinicians can feel more comfortable in prescribing higher doses, because any untoward reactions can be quickly observed and controlled. The higher initial doses will assist in more quickly reducing psychotic symptoms to a tolerable level.

In those patients with an unknown or unclear history of neuroleptic medications, the second-generation antipsychotics olanzapine, risperidone, quetiapine, ziprasidone, and aripiprazole are generally recommended as first-line treatments (66,67). Clozapine, given its side effects, need for authorization, and the laboratory data required before prescribing, should not be given first line in emergency settings except as continuation of outpatient treatment. Because of their side effect potential, first-generation antipsychotics such as haloperidol, fluphenazine, and thiothixene should only be given to patients in whom there is a clear history of efficacy and tolerability for these agents. Recommended dosages can be found in Table 20.2.

With significant anxiety, restlessness, and/or discomfort of the individual, the authors recommend adding oral lorazepam 0.5 to 2 mg or clonazepam 0.5 to 1 mg to the initial antipsychotic dose. Extrapyramidal side effects are more common with high-potency neuroleptics (haloperidol, fluphenazine) and atypical antipsychotics with more dopamine-blocking potential (risperidone). It is prudent to add oral diphenhydramine 25 to 50 mg or oral benztropine mesylate 1 to 2 mg to these agents. With regard to working with emergency psychiatry patients, always monitor for akathisia secondary to antipsychotic usage, because emerging akathisia is a risk factor for assault and may result in future noncompliance.

TABLE 20.2 Initial Oral Dose Ranges for First-Line Antipsychotics

Drug	Dose Range (mg)
Olanzapine	5-20
Risperidone	1-4
Quetiapine	200-600
Ziprasidone	60-80
Aripiprazole	7.5-30

A benzodiazepine as described previously will treat akathisia more quickly than a beta-blocker.

Although several antipsychotic medications can be given in parenteral forms, it is preferable, when possible, to give medications orally. This will assist in future compliance and in creating a therapeutic alliance with patients, who may be less inclined to trust and work with physicians who have subjected them to injections (67). Although intramuscular neuroleptics are indicated for the treatment of agitation, there will be antipsychotic effects as well; however, these are not intended as replacement therapy for oral antipsychotics. Instead, efforts to engage the patient into voluntarily taking oral medications should always be a priority.

Criteria for Hospitalization

Patients with acute, unresolvable symptoms of psychosis leading to suicidal or homicidal ideation, whose symptoms do not show a course toward prompt resolution in the emergency setting, should invariably be admitted for psychiatric hospitalization. Similarly, patients with persistent command auditory hallucinations telling them to hurt themselves or others should be admitted, even if they have no intent of responding to the commands (68). Patients whose suicidality, thoughts of hurting others, or command hallucinations have dissipated may be candidates for lower levels of care after a period of observation, if the clinician determines the patient is truly no longer at an increased risk.

In the absence of dangerousness, mere symptoms of psychosis do not necessarily indicate a need for hospitalization. Many patients with hallucinations or disorganization can be treated as outpatients if there is a good follow-up plan of psychiatric care and an appropriate level of housing in place. However, patients who are very disorganized or catatonic and unable to adequately care for themselves, or unable to avail themselves of services and housing, likely will need inpatient stabilization.

Criteria for Discharge

Patients whose symptoms of psychosis are relieved or are no longer causing the patient pronounced distress, and who show no evidence of being a danger to themselves or others, may be able to be discharged. Ideally, this should happen with a strong discharge plan that includes a prompt appointment with the outpatient psychiatrist and case manager, if applicable. Patients with good follow-up plans are far less likely to be readmitted than patients without adequate aftercare (69).

Appropriate housing can also help ensure stability for a patient and reduce recidivism. Homeless patients have higher numbers of visits per capita to psychiatric EDs than do domiciled individuals (70). At the time of stabilization of psychotic symptoms, if a patient does not have a secured living situation, involvement of social service personnel should be requested.

Interventions for the Difficult-to-Treat or Treatment-Resistant Patient

Medication Noncompliance

A patient with acute symptoms of psychosis might be paranoid, suspicious, or otherwise reluctant to take medications. In these instances, directed counseling from the physician using clear, short, and supportive phrases concerning the benefits and risks of the medication may be enough to overcome the fears. If not, and a patient refuses to consent to appropriate psychiatric medications, injectable forms of several antipsychotic medications may be considered for use. Although indicated for agitation, these medications will also build to serum concentrations with antipsychotic effect. Laws in municipalities differ on the ability to administer parenteral medications against a patient's will, in some cases only permitting it when there is clear danger to self or others or only with a judge's order.

When a patient has consented to medications but is suspected of cheeking or otherwise being deceptive about medication intake, rapid-dissolving tablet formulations or liquid versions of medications, which make it more difficult to feign compliance, should be prescribed.

Substance Abuse Comorbidity

The abuse of intoxicants in patients with chronic psychotic illnesses is pronounced and frequently leads to emergency psychiatric contacts (71). In the emergency setting, it is often difficult to clarify which psychotic symptoms derive from the intoxicant and which are underlying and chronic.

In such cases, where a patient has a known history of a psychotic illness and is presently under the influence of stimulants (cocaine, amphetamines, cathinones), it is prudent to begin treatment of both situations promptly. In general, it is effective to restart the patient's neuroleptic medication with the addition of a benzodiazepine, usually lorazepam or clonazepam. It is best to allow a period of time for the patient to detoxify from the substance abuse and then reevaluate his or her mental status prior to making a decision about hospitalization.

For comorbid patients who have improved enough with sobriety for discharge, emphatic counseling should be provided as to the inadvisability of abusing substances in the face of mental illness. Substance abuse treatment and 12-step program information should be given to the patient, as well as ensuring proper follow-up with the outpatient psychiatrist. The emergency professional should also take the time to help identify triggers for substance abuse and clearly identify options, including addresses, phone numbers, and bus routes to facilities, in the case of imminent relapse.

Medication-Seeking and Malingering Patients

On occasion, clinicians may encounter patients who may be inventing or exaggerating symptoms of psychosis for secondary gain, typically to obtain unnecessary medications or find a safe place to sleep for the night. In these situations, it behooves the clinician to observe the patient for an extended period and judge behaviors outside of the direct interview setting. A patient who is truly hallucinating or acutely psychotic will likely maintain the same affect and behaviors whether or not he or she believes others to be watching, whereas a malingering patient may not. Persons feigning psychosis usually exaggerate hallucinations and delusions but will be free of thought disorder, which is difficult to feign. The malingerer also has difficulty feigning relatedness, concrete thinking, and blunted affect. Obtaining as much past history and collateral information as possible can further help clinicians evaluate the truthfulness of the patient (72).

Medications, especially those with abuse potential, should be used with trepidation in patients suspected of feigning symptoms of psychosis. Administration of these medications will only enable drug-seeking behavior. It is sensible to substitute nonsteroidal anti-inflammatory agents for requested opiates and diphenhydramine or hydroxyzine instead of benzodiazepines until a complete evaluation can be done. A full discussion of treatment of malingering and factitious disorders can be found in Chapter (30 fill when chapter numbers known).

SPECIAL FOCUS: FIRST EPISODE OF PSYCHOSIS

Presentation

Patients who develop a new-onset psychotic disorder frequently end up in an emergency setting and require a comprehensive evaluation. When such a patient experiences a first psychotic episode, both patient and family are usually quite distressed by the experience.

The presentations can be quite varied. In some cases, the patient first comes to the attention of law enforcement because of violent or bizarre behavior in public. At other times, concerned family members or friends may bring the patient to the ED because of increasingly unusual behavior, such as talking to imaginary people, voicing paranoid delusions, and socially withdrawing from significant others.

Evaluation

Once in the ED, evaluation of the need for immediate intervention is required. If there is a significant risk for violence or disorganized behavior that may place the patient or others at risk for harm, the patient may need to be emergently medicated, secluded, or restrained. Once safety has been established, then the comprehensive evaluation of the patient can begin.

If the patient is able to communicate clearly, a detailed history should be taken, including information about onset of symptoms, changes in behavior, and recent alcohol and substance abuse, as well as questions about any intake of unusual foods, herbal medicines, or vitamin formulations. A suicide and violence risk assessment is mandatory. If the patient is mute or too disorganized, then collateral information from family members is very important. They may shed light on such issues as family history of psychotic illness, past medical problems, premorbid functioning versus current functioning, substance abuse, the time line of behavioral changes, the nature of the behavioral changes, and recent suicidal and violent ideation and behavior.

One must keep an open mind when evaluating a patient with an apparent first episode of psychosis. Schizophrenia should not be immediately placed at the top of the differential diagnosis list. A thorough evaluation must include a medical history and a physical examination that includes a neurologic examination. A battery of laboratory tests should include a chemistry panel (electrolytes, blood urea nitrogen, creatinine, calcium, and liver function tests), complete blood count, urinalysis, toxicology screen, thyroid function tests, and a test for syphilis. If there are any findings of concern on the neurologic examination, a brain scan (computerized axial tomography or magnetic resonance imaging) should be performed immediately (73).

Once medical problems and substances have been ruled out as possible causes, then serious consideration of diagnosing the patient with a psychiatric disorder is warranted. If mood symptoms are present, then the diagnoses bipolar disorder, schizoaffective disorder, and major depression with psychotic features will be part of the differential diagnosis. If the mood component is minimal, then diagnoses such as schizophrenia and delusional disorder should be considered.

Patients who experience their first psychotic episode and later go on to be diagnosed with schizophrenia will often have gone through a prodromal phase. Therefore, psychiatric emergency service (PES) staff should obtain from the patient and collaterals whether prodromal features were present, including social withdrawal, impairment in role functioning, peculiar behavior, poor hygiene, blunted or inappropriate affect, vague or odd manner of speech, odd or bizarre ideation, unusual perceptual experiences, lack of interest or initiative, anxiety, disturbance of sleep, suspiciousness, and irritability (74,75). Another key component of the onset of schizophrenia is the comorbidity of substance abuse. Studies have shown that patients with recent onset of schizophrenia have an increased risk of problems with alcohol and substance abuse, particularly cannabis and psychostimulants (76). It is not clear whether the substance abuse predisposes the patient to schizophrenia or whether schizophrenia places a patient at higher risk for abusing substances.

Intervention and Treatment

Patients with a first psychotic episode are at an elevated risk for suicidal behavior both before and after their first presentation (77). Patients who go on to be diagnosed specifically with schizophrenia have a significantly increased risk of suicide attempts, with a lifetime risk of mortality from suicide of 5% (78). In addition, the lifetime prevalence for suicide attempts in those with a diagnosis of schizophrenia was 39.2%, as opposed to only 2.8% of those without the illness (79). A careful suicide risk assessment that includes collateral information from significant others may reveal information leading to timely and appropriate care, perhaps saving patients from life-threatening suicidal behavior.

Another potential benefit of early intervention is that the patient begins to receive psychiatric treatment promptly. Although it has not been definitively proven that patients who start pharmacologic treatment earlier rather than later have better long-term outcomes, it is an opportunity to immediately start reducing the severity of the patient's symptoms and hence reduce the distress of both the patient and the patient's family.

CONCLUSION

Psychosis is a common presenting problem in the PES. The etiology of psychosis is often multifactorial, involving one or more medical, substance use, and primary psychiatric diagnoses. If psychotic symptoms are present, the emergency psychiatrist must be able to recognize when these are caused by delirium, complicated withdrawal states, or the presence of new neurologic deficits and be prepared to take necessary steps to ensure patient safety and wellness. Challenges in the rapid assessment and treatment of the patient with psychosis in emergency settings include forming a collaborative and therapeutic working relationship, calming accompanying agitation with the least restrictive interventions, and recognizing possible malingering. Although an often difficult task, stabilizing acute exacerbations of psychosis in a swift and benign way greatly benefits patients and all involved in their care.

REFERENCES

1. Forster, P. L., Buckley, R., & Phelps, M. A. (1999). Phenomenology and treatment of psychotic disorders in the psychiatric emergency service. *Psychiatric Clinics of North America, 22*(4), 735–754.
2. Frame, D. S., & Kercher, E. E. (1991). Acute psychosis. Functional versus organic. *Emergency Medicine Clinics of North America, 9*(1), 123–136.
3. Richards, C. F., & Gurr, D. E. (2000). Psychosis. *Emergency Medicine Clinics of North America, 18*(2), 253–262.
4. McKetin, R., McLaren, J., Lubman, D., et al. (2006). The prevalence of psychotic symptoms among methamphetamine users. *Addiction, 101*(10), 1473–1478.
5. McGuire, P. K., Cope, H., & Fahy, T. A. (1994). Diversity of psychopathology associated with use of 3,4-methylenedioxymethamphetamine ("Ecstasy"). *British Journal of Psychiatry, 165*(3), 391–395.
6. Landabaso, M. A., Iraurgi, I., Jiménez-Lerma, J. M., et al. (2002). Ecstasy-induced psychotic disorder: Six-month follow-up study. *European Addiction Research, 8*(3), 133–140.
7. Vecellio, M., Schopper, C., & Modestin, J. (2003). Neuropsychiatric consequences (atypical psychosis and complex-partial seizures) of ecstasy use: Possible evidence for toxicity-vulnerability predictors and implications for preventative and clinical care. *Journal of Psychopharmacology, 17*(3), 342–345.
8. Lowenstein, D. H., Massa, S. M., Rowbotham, M. C., et al. (1987). Acute neurologic and psychiatric complications associated with cocaine abuse. *American Journal of Medicine, 83*(5), 841–846.
9. Manschreck, T. C., Laughery, J. A., Weisstein, C. C., et al. (1988). Characteristics of freebase cocaine psychosis. *Yale Journal of Biology and Medicine, 61*(2), 115–122.
10. Brady, K. T., Lydiard, R. B., Malcolm, R., et al. (1991). Cocaine-induced psychosis. *The Journal of Clinical Psychiatry, 52*(12), 509–512.
11. Weinstein, A. M., Rosca, P., Fattore, L., & London, E. D. (2017). Synthetic cathinone and cannabinoid designer drugs pose a major risk for public health. *Front Psychiatry, 8*(156), 1–11.
12. McCarron, M. M., Schulze, B. W., Thompson, G. A., et al. (1981). Acute phencyclidine intoxication: Clinical patterns, complications, and treatment. *Annals of Emergency Medicine, 10*(6), 290–297.
13. Pope, H. G., & Katz, D. L. (1988). Affective and psychotic symptoms associated with anabolic steroid use. *American Journal of Psychiatry, 145*(4), 487–490.
14. Pope, H. G., & Katz, D. L. (1990). Homicide and near-homicide by anabolic steroid users. *The Journal of Clinical Psychiatry, 51*(1), 28–31.
15. Maruff, P., Burns, C. B., Tyler, P., et al. (1998). Neurological and cognitive abnormalities associated with chronic petrol sniffing. *Brain, 121*(10), 1903–1917.
16. Ehrenpreis, J. E., DesLauriers, C., Lank, P., Armstrong, P. K., & Leikin, J. B. (2014). Nutmeg poisonings: A retrospective review of 10 years experience from the Illinois Poison Center, 2001–2011. *Journal of Medical Toxicology, 10*(2), 148–151.
17. Maglione, M., Miotto, K., Iguchi, M., et al. (2005). Psychiatric effects of ephedra use: An analysis of Food and Drug Administration reports of adverse events. *American Journal of Psychiatry, 162*, 189–191.
18. Stevinson, C., & Ernst, E. (2004). Can St. John's wort trigger psychoses? *International Journal of Clinical Pharmacology and Therapeutics, 42*(9), 473–480.
19. Martinak, B., Bolis, R. A., Black, J. R., Fargason, R. E., & Birur, B. (2017). Dextromethorphan in cough syrup: The poor man's psychosis. *Psychopharmacology Bulletin, 47*(4), 59–63.
20. Greenberg, D. M., & Lee, J. W. (2001). Psychotic manifestations of alcoholism. *Current Psychiatry Reports, 3*(4), 314–318.
21. Ismail, M. F., Doherty, K., Bradshaw, P., et al. (2018). Symptom-triggered therapy for assessment and management of alcohol withdrawal syndrome in the emergency department shortstay clinical decision unit. *Emergency Medicine Journal, 36*(1), 18–21.
22. Oakley, H. F. (1980). Psychiatric emergencies in endocrine and metabolic disease. *Clinics in Endocrinology and Metabolism, 9*(3), 615–624.
23. Bell, D. S., & Cutter, G. (1994). Characteristics of severe hypoglycemia in the patient with insulin-dependent diabetes. *Southern Medical Journal, 87*, 616–620.
24. Heinrich, T. W., & Grahm, G. (2003). Hypothyroidism presenting as psychosis: Myxedema madness revisited. *Primary Care Companion to The Journal of Clinical Psychiatry, 5*(6), 260–266.
25. Brownlie, B. E., Rae, A. M., Walshe, J. W., et al. (2000). Psychoses associated with thyrotoxicosis—"thyrotoxic psychosis". A report of 18 cases, with statistical analysis of incidence. *European Journal of Endocrinology, 142*(5), 438–444.

26. Gertner, J. M., Hodsman, A. B., & Neuberger, J. N. (1976). 1-Alpha-hydroxycholecalciferol in the treatment of hypocalcaemic psychosis. *Clinical Endocrinology, 5*(5), 539–543.

27. Ang, A. W., Ko, S. M., & Tan, C. H. (1995). Calcium, magnesium, and psychotic symptoms in a girl with idiopathic hypoparathyroidism. *Psychosomatic Medicine, 57*(3), 299–302.

28. Joborn, C., Hetta, J., Palmér, M., et al. (1986). Psychiatric symptomatology in patients with primary hyperparathyroidism. *Upsala Journal of Medical Sciences, 91*(1), 77–87.

29. Hirsch, D., Orr, G., Kantarovich, V., et al. (2000). Cushing's syndrome presenting as a schizophrenia-like psychotic state. *Israel Journal of Psychiatry and Related Sciences, 37*(1), 46–50.

30. Saad, M. F., Adams, F., Mackay, B., et al. (1984). Occult Cushing's disease presenting with acute psychosis. *American Journal of Medicine, 76*(4), 759–766.

31. Bochner, F., Burke, C. J., Lloyd, H. M., et al. (1979). Intermittent Cushing's disease. *American Journal of Medicine, 67*(3), 507–510.

32. Ananth, J., Swartz, R., Burgoyne, K., et al. (1994). Hepatic disease and psychiatric illness: Relationships and treatment. *Psychotherapy and Psychosomatics, 62*(3–4), 146–159.

33. Sewell, D. D. (1996). Schizophrenia and HIV. *Schizophrenia Bulletin, 22*, 465–473.

34. Sewell, D. D., Jeste, D. V., Atkinson, J. H., et al. (1994). HIV-associated psychosis: A study of 20 cases. San Diego HIV Neurobehavioral Research Center Group. *American Journal of Psychiatry, 151*(2), 237–242.

35. Allen, M., et al. (2014). Psychosis in neurosyphilis: An association of poor prognosis. *General Hospital Psychiatry, 36*, 361.e5–361.e6.

36. Daif, A., Obeid, T., Yaqub, B., et al. (1992). Unusual presentation of tuberculous meningitis. *Clinical Neurology and Neurosurgery, 94*(1), 1–5.

37. Jebaraj, P., Oommen, M., Thopuram, P., et al. (2005). Tuberculous meningitis masked by delirium in an alcohol-dependent patient: A case report. *Acta Psychiatrica Scandinavica, 112*(6), 478–479.

38. Johnson, F. Y., & Naraqui, S. (1993). Manic episode secondary to cryptococcal meningitis in a previously healthy adult. *Papua New Guinea Medical Journal, 36*(1), 59–62.

39. Sa'adah, M. A., Araj, G. F., Diab, S. M., et al. (1995). Cryptococcal meningitis and confusional psychosis. A case report and literature review. *Tropical and Geographical Medicine, 47*(5), 224–226.

40. Duke, T., & Mai, M. (1999). Meningitis or madness: A delicate balance. *Journal of Paediatrics and Child Health, 35*(3), 319–320.

41. Alao, A. O., & Yolles, J. C. (1998). Isoniazid-induced psychosis. *Annals of Pharmacotherapy, 32*(9), 889–891.

42. Stangeland, H., Orgeta, V., & Bell, V. (2018). Poststroke psychosis: A systematic review. *Journal of Neurology, Neurosurgery, and Psychiatry, 89*(8), 879–885.

43. Sato, T., Takeichi, M., Abe, M., et al. (1993). Frontal lobe tumor associated with late-onset seizure and psychosis: A case report. *The Japanese Journal of Psychiatry and Neurology, 47*(3), 541–544.

44. Lisanby, S. H., Kohler, C., Swanson, C. L., et al. (1998). Psychosis secondary to brain tumor. *Seminars in Clinical Neuropsychiatry, 3*(1), 12–22.

45. Madhusoodanan, S., Ting, M. B., Farah, T., et al. (2015). Psychiatric aspects of brain tumors: A review. *World Journal of Psychiatry, 5*(3), 273–285.

46. Clancy, M. J., Clarke, M. C., Connor, D. J., et al. (2014). The prevalence of psychosis in epilepsy; a systematic review and meta-analysis. *BMC Psychiatry, 14*, 75.

47. Kanner, A. M., & Rivas-Grajales, A. M. (2016). Psychosis of epilepsy: A multifaceted neuropsychiatric disorder. *CNS Spectrums, 21*(3), 247–257.

48. Maguire, M., Singh, J., & Marson, A. (2018). Epilepsy and psychosis: A practical approach. *Practical Neurology, 18*(2), 106–114.

49. Olson, K. R. (1984). Carbon monoxide poisoning: Mechanisms, presentation, and controversies in management. *The Journal of Emergency Medicine, 1*(3), 233–243.

50. Ropacki, S. A., & Jeste, D. V. (2005). Epidemiology of and risk factors for psychosis of Alzheimer's disease: A review of 55 studies published from 1990 to 2003. *American Journal of Psychiatry, 162*(11), 2022–2030.

51. Miller, B. L., Lesser, I. M., Boone, K., et al. (1989). Brain white-matter lesions and psychosis. *British Journal of Psychiatry, 155*, 73–78.

52. Mourik, J. C., Rosso, S. M., Niermeijer, M. F., et al. (2004). Frontotemporal dementia: Behavioral symptoms and caregiver distress. *Dementia and Geriatric Cognitive Disorders, 18*(3–4), 299–306.

53. Mowadat, H. R., Kerr, E. E., & StClair, D. (1993). Sporadic Pick's disease in a 28-year-old woman. *British Journal of Psychiatry, 162*, 259–262.

54. Waddington, J. L., Youssef, H. A., Farrell, M. A., et al. (1995). Initial "schizophrenia-like" psychosis in Pick's disease: Case study with neuroimaging and neuropathology, and implications for frontotemporal dysfunction in schizophrenia. *Schizophrenia Research, 18*(1), 79–82.

55. Ballard, C. G., O'Brien, J. T., Swann, A. G., et al. (2001). The natural history of psychosis and depression in dementia with Lewy bodies and Alzheimer's disease: Persistence and new cases over 1 year of follow-up. *The Journal of Clinical Psychiatry, 62*(1), 46–49.

56. Ballard, C. G., Jacoby, R., Del Ser, T., et al. (2004). Neuro-pathological substrates of psychiatric symptoms in prospectively studied patients with autopsy-confirmed dementia with Lewy bodies. *American Journal of Psychiatry, 161*(5), 843–849.

57. Appenzeller, S., Cendes, F., & Costallat, L. T. (2007). Acute psychosis in systemic lupus erythematosus. *Rheumatology International, 28*(3), 237–243.

58. Hajighaemi, F., Etemadifar, M., & Bonakdar, Z. S. (2016). Neuropsychiatric manifestations in patients with systemic lupus erythematosus: A study from Iran. *Advanced Biomedical Research, 5*, 43.

59. Alpert, O., Marwaha, R., & Huang, H. (2014). Psychosis in children with systemic lupus erythematosus: The role of steroids as both treatment and cause. *General Hospital Psychiatry, 36*, 549–554.

60. Bost, C., Pacual, O., & Honnorat, J. (2016). Autoimmune encephalitis in psychiatric institutions: Current perspectives. *Neuropsychiatric Disease and Treatment, 12*, 2775–2787.

61. Fiseković, S., & Burnazović, L. (2005). Clinical features in emergency psychiatric conditions. *Psychiatria Danubina, 17*(3–4), 197–200.

62. Benvenuti, A., Rucci, P., & Ravani, L. (2005). Psychotic features in borderline patients: Is there a connection to mood dysregulation? *Bipolar Disorder, 7*(4), 338–343.

63. Arnone, D., Patel, A., & Tan, G. (2006). The nosological significance of Folie à Deux: A review of the literature. *Annals of General Psychiatry, 5*, 11.

64. Agid, O., Kapur, S., Arenovich, T., et al. (2003). Delayed-onset hypothesis of antipsychotic action: A hypothesis tested and rejected. *Archives of General Psychiatry, 60*, 1228–1235.

65. Kapur, S., Arenovich, T., Agid, O., et al. (2005). Evidence for onset of antipsychotic effects within the first 24 hours of treatment. *American Journal of Psychiatry, 162*(5), 939–946.

66. Lehman, A., Lieberman, J., Dixon, L., et al. (2004). *Practice guideline for the treatment of patients with schizophrenia* (2nd ed.). Washington, DC: American Psychiatric Association.

67. Yildiz, A., Sachs, G. S., & Turgay, A. (2003). Pharmacological management of agitation in emergency settings. *Emergency Medicine Journal, 20*, 339–346.

68. Jacobs, D., Baldessarini, R., Conwell, Y., et al. (2003). *Practice guideline for the assessment and treatment of patients with suicidal behaviors.* Washington, DC: American Psychiatric Association.

69. Nelson, E. A., Maruish, M. E., & Axler, J. L. (2001). Effects of discharge planning and compliance with outpatient appointments on readmission rates. *Psychiatric Services, 51*(7), 885–889.

70. McNiel, D. E., & Binder, R. L. (2005). Psychiatric emergency service use and homelessness, mental disorder and violence. *Psychiatric Services, 56*, 699–704.

71. Galanter, M., Castaneda, R., & Ferman, J. (1988). Substance abuse among general psychiatric patients: Place of presentation, diagnosis, and treatment. *American Journal of Drug and Alcohol Abuse, 14*(2), 211–235.

72. Resnick, P. J., & Knoll, J. (2005). Faking it: How to detect malingered psychosis. *Current Psychiatry, 4*(11), 13–25.

73. Sheitman, B. B., Lee, H., Strous, R., et al. (1997). The evaluation and treatment of first-episode psychosis. *Schizophrenia Bulletin, 23*(4), 653–661.

74. Jackson, H. J., McGorry, P. D., & Dudgeon, P. (1995). Prodromal symptoms of schizophrenia in first-episode psychosis: Prevalence and specificity. *Comprehensive Psychiatry, 36*(4), 241–250.

75. Yung, A. R., & McGorry, P. D. (1996). The prodromal phase of first-episode psychosis: Past and current conceptualizations. *Schizophrenia Bulletin, 22*(2), 353–370.

76. Barnes, T. R., Mutsatsa, S. H., Hutton, S. B., et al. (2006). Comorbid substance use and age at onset of schizophrenia. *British Journal of Psychiatry, 188*, 237–242.

77. Clarke, M., Whitty, P., Browne, S., et al. (2006). Suicidality in first episode psychosis. *Schizophrenia Research, 86*(1–3), 221–225.

78. Palmer, B. A., Pankratz, V. S., & Bostwick, J. M. (2005). The lifetime risk of suicide in schizophrenia: A reexamination. *Archives of General Psychiatry, 62*, 247–253.

79. Fuller-Thomson, E., & Hollister, B. (2016). Schizophrenia and suicide attempts: Findings from a representative community-based Canadian sample. *Schizophrenia Research and Treatment, 2016*, 1–11.

21

Depression

Flávio Casoy, Kaitlyn Garcia

Major depressive disorder (MDD) and related illness are the most common psychiatric illnesses in the general population and add significantly the global burden of morbidity and mortality. Depression is different from usual changes in mood or brief reactions to adversities in everyday life. According to the World Health Organization (WHO), more than 300 million people are affected worldwide. Particularly when people have repeated episodes, long-lasting episodes, or episodes with moderate or severe intensity, depression can severely hinder individuals' ability to function at work, in school, and in their relationships. In its worst form, depression can lead to suicide. According to the WHO, almost 800,000 people die by suicide each year and it is the second leading cause of death in 15- to 29-year-olds (1). In the United States, 45,000 people died by suicide in 2016 and suicide rates went up by more than 30% since 1999; however, more than half of US suicides are completed by people who did not have a known psychiatric illness, demonstrating suicide is multifactorial and there is widespread underdiagnosis of mental illness (2). Given the common relatively early age of onset of depression, this illness has an extremely significant social cost. Interference with social functioning results in more common early termination of education, inability to marry or remain in a stable relationship (and therefore loss of associated economic stability), adolescent childbearing, and difficulty finding or maintaining employment (with resultant loss of productivity and financial dependence on others) (3).

The emergency department (ED) and psychiatric emergency services are common points of entry into the mental health system for individuals with depression. Because of the fragmented and sparse nature of community mental health resources and due to the significant functional impairment caused by depression, it is common for the first point of contact to be during a crisis. It is important for professionals in emergency settings to be familiar with depression, given its widespread prevalence and associated morbidity and mortality. In medical settings, depression is often comorbid in patients with chronic medical conditions who routinely return to the ED for decompensation of their medical illnesses (4). This chapter will discuss depression in the emergency setting and its evaluation, diagnosis, and treatment.

EPIDEMIOLOGY

In a recent national survey of over 36,000 adults, the lifetime prevalence of MDD in the United States is one in five; women have twice the risk of developing at least one lifetime major depressive episode (MDE) then men. The 12-month prevalence was 10%. Most cases were moderate or severe and associated with significant functional impairment (5).

Rates of ED utilization for mental health problems have been increasing; 6.3% of all ED visits are related to mental health problems, 17% of which are due to mood disorders (6). In studies that assess all ED patients for depression, rates of depression vary from 20% to 30% (7–9). This is likely a low estimate, given the fact that the accuracy of depression recognition by nonpsychiatric physicians is generally low (10). In pediatric EDs, 3.3% of all visits were for psychiatric-related causes. ED visits for psychiatric causes tend to have longer lengths of stay (11,12).

From 1993 to 2008, visits to EDs for suicide attempts and self-inflicted injury doubled in frequency. Thirty-four percent of all attempted suicides and self-inflicted injury visits were coded for depressive disorders. Fifty-four percent of attempted suicides were coded with any mental health problems. Women present to EDs slightly more frequently than men for suicidal attempts or gestures (13), although men complete suicide much more often than women (14).

PRESENTING FEATURES

MDD exists on a spectrum from mild to severe. In its mildest forms, the patient does meet the standard criteria, but barely, and the symptoms are distressing, but manageable and result in only mild impairment in social or occupational functioning. In its most severe form, the symptoms are unmanageable and severely interfere with patients' ability to function. Risk of suicide increases with severity of MDEs (15). Researchers have commonly cited that approximately 15% of individuals with depression complete suicide; however, this rate is complicated by widespread underdiagnosis and incorrect diagnosis of depression (16,17).

MDD is significantly associated with many different chronic physical disorders, including arthritis, asthma, cancers, cardiovascular disease, diabetes, hypertension, chronic respiratory disorders, and chronic pain (Table 21.1) (3). MDD is also very highly associated with substance use disorders (18).

Individuals with depression are at significantly higher risk for suicide. In a systematic review of case reports and case series in the United Kingdom, authors found that more than half of people who die by suicide have depression when their lives are retrospectively reviewed (although they may not have been diagnosed while alive) (14,19). It is clear that the suicide risk for individuals with depression is many times that of the general population (20–22). Considering the growing substance use disorder epidemics in the United States and the increasing rates of suicide, it is very likely that the overall risk of suicide in patients with depression is growing (23).

While depressed mood is considered the fundamental feature of depression, it is possible for individuals to present without depressed mood. Patients may initially deny depressed mood but then become more forthcoming in interview with closer questioning. In other individuals who report feeling "blah," or not having any feelings, or feeling anxious, sad, or depressed, mood may be inferred from their facial expression (15). Individuals may deny changes in mood but report somatic complaints, such as body aches, fatigue, breathing problems, headaches, and upset stomach (15, 24). Others may externally demonstrate their sad mood as irritability or low tolerance for frustration (15). The heterogeneous presentation of patients on first arrival suggests that all patients who present to psychiatric emergency services or medical ED should be screened for depression, given the significant impact untreated depression has on ability to function. In medical ED settings, all patients should be screened for depression, given the frequent somatic complaints of depressed patients and because medically ill patients with comorbid depression have worse overall outcomes (4).

Both psychiatric and medical comorbidities are common in individuals with MDD. There has not been an updated National Comorbidity Survey since the release of Diagnostic and Statistical Manual of Mental Disorders, 5th Edition (DSM-5), but the 2003 replication shows most lifetime and 12-month cases of MDD had other comorbid psychiatric disorders, with prevalence rates of 72.1% and 78.5%, respectively (25). The National Epidemiologic Survey on Alcohol and Related Conditions III conducted using DSM 5 criteria in 2012 to 13 confirmed

TABLE 21.1 Prevalence of Chronic Serious Medical Illnesses and Depression (4)

Illness	Prevalence of Major Depression (Percent)
Diabetes	11-15
Coronary artery disease	15-23
Human immunodeficiency virus	4-23
Stroke	9-31
Parkinson	20-30
Multiple sclerosis	16-30

Reprinted from Katon, W., Ciechanowski, P. (2002). Impact of major depression on chronic medical illness. *Journal of Psychosomatic Research, 53*(4), 859–863. Copyright © 2002 Elsevier. With permission.

significant comorbidity of other psychiatric illnesses in MDD, with lifetime comorbidity prevalence for alcohol use disorder 40.8%, for generalized anxiety disorder 20.5%, for posttraumatic stress disorder 16.3%, and for borderline personality disorder 26.6% among others (25). A separate study found 84.4% of individuals with posttraumatic stress disorder meet criteria for MDD (26).

With improving public attitudes toward cannabis, more people are trying to self-manage depression with cannabis use, despite lack of evidence that cannabinoids are effective for depression. There is evidence that cannabis worsens the course of depressive disorders. Individual with substance use disorders are less likely to access or complete treatment for depression. Dual-diagnosis treatment for individuals with depression and substance use disorders is more effective for these individuals than either treatment alone (5). In emergency settings, there needs to be adequate screening for both depression and substance use disorders to ensure correct referrals.

Depression with psychotic features has traditionally been considered a severe type of depression. These individuals generally have delusions or hallucinations that are congruent with their depressed mood; these often include themes of personal inadequacy, guilt, disease, death, nihilism, or deserved punishment. It is possible for individuals to present with delusions that are not mood congruent. In these cases, it is important to determine if these psychotic symptoms preceded the major mood episode because this could indicate a different diagnosis (15). It is estimated that one in four patients repeatedly admitted for depression in the United States has psychotic features (27). This is a widely cited number since 1984, and new estimates have not been reported (28). However, there are more recent meta-analyses with data from studies around the world that roughly confirm this figure. Patients with psychotic depression have twice the suicide risk of patients with nonpsychotic depression (29).

IMMEDIATE INTERVENTIONS

Patients who present with depression, with suicidal ideation, or who recently made a gesture or attempt must be immediately triaged and assessed. Two issues must be addressed immediately. First,

the responsible clinician must assess for suicide risk to determine if the person may be left alone while undergoing the evaluation. Second is assessing for underlying medical condition or physiologic effect of a substance that may mimic symptoms of depression. This is critical since some conditions may be life-threatening.

Clerical and other ancillary staff in triage should be given clear protocols on how to alert responsible nursing or physician staff for the need to assess risk. Dangerous items in the environment or in the patient's possession should be removed and secured. Staff may give patients validated depression screening instruments, but these are not substitutes to a clinical assessment by psychiatrists or other mental health professionals who have training in conducting suicide risk assessments.

As soon as possible upon arrival, vital signs should be evaluated to determine if there may be any life-threatening underlying conditions. Most concerning is delirium from a yet unrecognized medical condition. While delirium is associated with psychomotor agitation and confusion, it can also present with decreased motivation, psychomotor retardation, and depressed mood. Without investigation, confusion and altering levels of consciousness may not be readily apparent. This is particular the case in patients who have experienced a rapid or sudden change in their mood or who do not have any prior psychiatric history. In individuals with chronic medical problems, careful assessment is needed to determine if psychiatric symptoms are due to an exacerbation of underlying medical problems. See Chapter 24 for a more complete discussion of delirium.

Evaluation of depressed patients in emergency settings requires the evaluator to quickly establish trust and rapport with the patient. Emergency settings are often chaotic and frightening. Evaluators may be accustomed to the setting, but patients are often not. Care must be taken to help assure the patient of safety and confidentiality, and the interview should occur in a setting where there will not be constant interruptions. Often patients present with hopelessness about the future and treatment. Evaluators should speak to the patient's affect to help the patient feel seen but also try to convey hope that depression is treatable and the staff are committed to helping the patient. The quality and nature of the interaction in the emergency setting can help set the stage for a successful inpatient psychiatric admission and increase the odds that the patient engages in outpatient treatment.

Clinical staff must follow state laws and hospital policy to ensure the least restrictive means of ensuring the patient's safety while the assessment is pending. This may range from direct one-to-one staff observation to housing the patient in a locked portion of the facility with security at the door to employing emergent medications or even restraints. Staff should always employ the least restrictive method as methods that are excessively heavy-handed can irreparably undermine the possibility of a therapeutic alliance and an effective assessment and intervention. Addressing the patient's concerns, involving family when possible, reassuring the patient's fears, and calmly reminding the patient the staff's concern for her safety and desire to help are the most effective means of ensuring cooperation through the assessment.

EVALUATION

After the initial phase of determining acute risk and ensuring medical stabilization, the next stage in the evaluation of depression is a detailed interview with the patient to collect information regarding history of current episode (including onset, duration, intensity, progression, modifying factors, functional impairment, current treatment and response, changes to treatment, and risky behaviors); history of prior episodes; prior treatments; psychiatric comorbidities; medical history; and prior suicide attempts. The interview should be natural and conversational, and the patient should be able to describe symptoms in her own words with the interviewer asking for clarifications and follow-up questions as needed. The interview should also include questions about family history, history of violence, usual day-to-day activities, social history (demographic data, marital and parenting status, employment, education, living situation, financial resources, and social supports), substance use, and involvement in legal system. Symptoms that are not consistent with MDD should increase suspicion for an alternative diagnosis or a comorbid diagnosis.

A mental status examination (MSE) is a critical and fundamental part of the assessment. It provides a picture of the patient at the time of the assessment and helps track the progression of the illness throughout treatment. The MSE typically starts by gathering information about the patient's appearance. This includes observations about grooming, hygiene, dress, posture during assessment, and eye contact. Individuals with depression can present with poor grooming or hygiene due to decreased energy or motivation. They may avert their eyes. The MSE also includes an assessment of behavior such as ability to cooperate in the interview and attitude toward assessment. Poor frustration tolerance and irritability readily become apparent. Critical diagnostic information can be gathered this way even before the start of the interview. The MSE also includes an assessment of the volume, pace, and quality of the patient's speech. Depressed patients often speak slowly in a low voice and in a monotone rhythm. Depressed individuals can have marked psychomotor retardation or agitation. This is readily apparent in the MSE. A key feature of the MSE is asking for the patient's description of her mood. At times it may be necessary to probe, given patients often describe their mood with descriptors that do not apply to mood, such as "tired" or "overworked." It is common for depressed patients to feel sad, anxious, and irritable. Some patients are unable to report a mood. Where mood is a symptom we elicit from the patient, affect is a sign we observe. Affect describes the reactivity of the patient's facial muscles and expressions to her internal experience of mood or the topic of conversation. We note whether the affect is congruent with the topic of conversation and with the patient's reported mood. We also note the range of the affect. Does it react appropriately or is it constricted in range? Depressed patients often have decreased reactivity of affect and sometimes have no facial expression at all. We describe the absence of affect as a "flat" affect. It is also important to comment on the quality of the affect, that is, what is the mood that the patient appears to be experiencing. Depressed patients often have a dysthymic affect. This is difficult to do when the affect is flat. It is important to assess the patient's thought process. Often depressed patients have thought blocking or a general paucity of thought. It is interesting to know if their thoughts are overall linear or if they have loosening of associations or disorganized thinking. Disorganized thought would raise suspicion for alternate diagnoses. The MSE also assesses the content of the thought. Is the patient experiencing hallucinations or delusions? This would suggest a more severe depression or an alternate diagnosis. Does the patient have anxious ruminations? Does she have intrusive traumatic memories? Critically, does the patient have suicidal or homicidal ideation? A fundamental portion of the MSE is to assess orientation. If the patient is not oriented to herself, to the place, time, or situation, this would suggest she may be experiencing delirium. Short-term memory impairment suggests difficulty with concentration and memory formation. A rough assessment of the patient's overall intellectual ability is helpful in determining what level of care the patient requires, given the symptoms that may be present. A developmentally delayed patient will need much more support than a patient of average cognitive resources. Insight reflects the patient's understanding of her illness and the impact of her illness on other aspects of her life. Judgment refers to the ability of the patient to take actions that are consistent with her overall plan and best interest and whether the patient can assess the consequences of her actions. The MSE is also helpful in determining if the patient is a trustworthy historian.

If the family is present or available over the telephone, obtaining a detailed recent history of the patient's symptoms, a psychiatric and medical history, recent lifestyle changes, a list of the patient's medications, and any concerns the family may have is exceedingly helpful in determining the patient's diagnosis, risk, and disposition. Indirect information from other sources such as outpatient providers, friends, roommates, coworkers, police officers, emergency medical services (EMS) technicians, and so on can also be very helpful. Confidentiality laws must be observed in obtaining indirect information, but sometimes breach of confidentiality may be necessary in situations where the patient's safety is at risk.

Since suicidal ideation is a common presenting feature of major depression and suicide attempts or gestures are frequent reasons patients are brought to emergency settings, a suicide risk assessment should be completed on every patient who presents with depression. There are both fixed and modifiable risk factors for self-harm that contribute to both overall acute and chronic risk. Completing a suicide risk assessment is a fundamental component of assessing depression in emergency settings. There are certain nonmodifiable factors that increase both acute and chronic risk of self-harm. These include male gender, age over 65 years, history of childhood maltreatment, family history of suicide, history of prior suicide attempts, and unrelenting pain or other medical illnesses (14, 30). There are also racial and ethnic differences in risk, but these vary geographically (14). Modifiable factors can change with treatment. These include severity of depressive illness, untreated or undertreated comorbid psychiatric disorders, access to means, current intention or plan to kill self, history of impulsive behavior, substance use, life stressors, subjective experience of hopelessness, presence of a personality disorder, recent discharge from a psychiatric hospital, and medical illnesses (14, 30). Additionally, protective factors such as engagement with treatment, work and family, and plans for the future need to be considered. These different risk and protective factors, along with the clinical experience and judgment of psychiatrist, guide the determination of the patient's imminent and chronic risk of self-harm. A determination of level of care is based on this risk assessment. There are validated tools that can help guide the determination of acute risk of self-harm. The most widely used tool is the Columbia-Suicide Severity Rating Scale (C-SSRS) (31). Many emergency settings incorporate the C-SSRS into their electronic medical records and have staff who do not specialize in mental health ask the questions as part of systematic screening of all patients. Screening tools such as the C-SSRS are very helpful, but they cannot replace seasoned clinical judgment by well-trained professionals and a careful consideration of each patient's particular history, subjective experience, and situation. Chapter 31 covers suicide risk assessment in detail.

Disruption in mood can be attributed to many different psychiatric or medical illnesses as well as medications and substances of abuse. It is important to develop a broad differential diagnosis early in the presentation to ensure accuracy in the diagnosis and subsequent treatment (see Tables 21.2-21.5 for detailed differential diagnosis information).

TABLE 21.2 Psychiatric Differential Diagnosis for Depressed Mood (15)

Major Depressive Disorder
Persistent depressive disorder
Cyclothymic disorder
Bipolar disorder (type I or II), most recent or current episode depressed
Adjustment disorder with depressed mood
Posttraumatic stress disorder
Generalized anxiety disorder
Obsessive compulsive disorder
Panic Disorder
Minor or major neurocognitive disorders
Delirium
Anorexia nervosa
Bulimia nervosa
Other eating disorders
Schizophrenia
Schizoaffective disorder
Alcohol use disorder (or intoxication, withdrawal)
Cannabis use disorder (or intoxication, withdrawal)
Opioid use disorder (or intoxication, withdrawal)
Cocaine use disorder (or intoxication, withdrawal)
Stimulant use disorder (eg., methamphetamine, or intoxication, withdrawal)
Synthetic cannabinoid use disorder (or intoxication, withdrawal)
Other drug use disorders
Borderline personality disorder
Dependent personality disorder
Narcissistic personality disorder
Other personality disorders

As mentioned previously, medical illnesses can mimic depression or have worse outcomes due to depression. Patients who present with depression or suicidal ideation should have a cursory physical and neurological examination and, if clinically indicated, undergo a battery of laboratory examinations including complete blood count with differential, comprehensive metabolic panel, thyroid function test, urinalysis, and urine toxicology screen. When appropriate, patients should also have a urine pregnancy test, therapeutic drug serum levels, lipid levels, hemoglobin-A1c, human immunodeficiency virus (HIV), hepatitis, or other sexually transmitted disease (STD) testing.

TABLE 21.3 Lifestyle and Social Differential Diagnosis

Relational problems and breakups
Bereavement
Occupational or academic problems
Economic problems
Other phase of life or acculturation problems
Involvement with legal system
Lack of housing or access to adequate food
Problems related to abuse or neglect, victimization, or discrimination

TABLE 21.4 Medical Differential Diagnosis (32–34)

Neoplasm—primary cerebral, primary abdominal, metastasis, paraneoplastic syndromes
Trauma—head trauma, pain
Infectious—human immunodeficiency virus (HIV), infectious mononucleosis, viral hepatitis, influenza, viral pneumonia, toxoplasmosis, tertiary syphilis, Lyme disease, specific infections, sepsis
Cardiac—myocardial infarct, coronary artery disease, congestive heart failure
Neurological—multiple sclerosis, Parkinson disease, epilepsy, sleep apnea, cerebrovascular infarction, Huntington disease
Endocrine-metabolic—hypothyroidism or hyperthyroidism, hyperparathyroidism, hypopituitarism, Addison disease, Cushing syndrome, diabetes
Nutritional—vitamin B12 deficiency, folic acid deficiency
Inflammatory—rheumatoid arthritis, systemic lupus erythematosus
Respiratory—asthma, chronic obstructive pulmonary disease, cystic fibrosis

DIAGNOSIS

Diagnosis of major depression is made in accordance with the DSM-5 criteria (15). Symptoms have to be present for most of the day in a contiguous 2-week period and lead to a decrease in functioning. The DSM-5 differentiates between an MDE and MDD. An MDE can occur in MDD, but also in bipolar disorder. MDD can be diagnosed when the patient has had at least one MDE. However, an MDE or MDD cannot be diagnosed if the symptoms are due to the physiological effects of a substance or a nonpsychiatric condition or if they can be better accounted for by another condition, such as bereavement or situational problem. If the patient has had at any point in his life a manic or hypomanic episode, then the diagnosis of MDD is excluded. It is not possible for bipolar and MDD to be comorbid. If the patient has ever had a manic or hypomanic episode, the diagnosis is always bipolar disorder even

if he currently presents with an MDE. Suicidality is a common presentation to emergency settings, but not all suicidal patients can be diagnosed with depression. Individuals who have not met the 2-week time course specified in the DSM-5 also cannot be diagnosed with MDD.

DISPOSITION AND TREATMENT

Given the general scarcity of inpatient beds and patchwork and inconsistent nature of outpatient programs available to patients because of insurance status, emergency settings have become a critical stopgap for many patients with depression who are unable to access alternate services.

Inpatient psychiatric hospitalization should be considered for patients deemed to be at high risk of self-harm or for patients who are so impaired that they are unable to adequately care for themselves without significant structured staff support. Inpatient hospitals are best situated to alter acute

TABLE 21.5 Pharmacological Differential Diagnosis (32, 35)

Neurological/psychiatric—amantadine, anticholinesterases, antipsychotics, baclofen, barbiturates, benzodiazepines, bromocriptine, carbamazepine, disulfiram, levodopa, phenytoin, ethosuximide
Antibacterial/antifungal—ampicillin, griseofulvin, metronidazole, trimethoprim
Anti-inflammatory/analgesics—corticosteroids, indomethacin, opioids
Antineoplastics—vincristine, vinblastine, asparaginase, azathioprine, bleomycin, hexamethylamine
Cardiovascular—clonidine, alpha-methyldopa, digitalis, propranolol, reserpine
Gastrointestinal—cimetidine, ranitidine
Other—naltrexone, oral contraceptives

risk factors for self-harm. Patients who develop psychotic symptoms often do require an inpatient admission because their disconnection from reality places them at higher risk for self-harm and inability to care for themselves, even if this is not verbalized. An inpatient admission should also be considered for patients who present with irrational medication regimens or who have had numerous unsuccessful adequate medication trials so the hospital can refer them to electroconvulsive therapy. If patients present with chronic symptoms or if all their risk factors for self-harm are chronic in nature, an inpatient admission can generally do little to alter the course of their illness.

When available, partial hospital programs, day treatment programs, intensive outpatient programs, and psychosocial clubhouses are often an excellent alternative to an inpatient admission because they provide the intensive therapeutic support in a less restrictive environment. In addition, referral to outpatient mental health services is very important to ensure the patient stabilizes and receives treatment for chronic risk factors. It is important to involve family members and friends in the disposition decision as they often have to take responsibility to ensure the patient adheres to treatment. If the family is unable to help the patient navigate starting outpatient treatment, then the patient may need to go to a psychiatric hospital. Families are also critical in ensuring any guns, ammunition, knives, and other dangerous objects are removed from the home and secured. Having a gun at home significantly increases the risk of completing suicide (36).

In communities with scarce availability of outpatient mental health or where the only available referral is to a primary medical doctor, then the bar for an inpatient admission should generally be lowered. It is important that the disposition matches the patient's risk for self-harm and severity of symptoms, but in communities where there are few options, then more patients likely have to be referred to an inpatient hospital. Leadership of emergency settings should create and maintain relationships with local mental health authorities to ensure that adequate discharge options are available to their patients. It is common for emergency settings to only give a referral telephone number to a patient without knowing if that number truly provides access (37).

Patients who are actively suicidal or whose depression is so impairing that they are unable to make reasonable decisions may have to be hospitalized involuntarily if local clinical staff worry their depression results in their not having capacity to voluntarily enter a hospital. Laws surrounding involuntary holds are different in each US state and Canadian province. Physicians in ED settings need to become familiar with local laws and hospital policy.

Given that depression may present with irritable mood or anxious distress and that it is often comorbid with anxiety disorders, evaluators may need to pharmacologically treat significant anxiety, irritability, or agitation prior to or in the course of the evaluation to help the patient successfully complete the evaluation. These are generally treated with low-dose benzodiazepines such as 1 to 2 mg of lorazepam or a low-dose slightly sedating antihistamine such as 25 to 50 mg hydroxyzine. Additionally, given the high comorbidity between substance use disorders and depression, acute withdrawal must be addressed urgently. For severe agitation in depression, mixed states, or intoxication, physicians may need to use a combination of lorazepam with a typical or atypical antipsychotic. In patients who present with depression with catatonic features, a lorazepam challenge is the best way to help "free" the patient from catatonia. There has been excitement over administering ketamine in emergency settings for rapid resolution of suicidal ideations. There have been several randomized controlled trials where patients are treated with 0.5 mg/kg over 45 minutes. There have been both positive and negative studies. At this point there is not sufficient evidence to suggest the routine use of ketamine in emergency settings (38). However, with the recent FDA approval of an intranasal formulation of esketamine, this treatment may become more common in inpatient and outpatient psychiatric settings, but as of this writing, no clear best practices have emerged in the use of this new medication.

The first-line treatment for depression is combined psychotherapy and a selective serotonin reuptake inhibitor (SSRI) or serotonin-norepinephrine reuptake inhibitors (SNRIs) (39). In patients who are treatment-naive, education in emergency settings is very important to help ensure adherence. A patient should be educated that antidepressants do not work immediately and can, in fact, take several weeks to start working. Patients should be told the possible side effects of the medication and risk for taking inconsistently. Given the difficulty of accessing outpatient care, it is helpful to start pharmacological treatment from the ED with instructions for the patient to return in case of worsening symptoms or possible medication adverse reactions. In settings where there is ready access to outpatient psychiatry, emergency staff can defer the decision of which medication to start to the outpatient clinical staff. Care should be given to prescribe medications that are affordable to the patient. For patients who are already on complex regimens, who have an accessible outpatient psychiatrist, or who have tried several medications, it may be best to defer to the outpatient mental health team. SSRIs and SNRIs should be used with extreme care (and probably not started in the ED) in any patient with a history of manic or hypomanic episode, even if currently in a depressive episode, as these medications could trigger a manic episode. There is no evidence to use a benzodiazepine as a first-line treatment for depression.

CONCLUSION

Depression is common, and it can be fatal. In emergency settings, completing a detailed suicide risk assessment and ruling out medical or drug-related causes of depression are the first steps when assessing depressed patients. Given depression is both underdiagnosed and undertreated, ED clinicians should consider it in patients with vague somatic complaints or who have chronic medical illnesses. Providing patient education about depression, referring patients to the most appropriate level of care, and starting an antidepressant in settings with difficult access to outpatient mental health are the most important interventions for patients who do not require an inpatient psychiatric admission.

REFERENCES

1. WHO. (2018). *Depression: Fact sheets*. Retrieved December 22, 2018, from https://www.who.int/news-room/fact-sheets/detail/depression.

2. CDC. (2018). Suicide rising across the U.S. *Vital Signs*. Retrieved from https://www.cdc.gov/vitalsigns/suicide/index.html.

3. Kessler, R. C. (2012). The costs of depression. *Psychiatric Clinics of North America, 35*(1), 1–14.

4. Katon, W., & Ciechanowski, P. (2002). Impact of major depression on chronic medical illness. *Journal of Psychosomatic Research, 53*(4), 859–863.

5. Hasin, D. S., et al. (2018). Epidemiology of adult DSM-5 major depressive disorder and its specifiers in the United States. *JAMA Psychiatry, 75*(4), 336–346.

6. Larkin, G. L., et al. (2005). Trends in U.S. emergency department visits for mental health conditions, 1992–2001. *Psychiatric Services, 56*(6), 671–677.

7. Hoyer, D., & David, E. (2012). Screening for depression in emergency department patients. *The Journal of Emergency Medicine, 43*(5), 786–799.

8. Booth, B. M., et al. (2011). Substance use, depression, and mental health functioning in patients seeking acute medical care in an inner-city ED. *The Journal of Behavioral Health Services & Research, 38*(3), 358–372.

9. Boudreaux, E. D., Clark, S., & Camargo, C. A., Jr. (2008). Mood disorder screening among adult emergency department patients: A multicenter study of prevalence, associations and interest in treatment. *General Hospital Psychiatry, 30*(1), 4–13.

10. Cepoiu, M., et al. (2008). Recognition of depression by non-psychiatric physicians—A systematic literature review and meta-analysis. *Journal of General Internal Medicine, 23*(1), 25–36.

11. Zhu, J. M., Singhal, A., & Hsia, R. Y. (2016). Emergency department length-of-stay for psychiatric visits was significantly longer than for nonpsychiatric visits, 2002–11. *Health Affairs, 35*(9), 1698–1706.

12. Mahajan, P., et al. (2009). Epidemiology of psychiatric-related visits to emergency departments in a multicenter collaborative research pediatric network. *Pediatric Emergency Care, 25*(11), 715–720.

13. Ting, S. A., Sullivan, A. F., et al. (2012). Trends in US emergency department visits for attempted suicide and self-inflicted injury, 1993–2008. *General Hospital Psychiatry, 34*(1), 557–565.

14. Hawton, K., & van Heeringen, K. (2009). Suicide. *Lancet, 373*(9672), 1372–1391.

15. American Psychiatric Association. (2013). *Diagnostic and statistical manual of mental disorders: DSM-5™* (5th ed.). Arlington, VA: American Psychiatric Association.

16. Guze, S. B., & Robins, E. (1970). Suicide and primary affective disorders. *British Journal of Psychiatry, 117*(539), 437–438.

17. Oquendo, M. A., Malone, K. M., & Mann, J. J. (1997). Suicide: Risk factors and prevention in refractory major depression. *Depression & Anxiety, 5*(4), 202–211.

18. Lai, H. M., et al. (2015). Prevalence of comorbid substance use, anxiety and mood disorders in epidemiological surveys, 1990-2014: A systematic review and meta-analysis. *Drug and Alcohol Dependence, 154*, 1–13.

19. Cavanagh, J. T. O., Carson, A. J., et al. (2003). Psychological autopsy studies of suicide: A systematic review. *Psychological Medicine, 33*(3), 395–405.

20. Monk, M. (1987). Epidemiology of suicide. *Epidemiologic Reviews, 9*(1), 51–69.

21. Harris, E. C., & Barraclough, B. (1997). Suicide as an outcome for mental disorders. *The British Journal of Psychiatry, 170*(3), 205–228.

22. Kowalenko, T., & Khare, R. K. (2004). Should we screen for depression in the emergency department? *Academic Emergency Medicine, 11*(2), 177–178.

23. Rockett, I. R. H., Caine, E. D., et al. (2019). Mortality in the United States from self-injury surpasses diabetes: A prevention imperative. *BMJ Injury Prevention, 25*, 331–333.

24. Kumar, A., et al. (2004). A multicenter study of depression among emergency department patients. *Academic Emergency Medicine, 11*(12), 1284–1289.

25. Kessler, R. C., et al. (2003). The epidemiology of major depressive disorder: Results from the National Comorbidity Survey Replication (NCS-R). *JAMA, 289*(23), 3095–3105.

26. Spinhoven, P., et al. (2014). Comorbidity of PTSD in anxiety and depressive disorders: Prevalence and shared risk factors. *Child Abuse & Neglect, 38*(8), 1320–1330.

27. Schatzberg, A. F. (2003). New approaches to managing psychotic depression. *The Journal of Clinical Psychiatry, 64*(Suppl. 1), 19–23.

28. Coryell, W., Pfohl, B., & Zimmerman, M. (1984). The clinical and neuroendocrine features of psychotic depression. *The Journal of Nervous and Mental Disease, 172*(9), 521–528.

29. Gournellis, R., et al. (2018). Psychotic (delusional) depression and suicidal attempts: A systematic review and meta-analysis. *Acta Psychiatrica Scandinavica, 137*(1), 18–29.

30. Hawton, K., Casanas, C., et al. (2013). Risk factors for suicide in individuals with depression: A systematic review. *Journal of Affective Disorders, 147*(1), 17–28.

31. The Columbia Protocol for Your Setting. The Columbia Lighthouse Project: Identify Risk, Prevent Suicide. Retrieved December 23, 2018, from http://cssrs.columbia.edu/the-columbia-scale-c-ssrs/cssrs-for-communities-and-healthcare/#filter=.healthcare.english.

32. Akiskal, H. S. (2017). Mood disorders: Clinical features. In Sadock, B. J., Sadock, V. A., & Ruiz, P. (Eds.), *Kaplan & Sadock's comprehensive textbook of psychiatry*. Philadelphia, PA: Wolters Kluwer.

33. Shapiro, P. A., & Critchfield, A. R. (2017). Cardiovascular disorders. In Sadock, B. J., Sadock, V. A., & Ruiz, P. (Eds.), *Kaplan & Sadock's comprehensive textbook of psychiatry*. Philadelphia, PA: Wolters Kluwer.

34. Ritz, T., Werchan, C. A., & Brown, E. S. (2017). Respiratory disorders. In Sadock, B. J., Sadock, V. A., & Ruiz, P. (Eds.), *Kaplan & Sadock's comprehensive textbook of psychiatry*. Philadelphia, PA: Wolters Kluwer.

35. Milner, K. K., Florence, T., & Glick, R. L. (1999). Mood and anxiety syndromes in emergency psychiatry. *Psychiatric Clinics of North America, 22*(4), 755–777.

36. Anglemyer, A., Horvath, T., & Rutherford, G. (2014). The accessibility of firearms and risk for suicide and homicide victimization among household members: A systematic review and meta-analysis. *Annals of Internal Medicine, 160*(2), 101–110.

37. Rhodes, K. V., et al. (2009). Referral without access: For psychiatric services, wait for the beep. *Annals of Emergency Medicine, 54*(2), 272–278.

38. Ionescu, D. F., Bentley, K. H., et al. (2019). Repeat-dose ketamine augmentation for treatment-resistant depression with chronic suicidal ideation: A randomized, double blind, placebo controlled trial. *Journal of Affective Disorders, 243*(1), 516–524.

39. Yatham, L. N., & Kennedy, S. H. (2017). Mood disorders: Pharmacological treatment of depression and bipolar disorders. In Sadock, B. J., Sadock, V. A., & Ruiz, P. (Eds.), *Kaplan & Sadock's comprehensive textbook of psychiatry*. Philadelphia, PA: Wolters Kluwer.

22

Mania and Mixed States

Alan C. Swann

Mania is a behavioral syndrome that can be life-threatening or life-ruining. Many medical conditions can cause or contribute to mania (1,2). Bipolar disorder is defined as the cause of primary mania. Successful management of mania requires identification of causal and contributory factors and of complications (medical, social, and legal), and definitive steps toward stabilization of behavior. Some aspects of treatment are specific to the cause of the manic episode; others are more generally related to severe agitation associated with the manic syndrome.

PRESENTING CLINICAL FEATURES

Classic mania would appear easy to recognize. Mania can also occur in the context of other psychiatric disturbances, including mixed states in which syndromal depression is present (3). Further, mania can present diagnostic challenges because it can have many medical causes in addition to bipolar disorder and because it can lead to medical complications (1,2). Elements of manic and depressive states can combine in the same episodes, and the severity of either can fluctuate (4,5). Finally, even when the presence of acute mania is recognized, it can be clinically challenging to treat the patient effectively while dealing with the many problems that mania can generate.

The Manic Syndrome
Components of the Manic State

More than a disturbance of affect, mania is a pervasive syndrome encompassing potentially drastic changes in content and form of thought, physical activity, and behavior. Table 22.1 summarizes the components of mania.

Diagnostic Criteria for a Manic Episode and Their Relevance

Table 22.2 shows the Diagnostic and Statistical Manual of Mental Disorders, 5th Edition (*DSM-5*)

diagnostic criteria for a manic episode (6). The symptomatic criteria mean, essentially, that the patient is experiencing a pervasive disturbance of affect, thought, physical function, and behavior. The duration and severity requirements improve the reliability of diagnosis. Criteria for hypomania are more problematic. A duration requirement of 2 days may have more validity than the generally accepted 4 days (7).

Common Presentations of Mania
Classic Mania

Classic mania is generally defined as a manic episode without prominent depressive or psychotic features. These episodes also are considered not to be associated with rapid changes to other mood states. The patient may exhibit increased goal-directed hyperactivity, euphoric affect, grandiosity, rapid speech that is hard to interrupt, and racing thoughts. Even the most infectiously euphoric patient, however, is likely to become irritable in the face of delay or interference.

Psychotic Manic States

About half of manic episodes are associated with delusions or hallucinations or both (8,9). These episodes generally entail more severe functional impairment than do episodes without psychotic features (10). Delusions and hallucinations are usually mood congruent but can also be mood incongruent. Mood-incongruent delusions are associated with more severe, longer-term psychosocial impairment (11).

Mixed States

Manic episodes can have prominent depressive features. In DSM-5, there is a mixed state specifier whereby either a manic or depressive episode is considered to have mixed features if at least three nonoverlapping symptoms from the

TABLE 22.1 Components of the Manic Syndrome

Mood/affect	Euphoria, irritability, impatience, time pressure In mixed states: depression, anxiety
Cognition	Form: racing thoughts, flight of ideas, distractibility Content: grandiose, paranoid; delusions/hallucinations in about 50%
Physical	Increased motor activity; decreased need for sleep
Behavior	Increased goal-directed behavior commensurate with affective and cognitive disturbances Interpersonal distortions: "manic game," excessively intrusive, competitive

Information from Swann, A. C., Janicak, P. L., Calabrese, J. R., et al. (2001). Structure of mania: Depressive, irritable, and psychotic clusters with different retrospectively-assessed course patterns of illness in randomized clinical trial participants. *Journal of Affective Disorders, 67*(1–3), 123–132 and Janowsky, D. S., Leff, M., & Epstein, R. S. (1970). Playing the manic game: Interpersonal maneuvers of the acutely manic patient. *Archives of General Psychiatry, 22*, 252–261.

TABLE 22.2 Diagnostic Criteria for a Manic Episode

Component	Criteria
Primary affective symptom	Distinct period of abnormally and persistently elevated, expansive, or irritable mood, and abnormally and persistently goal-directed behavior or energy, lasting at least 1 week and present most of the day, nearly every day.
Syndromal criteria	At least three of seven specified manic symptoms (inflated self-esteem/grandiosity, decreased need for sleep, more talkative than usual or pressured speech, flight of ideas/racing thoughts, distractibility, increased goal-directed activity/psychomotor agitation, excessive involvement in activities with high potential for painful consequences) or at least four if predominant mood is irritable.
Distress or impairment	Severe enough to cause marked impairment in social or occupational functioning, hospitalization, or psychosis
Caused by bipolar disorder	Not due to physiologic effects of a substance or another medical illness. A manic episode that emerges during antidepressant treatment but persists at fully syndromal level beyond the physiological effect of that treatment is sufficient evidence for a manic episode.
Mixed states	The former criteria for a mixed state have been replaced by the mixed state specifier, whereby either a depressive or manic episode is considered to have mixed features if certain symptoms from the other mood state are also present.

Information from American Psychiatric Association. (1995). *Diagnostic and statistical manual of mental disorders* (5th ed., pp. 328–335). Washington, DC: American Psychiatric Association.

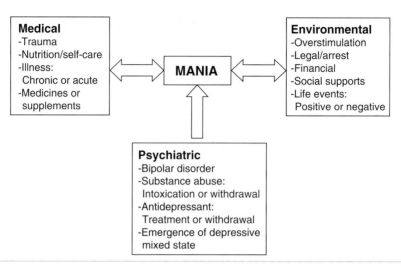

FIGURE 22.1 • Interactions in Manic Episodes. Note the bidirectional relationship between mania and medical and environmental factors. These can contribute to or precipitate a manic episode, can be consequences of manic episodes, or both.

other mood state are present for at least 7 days (6). There appears to be a continuum of mixed states across depression and mania (4,5,12-14). Severity of depression or mania can fluctuate during the episode (13). Mixed episodes are challenging for the following reasons:

1. Patients susceptible to mixed episodes usually have a severe course of illness with greater likelihood of substance use disorders, anxiety disorders, trauma, neurologic insults, and medical disorders compared with patients without mixed episodes (4,5,14).
2. The combination of mania, with its activation and impulsivity, and depression, with its hopelessness, is dangerous, with potential for suicide and violent behavior (15,16).
3. Mood lability (13) and severe agitation (17) in mixed states can make these patients unpredictable and difficult to manage clinically and underscore the misery that these patients may experience.
4. Mixed episodes are harder to treat, on average, than nonmixed episodes (18-20).

Contexts of Manic Episodes: Medical, Social, and Legal

Patients in manic episodes are often in trouble. Mania engenders interpersonal conflict, poorly considered financial and legal decisions, and indiscretions (21,22). Further, patients in manic

episodes tend to neglect their health. Figure 22.1 summarizes the manner in which mania can produce clinical and social consequences that complicate its emergency treatment.

Bipolar Disorder and Secondary Mania

Mania is a nonspecific syndrome with many medical and pharmacologic causes (1,2). Table 22.3 briefly summarizes some conditions that can contribute to manic episodes. Patients with bipolar disorder are more susceptible to mania of any cause, primary or secondary, than are individuals who do not have bipolar disorder (2). This especially holds for patients susceptible to mixed states (16). Mania is a prominent potential cause of catatonia, especially if other medical or psychiatric disorders are also present (23,24). Therefore, the clinician must be alert for both contributors to and effects of manic episodes in bipolar disorder. Mental status examination alone is not likely to distinguish episodes with organic features (25). Figure 22.1 summarizes this schematically.

Behavioral and Interpersonal Problems in Mania: The "Manic Game"

Individuals who are experiencing manic episodes present interpersonal challenges to the emergency clinician. Cognitive disorganization, the

TABLE 22.3 Some Factors That Can Cause or Contribute to Manic Syndromes

| **Psychiatric** |
| Bipolar disorder |
| Schizophrenia |
| Schizoaffective disorder |
| **Substance-related** |
| Stimulant intoxication |
| Alcohol and/or sedative withdrawal |
| Nicotine withdrawal |
| **Nonpsychiatric medical** |
| Collagen vascular and other inflammatory diseases |
| Infections, including HIV |
| Head trauma |
| Endocrine disorders, especially thyrotoxicosis |
| Cancers, including small-cell carcinoma |
| **Pharmacologic** |
| Drugs influencing monoaminergic function: antidepressants, stimulants, antiparkinsonian agents |
| Withdrawal of antidepressant treatment |
| Corticosteroids |
| Supplements, including testosterone, DHEA, ginseng |
| Some antibiotics, including antiretroviral agents |
| **Environmental** |
| Sleep deprivation |
| Stressors or situational changes, possibly especially those disrupting social and/or sleep–activity rhythms |
| Overstimulation |

DHEA, dehydroepiandrosterone; HIV, human immunodeficiency virus.
Information from Dunner, D. L. (1992). Differential diagnosis of bipolar disorder. *Journal of Clinical Psychopharmacology*, *12*(1 Suppl. I), 7S–12S; Krauthammer, C., & Klerman, G. L. (1978). Secondary mania: Manic syndromes associated with antecedent physical illnesses or drugs. *Archives of General Psychiatry*, *35*, 1333–1339; and McIntyre, J. S. (1979). Mania: The common symptom of several illnesses. *Postgraduate Medicine*, *66*(1), 145–149.

characteristic cognitive distortions of mania, and disinhibited goal-directed hyperactivity make it difficult to interview manic patients (26). The patient is likely to construct a wall of words that reduces, rather than facilitates, communication. In addition, patients who are manic exhibit a constellation of interpersonal maneuvers that can lead to escalation of their symptoms and can be severely disruptive (27). These interpersonal maneuvers, called "the manic game" by Janowsky

et al. (27), include manipulation of self-esteem by flattery and devaluation, splitting, testing limits, eliciting anger, and projecting responsibility, and stem largely from the fear of losing control that is pervasive in manic episodes. This difficult aspect of behavior is pervasive in home, social, and work situations and contributes to social and occupational problems and loss of support systems. It is imperative to behave in a consistent manner and not to yield to temptations to please or to compete with the patient. The patient should also be protected as effectively as possible against overstimulation. Interpersonal inconsistency is a particularly harmful variety of overstimulation in mania.

IMMEDIATE INTERVENTIONS FOR ACUTE PRESENTATIONS

Ensuring Safety of the Patient

Physical

Patients in manic episodes are in danger of accidents and trauma, including provocation (intentional or unintentional) of attacks by others. Patients who are in mixed states, or who have labile affect, are also at risk for suicide because their severe impulsivity and overactivity can combine with depressed mood or hopelessness (16,28). Mixed features can emerge in an episode that originated as "pure" mania or depression (29,30). In a sufficiently impulsive and hyperactive patient, it only takes relatively mild depression to confer risk for suicide, and such patients are more likely than others to make violent attempts, with severity that may be out of proportion to the apparent wish to die (28,31,32).

Social

Mania is associated with potential for severe social, legal, economic, and occupational disruption (21,22). One should never underestimate the likelihood that a patient has carried out, or soon will carry out, an act that has the potential to ruin his or her life. The clinician must also assume that, whatever he or she knows about the episode, there is generally more going on. For example, indiscretions carried out while manic can lead others to seek revenge on the patient. Hospitals and waiting rooms are not immune from such disturbances.

Medical

As shown in Figure 22.1, mania can be caused by medical disorders or their treatment. In addition, manic episodes can have medical complications that are emergencies in their own right, including trauma, intoxication with drugs of abuse (or prescribed drugs), and withdrawal from drugs, especially alcohol (33). Patients may also neglect to take care of concurrent medical problems and can neglect basic health, leading to dehydration, malnourishment, or exhaustion.

Ensuring Safety of the Staff

Individuals, even if otherwise peaceable and friendly, may have the potential to be severely assaultive when manic (34,35). It may not take much to set off a manic patient. Staff must behave toward the patient in a predictable, consistent, firm, and respectful manner, taking into account the interpersonal distortions that often accompany mania. This is helped by definitive and rapid pharmacologic treatment as soon as it is safe to do so. Finally, staff must be aware of enemies that the patient may have made during the episode.

Initial Management of Overstimulation and Severe Agitation

Table 22.4 summarizes measures for the management of overstimulation and agitation in mania. These include complementary pharmacologic and nonpharmacologic strategies.

Management of Interpersonal Conflict in Mania

The potential for interpersonal conflict can be diminished, and conflict can be reduced, by attention to the interrelated aspects of mania that lead to conflict: fear of loss of control, fear of inferiority (leading to excessive competitiveness), lack of boundaries, and time pressure or impatience (27). It is important to remove sources of overstimulation and to institute treatment as soon as possible. This must be done in a manner that does not provoke further conflict. The interview must be conducted in a manner that provides the structure and boundaries that the patient lacks but that respects the patient's sense of time (26). The clinician must behave in a manner that is friendly and respectful, yet firm, and must avoid getting into arguments or into the competitive and other traps that are inherent in the "manic game" (27). When possible, patients can be given choices as long as the clinician controls the alternatives (eg, whether the patient would prefer medicine as a liquid or an injection). Sometimes it is possible to find something about the patient's condition that he or she does not like; this can provide an avenue to initial treatment.

TABLE 22.4 Management of Overstimulation and Severe Agitation in Emergency Settings

Pharmacologic
Antipsychotic agents (conventional or atypical)
Antipsychotic agents combined with benzodiazepines
Nonpharmacologic
Consistent, predictable interpersonal behavior
Reduction in environmental noise and unpredictability

Information from Allen, M. H., Currier, G. W., Carpenter, D., et al. (2005). Treatment of behavioral emergencies 2005. *Journal of Psychiatric Practice*, *11*(Suppl. I), 5–108 and Allen, M. H., Currier, G. W., Hughes, D. H., et al. (2001). The expert consensus guideline series. Treatment of behavioral emergencies. *Postgraduate Medicine*, special Report, 1–88.

Addressing Potential Medical Emergencies

Mania can conceal medical emergencies. These can include traumatic injuries (36), intoxication with stimulants (37), and withdrawal from alcohol or sedatives or both (33). In addition, secondary mania can be associated with acute medical conditions, such as thyrotoxicosis (2). Although it may be difficult to examine a patient or carry out laboratory investigations, careful evaluation and vital signs can provide valuable information. It can be difficult to address, or even to detect, the medical problems until manic symptoms are at least partially treated. Therefore, it is valuable to (a) make maximal efforts to obtain information about the patient, including recent activities, drug ingestions, and medical history, from any reliable informants that can be located, (b) obtain toxicology screens and breathalyzer tests as soon as possible, and (c) use initial treatments that can reduce manic agitation without unnecessarily compromising other potential medical problems—for example, using anticonvulsant treatments with antimanic effects if potential alcohol withdrawal is suspected (38).

EVALUATION

Assessing the Presenting Situation

It is helpful to determine under what conditions, and by whom, the patient was brought to the emergency department. Although this can be difficult in a busy facility, the clinician or a colleague should always try to interview anyone who arrived with the patient, whether a police officer, friend, relative, or ambulance driver (26).

General Principles of Evaluation of Manic Patients

Because they are difficult to interview and examine, patients experiencing manic episodes are a challenge to evaluate. This challenge is exacerbated by the complex situations that manic episodes can generate. Therefore, one must obtain information from as many sources as possible. These sources include whoever brought the patient in, anyone who referred the patient, someone who lives with the patient, and the patient's physician or clinician. It may well not be possible to contact all these individuals, or some may not exist, but it is important to take pains to contact as many of them as possible. It may be necessary to delegate a colleague to do so. Further principles are to take nothing for granted and to assume that the patient's actual situation is more complicated than it appears (39).

Potential for Homicide, Suicide, or Other Serious Harm

As described earlier, manic episodes hold the potential for harm to others (34); harm to self, including suicide (16); provocation of harm by others (including "suicide by cop" (40)); and accidents (41). These potentials can be reduced by remaining vigilant, minimizing overstimulation, addressing the interpersonal problems inherent in mania (27), and instituting prompt pharmacologic treatment (39). Mood lability or fluctuating mixed features exacerbates these risks.

DIAGNOSIS AND DIFFERENTIAL DIAGNOSIS

Differential Diagnosis of the Acute Manic Syndrome

The manic syndrome has many potential medical causes (1,2). Bipolar disorder does not confer immunity to any of these causes, and, in fact, makes it easier for other medical conditions to elicit manic syndromes. Therefore, one should always be alert to the potential contribution of one of the conditions in Table 22.3, even when one knows that a patient has bipolar disorder.

Mania and Substance Abuse

Substance abuse is a common complication of bipolar disorder. Susceptibility to substance abuse can be increased by manic or mixed states in a state-dependent manner (42). Conversely, substance abuse or withdrawal can increase the likelihood or severity of a manic episode (2). Table 22.5 summarizes some prominent relationships between substance use disorders and mania.

Mania and Medical Problems

Table 22.3 summarizes medical problems commonly associated with manic episodes. Acute medical problems, such as thyrotoxicosis, can precipitate manic episodes that can potentially be treated by addressing the medical problem. Other medical problems, such as multiple sclerosis or collagen vascular diseases, can precipitate manic episodes that must be treated in their own right in parallel to treatment of the underlying illness.

Treatment of medical problems can also precipitate or exacerbate mania. For example, patients with collagen vascular or inflammatory disorders may experience a manic episode as a result of the illness or as a result of the corticosteroids used to treat the illness; risk for corticosteroid-induced mania is increased in individuals with personal or family histories of mood disorders (43-45).

Identifying Consequences of Mania That Require Intervention

Consequences of mania, including trauma, neglect of underlying medical problems, and substance-related problems, may need intervention, sometimes on an emergency basis. These

TABLE 22.5 Interactions Between Substance and Alcohol Abuse and Mania

Mania increases substance abuse	Increased reward-related behavior: stimulants, alcohol, nicotine Self-treatment: alcohol, nicotine
Substance abuse increases manic symptoms	Stimulant intoxication Alcohol/sedative withdrawal Nicotine withdrawal
Substance abuse alters course of illness	More unstable course of illness and treatment response Treatment response in manic episodes Increased susceptibility to antidepressant-induced destabilization

Information from Henry, C., Bellivier, F., Sorbara, F., et al. (2001). Bipolar sensation seeking is associated with a propensity to abuse rather than to temperamental characteristics. *European Psychiatry, 16*(5), 289–292; Reich, L. H., Davis, R. K., & Himmelhoch, J. M. (1974). Excessive alcohol use in manic-depressive illness. *American Journal of Psychiatry, 131*, 83–86; Gonzalez-Pinto, A., Gutierrez, M., Ezcurra, J., et al. (1998). Tobacco smoking and bipolar disorder. *The Journal of Clinical Psychiatry, 59*(5), 225–228; Krauthammer, C., & Klerman, G. L. (1978). Secondary mania: Manic syndromes associated with antecedent physical illnesses or drugs. *Archives of General Psychiatry, 35*, 1333–1339; Goldberg, J. F., Garno, J. L., Leon, A. C., et al. (1999). A history of substance abuse complicates remission from acute mania in bipolar disorder. *The Journal of Clinical Psychiatry, 60*(11), 733–740; and Manwani, S. G., Pardo, T. B., Albanese, M. J., et al. (2006). Substance use disorder and other predictors of antidepressant-induced mania: A retrospective chart review. *The Journal of Clinical Psychiatry, 67*(9), 1341–1345.

TABLE 22.6 Pharmacologic Treatments for Mania in Emergency Settings

Class	Routes of Administration	Remarks
Antipsychotic	Oral, liquid, intramuscular	Conventional or atypical agents appear effective; choice based on clinical feasibility balanced with tolerability
Anticonvulsant	Oral, intravenous, liquid	*Initial:* Divalproex, oral loading or intravenous *Restoration:* Recently discontinued treatments that were effective
Lithium	Oral	Restoration if recently discontinued
Benzodiazepine	Oral, intramuscular	Adjunct to antipsychotic
Antinoradrenergic	Oral	Alpha-2 agonist or beta-antagonist Adjunct to antipsychotic

Reprinted with permission from Allen, M. H., Currier, G. W., Carpenter, D., et al. (2005). Treatment of behavioral emergencies 2005. *Journal of Psychiatric Practice*, *11*(Suppl. 1), 5–108.

conditions have been summarized earlier in the chapter. Effective management of the behavioral manic syndrome can make these conditions easier to detect and manage.

MANAGEMENT OF ACUTE MANIA IN THE EMERGENCY SETTING

Criteria for Hospitalization

Generally, hospitalization should be considered if patients' symptoms constitute a danger to themselves or others, if patients are unable to care for themselves otherwise, if patients are likely to do something that will ruin their lives because of the episode before the episode can be treated, or if there is the strong possibility of a serious medical condition that, because of the patient's manic syndrome, cannot be safely evaluated or treated on an outpatient basis. Evaluations should focus on establishing whether hospitalization is necessary as efficiently as possible.

The decision to hospitalize is a function of the severity of symptoms, their trajectory, and the quality of the patient's support system. In this regard, it is important to be aware of the potential that the support system may already be strained to the breaking point and will be needed during the patient's recuperation.

Treatment Within the Emergency Setting

Pharmacologic Treatments

Pharmacologic treatments are summarized in Table 22.6. They have two roles: early symptom reduction that fosters the safety of the patient and others, and more definitive treatment of the manic episode. Emergency psychopharmacologic treatment of mania has been reviewed (39,46,47). Table 22.6 also gives information about modes of administration. Conventional capsules or tablets have the potential disadvantages of not working as quickly as other dosage forms and of being harder to administer reliably. Liquid forms can be easier to administer in emergency settings, although patients can spit them out or can surreptitiously put absorbent materials into their mouths. Liquid medicines can, in some cases, work as rapidly as parenteral medicines. Intramuscular injections can work quickly and be reliably administered but are more invasive than other forms. Intravenous administration can produce rapid results and precise dose titration (48), but it can be difficult to give an intravenous injection to someone who is manic.

Antipsychotic Treatments

Antipsychotic treatments are effective in rapidly reducing overstimulation and agitation;

TABLE 22.7 Nonpharmacologic Strategies for Manic Episodes in Emergency Settings

Obtain information	Whoever lives with the patient Family Whoever referred or brought the patient in Physicians or therapists who have treated the patient
Support	Provide information for family or significant others about advocacy groups, other sources of support, and characteristics and treatment of bipolar disorder
Treatment	Strategies to reduce overstimulation (see Table 22.4)
Groundwork for follow-up	Contact patient's current clinician and/or facility to which the patient is being referred Ensure that continued treatment and monitoring will be available Ensure that significant others understand and, if possible, can participate in follow-up

many have been approved to treat manic or mixed states (49-51). Antimanic effects appear to characterize antipsychotics in general, as a class (51). Akathisia, especially with higher-potency antipsychotics, can exacerbate manic or mixed states.

Mood-Stabilizing Treatments

Mood-stabilizing treatments, including lithium and anticonvulsant treatments such as valproate preparations or carbamazepine, are useful in treating manic episodes, as well as impulsive aggression (52,53). However, their onset of action, with the exception of orally loaded or intravenous valproate (48,54), is too slow for emergency purposes. An exception is when the clinician finds that an episode was likely to have been precipitated by interruption in taking a mood-stabilizing treatment (55). Lithium levels can also decline, due to increased renal clearance, during hypomania or mania, so if a patient is taking lithium, it can be worthwhile to check the lithium level and increase the dose if necessary (56).

Identifying Treatments That May Be Making the Patient Worse

Many treatments, such as antidepressants, stimulants, catecholaminergic drugs such as decongestants, corticosteroids, and even dietary supplements such as ginseng or dehydroepiandrosterone (DHEA), can precipitate or exacerbate mania (see Tables 22.3 and 22.5) (57-59).

Interaction Between Emergency and Ongoing Treatment

Many treatments that acutely improve behavioral problems associated with manic syndromes may be useful components in the eventual resolution of the episode and in longer-term treatment (39). Other treatments, such as lithium, are useful in longer-term treatment but have little use in emergency settings unless a patient is known to have discontinued lithium recently (55). Whenever possible, any treatment that is likely to be continued after emergency treatment should be discussed with the physician who will be caring for the patient at that time. When this is not feasible or possible, the best acute treatment for the circumstances must be instituted.

Nonpharmacologic Principles

Nonpharmacologic strategies are summarized in Table 22.7. These include adherence to the principles of reducing overstimulation and managing the characteristic interpersonal problems of mania (26,27). In addition, whenever possible, it is necessary to use the emergency intervention as a means of educating significant others about the patient's illness and improving the continuity of the patient's treatment.

Preventing Escalation

The principles of preventing escalation are summarized in Table 22.8. These include addressing the interpersonal problems of mania and their

TABLE 22.8 Preventing Escalation

Address overstimulation (see Table 22.4)	Begin as soon as possible
Address interpersonal distortions	Monitor results
Vigorous pharmacologic treatment (see Table 22.6)	If results are not satisfactory: Be prepared to make changes, reevaluate diagnoses, and be alert to the possibility of additional substance-related, medical, legal, or social problems
Address environmental circumstances	Consistent behavior by staff Monitor or restrict outside contacts, including cell phone
Identify and enlist potential allies who can facilitate communication and participation in treatment	

underlying mechanisms (27), instituting early and effective pharmacologic treatment (39), and educating staff in the principles of interacting with patients who are manic (26). Escalation often occurs when interpersonal maneuvers of the manic patient lead to successful testing of limits, confirming the patient's fear that there is no effective structure (27). All personnel who interact with potentially manic patients should behave in a consistent manner.

Interventions for the Difficult-to-Treat or Treatment-Resistant Patient

Pharmacologic Treatments

Severe agitation may require synergistic combinations of treatments or more rapid dosage forms. The most basic synergistic treatment combination is that of an antipsychotic medicine with a benzodiazepine (39,60) or, perhaps, a loading dose of a valproate preparation (54).

Mobilizing Potential Allies

The emergency evaluation requires information from as many sources as possible. This provides the opportunity to contact and mobilize individuals who will be potential allies during and after treatment of the acute episode.

Reassessing the Diagnosis

One should always be open to the fact that an apparent primary manic episode has been precipitated or exacerbated by another medical condition

(2). The potential for receiving unexpected new information about a patient exists at all times. The dictum of taking nothing for granted cannot be overemphasized. One must be particularly alert for unusual response, lack of response, or intolerance to medicines.

Limits of Emergency Treatment

As soon as it is possible to discern that a patient is not going to stabilize under emergency conditions, that a patient is likely to have medical problems that cannot be immediately characterized or that a patient is likely to overtax the resources of the emergency services, thereby compromising other patients, steps should be taken to transfer the patient to a more appropriate facility. In the case of mania, the safest assumption is that this will be the case, so the possibility should be considered from an early stage of treatment.

SUMMARY

The manic syndrome is a potentially severe condition. It can be caused by a variety of medical conditions, including bipolar disorder. Potential causes can interact. In addition, mania generates potential complications such as traumatic injuries and exacerbations of substance use. Potential interactions between mania and substance abuse or withdrawal are important. Emergency management involves vigilant observation, efficient gathering of information from all possible sources, effective management of overstimulation and the interpersonal problems associated with mania, and prompt, effective pharmacologic treatment. Because resolution of the episode will not take place until later and some of the most valuable long-term treatments are not useful in emergency settings, attempts must be made to coordinate emergency treatment with other phases of treatment.

REFERENCES

1. Dunner, D. L. (1992). Differential diagnosis of bipolar disorder. *Journal of Clinical Psychopharmacology, 12*(1 Suppl. l), 7S–12S.
2. Krauthammer, C., & Klerman, G. L. (1978). Secondary mania: Manic syndromes associated with antecedent physical illnesses or drugs. *Archives of General Psychiatry, 35*, 1333–1339.
3. Swann, A. C., Janicak, P. L., Calabrese, J. R., et al. (2001). Structure of mania: Depressive, irritable, and psychotic clusters with different retrospectively-assessed course patterns of illness in randomized clinical trial participants. *Journal of Affective Disorders, 67*(1–3), 123–132.
4. Swann, A. C., Lafer, B., Perugi, G., Frye, M. A., Bauer, M., Bahk, W.-M., Scott, J., Ha, K., & Suppes, T. (2013). Bipolar mixed states: An International Society for Bipolar Disorders Task Force report of symptom structure, course of illness, and diagnosis. *American Journal of Psychiatry, 170*, 31–42.
5. Swann, A. C., Steinberg, J. L., Lijffijt, M., & Moeller, F. G. (2009). Continuum of depressive and manic mixed states in patients with bipolar disorder: Quantitative measurement and clinical features. *World Psychiatry, 8*, 166–172.
6. American Psychiatric Association. (2013). *Diagnostic and statistical manual of mental disorders* (5th ed.). Washington, DC: American Psychiatric Association.
7. Judd, L. L., & Akiskal, H. S. (2003). The prevalence and disability of bipolar spectrum disorders in the US population: Re-analysis of the ECA database taking into account subthreshold cases. *Journal of Affective Disorders, 73*(1–2), 123–131.
8. Breslau, N., & Meltzer, H. Y. (1988). Validity of subtyping psychotic depression: Examination of phenomenology and demographic characteristics. *American Journal of Psychiatry, 145*, 35–40.
9. Rosenthal, N. E., Rosenthal, L. N., Stallone, F., et al. (1979). Psychosis as a predictor of response to lithium maintenance treatment in bipolar affective disorder. *Journal of Affective Disorders, 1*(4), 237–245.
10. Swann, A. C., Daniel, D. G., Kochan, L. D., et al. (2004). Psychosis in mania: Specificity of its role in severity and treatment response. *The Journal of Clinical Psychiatry, 65*(6), 825–829.
11. Strakowski, S. M., Williams, J. R., Sax, K. W., et al. (2000). Is impaired outcome following a first manic episode due to mood-incongruent psychosis? *Journal of Affective Disorders, 61*(1–2), 87–94.
12. Akiskal, H. S., & Benazzi, F. (2003). Family history validation of the bipolar nature of depressive mixed states. *Journal of Affective Disorders, 73*(1–2), 113–122.
13. Turvey, C. L., Coryell, W. H., Solomon, D. A., et al. (1999). Long-term prognosis of bipolar I disorder. *Acta Psychiatrica Scandinavica, 99*(2), 110–119.
14. Himmelhoch, J. M., & Garfinkel, M. E. (1986). Sources of lithium resistance in mixed mania. *Psychopharmacology Bulletin, 22*, 613–620.
15. Akiskal, H. S., Benazzi, F., Perugi, G., et al. (2005). Agitated "unipolar" depression re-conceptualized as a depressive mixed state: Implications for the antidepressant-suicide controversy. *Journal of Affective Disorders, 85*(3), 245–258.
16. Dilsaver, S. C., Chen, Y. R., Swann, A. C., et al. (1995). Suicidality in patients with pure and depressive mania. *American Journal of Psychiatry, 151*, 1312–1315.
17. Swann, A. C., Secunda, S. K., Katz, M. M., et al. (1993). Specificity of mixed affective states: Clinical comparison of mixed mania and agitated depression. *Journal of Affective Disorders, 28*, 81–89.
18. Swann, A. C., Bowden, C. L., Morris, D., et al. (1997). Depression during mania: Treatment response to lithium or divalproex. *Archives of General Psychiatry, 54*, 37–42.
19. Dilsaver, S. C., Swann, A. C., Shoaib, A. M., et al. (1993). Mixed mania associated with nonresponse to antimanic agents. *American Journal of Psychiatry, 150*, 1548–1551.
20. Swann, A. C., Secunda, S. K., Katz, M. M., et al. (1986). Lithium treatment of mania: Clinical characteristics, specificity of symptom change, and outcome. *Psychiatry Research, 18*, 127–141.
21. Calabrese, J. R., Hirschfeld, R. M., Reed, M., et al. (2003). Impact of bipolar disorder on a U.S. community sample. *The Journal of Clinical Psychiatry, 64*(4), 425–432.
22. Swann, A. C., Lijffijt, M., Lane, S. D., Kjome, K. J., Steinberg, J. L., & Moeller, F. G. (2011). Criminal conviction, impulsivity, and course of illness in bipolar disorder. *Bipolar Disorders, 13*, 173–181.

23. Braunig, P., Kruger, S., & Shugar, G. (1998). Prevalence and clinical significance of catatonic symptoms in mania. *Comprehensive Psychiatry, 39*(1), 35–46.

24. Fink, M., & Taylor, M. A. (2001). The many varieties of catatonia. *European Archives of Psychiatry and Clinical Neuroscience, 251*(Suppl. 1), 8–13.

25. Johnstone, E. C., Cooling, N. J., Frith, C. D., et al. (1988). Phenomenology of organic and functional psychoses and the overlap between them. *British Journal of Psychiatry, 153*, 770–776.

26. Mackinnon, R. A., Buckley, P. J., & Michels, R. (2006). *The psychiatric interview in clinical practice*. Washington, DC: American Psychiatric Press.

27. Janowsky, D. S., Leff, M., & Epstein, R. S. (1970). Playing the manic game: Interpersonal maneuvers of the acutely manic patient. *Archives of General Psychiatry, 22*, 252–261.

28. Swann, A. C., Dougherty, D. M., Pazzaglia, P. J., et al. (2005). Increased impulsivity associated with severity of suicide attempt history in patients with bipolar disorder. *American Journal of Psychiatry, 162*(9), 1680–1687.

29. Kotin, J., & Goodwin, F. K. (1971). Depression during mania: Clinical observations and theoretical implications. *American Journal of Psychiatry, 129*, 55–62.

30. Swann, A. C., Moeller, F. G., Steinberg, J. L., Schneider, L., Barratt, E. S., & Dougherty, D. M. (2007). Manic symptoms and impulsivity during bipolar depressive episodes. *Bipolar Disorders, 9*, 206–212.

31. Peterson, L. G., Peterson, M., O'Shanick, G., et al. (1985). Violent suicide attempts: Lethality of method vs intent. *American Journal of Psychiatry, 142*, 228–231.

32. Simon, T. R., Swann, A. C., Powell, K. E., et al. (2001). Characteristics of impulsive suicide attempts and attempters. *Suicide and Life-Threatening Behavior, 32*(Suppl. 1), 30–41.

33. Lubman, A., Emrich, C., Mosimann, W., et al. (1983). Altered mood and norepinephrine metabolism following withdrawal from alcohol. *Drug and Alcohol Dependence, 12*, 3–13.

34. Binder, R. L., & McNiel, D. E. (1988). Effects of diagnosis and context on dangerousness. *American Journal of Psychiatry, 145*, 728–732.

35. Buchanan, A., Reed, A., Wessely, S., et al. (1993). Acting on delusions. II: The phenomenological correlates of acting on delusions. *British Journal of Psychiatry, 163*, 77–81.

36. McAllister, T. W. (1992). Neuropsychiatric sequelae of head injuries. *Psychiatric Clinics of North America, 15*, 395–413.

37. Sherwood, B. E., Suppes, T., Adinoff, B., et al. (2001). Drug abuse and bipolar disorder: Comorbidity or misdiagnosis? *Journal of Affective Disorders, 65*(2), 105–115.

38. Myrick, H., Brady, K. T., & Malcolm, R. (2000). Divalproex in the treatment of alcohol withdrawal. *American Journal of Drug and Alcohol Abuse, 26*(1), 155–160.

39. Allen, M. H., Currier, G. W., Carpenter, D., et al. (2005). Treatment of behavioral emergencies 2005. *Journal of Psychiatric Practice, 11*(Suppl. l), 5–108.

40. Bresler, S., Scalora, M. J., Elbogen, E. B., et al. (2003). Attempted suicide by cop: A case study of traumatic brain injury and the insanity defense. *Journal of Forensic Sciences, 48*(1), 190–194.

41. Baldessarini, R. J. (2002). Treatment research in bipolar disorder: Issues and recommendations. *CNS Drugs, 16*(11), 721–729.

42. Reich, L. H., Davis, R. K., & Himmelhoch, J. M. (1974). Excessive alcohol use in manic-depressive illness. *American Journal of Psychiatry, 131*, 83–86.

43. Brown, E. S., Suppes, T., Khan, D. A., et al. (2002). Mood changes during prednisone bursts in outpatients with asthma. *Journal of Clinical Psychopharmacology, 22*(1), 55–61.

44. Couturier, J., Steele, M., Hussey, L., et al. (2001). Steroid-induced mania in an adolescent: Risk factors and management. *The Canadian Journal of Clinical Pharmacology, 8*(2), 109–112.

45. Minden, S. L., Orav, J., & Schildkraut, J. J. (1988). Hypomanic reactions to ACTH and prednisone treatment for multiple sclerosis. *Neurology, 38*, 1631–1634.

46. Allen, M. H., Currier, G. W., Hughes, D. H., et al. (2001). The expert consensus guideline series. Treatment of behavioral emergencies. *Postgraduate Medicine*, Special Report, 1–88.

47. Swann, A. C. (1999). Treatment of aggression in patients with bipolar disorder. *The Journal of Clinical Psychiatry, 60*(Suppl. 15), 25–28.

48. Grunze, H., Erfurth, A., Amann, B., et al. (1999). Intravenous valproate loading in acutely manic and depressed bipolar I patients. *Journal of Clinical Psychopharmacology, 19*(4), 303–309.

49. Gerlach, J., & Larsen, E. B. (1999). Subjective experience and mental side-effects of antipsychotic treatment. *Acta Psychiatrica Scandinavica, 99*(Suppl. 395), 113–117.

50. Kinghorn, W. A., & McEvoy, J. P. (2005). Aripiprazole: Pharmacology, efficacy, safety and tolerability. *Expert Review of Neurotherapeutics, 5*(3), 297–307.

51. Butler, M., Urosevic, S., Desai, P., et al. (2018). *Treatment for bipolar disorder in adults: A systematic review*. Appendix E, Antipsychotics for mania. Comparative Effectiveness Review, No. 208. Rockville, MD: Agency for Healthcare Research and Quality. Retrieved from https://www.ncbi.nlm.nih.gov/books/NBK532182/.

52. Hollander, E., Tracy, K. A., Swann, A. C., et al. (2003). Divalproex in the treatment of impulsive aggression: Efficacy in cluster B personality disorders. *Neuropsychopharmacology, 28*(6), 1186–1197.

53. Steiner, H., Petersen, M. L., Saxena, K., et al. (2003). Divalproex sodium for the treatment of conduct disorder: A randomized controlled clinical trial. *The Journal of Clinical Psychiatry, 64*(10), 1183–1191.

54. McElroy, S. L., Keck, P. E., Jr., Stanton, S. P., et al. (1996). A randomized comparison of divalproex oral loading versus haloperidol in the initial treatment of acute psychotic mania. *The Journal of Clinical Psychiatry, 57*, 142–146.

55. Suppes, T., Baldessarini, R. J., Faedda, G. L., et al. (1991). Risk of recurrence following discontinuation of lithium treatment in bipolar disorder. *Archives of General Psychiatry, 48*(12), 1082–1088.

56. Greenspan, K., Goodwin, F. K., Bunney, W. E., et al. (1968). Lithium ion retention and distribution. Patterns during acute mania and normothymia. *Archives of General Psychiatry, 19*(6), 664–673.

57. Lake, C. R. (1991). Manic psychosis after coffee and phenylpropanolamine. *Biological Psychiatry, 30*, 401–404.

58. Maglione, M., Miotto, K., Iguchi, M., et al. (2005). Psychiatric effects of ephedra use: An analysis of Food and Drug Administration reports of adverse events. *American Journal of Psychiatry, 162*(1), 189–191.

59. Steel, Z., & Blaszczynski, A. (1998). Impulsivity, personality disorders and pathological gambling severity. *Addiction, 93*(6), 895–905.

60. Garza-Trevino, E. S., Hollister, L. E., Overall, J. E., et al. (1989). Efficacy of combinations of intramuscular antipsychotics and sedative-hypnotics for control of psychotic agitation. *American Journal of Psychiatry, 146*(12), 1598–1601.

23

Anxiety

Jagoda Pasic, Paul Zarkowski

Anxiety disorders are the most prevalent mental health disorders in the United States, with lifetime prevalence of 29% and 12-month prevalence of 18% (1). According to the data from the National Hospital Ambulatory Medical Care Survey, anxiety-related visits account for 16% of all mental health visits among patients presenting in the emergency departments (EDs) (2).

PRESENTING CLINICAL FEATURES

Anxiety is a symptom of many clinical syndromes of diverse etiology and manifestations. The symptoms may be relatively constant or develop quickly over minutes. Patients subjectively experience anxiety as a diffuse, unpleasant, vague sense of apprehension and uneasiness and may include a variety of *psychological symptoms*: anger, irritability, inability to focus and fear of being outside oneself (depersonalization), losing control, or impending death. These symptoms are often accompanied by a varying degree of autonomic symptoms (*physical symptoms*) ranging from, perspiration, palpitations to severe chest pain, choking, and shortness of breath. Anxiety can be associated with other symptom clusters including neurologic; tremor, dizziness, blurred vision, light-headedness, numbness, tingling muscle tension, and chills or gastrointestinal; nausea, cramps, abdominal pain, vomiting, or diarrhea. Palpitations, for example, are the most common symptom of panic attacks in patients who are presenting in medical settings (3). Anxiety can be an intensely negative experience and it may cause extreme subjective distress. Recurrent anxiety can become disabling and the person may avoid places where attacks occurred or restrict his or her normal activities and become housebound (*behavioral symptoms*). Anxiety symptoms can result from many physical, medical, and psychiatric disorders.

Depending on the severity of symptoms, patients with anxiety present in different care settings. Only 26% of panic attack patients initially seek care in a mental health setting. Patients with predominantly somatic symptoms seek help from nonpsychiatric physicians, most often in the primary care settings (35%) (4). 32% of patients with a severe anxiety attack present in the ED with chest pain, shortness of breath, tachycardia, and fear of a myocardial infarction (MI) or death. 25% of patients who present to an ED with chest pain meet criteria for panic disorder, although 98% are undiagnosed on arrival (5). Many patients with an acute anxiety attack will have resolution of their symptoms before arrival at the ED. However, some patients may continue to have anxiety symptoms that persist for hours and may lead to multiple ED visits. A recent study reported high prevalence of abnormal anxiety symptoms (47%) in patients with low-risk chest pain, and such patients have an increased risk of multiple ED return visits (6).

IMMEDIATE INTERVENTIONS FOR ACUTE PRESENTATIONS

The first intervention for an anxious patient should be to demonstrate genuine concern and to assess patient safety. The physician must consider the risks of serous medical events, such as MI or hypoxia. Immediate interventions include monitoring of vital signs and evaluating need for oxygen. If the vital signs and initial physical examination do not indicate a life-threatening event, the physician can offer reassurance while proceeding with the evaluation. A calming, reassuring approach may be effective in decreasing discomfort and anxiety level. Patients may require pretreatment with medications before finishing the evaluation or obtaining a complete history.

EVALUATION

The initial evaluation begins with the *current complaint* including the course, intensity, and duration of symptoms. The patient needs to be asked about environmental triggers, such as stressful life events and sleep deprivation. Associated cognitive elements, including obsessions, ruminations, worries, and particularly, suicidal ideations need to be assessed ("see Criteria for Hospitalization below").

The important elements of *history* include age of onset of anxiety, family history of anxiety, childhood antecedents, resultant avoidance, and traumatic events. The medical history should focus on conditions associated with anxiety and frequent ED visits, eg, asthma and chronic obstructive pulmonary disease (COPD) exacerbation. All medications need to be reviewed, including over-the-counter (OTC) medications. Cold remedies may cause acute anxiety symptoms in a vulnerable patient. Previous medication trials should be reviewed in order to establish if acute anxiety symptoms are secondary to initiation or discontinuation of selective serotonin reuptake inhibitor (SSRI), side effects to current treatment, or poor treatment response. Recreational drugs, particularly stimulants and alcohol, caffeine consumption, smoking, and vaping, all need to be carefully ascertained in history because of high incidence of substance use in the ED population.

A thorough *physical examination* should be performed in all patients presenting with acute anxiety symptoms. There is a considerable overlap between physical symptoms of acute anxiety and serious medical conditions, such as cardiovascular (eg, angina and MI), respiratory (eg, COPD), endocrine (hyperthyroidism), hematologic (eg, anemia), and neurological (eg, seizures) diseases.

A number of *laboratory tests* should be performed, depending on the symptom presentation and associated physical symptoms. The following laboratory tests are recommended: toxicology screen, complete blood count (CBC), electrolytes, glucose, BUN/Cr, thyroid-stimulating hormone (TSH), T4-free, T3 and T3-uptake, and ECG if the patient has cardiac symptoms or is older than 40 years. Other tests should be directed by clinical suspicion. For example, patients with cardiac symptoms should have serial cardiac enzymes

taken to rule out MI and echocardiography for suspected mitral valve prolapse. Patients with prominent respiratory symptoms may need to have a chest X-ray, blood gases, and V-Q scan to rule out pulmonary embolism (PE); for suspected seizures, EEG would be indicated.

DIAGNOSIS/DIFFERENTIAL DIAGNOSIS

Medical Disorders

Diagnosis of primary anxiety requires differentiation from medical disorders. The difficulty with the differential diagnosis of acute anxiety presentation is that patients typically have symptoms across multiple organ systems, hence it can be a complex differential. Factors suggesting a medical etiology include onset late in life, absence of an initial life event or precipitating event, absence of avoidance or fear, and absence of childhood antecedents or family history. Poor response to trials of antipanic or antidepressant medications may be suggestive of an underlying medical disorder. Previous systematic reviews and meta-analysis have supported a connection between panic disorder and cardiac disorders, but the heterogeneity relating to methodology has made conclusions not unequivocal. However, the most recent updated systematic review highly supports this relationship (7).

Psychiatric Disorders
Primary Anxiety Disorders

Panic attacks or intense anxiety develop suddenly and can occur at any time, even during sleep. Classically it is associated with fear of impending doom or loss of control, with symptoms of autonomic arousal and intense need to flee from the situation in which the attack occurred. An attack usually peaks within 10 minutes, but some symptoms may last much longer. Although panic attack is not a separate DSM disorder, it is prerequisite to a diagnosis of *panic disorder*. 90% of panic disorder patients believe that they suffer from a serious physical disorder, so they seek help in the general medical system. Such patients often undergo expensive cardiac workups, but they receive neither a diagnosis of panic disorder nor treatment for the disorder. An additional challenge in making the right diagnosis is that patients with chest pain that is significant enough to warrant testing for coronary artery disease (CAD) are as likely to have panic disorder and no CAD (22%) as they are to have CAD and no panic disorder (18%) (8). Furthermore, cardiac patients tend to have an increased prevalence of panic disorder and significantly greater mean ED visits in 12 months than patients with CAD and no panic disorder (9). Of interest, one recent study developed a brief seven-item clinician rating scale, which proposes to be used in the ED to distinguish between patients with panic attacks or panic disorder and those with cardiac disorders. They noted that the presence of panic attacks does not rule in or rule out the presence of cardiac disorders, but it does help with the recognition of panic attacks in the context of panic disorder (10).

Patients with prominent psychological or behavioral components of anxiety in addition to physical symptoms are more likely to be referred for a psychiatric evaluation. Such patients typically present with intense irritability, sense of impending doom or loss of control, uncontrolled worrying, or limited functioning due to avoidance. In addition, patients with repeated, unresolved attacks clinically present with a sense of hopelessness, dysphoria and ultimately, with suicidal ideation.

Patients with *specific phobia* fear and avoid specific situations, eg, airplanes, heights, or objects, eg, snakes, dogs. Exposure to the feared stimuli consistently induces intense anxiety with a panic attack–like reaction. Patients rarely seek care in the ED because of relatively intact insight into the origin of their anxiety symptoms.

Patients with *social phobia* are fearful of social or performance situations, such as public speaking in which humiliation or embarrassment might occur. Exposure to such situations almost invariably provokes anxiety, which may take a form of panic attacks, but unlike patients with panic disorder, patients with social phobia recognize that the fear is excessive or unreasonable. Though patients with social phobia may present often in ED with panic attacks (23%), they are almost three times less likely than panic disorder patients to present in cardiology clinics (46% vs 16%) or undergo excessive medical workup (11).

Patients with *obsessive compulsive disorder* (OCD) suffer from recurrent, intrusive, senseless, and distressing thoughts (*obsessions*) or the need to repeat certain stereotypical behaviors or rituals to reduce anxiety and distress (*compulsions*). Patients with uncomplicated OCD generally do not present in the ED. However, with their underlying susceptibility to anxiety, an ED visit can be precipitated by exaggerated anxiety due to OTC medications (cold remedies), medical conditions (asthma), excessive caffeine and nicotine use, and other substance use. Of all anxiety disorders, OCD has the lowest rate of seeking medical care through the ED (16%) (11).

Patients with *posttraumatic stress disorder* (PTSD) and *acute stress disorder* develop anxiety symptoms after exposure to actual or threatened death or serious or sexual violence either by direct experience, learning of trauma to a person close to them, or repeated or extreme exposure to aversive details. These patients may startle easily, become emotionally numb, lose interest in things they used to enjoy, have trouble feeling affectionate, be irritable, angry, hypervigilant, and reexperience traumatic event in recurrent intrusive recollections, dreams, or flashbacks. PTSD and acute stress disorder differ by the duration of symptoms more or less than a month. PTSD was initially associated with war veterans, but it can result from a variety of traumatic events, such as natural disasters due to floods or earthquakes, bombing, child abuse, rape, mugging, shooting, and car/plane/train accidents. Victims of recent trauma may present in the ED in a crisis like state of anxiety and agitation. There is evidence that panic attacks occur in 53% to 90% of trauma survivors during the traumatic experience, and half of them report recurrent panic attacks post trauma (12). PTSD patients typically experience panic attacks during exposure to triggers that evoke recall of the original traumatic event. About 15 % of Americans will experience a serious physical or sexual assault, and a high number of them will develop an acute stress disorder. PTSD will develop in about 30% to 50% of those exposed (13). Hence, appropriate diagnosis and treatment initiation for patients with acute stress disorder and PTSD in the ED are important considerations for secondary prevention of PTSD.

Patients who experience excessive worry and anxiety and have symptoms of restlessness or feeling keyed up or on edge, being easily fatigued, irritable, with poor concentration, muscle tension, and sleep disturbance may be given a diagnosis of *generalized anxiety disorder* (GAD). Chronic GAD can be demoralizing and frequently the cause of disturbed social and occupational functioning. Though GAD patients most often have a chronic course, they occasionally have panic attacks that can lead to ED visits. Patients with GAD have high rates of seeking care through the ED (28%) and urgent care (31%) (11). GAD diagnosis in the ED is most often encountered in the context of comorbid disorders, such as major depression, dysthymic disorder, social and simple phobias, substance-related disorders, and personality disorders.

Anxiety Secondary to Another Primary Psychiatric Disorder

Although primary anxiety disorders are often comorbid with other psychiatric disorders, anxiety can also be an associated feature of another primary psychiatric disorder. The symptoms of anxiety may temporarily become the primary focus of clinical attention in the ED but should not distract the clinician from arriving at the most accurate diagnosis.

Anxiety commonly accompanies *major depression*, and anxious distress can be added as a specifier in the DSM-5. 45% of the patients in the STAR-D trial for the treatment of major depression indicated the presence of moderate anxiety symptoms on the Hamilton Depression Rating Scale (HAM-D) (14). Insomnia, fatigue, and difficulty concentrating are common to both primary anxiety and affective disorders. The presence of anhedonia and persistent depressed mood are important differentiating symptoms.

Anxiety frequently accompanies *bipolar disorder*. The pressured speech and increased activity of acute mania may be difficult to differentiate in the ED from the restlessness and psychomotor agitation of a primary anxiety disorder. Inflated self-esteem, grandiosity, and increased involvement in pleasurable but dangerous activities are important differentiating signs.

Anxiety commonly co-occurs with *psychosis* and is listed as an associated feature of schizophrenia by the DSM-5. The degree of worry, fear, and physical manifestations of nervousness is commonly included in the assessment of severity of psychosis (Brief Psychiatric Rating Scale—BPRS). 62% of patients with schizophrenia report symptoms that meet the DSM-5 criteria for a comorbid anxiety disorder, most commonly OCD and social anxiety. Measures of suspiciousness and paranoia often mirror symptoms of panic and social anxiety (15). Assessment of reality testing and level of insight is important for differentiating psychosis from primary anxiety disorders. Irregular speech should be closely monitored for the presence of a formal thought disorder. Schizophrenia may also be differentiated by the presence of affective flattening, alogia, or avolition.

Anxiety is frequently associated with *cognitive disorders*. Symptoms of anxiety were reported by 25% of patients with mild cognitive impairment and 35% with mild Alzheimer disease (16). In a separate study, the severity of anxiety was correlated with decreasing function as measured by the loss of skills of daily living (17). The Mini-Mental Status Examination and clock face drawing are useful screening tests for estimating cognitive function and should be performed routinely in the ED. Both tests may miss subtle signs of early cognitive loss in high-functioning individuals.

Persistently high levels of anxiety about health or medical symptoms is one of the criteria for *somatic symptom disorder* in the DSM-5. Patients with this disorder may be over represented in ED because of their distressing and long-standing medical complaints, greater than 6 months by definition. Panic disorder may be distinguished by the clustering of symptoms around discrete periods of panic. GAD may be differentiated by the expanded scope of worries beyond physical health.

Anxiety can be a prominent symptom of all phases of *substance-related disorders* including intoxication and withdrawal, for mild to severe severity, for most substances listed in the DSM-5. Among patients presenting to a busy urban psychiatric emergency service (PES), 20% tested positive for THC, 18% for cocaine, 9.5% for benzodiazepines, 9% for opiates, and 7% for amphetamines

(18). In a separate sample, 25% had positive blood alcohol levels and 16% had BAL (blood alcohol level) readings above 0.10% (19). Symptoms of anxiety related to substance use or withdrawal can be difficult to distinguish from those arising from a primary anxiety disorder. Lab tests including, blood alcohol and urine toxicology screens are crucial. Physical signs indicative of substance use include charcoal burns on the fingers for smoking cocaine, needle tracks for IV drugs, and conjunctival injection for tetrahydrocannabinol (THC).

Adjustment disorder is an exaggerated response to psychosocial stress that does not meet the criteria for another primary anxiety disorder. The diagnosis (with anxiety or with mixed anxiety and depressed mood) is given when a patient presents with nervousness, worry, or jitteriness that developed in response to an identifiable stressor. Patients with adjustment disorder with anxiety may suffer marked distress that causes significant impairment of functioning and may lead to an ED visit. One study of emergency room visits found that 13% of adults and 42% of adolescents were diagnosed as having adjustment disorder (20). Adjustment disorder with anxious mood can be difficult to differentiate from other anxiety disorders or personality disorders. Particular care must be taken to distinguish between the reasonable, expected response to psychosocial stressors, and the inordinate response that may indicate the diagnosis of adjustment disorder.

Anxiety Secondary to Personality Disorders

Comorbidity between anxiety disorders and personality disorders is as high as 65%, with borderline personality disorder (BPD) as the most common. Patients with BPD can manifest intense anxiety that can lead to their presentation in the ED. Comorbid borderline personality has been shown to increase the clinical severity of panic disorder. It is virtually impossible to distinguish panic attacks from the stress-induced fragmentation of identity that occurs in patients with BPD (21). There is a considerable overlap between BPD and PTSD. Rates of current PTSD in individuals with BPD range between 25% and 56%, compared with about 10% lifetime rates of PTSD in the general population (22).

MANAGEMENT

Criteria for Hospitalization

In patients with severe symptoms not responding to pharmacological and/or nonpharmacological intervention, hospitalization should be considered. The critical factors favoring hospitalization include a significant level of patient distress, lack of social support, poor problem-solving skills, and deficient coping mechanisms. As in other psychiatric disorders, the threshold for hospitalization includes grave disability and significant threat of harm to self or others.

The presence of a anxiety disorder increases the risk of suicidal thoughts and behaviors. In a large sample of patients with one or more anxiety disorders drawn from primary care clinics, 16% endorsed suicidal ideation in the past month, with 18% reporting at least one suicide attempt during their lifetime (23). After controlling for sociodemographic factors, axis I and II disorders, the presence of any anxiety disorder significantly increases the risk of suicide attempts, with PTSD and panic disorder associated with the highest risk (24). Specifically, the presence of panic disorder, but not panic attacks, was significantly correlated with more suicide attempts within the past year after controlling for demographic factors and comorbid illness (25). Patients with any primary anxiety disorder were 3.6 times more likely to attempt suicide after controlling for sociodemographic factors and other mental illnesses (26). Negative prognostic factors include therapeutic hopelessness and discomfort from severe anxiety.

Although the presence of psychosis, mania, and substance abuse increases the risk of violent behavior, the presence of uncomplicated anxiety disorders has not been shown to increase the risk of violence. Severity of anxiety symptoms was found to be unrelated to homicidal ideation and intent in a group of patients with primary anxiety disorders. Male gender was the only significant independent predictor of violent ideation in this patient group when controlling for substance abuse and legal problems (27). Patients with uncomplicated primary anxiety disorders rarely require hospitalization on the basis of danger to others.

Patients with anxiety disorders may experience significant impairment in social and occupational functioning to the degree that they are unable to perform their usual daily activities. 32% to 43% of patients report their anxiety symptoms made it "very or extremely difficult" to do their work, to take care of things at home, or to get along with other people (28). However, patients with uncomplicated illness are rarely disabled to the degree that they are unable to meet their basic physical needs or provide for their own safety. For this reason, psychiatric hospitalization is rarely indicated on the basis of grave disability. Comorbid affective, psychotic, or substance-related illness may severely interfere with basic functioning and significantly contribute to the grounds for hospitalization.

Criteria for Diversion

Selected patients with severe symptoms may be considered for diversion from hospital-based inpatient care to alternative care settings. The specific criteria for diversion will vary based on which services and care settings are available in any given community. Generally, the criteria for placement in a diversion bed are the same as for psychiatric hospitalization but with the risk of harm at a lower level of imminence. Diversion beds usually offer 24-hour staff to dispense but not prescribe medication and an opportunity to be engaged with agencies to arrange ongoing community-based care. Only patients with a reasonable level of cooperation with treatment and lower risk of harm to self or others should be placed in diversion beds.

Treatment Within the Emergency Setting

Behavioral and Psychological Intervention

Relaxation procedures may be effective for persistent symptoms of panic after ruling out the presence of a life-threatening condition. The patient is instructed to focus on deep slow breathing. If hyperventilation continues after a trial of directed breathing, breathing into a paper bag may be helpful. The patient is instructed to take 6 to 12 natural breaths and breathe back into a paper bag held over mouth and nose. This intervention will raise pCO_2 and slow the respiration rate. Other nonpharmacological measures include instructing the patient to tense and relax large groups of muscle and diverting conversation (29).

If during the assessment, the presence of an acute traumatic precipitating factor is detected, then the coping mechanisms of the patient should be assessed further. Brief supportive psychological intervention has been shown to be effective (30).

Acute Pharmacological Treatment

Benzodiazepines

Acute pharmacologic treatment may be indicated in cases involving high levels of discomfort and prolonged duration of panic symptoms. Benzodiazepines are the emergency medications of choice. Unlike chronic use, acute use of benzodiazepines is safe and reliable and does not risk dependency or withdrawal. However, the benefits of benzodiazepine use in the ED must be balanced against the risk of reinforcing help-seeking behavior from the ED and preventing patients from developing other therapeutic options to deal with panic symptoms.

There are many different protocols for the treatment of panic attacks using benzodiazepines, and most EDs and PES vary in their choices. Most common options include alprazolam (0.25-1 mg po), lorazepam (0.5-2 mg po), diazepam (2-10 mg po), and clonazepam (0.5-2 mg po). Lorazepam and diazepam are available for intramuscular and intravenous use and are reserved for more severe panic attacks or when medical conditions create a life-threatening situation, eg, MI, arrhythmias, hypoxia. Patients treated with benzodiazepines should be closely monitored for respiratory depression, oversedation, and rebound anxiety. Benzodiazepines may produce paradoxical anxiety and disinhibition in a small subset of patients.

Other Agents

Because of benzodiazepines' high-abuse potential, some EDs/PES favor hydroxyzine (25 to 50 mg po or IM). A meta-analysis of five random controlled trials suggested that hydroxyzine was as effective as benzodiazepines for managing GAD. A high risk of bias in the studies prevented the authors from supporting hydroxyzine as first-line treatment (31). However the increased sedation and drowsiness with hydroxyzine makes it particularly useful for managing the acute symptoms of GAD, including insomnia, in the ED. There have been no controlled studies of hydroxyzine in panic attacks patients, but case studies and our clinical experience suggest it may be useful (32).

Beta-blocker medications are another option for patients with panic attacks, acute stress disorder, and PTSD. They ease anxiety and some physical symptoms such as tremulousness, palpitations, and tachycardia. Beta-blockers are not addictive and do not cause drowsiness. Propranolol (10 mg to 40 po) acts centrally and is most commonly used. Preliminary data suggested that propranolol given within 6 hours of a traumatic event may be effective in preventing subsequent development of PTSD (33). A subsequent meta-analysis failed to support the efficacy of propranolol to prevent PTSD. This review included a larger negative retrospective chart review along with four prospective trials showing various degrees of benefit (34).

Although atypical antipsychotics have been of interest in the treatment of anxiety disorders, there are few well-designed clinical trials to support their use in primary anxiety disorders. Quetiapine (300-600 mg/d) was shown to be effective in the treatment of anxiety symptoms in patients with bipolar disorder (35). The empirical use of quetiapine (25-100 mg po) as a PRN medicine for anxiety on inpatient psychiatry units supports its efficacy for the acute management of panic attacks, yet an 8-week trial of augmentation with quetiapine XR 150 mg failed to show an advantage over placebo in the management of SSRI-resistant panic disorder (36). Concern over the side-effect profile of antipsychotic agents limits their use for augmentation or monotherapy for primary anxiety disorders.

Gabapentin has been used as an off-label agent in a variety of anxiety disorders including GAD, social phobia, PTSD, panic disorder, and anxiety associated with bipolar disorder and substance use (37). Although there are no controlled studies supporting the use of gabapentin in the treatment of acute anxiety in the ED, a trial with a low dose (100-600 mg) might be useful for patients with comorbid anxiety and substance use (38). Valproic acid (250-500 mg) could be another nonbenzodiazepine option though there are no studies to support its use in acute anxiety.

Antidepressants are first-line agents in the long-term treatment of anxiety disorders. However, they are not suitable for the management of acute anxiety in the ED because of delay in onset of action. An exception is trazodone. Trazodone (25-50 mg) can be an effective anxiolytic in the elderly without causing significant cognitive impairment because of its low anticholinergic activity.

Patient Education

Patient education is an essential part of the acute treatment of patients with panic attacks. Once the diagnosis of panic attack is made, it should be shared with the patient and family. The patient should receive reassurance that panic attacks are not imminently life-threatening but can have serious long-term consequences if not treated. Prior to discharge from our ED, patients suffering from recurrent panic attacks are encouraged to develop alternative strategies in dealing with their attacks and write these strategies on a 3 × 5 index cards that they take home as a "fire drill" card to remind them what to do when the attacks occur.

Referral for Outpatient Treatment

In addition to immediate interventions, as discussed above, it may sometimes be appropriate to start outpatient medications in the ED. In such cases, patients may be provided with a short supply of hydroxyzine (50 mg tid, or qid) and a referral to either a primary care doctor or to a mental health clinic. Ideally, patients with panic attacks should be referred to a psychiatrist for evaluation because panic attacks are often comorbid with other psychiatric and substance-related disorders, significantly increasing case complexity. Patients with alcohol-related disorders and anxiety most often benefit from referral to a co-occurring disorders program.

Though there are no established evidence-based treatments for anxiety in the context of adjustment disorder, the ultimate goals of treatment are to mobilize the patient's stress-coping mechanisms and to prevent adjustment disorder from developing into chronic conditions, such as GAD or major depression. Hence, patients presenting in ED with adjustment disorders should be referred for psychiatric follow-up.

Medications that could be considered for longer-term treatment such as SSRI/SNRI (serotonin and norepinephrine reuptake inhibitor), benzodiazepines, tricyclic antidepressants (TCAs)/monoamine oxidase inhibitors (MAOIs), and buspirone are not started typically in the ED unless outpatient mental health services are readily available. One ED study showed good results with paroxetine initiation in patients diagnosed with panic disorder (39). We have had a good experience using a protocol which consists of 1 to 3 day supply of medication and a "next day" mental health appointment. Although cognitive behavioral therapy (CBT) is proven as an effective treatment for a variety of anxiety disorders (40), referrals from the ED are limited by the relative scarcity of CBT therapists in community mental health settings and other insurance-related issues.

Interventions for the Difficult-to-Treat or Treatment-Resistant Patient

Delay in establishing an accurate diagnosis, delay in onset of treatment, and failure of primary care settings to appropriately address patients' needs (5), along with high recurrence rates and poor response to treatment, render anxiety disorders at high risk for treatment resistance (37). Interventions lay in establishing a proper diagnosis and making a referral to an appropriate care setting. Some patients will warrant immediate intervention including hospitalization, and some patients may be referred for outpatient follow-up with various pharmacological strategies started in the ED. With appropriate outpatient follow-up or admission to psychiatric unit, antidepressant agents (such as SSRI or SNRI) may be prescribed. The potential side effects and delayed benefits from antidepressants should be included in the informed consent process. A combination treatment may include addition of agents such as clonazepam (because of long half-life and less potential for subclinical withdrawal), hydroxyzine (because of nonaddicting properties), anticonvulsants, particularly with GABAergic properties (gabapentin, pregabalin, tiagabine), and atypical antipsychotic agents (quetiapine, olanzapine). ED-specific nonpharmacological interventions include *exposure instruction* (41), *case management–based intervention* (42), and *brief face-to-face contact with mental health representatives* (30). These interventions have shown a statistically significant reduction of ED utilization in patients with anxiety disorders.

High comorbidity of anxiety disorders with substance abuse, bipolar disorder, and personality disorders creates a considerable treatment challenge. About 20% of patients with bipolar disorder have a lifetime diagnosis of panic disorder. Use of antidepressants in refractory panic patients with a bipolar diathesis may lead to increased cycling and agitation. Such patients should be considered for anticonvulsant and benzodiazepine therapy in place of standard antidepressant treatment. Second-generation antipsychotics, such as quetiapine and olanzapine, have been suggested as alternative treatments for patients with comorbid anxiety and bipolar disorder (43).

As for the substance-related disorders, commonly abused substances in anxiety patients include nicotine, alcohol, cocaine, and cannabis. Each substance may precipitate an acute anxiety attack and lead to treatment resistance and failure. Pharmacological treatment of comorbid anxiety disorder and substance abuse may be hampered by the fact that some antiaddictive medications, eg, bupropion and naltrexone, may trigger further panic attacks. Finally, patients may be undertreated because of clinician's reluctance to prescribe addicting medications such as benzodiazepines because of substance abuse history and drug-seeking behaviors. Appropriate medication management with attention to chemical dependency issues is crucial. Co-occurring disorders programs are very helpful in this population.

The combination of an anxiety disorder and comorbid BPD may present challenges to the clinician working in the ED. There are no placebo controlled studies in this patient group, however injectable atypical antipsychotic agents (olanzapine and ziprasidone) are effective in BPD patients in acute crisis with agitation. In addition, oral aripiprazole, quetiapine, and olanzapine are effective in the treatment of agitation in patients with BPD (44).

Transcultural and minority issues may present a challenge to ED clinicians and contribute to treatment resistance of anxiety disorders. These issues are poorly studied in the literature but are often encountered by ED clinicians because of high rates of urban and refugee-related PTSD. Awareness of cross-cultural issues is important for effective treatment of this population (45).

REFERENCES

1. Kessler, R. C., Chiu, W. T., Demler, O., Merikangas, K. R., & Walters, E. E. (2005). Prevalence, severity, and comorbidity of 12-month DSM-IV disorders in the National Comorbidity Survey Replication. *Archives of General Psychiatry, 62*(6), 617–627. Erratum in: Merikangas, K. R. (2005). *Archives of General Psychiatry, 62*(7), 709.

2. Smith, R. P., Larkin, G. L., & Southwick, S. M. (2008). Trends in U.S. emergency department visits for anxiety-related mental health conditions, 1992–2001. *The Journal of Clinical Psychiatry, 69*(2), 286–294.

3. Barsky, A. J., Cleary, P. D., Sarnie, M. K., & Ruskin, J. N. (1994). Panic disorder, palpitations, and the awareness of cardiac activity. *The Journal of Nervous and Mental Disease, 182*, 63–71.

4. Katerndahl, D. A., & Realini, J. P. (1995). Where do panic attack sufferers seek care? *The Journal of Family Practice, 40*, 237–243.

5. Fleet, R. P., Dupuis, G., Marchand, A., Burelle, D., Arsenault, A., & Beitman, B. D. (1996). Panic disorder in emergency department chest pain patients: Prevalence, comorbidity, suicide ideations, and physician recognition. *American Journal of Medicine, 101*, 371–380.

6. Musey, P. I., Jr., Patel, R., Fry, C., Jimenez, G., Koene, R., & Kline, J. (2018). Anxiety associated with increased risk for emergency department recidivism in patients with low-risk chest pain. *American Journal of Cardiology, 122*(7), 1133–1141.

7. Caldirola, D., Schruers, K. R., Nardi, A. E., DeBerardis, D. D., Fornaro, M., & Perna, G. (2016). Is there cardiac risk in panic disorder? An updated systematic review. *Journal of Affective Disorders, 194*, 38–49.

8. Lynch, P., & Galbraith, K. M. (2003). Panic in the emergency room. *The Canadian Journal of Psychiatry, 48*, 361–366.

9. Korczak, D. J., Goldstein, B. I., & Levitt, A. J. (2007). Panic disorder, cardiac diagnosis and emergency department utilization in an epidemiologic community sample. *General Hospital Psychiatry, 29*(4), 335–339.

10. Sung, S. C., Rush, A. J., Ernest, A., Lim, L. E. C., Pek, M. P. P., Choi, J. M. F., Ng, M. P. K., & Ong, M. E. H. (2018). A brief interview to detect panic attacks and panic disorder in emergency department patients with cardiopulmonary complaints. *Journal of Psychiatric Practice, 24*, 32–44.

11. Deacon, B., Lickel, J., & Abramowitz, J. S. (2007). Medical utilization across the anxiety disorders. *Journal of Anxiety Disorders, 22*(2), 344–350.

12. Bryant, R. A., & Panasetis, P. (2001). Panic symptoms during trauma and acute stress disorder. *Behaviour Research and Therapy, 39*, 961–966.

13. Kessler, R. C., Sonnega, A., Bromet, E., Hughes, M., & Nelson, C. B. (1995). Posttraumatic stress disorder in the National Comorbidity Survey. *Archives of General Psychiatry, 52*, 1048–1060.

14. Fava, M., Rush, A. J., Alpert, J. E., Carmin, C. N., Balasubramani, G. K., Wisniewski, S. R., Trivedi, M. H., Biggs, M. M., & Shores-Wilson, K. (2006). What clinical and symptom features and comorbid disorders characterize outpatients with anxious major depressive disorder: A replication and extension. *The Canadian Journal of Psychiatry, 51*, 823–835.

15. Huppert, J. D., & Smith, T. E. (2005). Anxiety and schizophrenia: The interaction of subtypes of anxiety and psychotic symptoms. *CNS Spectrums, 10*, 721–731.

16. Hwang, T. J., Masterman, D. L., Ortiz, F., Fairbanks, L. A., & Cummings, J. L. (2004). Mild cognitive impairment is associated with characteristic neuropsychiatric symptoms. *Alzheimer Disease and Associated Disorders, 18*, 17–21.

17. Teri, L., Ferretti, L. E., Gibbons, L. E., Logsdon, R. G., McCurry, S. M., Kukull, W. A., McCormick, W. C., Bowen, J. D., & Larson, E. B. (1999). Anxiety of Alzheimer's disease. *The Journals of Gerontology. Series A, Biological Sciences and Medical Sciences, 54*, M348–M352.

18. Zarkowski, P., Pasic, J., Russo, J., & Roy-Byrne, P. (2007). Excessive tearfulness: Diagnostic sign for cocaine-induced depression. *Comprehensive Psychiatry, 48*, 252–256.

19. Teplin, L. A., Abram, K. M., & Michaels, S. K. (1989). Blood alcohol level among emergency room patients: A multivariate analysis. *Journal of Studies on Alcohol, 50*, 441–447.

20. Hillard, J. R., Slomowitz, J., & Levi, L. S. (1987). A retrospective study of adolescents' visits to a general hospital psychiatric emergency service. *The American Journal of Psychiatry, 144*, 432–436.

21. Tesar, G. E., & Rosenbaum, J. F. (1994). The anxious patient. In Hyman, S. E., & Tesar, G. E. (Eds.), *Manual of psychiatric emergencies* (pp. 129–142). Boston, MA: Little, Brown and Company.

22. Bolton, E. E., Mueser, K. T., & Rosenberg, S. D. (2006). Symptom correlations of posttraumatic stress disorder in clients with borderline personality disorder. *Comprehensive Psychiatry, 47*, 357–361.

23. Bomyea, J., Lang, A. J., Craske, M. G., Chavira, D., Sherbourne, C. D., Rose, R. D., Golinelli, D., Campbell-Sills, L., Welch, S. S., Sullivan, G., Bystritsky, A., Roy-Byrne, P., Murray, B., & Stein, M. B. (2013). Suicidal ideation and risk factors in primary care patients with anxiety disorders. *Psychiatry Research, 209*, 60–65.

24. Nepon, J., Belik, S. L., Bolton, J., & Sareen, J. (2010). The relationship between anxiety disorders and suicide attempts: Findings from the National Epidemiologic Survey on Alcohol and Related Conditions. *Depression and Anxiety, 27*(9), 791–798.

25. Goodwin, R., & Roy-Byrne, P. P. (2006). Panic and suicide ideation and suicide attempts: Results from the National Comorbidity Survey. *Depression and Anxiety, 23*, 124–132.

26. Sareen, J., Cox, B. J., Afifi, T., de Graaf, R., Asumndson, G. G., ten Have, M., & Stein, M. (2005). Anxiety disorders and risk for suicidal ideation and suicide attempts. *Archives of General Psychiatry, 62*, 1249–1257.

27. Schwartz, R. C., Wendling, H. M., & Guthrie, H. K. (2005). Examining anxiety as a predictor of homicidality. *Journal of Interpersonal Violence, 20*, 848–854.

28. Kroenke, K., Spitzer, R. L., Williams, J. B., Monahan, P. O., & Löwe, B. (2007). Anxiety disorders in primary care: Prevalence, impairment, comorbidity, and detection. *Annals of Internal Medicine, 146*, 317–325.

29. Merritt, T. C. (2000). Recognition and acute management of patients with panic attacks in the emergency department. *Emergency Medicine Clinics of North America, 18*, 289–300.

30. Dyckman, J. M., Rosenbaum, R. L., Hartmeyer, R. J., & Walter, L. J. (1999). Effects of psychological intervention on panic attack patients in the emergency department. *Psychosomatics, 40*, 422–427.

31. Guaiana, G., Barbui, C., & Cipriani, A. (2010). Hydroxyzine for generalized anxiety disorder. *The Cochrane Database of Systematic Reviews,* (12), CD006815.

32. Iskandar, J. W., Griffeth, B., & Rubio-Cespedes, C. (2011). Successful treatment with hydroxyzine of acute exacerbation of panic disorder in a healthy man: A case report. *The Primary Care Companion for CNS Disorders, 13*(3), PCC.10l01126.

33. Pitman, R. K., Sanders, K. M., Zusman, R. M., Healy, A. R., Cheema, F., & Lasko, N. B. (2002). Pilot study of secondary prevention of posttraumatic stress disorder with propranolol. *Biological Psychiatry, 51*, 189–192.

34. Argolo, F. C., Cavalcanti-Ribeiro, P., Netto, L. R., & Quarantini, L. C. (2015). Prevention of posttraumatic stress disorder with propranolol: A metaanalytic review. *Journal of Psychosomatic Research, 79*(2), 89–93.

35. Calabrese, J. R., Keck, P. E., Jr., Macfadden, W., Minkwitz, M., Ketter, T. A., Weisler, R. H., Cutler, A. J., McCoy, R., Wilson, E., & Mullen, J. (2005). A randomized, double-blind, placebo-controlled trial of quetiapine in the treatment of bipolar I or II depression. *American Journal of Psychiatry, 162*(7), 1351–1360.

36. Goddard, A. W., Mahmud, W., Medlock, C., Shin, Y.-W., & Shekhar, A. (2015). A controlled trial of quetiapine XR coadministration treatment of SSRI-resistant panic disorder. *Annals of General Psychiatry, 14*, 26–32.

37. Pollack, M. H., Matthews, J., & Scott, E. L. (1998). Gabapentin as a potential treatment for anxiety disorders. *The American Journal of Psychiatry, 155*, 992–993.

38. Verduin, M. L., McKay, S., & Brady, K. T. (2007). Gabapentin in comorbid anxiety and substance use. *The American Journal on Addictions, 16*, 142–143.

39. Wulsin, L. L. T., Storrow, A., Evans, S., Dewan, N., & Hamilton, C. (2002). A randomized, controlled trial of panic disorder treatment initiation in an emergency department chest pain center. *Annals of Emergency Medicine, 39*, 139–143.

40. Otto, M. W., Smits, J. A., & Reese, H. E. (2004). Cognitive-behavioral therapy for the treatment of anxiety disorders. *The Journal of Clinical Psychiatry, 65*(Suppl. 5), 34–41.

41. Swinson, R. P., Soulios, C., Cox, B. J., & Kuch, K. (1992). Brief treatment of emergency room patients with panic attacks. *The American Journal of Psychiatry, 149*, 944–946.

42. Kolbasovsky, A., Reich, L., Futterman, R., & Meyerkopf, N. (2007). Reducing the number of emergency department visits and costs associated with anxiety: A randomized controlled study. *The American Journal of Managed Care, 13*, 95–102.

43. Gao, K., Muzina, D., Gajwani, P., & Calabrese, J. R. (2006). Efficacy of typical and atypical antipsychotics for primary and comorbid anxiety symptoms or disorders: A review. *The Journal of Clinical Psychiatry, 67*, 1327–1340.

44. Grootens, K. P., & Verkes, R. J. (2005). Emerging evidence for the use of atypical antipsychotics in borderline personality disorder. *Pharmacopsychiatry, 38*, 20–23.

45. Pasic, J., Poeschla, B., Boynton, L., & Nejad, S. (2010). Cultural issues in emergency psychiatry: Focus on Muslim patients. *Primary Psychiatry, 17*(7), 37–43.

24

Delirium

Karen M. Lommel, Nicole S. Parrish, Benjamin T. Griffeth

Delirium is a complex, often reversible, but potentially lethal disorder that can occur in patients both young and old. Delirium often goes undetected by even skilled practitioners because of the waxing and waning nature of the illness. The patient can look very different at the time of the interview and physician examination in comparison to prior to arrival or just a few hours later after they leave the emergency department (ED) and return home with family. Given the fluctuations often seen in the mental status examination, it is necessary to obtain as much family collateral as possible early in the evaluation process to determine the patient's baseline cognition and functioning. After delirium has been recognized as the cause of the clinical presentation, clinicians must work quickly to treat the underlying etiology to prevent adverse outcomes, including death. This chapter will guide the reader through this complex condition by first providing the epidemiology and etiology of delirium followed by exploration of the disorder, starting with the clinical presentation of delirium and working through to diagnosis and treatment of the many causes of this complex disorder. The focus will remain on the role of the emergency psychiatrist in recognition of delirium and assisting emergency medicine providers in determining appropriate treatment and disposition of the patient.

EPIDEMIOLOGY AND OUTCOMES

Delirium is a common clinical syndrome of acutely altered consciousness with altered cognition presenting with a fluctuating course. It is present in 7% to 20% of patients presenting to EDs (1). It is considered a medical emergency because of the elevated rates of morbidity and mortality involved with the diagnosis. Rates of mortality range from a risk ratio of 1.95 to 4.91 based on the length of observation

following the diagnosis and the underlying medical conditions that led to delirium (2-5). Unfortunately, patients with longer periods of mechanical ventilation, prolonged intensive care units stays, and overall hospitalization are more likely to be discharged to nursing homes or other institutions (3-5).

ETIOLOGY

Delirium represents a brain dysfunction analogous to acute kidney injury. The dysfunction of an end-organ system, in this case the brain, is often due to illness or injury located elsewhere in the body. Delirium is more common in those with underlying brain compromise such as neurocognitive disorders. Although having a neurocognitive disorder, visual impairment, urinary catheterization, and low albumin levels are independently associated with delirium overall, multiple simultaneous etiologies are common (2).

The specific etiology of delirium remains unknown, but certain factors are common with all patients experiencing delirium. Diffuse cognitive impairments are seen with attentional deficits and disorientation, memory impairment, slowed or impaired executive function, and disturbance of the sleep-wake cycle. Electroencephalogram (EEG) findings support this global impact on the brain as noted by the ubiquitous finding of diffuse slowing including triphasic delta waves. Other causes of global change to oxygenation, glucose level, or physical arrangement of the brain have the greatest likelihood of initiating onset of delirium.

Several neurotransmitters have been implicated in the development and continuation of delirium. Acetylcholine reduction, whether due to anticholinergic drugs or due to decreased synthesis, as well as thiamine deficiency or hypoglycemia, commonly manifests as delirium. Studies of cerebrospinal fluid of patients with delirium consistently show alterations of endorphins, gamma-aminobutyric acid (GABA), norepinephrine, and serotonin among others (6). A closer look at possible causes and contributors to this disease will be explored when we examine how to create a differential diagnosis in suspected cases of delirium later in this chapter.

EVALUATION OF THE PATIENT

Delirium presents as an acute alteration in consciousness that is usually characterized by reduced awareness of the surrounding environment. This alteration in consciousness is accompanied with alterations of cognition. The Diagnostic and Statistical Manual of Mental Disorders, 5th Edition (DSM-V) describes delirium as a disturbance in attention and awareness that develops over a short period of time and is associated with cognitive deficits (6).

Associated clinical features can include psychomotor hyperactivity or hypoactivity, sleep-wake disruption, perceptual disturbance (illusions and hallucinations), and altered neurological function (autonomic instability, myoclonic jerking, and dysarthria) (7). EEG often shows diffuse slowing unless the delirium is related to alcohol or benzodiazepine withdrawal. Unfortunately, these various manifestations can be difficult to distinguish from other psychiatric illness, such as mania, schizophrenia, or neurocognitive disorders such as dementia.

Studies suggest that the majority of cases of delirium in the elderly are overlooked in the ED setting. Delirium can be missed quite often with some studies suggesting the maximum detection rate by the ED providers of cases of delirium across all patient age groups to be as low as 24% (1). Many emergency physicians are familiar with the "classic" form of delirium (hyperactive) but less aware of hypoactive or mixed presentation. The emergency physician needs to be an astute clinician and consultant to determine the presence of hypoactive delirium (often confused for severe depression or early catatonia). The DSM-V describes the following three subtypes of delirium

which demonstrate how differently patients may present (7).

- Hyperactive: These individuals may be agitated and refuse to cooperate with medical care.
- Hypoactive: These individuals may be sluggish and lethargic.
- Mixed level of activity: These individuals may have a normal level of psychomotor activity even though attention and awareness are disturbed. They may also have rapidly fluctuating activity levels.

The initial approach to assessing the delirious patient is much like any other patient assessment. The emergency physician may request early consultation for a patient with a known psychiatric illness prior to ruling out delirium. Each of these core areas of the assessment will yield clues to not only the presence of delirium, but to a possible underlying cause (3). After discussion with emergency medicine provider, the emergency psychiatrist should ask the following questions:

Do we know the patient's cognitive baseline?

Do we have a clear understanding of the events leading up to this moment?

Has this patient ever had anything like this happen before?

Are there new medications on board recently; or herbal medications/illicit substances?

As well known to the psychiatrist, The Mini-Mental Status Examination (MMSE) is currently the most widely used tool across medical specialties for this purpose. However review of the literature indicates that although it is a fast tool for the ED, the specificity is only 38% (1). Newer tools such as the DTS (Delirium Triage Screen) and RAS (Richmond Agitation and Sedation Scale) may be better tools. However, these have not been compared to the MMSE or each other in research trials as of yet (8). After one of these initial screening tools is utilized and the suspicion for delirium remains high, most providers in the ED use the CAM: Confusion Assessment Method or the bCAM: Brief Confusion Assessment Method. The CAM is currently the most common of the two, and according to several systematic reviews, it has a sensitivity of 93% to 100% and a specificity of 90% to 95% (9-11). The benefit of the CAM is that it only takes about 5 minutes to administer and bCAM takes as little as 2 minutes

TABLE 24.1 Comparing Delirium and Dementia

	Delirium	Dementia
Onset	Abrupt	Insidious
Course	Fluctuating	Slow decline
Duration	Hours-weeks	Months-years
Attention, orientation	Impaired	Impaired in later stages
Speech	Incoherent, rapid/slowed	Word finding difficulties
Thoughts	Disorganized, delusions	Impoverished
Perceptions	Hallucinations	Present in later stages

Reprinted from Han, J. H., Wilson, A., & Ely, E. W. (2010). Delirium in the older emergency department patient: a quiet epidemic. *Emergency Medicine Clinics of North America, 28*(3), 611–631. Copyright © 2010 Elsevier. With permission.

(11,12). The bCAM is based on the DSM-V criteria listed earlier in this Chapter. Vanderbilt University School of Medicine published a comprehensive guide with sample questions (13).

Another common reason for consultation in the ED is to distinguish between delirium and dementia. It is important to note before moving on that dementia, delirium, and psychotic disorders can mimic each other. Also, they can present at the same time in the same patient. In fact, dementia is a major risk factor for delirium. Understanding the difference between dementia and delirium is an important skill required of all providers (Table 24.1).

DIFFERENTIAL DIAGNOSIS

After the emergency physician and consulting psychiatrist have finished the medical workup with complicated delirium patients, the two teams may need to explore all potential diagnoses, although this can be difficult in the busy ED setting when additional critically ill patients need attention. Performing a large number of tests is often not helpful for these patients. The provider should focus initial tests as much as possible on the clues gained from the initial assessment (4). Typical initial testing includes complete blood count (CBC), comprehensive metabolic panel (CMP), blood alcohol, thyroid-stimulating hormone (TSH) (some delay in results), urine drug screen, urinalysis, pulse oxygen saturation, chest radiograph, electrocardiogram (ECG), and less often venous blood gas

(VBG)/arterial blood gas (ABG). Other common tests are rapid plasma reagin (RPR), vitamin B12, and folate. Lumbar punctures and head imaging have typically shown to be low yield, and the clinician must rely on their clinical judgment as stroke, meningitis, and subarachnoid hemorrhage can be hiding behind the altered patient's confused state (9). Remembering the categories in the differential diagnosis of delirium including infections, substances, toxins, environmental insults, metabolic disturbances and deficiencies among others (Table 24.2), will provide the emergency medicine provider with a starting point to ensure all etiologies are considered. The emergency psychiatrist should also review this list to ensure psychiatric illnesses are not confused for delirium and vice versa.

It is important to note that a careful review of medications may point to an underlying instigator of the mental status change particularly in the elderly patient. Even when the patient is unable to tell you their prescriptions/herbals/over-the-counter medications and a care provider is not present, it is still important to note the list of medications associated with delirium (Table 24.3) so that current orders are carefully screened and these medications are avoided in the patient moving forward.

TREATMENT RECOMMENDATIONS

Capacity to make decisions is a key consideration for the patient with delirium and can prove to be challenging in this setting as many patients

TABLE 24.2 Differential Diagnosis of Delirium

Infection	Sepsis, pneumonia, HIV
Metabolic	Acidosis, alkalosis, electrolyte disturbance, hepatic failure, renal failure, thyroid, hyper/hypoglycemia
CNS	Hemorrhage, hydrocephalus, infection, seizures, stroke, tumor, metastases
Vascular	Hypertensive encephalopathy, arrhythmia, shock
Environmental	Hypo/hyperthermia
Heavy metals	Lead, manganese, mercury
Deficiencies	Vitamin B12, folate, niacin, thiamine
Hypoxia	Anemia, CO poisoning, COPD, pulmonary/cardiac failure
Trauma	Closed-head injury, heat stroke
Medication/toxins/substance related	Medications, illicit drugs, pesticides, solvents Alcohol, sedative-hypnotic withdrawal

COPD, chronic obstructive pulmonary disease; CNS, central nervous system; HIV, human immunodeficiency virus.

TABLE 24.3 Medications Associated With Delirium

Class of Drugs	Examples (not all Inclusive)
Sedatives/hypnotics	Benzodiazepines Barbiturates Sleeping medications
Narcotics	All, but especially meperidine
Anticholinergics	Antihistamines (diphenhydramine, hydroxyzine) Antispasmodics Antidepressants (amitriptyline, imipramine, doxepin) Neuroleptics (chlorpromazine, haloperidol, thioridazine)
Incontinence	Oxybutynin Hyoscyamine Atropine/scopolamine
Cardiac	Digitalis Antiarrhythmic (quinidine, procainamide, lidocaine) Antihypertensive
Gastrointestinal	H2-blockers (cimetidine, ranitidine, famotidine) Proton pump inhibitors Metoclopramide Herbal remedies (valerian root, St John's Wort kava kava)

will not be able to communicate effectively, or at all, with the provider and staff. By the time the emergency psychiatrist has been called to evaluate the patient, the emergency medicine provider will have addressed any life-threatening needs. Next, the provider must attempt to establish contact with next of kin, caregivers, or guardians to obtain appropriate consent and information about do-not-resuscitate (DNR) status, power of attorney, living will, and advanced directives. The emergency psychiatrist is trained in determining capacity and can be a valuable asset to emergency medicine colleagues.

There are times when physical restraint or seclusion is required to ensure safety of the patient and the staff. The role of physical restraints continues to be a controversial topic both in the literature and in practice. The best approach is to initially use verbal de-escalation, removal of activating stimuli, offering food or drink, a blanket, or other measures. It is essential to refrain from arguing with respect to reality testing with someone who is delirious or suffering from dementia. When these measures fail, the team must decide on pharmacological and or physical restraint options. It is important to remember that the experience for the delirious patient is distressing for them and the family members. Research indicates that close to 54% of patients recall what happened to them while they were delirious (14).

The goal is to first identify reversible causes of delirium and begin treatment as soon as possible. For example, the provider can work to treat underlying infections with antibiotics, evaluate for pain and treat appropriately, and assess for dehydration and initiate fluid replacement. The American Psychiatric Association (APA) guidelines summarized several common underlying causes of delirium and how to treat them. The key causes include hypoglycemia, hypoxia, hyperthermia/hypothermia, severe hypertension, alcohol intoxication/withdrawal, anticholinergics, urinary tract infection, stroke, pain, and dehydration.

Research is limited on nonpharmacological treatments; however, in common practice, several key practices exist across specialties. Some of these tactics can be implemented in the ED, even during the shorter duration of time present (in comparison to the inpatient setting). However, never underestimate the power of even small interventions.

Limit the number of visitors at one time.

Limit the number of new providers/nursing/staff who enter the patient room when possible.

As much as possible in the ED setting, maintain a calm and quiet environment.

Encourage a normal wake-sleep cycle and proper sleep hygiene by turning off lights at night and turning on lights during the day.

Reorient the patient often. Utilize white board, clock, and personal items/family pictures.

Ensure the patient has hearing aids or glasses if they normally wear such devices.

Review of the literature indicates limited evidence for the use of nonpharmacological practices to treat delirium. However, the efficacy of some interventions in preventing delirium in patients has been documented (6,15). Other interventions to both treat and prevent delirium include staff education, utilization of geriatric assessments and consults, nutrition monitoring, mobilization, assessing bowel and bladder function, and cognitive tasks such as crossword puzzles (6,16). As unusual as it may seem, some of these tasks can distract a patient awaiting ED evaluation and decrease the need for more aggressive intervention.

PHARMACOLOGICAL TREATMENT OPTIONS

Current recommendations from the literature suggest that pharmacological management should be reserved for severe agitation, any time delirium interferes with medical management, and with severe psychotic symptoms (17,18). The APA practice guidelines for delirium have not been updated and are not considered current. Therefore, we need to turn to the literature for updated information on the treatment of delirium and the common mistaken entity of dementia-related psychosis.

There are no medications that are FDA approved at this time for the treatment of delirium. Historically haloperidol and benzodiazepines have been most utilized off-label. Options now include these, as well as, several atypical antipsychotics, dexmedetomidine, melatonin, and there is promising research in the works regarding the use of ketamine. The patients' comorbid medical and psychiatric conditions will guide the emergency psychiatrist in recommending and utilizing the best agent.

A black box warning has been issued by the FDA to educate providers and patients of the increased risk of death in the elderly population with dementia with the use of antipsychotic medications. Caution must be exercised with slow and low dosing and close monitoring of the patient. The APA guidelines recommend starting low and titrating as tolerated and only as needed to achieve clinical improvement regardless of the patient age or medication used (18). Table 24.4 illustrates several examples of antipsychotic medication choices and common dosages. As with all antipsychotics, the provider must monitor for extrapyramidal syndrome (EPS) such as dystonia, akathisia, and tardive dyskinesia. Many providers also review the baseline ECG to monitor for risk of QT prolongation.

It is perplexing that many of the medications used to treat delirium are also the same medications listed as causes and contributors to delirium. For example, benzodiazepines and haloperidol should be carefully considered with this in mind. After haloperidol, lorazepam is often the next medication recommended even by experienced clinicians when formulating the next step in treatment of the agitated patient. Research suggests that a faster-acting medication, dexmedetomidine, may be a better alternative to sedation with benzodiazepines (20-22). Dexmedetomidine is an alpha-2 agonist that has been shown to prevent and treat delirium in the ICU and could be utilized in the ED setting but would take significant coordination between the psychiatrist and the emergency physician. Future research of the use of dexmedetomidine in the ED should look to compare important endpoints between its use and the use of traditional antipsychotics and benzodiazepine. This is not to say that benzodiazepines should fall off the list of potential treatments at this point,

TABLE 24.4 Common Pharmacological Interventions

Medication	Typical Dosage and Usual Route of Administration
Antipsychotics	
Haldol (haloperidol)	0.5-2.0 mg twice daily Oral, IV, IM, SQ available
Risperdal (risperidone)	0.5-1 mg twice daily Oral
Seroquel (quetiapine)	25-50 mg twice daily Oral
Abilify (aripiprazole)	5-30 mg once daily Oral
Zyprexa (olanzapine)	2.5-5 mg once daily Oral
Benzodiazepines	
Ativan (lorazepam)	0.5-1.0 mg q4 hours PRN Orally

Compiled from American Psychiatric Association. (2013). *Diagnostic and statistical manual of mental disorders: DSM-5.* Arlington, VA: American Psychiatric Association; Breitbart, W., & Alici, T. (2008). Agitation and delirium at the end of life: "We couldn't manage him." *JAMA, 300*(24), 2898–2904; Kalish, V., Gillham, J., & Unwin, B. (2014). Delirium in older persons: Evaluation and management. *American Family Physician, 90*(3), 150–158; Neufeld, K., Yue, J., Robinson, T., Inouye, S., & Needham, D. (2016). Antipsychotics for prevention and treatment of delirium in hospitalized adults: A systematic review and meta-analysis. *Journal of the American Geriatric Society, 64*(4), 705–714.

especially given the fact alcohol and benzodiazepine withdrawal is an important underlying cause of delirium and is generally treated with benzodiazepine protocols such as The Clinical Institute Withdrawal Assessment for Alcohol (CIWA) to prevent seizures and death in these patients.

Patients with a vulnerable neurological state such as those with dementia or traumatic brain injury (TBI) are often prescribed melatonin or Ramelteon, a melatonin receptor agonist, in hospital settings as these medications promote improved sleep-wake cycles. There is evidence that Ramelteon may help prevent delirium in hospitalized patients (23,24).

Treatment of delirium with ketamine in the ED is a controversial area that still requires much research. Preliminary studies suggest that ketamine is a safe and appropriate option especially for difficult-to-treat cases, as well as for initial treatment for hyperactive delirium. It has been suggested that there may be a decreased rate of intubation in hyperactive delirium patients treated with ketamine than for those who only receive other pharmacological interventions (25). For now, literature suggests that most clinicians are not yet comfortable utilizing this medication for these patients and this medication should remain as a second- or third-line agent until further research is published.

CONCLUSION

Patients who develop delirium have increased rates of prolonged hospital stays, decreased quality of life and increased morbidity and mortality. It is essential for the emergency psychiatrist to work together with the emergency medicine providers to ensure delirium is not dismissed as a psychiatric disorder without exploring the potential for underlying reversible causes. It is especially important for the emergency psychiatrist to help guide the emergency medicine providers in correct diagnosis with documentation of the differences between delirium and true psychiatric disorder. More importantly, the emergency psychiatrist may be the only one with the expertise to determine when there may be a psychiatric condition with co-occurring delirium. The key to decreasing morbidity and mortality is to work closely with the emergency medicine team for early detection and treatment of delirium.

REFERENCES

1. Barron, E. A., & Holmes, J. (2012). Delirium within the emergency care setting, occurrence and detection: A systematic review. *Emergency Medicine Journal, 30*(4), 263–268.
2. Ahmed, S., Leurent, B., & Sampson, E. L. (2014). Risk factors for incident delirium among older people in acute hospital medical units: A systematic review and meta-analysis. *Age and Ageing, 43*(3), 326–333.
3. Salluh, J., Wang, H., Schneider, E., Nagaraja, N., Yenokyan, G., Damluji, A., et al. (2015). Outcome of delirium in critically ill patients: Systematic review and meta-analysis. *BMJ, 350*, h2538.
4. Shi, Q., Presutti, R., Selchen, D., & Saposnik, G. (2012). Delirium in acute stroke: A systematic review and meta-analysis. *Stroke, 43*(3), 645–649.
5. Witlox, J., Eurelings, L. S. M., Jonghe, J. F. M. D., Kalisvaart, K. J., Eikelenboom, P., & Gool, W. A. V. (2010). Delirium in elderly patients and the risk of post-discharge mortality, institutionalization, and dementia. *JAMA, 304*(4), 443.
6. Kaplan, H. I., Sadock, B. J., & Sadock, V. A. (2000). *Comprehensive textbook of psychiatry*. Philadelphia, PA: Lippincott Williams & Wilkins.
7. American Psychiatric Association. (2013). *Diagnostic and statistical manual of mental disorders: DSM-5*. Arlington, VA: American Psychiatric Association.
8. LaMantia, M., Messina, F., Hobgood, C. D., & Miller, D. (2014). Screening for delirium in the emergency department: A systematic review. *Annals of Emergency Medicine, 63*(5), 551–560.
9. Gower, L., Gatewood, M., & Kang, C. (2012). Emergency department management of delirium in the elderly. *The Western Journal of Emergency Medicine, 13*(2), 194–201.
10. Mariz, J., Castanho, T., Teixeira, J., Sousa, N., & Santos, N. (2016). Delirium diagnostic and screening instruments in the emergency department: An up-to-date systematic review. *Geriatrics, 1*, 22.
11. Wong, C., Holroyd-Ledue, J., Simel, D., & Straus, S. (2010). Does this patient have delirium? Value of bedside instruments. *JAMA, 779*(7), 786.
12. Tamune, H., & Yasugi, D. (2017). How we can identify patients with delirium in the emergency department. A review of available screening and diagnostic tools. *American Journal of Emergency Medicine, 35*, 1332–1334.
13. Han, J. H. (2015). *Brief confusion assessment method (bCAM) instruction manual (Version 1)*. Vanderbelt University School of Medicine.

14. Breitbart, W., & Alici, T. (2008). Agitation and delirium at the end of life: "We couldn't manage him." *JAMA, 300*(24), 2898–2904.

15. Abraha, I., Trotta, F., Rimland, J., Cruz-Jentoft, A., Lozano-Montoya, I., Soiza, R., et al. (2015). Efficacy of non-pharmacological interventions to prevent and treat delirium in older patients: A systematic overview. The SENATOR project ONTOP series. *PLOS One, 10*(6), 1–31.

16. Hshieh, T., Yue, J., Oh, E., Puelle, M., Dowal, S., Travison, T., & Inouye, S. (2015). Effectiveness of multicomponent nonpharmacological delirium interventions: A meta-analysis. *JAMA Internal Medicine, 154*(4), 512–520.

17. Kalish, V., Gillham, J., & Unwin, B. (2014). Delirium in older persons: Evaluation and management. *American Family Physician, 90*(3), 150–158.

18. Trzepacz, P., Breitbard, W., Franklin, J., Levenson, J., Martini, D., & Wang, P. (2010). *Practice guidelines for the treatment of patients with delirium*. Washington, D.C: American Psychiatric Association.

19. Neufeld, K., Yue, J., Robinson, T., Inouye, S., & Needham, D. (2016). Antipsychotics for prevention and treatment of delirium in hospitalized adults: A systematic review and meta-analysis. *Journal of the American Geriatric Society, 64*(4), 705–714.

20. Maldonado, J. R. (2017). Acute brain failure: Pathophysiology, diagnosis, management, and sequelae of delirium. *Critical Care Clinics, 33*(3), 461–519.

21. Carrasco, G., Baeza, N., Cabre, L., Portillo, E., Gimeno, G., Manzanedo, D., & Calizaya, M. (2016). Dexmedetomidine for the treatment of hyperactive delirium refractory to haloperidol in non-intubated ICU patients: A non-randomized controlled trial. *Critical Care Medicine, 44*, 1295–1306.

22. Pandharipande, P. P., Ely, E. W., Arora, R. C., Balas, M. C., Boustani, M. A., et al. (2017). The intensive care delirium research agenda: A multinational, inter-professional perspective. *Intensive Care Medicine, 43*(9), 1329–1339.

23. Hatta, K., Kishi, Y., Wada, K., Takeuchi, T., Odawara, T., Usui, C., & Nakamura, H. (2014). Preventive effects of ramelteon on delirium: A randomized placebo-controlled trial. *JAMA Psychiatry, 71*, 397–403.

24. Mo, Y., Scheer, C. E., & Abdallah, G. T. (2016). Emerging role of melatonin and melatonin receptor agonists in sleep and delirium in intensive care unit patients. *Journal of Intensive Care Medicine, 31*(7), 451–455.

25. Cole, J., Moore, J., Nystrom, P., Orozco, B., Stellpflug, S., Kornas, R., et al. (2016). A prospective study of ketamine versus haloperidol for severe prehospital agitation. *Clinical Toxicology, 54*(7), 556–562.

25

Neurocognitive Disorders

Marc E. Agronin

PRESENTING CLINICAL FEATURES

Individuals with neurocognitive disorders (NCDs) are ubiquitous across medical and psychiatric settings and will often be the focus of psychiatric consultation. The fifth edition of the Diagnostic and Statistical Manual of Mental Disorders (DSM-5) replaced the term "dementia" with "major neurocognitive disorder" and broadened the definition to characterize an underlying brain disease that impairs cognition in one or more of the following domains: complex attention, executive function, learning and memory, perceptual motor skills, language, and social cognition (1). At present, there are an estimated 5.7 million Americans with Alzheimer disease alone, representing the majority of all individuals with NCDs (2). Vascular dementia and dementia with Lewy bodies are the next most common forms of NCDs, followed by frontotemporal dementia and then various NCDs associated with medical disease, substance use, or trauma (3). For the majority of affected individuals, NCDs are both progressive and irreversible.

Psychiatric emergencies with NCD patients typically involve one or more of the following conditions: delirium, agitation, psychosis, suicidal ideation, or failure to thrive. Although each of these conditions may have multiple causes, it is the presence of the NCD that incurs the vulnerability. These emergencies can present in many settings, including at home or in a long-term care facility, emergency department (ED), or an inpatient unit. Regardless of the setting, family caregivers—typically an older spouse or an adult daughter—who have shouldered the burden of whatever factors are driving the emergency are often present. These caregivers are critically important informants as well as partners in treatment and should always be engaged. They can help reduce the complexity of care for the NCD patient to a few basic elements.

Delirium, which is covered in detail in Chapter 24, is defined as an acute, transient alteration in brain function characterized by fluctuating levels of consciousness, distractibility, psychosis, and agitation. It most commonly occurs in older patients with NCDs and presents as a psychiatric emergency because of the risk of self-harm or harm to others as well as the increased rate of mortality in both the acute and recovery phases (4). The cause of delirium is multifactorial, reflecting the influence of predisposing factors (eg, NCD, substance abuse) and noxious insults (eg, infection, medications, surgery, sleep deprivation) on a vulnerable individual whose function becomes overwhelmed (5). The prevalence of delirium ranges from 8% to 17% of elderly ED patients to upwards of 50% of elderly medical inpatients, especially in ICU settings and after cardiac or orthopedic surgeries (5). Individuals with delirium are unable to fully attend to or cooperate with daily care and may engage in impulsive and unsafe behaviors as they attempt to deal with what they perceive to be an unfamiliar and frightening environment.

Acute agitation and psychosis associated with NCDs pose psychiatric emergencies because of the risk of self-harm or harm to others, either from physically aggressive behaviors or refusal to comply with necessary medications, hygiene, medical treatments, or hydration and nutrition. Up to 80% of individuals with NCDs will demonstrate one or more behavioral and psychological symptoms, including but not limited to various forms of agitation and psychotic symptoms such as paranoid delusions or hallucinations (6). These two types of symptoms often go hand in hand, especially when paranoia breeds fear and anger toward caregivers. Resultant behaviors include refusal to accept care and aggression toward caregivers who are perceived as threats.

Late-life depression is both a risk factor for all-cause NCDs and a common comorbid condition and may involve acute suicidal ideation (7). In general, rates of suicide are highest in older white men, with the presence of psychosocial losses and chronic illnesses such as dementia being major risk factors (8). Refusal to eat, drink, take medications, or comply with other aspects of daily care (eg, necessary blood draws or glucose checks, wound care) can lead to precipitous weight loss and overall cachexia in a condition known as *failure to thrive*. Depression is the most common cause, and the refusal to eat or drink may represent an indirect suicidal or life-threatening behavior. Other causes for failure to thrive include delirium, paranoia, dysphagia, pain, and apathy. Failure to thrive is a psychiatric emergency because continued weight loss and the lack of adequate nutrition and hydration can quickly become life-threatening in a frail individual (9).

IMMEDIATE INTERVENTIONS

Although thorough assessment should always precede treatment, psychiatric emergencies in the NCD patient often require immediate interventions because of imminent risk of harm. For states of delirium, agitation, and suicidal ideation, one-to-one monitoring is necessary to keep individuals from physically harming themselves or someone else and to restrict their range of travel and avoid unsafe situations. When a cognitively impaired individual living in the community needs more intensive monitoring and management than the 24-hour presence of a caregiver can provide, transfer to either an ED or a psychiatric unit should be considered. In nursing home or hospital settings, a 24-hour sitter, preferably someone with psychiatric training, may be sufficient. Keep in mind that even in an intensive care unit with constant monitoring, a cognitively impaired and delirious person with agitation can quickly pull out a tracheostomy or nasogastric tube, catheter, or drain if not watched closely and appropriately medicated (10). An individual with failure to thrive might need immediate transfer to an appropriate setting where he or she can receive intravenous hydration and perhaps even a feeding tube.

In these acute situations, clinicians should first attempt to communicate with the NCD patient on his or her level, providing reassurance and reorientation to person, place, and time. To the best of their ability, clinicians should try to eliminate environmental stresses such as over-stimulating lights or sounds and address unmet needs such as hunger, thirst, bladder or bowel pressure, pain, anxiety, fear, and boredom that might be triggering or exacerbating the disruptive behaviors. Acute agitation sometimes responds to verbal or physical distraction, such as changing the subject of conversation or taking the person to a quieter or more stimulating location, depending on the nature of the situation. The patient's ability to understand and respond to this communication and behavioral redirection will determine the next steps: If he or she cannot exercise some control over the behaviors and the risk of harm persists, then more restrictive measures must be considered.

Physical restraints are used for highly agitated individuals whose movements pose an imminent risk of self-harm or harm to others and who have not responded to other interventions. These restraints take many forms, including soft hand mitts to prevent self-injury, a vest or other form of physical barrier while sitting in a chair, or a netted enclosure attached to and surrounding a bed. The least restrictive method is always preferred, with constant monitoring and for the least amount of time possible. The use of such restraints has actually decreased in long-term care settings over the last decade, as it has become apparent that they may not always provide the degree of safety intended and can even exacerbate agitation and paranoia (10).

Psychotropic medications are used for immediate intervention for highly agitated individuals but will not work quickly for symptoms of psychosis, suicidal thinking, or failure to thrive. The goal is to select an appropriate medication for the target symptoms, administer an adequate dose in a manner that will bring quick results (ie, intramuscularly or intravenously), and then monitor for therapeutic response and side effects. More detailed use of these medications, including dosing strategies, is reviewed in a later section of this chapter.

EVALUATION

In the evaluation of the NCD patient during a psychiatric emergency, several basic clinical facts need to be ascertained as quickly as possible: the patient's baseline cognitive and functional status prior to the crisis (including the stage of cognitive impairment, ranging from mild to severe), the exact nature of the emergent change, and whether there is an imminent risk of harm. Because many NCD patients are not able to provide extensive or accurate history, the evaluation will require knowledgeable informants. If the patient resides in an assisted or long-term care facility, it is important to review any available records, with specific attention to medical history, laboratory findings, recent injury, and medication use as listed on an updated medication administration record.

Establishing rapport with cognitively impaired patients can be challenging, especially when they are in a state of acute confusion, agitation, or psychosis or are severely withdrawn. There are several rules of thumb: Approach the patient calmly, provide a clear but brief orientation to the nature of the interview and your role in it and inquire as to his or her concerns or needs. Make eye contact, smile, and do not rush questions. Make sure that the patient can hear and see you and find ways to overcome sensory limitations (eg, ensure patients have glasses or hearing aids available, if possible). With an uncooperative patient, ask for his or her help and do not threaten. Even highly agitated, paranoid, and confused patients can sense an insensitive, impatient, or disrespectful approach.

Once the nature of the problem has been determined, all available history gathered, and an introduction made, the next step is to conduct a focused mental status examination (MSE) that includes a cognitive screen. The MSE should note aspects of appearance, alertness, attention and concentration, speech and language, affect, mood, thought process and content, motoric behavior, abstract thinking, insight, and judgment. The cognitive screen is a quick, easily administered, and scored instrument that gathers data on various cognitive skills. The most popular screens include the Mini-Mental Status Examination (11), the Mini-Cog (12), and the clock drawing test (13,14). If an acutely agitated or confused dementia patient is not able to cooperate with any of these screens, the MSE will be based on observation.

The remainder of the evaluation of the patient will vary depending on the nature of the psychiatric emergency. Obvious delirium requires simultaneous medical and psychiatric evaluation; although if the psychiatrist sees the patient first, he or she should obtain vital signs and order a urinalysis and culture, a complete blood count, a fingerstick glucose level, and a basic chemistry profile without waiting for the internist. An MRI or CT scan of the brain is necessary whenever there has been recent head injury or when there is suspicion of an intracranial process. For the agitated and psychotic patient, an immediate pain assessment is necessary, as well as a urinalysis with culture and sensitivity, and a survey of the care environment to identify potential causes. With all psychiatric emergencies, a review of concurrent medical conditions and recent medication use may help identify a culprit that is causing altered mental status or behavioral changes. Major medical conditions that can cause these conditions are listed in Table 25.1. Medications that are common causes of mental status or behavioral changes include opioid analgesics, steroids, psychostimulants, antihistamines, and anticholinergic agents.

The acutely suicidal patient is most often depressed, which can result from both psychosocial stresses (eg, a recent move, the loss of a spouse or caregiver) as well as organic illness (eg, stroke, hypothyroidism, chronic pain). Always determine whether there is a past history of a mood disorder, and if so, what treatments have worked in the past. Basic laboratory studies to rule out metabolic causes include electrolytes, calcium, thyroid, renal and liver function tests, a complete blood count, and vitamin B12, and folate levels. NCD patients with failure to thrive are typically either depressed or suffering from severe apathy (9). In addition to the workup described for depression, a more thorough neurologic evaluation that includes a brain scan may reveal an underlying organic cause for an apathy syndrome (15).

DIFFERENTIAL DIAGNOSIS

Although the psychiatric emergencies described in this chapter occur commonly in cognitively impaired patients, a clinician encountering anyone of them should not assume the presence of an NCD without sufficient evidence. After all, older delirious and depressed patients can appear transiently cognitively impaired even when they do not have an actual NCD. Major clinical differences between delirium and NCDs are described

TABLE 25.1 Medical Problems Commonly Associated With Agitation, Psychosis, and Delirium

Infection
Acute renal, hepatic, or thyroid dysfunction
Sensory impairment or loss (blindness, deafness)
Metabolic disturbances
Acute neurologic events
Acute cardiac events
Acute pulmonary events
Occult malignancies (especially in central nervous system)
Occult bone fracture
Postoperative state
Substance intoxication or withdrawal

From Agronin, M. (2014). *Alzheimer's disease and other dementias: A practical guide* (3rd ed.). New York, NY: Routledge. Copyright © 2014 Mark E Agronin. Reproduced by permission of Taylor and Francis Group, LLC.

in detail in Chapter 24, but the provider should keep in mind that when the two conditions occur simultaneously, the most important clinical feature is the time course. Delirium has an acute onset and a waxing and waning course, whereas most NCDs have an insidious onset and either a static or a progressive course. For delirium superimposed upon a NCD, the clinician should look for an acute change in cognition and function relative to the baseline degree of impairment.

Conditions that also involve both cognitive and functional impairment in late life include intellectual delay and chronic schizophrenia. In contrast to an NCD, intellectual delay presents from birth, whereas schizophrenia typically begins in young adulthood. Given their degree of chronic impairment, they are almost always well documented in older individuals. Both conditions can produce the same psychiatric emergencies as dementia and will involve similar approaches to evaluation and management.

MANAGEMENT

Given the mental and physical vulnerability of a typical patient with moderate to severe cognitive impairment, one of the first questions in any psychiatric emergency should be whether the patient can be managed in the current setting. On the one hand, it is always best to keep the person in the most familiar environment, with consistent caregivers and daily routines. Transfer to more intensive medical or psychiatric settings not only runs the risk of precipitating increased confusion but also carries with it the risk of nosocomial infections and other iatrogenic conditions. However, there are several circumstances in which hospitalization is necessary. Delirium always has an emergent medical cause and should be managed in a hospital setting when it first presents. Medical causes for agitation or psychosis, such as a urinary tract infection, can sometimes be managed in a less intensive setting, but that is typically the decision of the internist and not the psychiatrist. Any psychiatric emergency in the cognitively impaired patient that involves recurrent physically assaultive behaviors, suicidal threats or gestures, or complete refusal to eat or drink for more than 48 hours that is believed secondary to psychiatric illness (such as major depression) should prompt transfer to an inpatient psychiatry unit—preferably a geriatric unit if available.

Sometimes, recurrent psychiatric emergencies in cognitively impaired patients are products of an environment without sufficient monitoring or structure or with a caregiver who is impaired. In such situations, there may be unsafe living conditions, lack of stimulation, poor management of medications, neglect, or even abuse of the NCD patient. Caregiving for these individuals can become overwhelming for anyone, especially for an older spouse who may be suffering from physical disability, cognitive impairment, or depression (3). Even under ideal conditions, progressive NCDs require an increasing intensity of supervision and hands-on care to prevent or mitigate medical or psychiatric issues that can precipitate a psychiatric crisis. When the clinician suspects that any of these conditions exist, the NCD patient may be better served by being transferred from home to a more structured living environment, such as an assisted living or a long-term care facility, or from an open unit to a locked memory care unit within a facility.

PHARMACOLOGIC TREATMENT

The use of psychotropic medications is inevitable for the psychiatric emergencies described in this chapter, always subject to the following maxim: *start low, go slow, but go*. The goals of pharmacologic treatment of delirium, agitation, and psychosis are similar, involving the selection of a single agent that will rapidly calm the patient without causing excessive sedation or other side effects. Several commonly used medications and their dosing strategies are listed in Table 25.2. The choice may depend on what has worked well in the past for the patient, excluding agents that have not been tolerated or that carry a high risk of interacting with existing medications or medical conditions. Despite the possibility of side effects such as sedation, dizziness, extrapyramidal rigidity, and increased risk for falls, the overall risk of injury to self or others due to not treating the patient may be far greater. In some cases, the use of specific pharmacologic agents may constitute palliative care, weighing the pain and suffering of the psychiatric symptoms in an end-stage NCD against the risks of side effects.

For the patient with suicidal ideation or failure to thrive due to depression, transfer to an inpatient psychiatric unit is necessary to monitor the patient and to initiate a selected antidepressant medication—or to revise medications that are not working. Clinical improvement may begin in several weeks but often requires 6 to 8 weeks for full effect. Commonly used antidepressants and their dosing strategies are listed in Table 25.3 (3,16,17). Severe appetite loss in failure

to thrive may improve with antidepressant therapy if depression is the underlying cause. When appetite loss is caused by apathy, psychostimulants such as methylphenidate (18) or modafinil (19) might help improve feeding behavior. Three commonly used medications to improve appetite are mirtazapine (20), dronabinol (21), and megestrol acetate (22). With any agent, these patients require an evaluation for dental, chewing, and swallowing problems, in addition to repeated attempts to improve feeding and nutritional supplementation (9). Once the patient has improved somewhat in an inpatient setting, he or she may be able to be safely returned to the previous setting as long as adequate supervision of behaviors and ongoing medication response is provided.

Psychiatric emergencies in dementia patients that do not respond readily to the clinical approaches previously described often turn out to actually be *medical* emergencies. Consider the following vignette:

An 85-year-old male nursing home resident with recurrent assaultive behaviors was not responding to behavioral redirection or antipsychotic medications. A basic medical evaluation, including urinalysis, was unrevealing. He was subsequently sent to the emergency department for medical clearance en route to a psychiatric unit, where he was found to be in atrial fibrillation. Treatment of the arrhythmia led to resolution of the behavioral problems.

Thus, resistant symptoms should prompt repeat medical evaluation, including comprehensive lab tests, urinalysis, chest radiograph, electrocardiogram, and a brain scan.

Persistent agitation or psychosis without a clear etiology can be quite challenging to treat, especially when psychotropic medications either do not work or cause excess sedation or other unacceptable side effects. The situation is even more complicated in dementia with Lewy bodies (DLB), in which psychosis is common, but nearly 50% of patients demonstrate sensitivity to antipsychotic medications characterized by acute decline in cognition and function, increased extrapyramidal symptoms, reduced alertness and drowsiness, and a significant increase in mortality over time (3,23). Although atypical antipsychotics may have a lower propensity than conventional antipsychotics to cause these reactions in DLB,

TABLE 25.2 Medications for Psychiatric Emergencies[a]

Strategy 1: Benzodiazepine		
Lorazepam (Ativan)	0.5 or 1 mg PO or IM	
Repeat as necessary after 30-60 min. PRN dosing every 4-12 h.		
Strategy 2: Antipsychotic[b]		
Risperidone (Risperdal)	0.25 or 0.5 mg (tablet, elixir, or orally dissolving M-tab)	*or*
Olanzapine (Zyprexa)	2.5 or 5 mg (tablet, orally dissolving Zydis, or IM)	*or*
Quetiapine (Seroquel)	25 or 50 mg (tablet)	*or*
Aripiprazole (Abilify)	2-5 mg (tablet, oral solution, IM)	*or*
Haloperidol (Haldol)	0.5 or 1 mg (tablet, oral solution, IM, IV)	
Repeat doses as necessary after 30-60 min.		
Strategy 3: Combine benzodiazepine with antipsychotic		
For severe or resistant agitation		
Strategy 4: Alternative agent		
Trazodone (Desyrel)	50 or 100 mg tablet	
Repeat as necessary after 30-60 min.		
Medications to avoid		
Short-acting benzodiazepines (triazolam, midazolam), antihistamines (diphenhydramine, hydroxyzine), chloral hydrate, low-potency conventional antipsychotics (chlorpromazine, thioridazine), and narcotic analgesics due to risk of oversedation, dizziness, ataxia, falls, confusion, and paradoxical agitation		

Based on table from Agronin, M. (2014). *Alzheimer's disease and other dementias: A practical guide* (3rd ed., p. 174). New York, NY: Routledge.
[a]None of the medications listed in this table have an FDA indication for agitation or psychosis associated with dementia. Their recommended use is based on clinical experience and research studies.
[b]Clinicians should be mindful of FDA warnings about the potential increased risk of cerebrovascular adverse events as well as increased mortality in patients with dementia-related psychosis treated with atypical antipsychotic agents.
BID, twice daily; IM, intramuscular; IV, intravenous; mg, milligrams; PO, by mouth; PRN, as needed; QAM, in the morning; QHS, at bedtime.

they should still be used with great caution (24). In DLB as well as complicated cases of delirium, an alternate strategy is the use of acetylcholinesterase inhibitors such as donepezil, rivastigmine, or galantamine (3,4,25).

In many cases, clinicians will simply not have sufficient past medical or psychiatric history to guide them in an emergent situation, perhaps because records are not available or an informant cannot be reached. Although this will certainly hamper diagnosis, most of the treatment approaches described in this chapter are still viable options. However, ongoing treatment should be modified, if necessary, once additional history is obtained.

Management may be complicated by certain legal issues, including the following:
• It is not certain whether the patient has the capacity to participate in medical decision-making.
• The patient is refusing transfer to an ED or inpatient unit.
• The patient is refusing to cooperate with treatment.
• The patient is under guardianship, but the guardian cannot be reached immediately.
• The caregiver or guardian is objecting to treatment recommendations.

When there is an immediate safety issue, the decision of the clinician must trump all of these concerns, especially when involuntary hospitalization

TABLE 25.3 Dosing for Recommended Antidepressants in Dementia

Antidepressant	Starting Dose	Range (mg/d)
Selective serotonin reuptake inhibitors		
Fluoxetine (Prozac)	5-10 mg	10-40
Sertraline (Zoloft)	12.5-25 mg	25-200
Paroxetine (Paxil, Pexeva)	5-10 mg	10-40
Paroxetine (Paxil CR)	12.5 mg	12.5-50
Citalopram (Celexa)	5-10 mg	10-40
Escitalopram (Lexapro)	5 mg	5-20
Other antidepressants		
Bupropion (Wellbutrin)		
Immediate release	37.5 or 50 mg BID	75-300
Sustained release (SR)	100 mg	100-300
Extended release (XR)	150 mg	150-450
Mirtazapine (Remeron)	7.5 or 15 mg QHS	15-45
Venlafaxine (Effexor)		
Immediate release	25 mg BID	75-225
Extended release (XR)	37.5-75 mg	75-225
Desvenlafaxine (Pristiq)	50 mg	50
Duloxetine (Cymbalta)	20 or 30 mg	30-60

From Agronin, M. (2014). *Alzheimer's disease and other dementias: A practical guide* (3rd ed., p. 190). New York, NY: Routledge. Copyright © 2014 Mark E Agronin. Reproduced by permission of Taylor and Francis Group, LLC. BID, twice daily; mg, milligrams; QAM, in the morning; QHS, at bedtime.

appears mandatory. The legal issues can then be addressed once the situation is safer. Sometimes emergent legal interventions are needed, such as for a patient refusing all food and water. In end-stage disease, hospice care may be appropriate. Perhaps the most difficult situation occurs when a caregiver or guardian actively obstructs the treatment. In these cases, the clinician may need to appeal to a protective services agency or to legal counsel when the obstruction of treatment appears to constitute neglect or abuse of the patient.

REFERENCES

1. American Psychiatric Association. (2013). *Diagnostic and statistical manual of mental disorders* (5th ed.). Washington, DC: American Psychiatric Association.
2. Alzheimer's Association. (2018). 2018 Alzheimer's disease facts and figures. *Alzheimer's & Dementia, 14*(3), 367–429. Retrieved from https://www.alz.org/media/HomeOffice/Facts%20and%20Figures/facts-and-figures.pdf.
3. Agronin, M. E. (2014). *Alzheimer's disease and other dementias: A practical guide* (3rd ed.). New York, NY: Routledge.
4. Hshieh, T. T., Inouye, S., & Oh, E. S. (2018). Delirium in the elderly. *Psychiatric Clinics of North America, 41*(1), 1–17.
5. Inouye, S. K., Westendorp, R. G. J., & Saczynski, J. S. (2014). Delirium in elderly people. *Lancet, 383*(9920), 911–922.
6. Davies, S. J. C., Burhan, A. M., Kim, D., et al. (2018). Sequential drug treatment algorithm for agitation and aggression in Alzheimer's and mixed dementias. *Journal of Psychopharmacology, 32*(5), 509–523.
7. Diniz, B. S., Butters, M. A., Albert, S. M., et al. (2013). Late-life depression and risk of vascular dementia and Alzheimer's disease: Systematic review and meta-analysis of community-based cohort studies. *British Journal of Psychiatry, 202*(5), 329–335.
8. Van Orden, K., & Conwell, Y. (2011). Suicides in late life. *Current Psychiatry Reports, 13*(3), 234–241.

9. Kumeliauskas, L., Fruetel, K., & Holtoyd-Leduc, J. M. (2013). Evaluation of older adults hospitalized with a diagnosis of failure to thrive. *Canadian Geriatrics Journal, 16*(2), 49–53.

10. Burk, R. S., Grap, M. J., Munro, C. L., et al. (2014). Predictors of agitation in the adult critically ill. *American Journal of Critical Care, 23*(5), 414–423.

11. Folstein, M. F., Folstein, S. E., & McHugh, P. R. (1975). Mini-mental state: A practical method for grading the cognitive state of patients for the clinician. *Journal of Psychiatric Research, 12*, 189–198.

12. Borson, S., Scanlan, J., Brush, M., et al. (2000). The Mini-Cog: A cognitive "vital signs" measure for dementia screening in multi-lingual elderly. *International Journal of Geriatric Psychiatry, 15*, 1021–1027.

13. Nishiwaki, Y., Breeze, E., Smeeth, L., et al. (2004). Validity of the clock-drawing test as a screening tool for cognitive impairment in the elderly. *American Journal of Epidemiology, 160*(8), 797–807.

14. Palsetia, D., Prasad Rao, G., & Tiwari, S. C. (2018). The clock drawing test versus mini-mental status examination as a screening tool for dementia: A clinical comparison. *Indian Journal of Psychological Medicine, 40*(1), 1–10.

15. Orr, W. B. (2011). Executive dysfunction in the elderly: From apathy to agitation. In Agronin, M. E., & Maletta, G. J. (Eds.), *Principles and practice of geriatric psychiatry* (2nd ed., pp. 659–674). Philadelphia, PA: Wolters Kluwer/Lippincott Williams & Wilkins.

16. Borson, S., & Thompson, D. (2011). Major depression and related disorders. In Agronin, M. E., & Maletta, G. J. (Eds.), *Principles and practice of geriatric psychiatry* (2nd ed., pp. 405–421). Philadelphia, PA: Wolters Kluwer/Lippincott Williams & Wilkins.

17. Orgeta, V., Tabet, N., Nilforooshan, R., & Howard, R. (2017). Efficacy of antidepressants for depression in Alzheimer's disease: Systematic review and meta-analysis. *Journal of Alzheimer's Disease, 58*(3), 725–733.

18. Nelson, J. C. (2015). The role of stimulants in late-life depression. *American Journal of Psychiatry, 172*(6), 505–507.

19. Schillerstrom, J. E., & Seaman, J. S. (2002). Modafinil augmentation of mirtazapine in a failure-to-thrive geriatric inpatient. *The International Journal of Psychiatry in Medicine, 32*(4), 405–410.

20. Segers, K., & Surquin, M. (2014). Can mirtazapine counteract the weight loss associated with Alzheimer disease? A retrospective open-label study. *Alzheimer Disease and Associated Disorders, 28*(3), 291–293.

21. Badowski, M. E., & Yanful, P. K. (2018). Dronabinol oral solution in the management of anorexia and weight loss in AIDS and cancer. *Therapeutics and Clinical Risk Management, 14*, 643–651.

22. Ruiz-García, V., López-Briz, E., Carbonell-Sanchis, R., et al. (2018). Megestrol acetate for cachexia–anorexia syndrome. A systematic review. *Journal of Cachexia, Sarcopenia and Muscle, 9*(3), 444–452.

23. Mayo, M. C., & Bordelon, Y. (2014). Dementia with Lewy bodies. *Seminars in Neurology, 34*(2), 182–188.

24. McKeith, I. G. (2011). Dementia with Lewy bodies. In Agronin, M. E., & Maletta, G. J. (Eds.), *Principles and practice of geriatric psychiatry* (2nd ed., pp. 333–342). Philadelphia, PA: Wolters Kluwer/Lippincott Williams & Wilkins.

25. Tampi, R. R., Tampi, D. J., & Ghori, A. K. (2016). Acetylcholinesterase inhibitors for delirium in older adults. *American Journal of Alzheimer's Disease & Other Dementias, 31*(4), 305–310.

26

Substance Use, Intoxication and Withdrawal

James. N. Kimball, Kelley-Anne C. Klein

At 11:45 PM, a 25-year-old college student was escorted into the emergency department (ED) by several police officers. Police were called because the young man was running and screaming about the "second coming of Jesus Christ." In the ED, the patient was agitated, with pressured speech, flight of ideas, hyperreligiosity, and extreme mood lability. His blood alcohol level was 0.292 mg/dL, and his urine toxicology screen was positive for benzodiazepines and cocaine. Previous records revealed that the patient had a remote history of mania and panic disorder. Because of agitation, he required physical restraints. He was combative in the ED and was treated with intramuscular antipsychotics. Medical staff monitored his vital signs while he slept in the ED for 8 hours. He then awoke and was calm. A mental status examination at that time revealed no evidence of mania, psychosis, or further agitation. His psychiatrist had seen him on the morning before ED presentation and noted that the patient was "normal." The psychiatrist corroborated the fact that the patient had had no exacerbation of mood or anxiety disorder in more than 2 years. The patient's psychiatric symptoms had been well controlled on clonazepam and valproate. Upon further examination, the patient was neither suicidal nor homicidal and was willing to see his psychiatrist. "I just partied too much last night," the patient apologetically explained. The psychiatrist believed he could be released to the care of his parents, who assured the ED staff that they would watch him and take him to see his psychiatrist that afternoon. His psychiatrist agreed with the treatment plan, and the patient was discharged from the ED (1).

This is a typical presentation in a contemporary psychiatric emergency service (PES). Drugs and alcohol complicate the clinical picture, and these substances can influence acute behavioral change. For example, a normally calm, quiet individual can seem manic, delirious, psychotic, or violently agitated under the influence of drugs or alcohol. Therefore, clinicians must be knowledgeable of the effects of acute intoxication and the signs and symptoms of drug or alcohol abuse, dependence, or withdrawal states (1).

Individuals with substance use disorders (SUDs) regularly access emergency care, with nearly half of all drug-related visits in the United States attributed to drug misuse or abuse (2,3). EDs disproportionately provide medical care for individuals with SUDs, thus offering access to over 20 million Americans aged 12 years and older who meet criteria for an SUD (4). Addictive drug and alcohol use are more common among those individuals who also have a psychiatric disorder than in the general population. For example, the lifetime prevalence of alcohol use disorder (AUD) in bipolar disorder is estimated to be around 35% (5); the prevalence of SUDs is 25.1 % in schizophrenia (6). As such, it should be expected that clinicians seeing patients with psychiatric disorders in the ED should also recognize comorbid substance abuse in their evaluation of the psychiatric patient.

ALCOHOL INTOXICATION

Ethanol intoxication is common among patients requiring emergency care and has been increasing (7). However; intoxication is rarely the primary reason for acute presentation. In one study, ethanol was detected in 15% to 40% of unselected ED patients (8). Acute agitation in the setting of alcohol intoxication is commonly encountered in the ED (9). Signs and symptoms of acute ethanol

TABLE 26.1 Signs and Symptoms Of Alcohol Intoxication Vary By Individual, These Are the Most Common in Correlation With BAC.

BAC Range	Common signs and Symptoms
0.01%-0.10%	Euphoria and mild deficits in coordination, attention, and cognition
0.10%-0.20%	Greater deficits in coordination and psychomotor skills, decreased attention, ataxia, impaired judgment, slurred speech, and mood variability
0.20%-0.30%	Lack of coordination, incoherent thoughts, confusion, nausea, and vomiting
Greater than 0.30%	Stupor and loss of consciousness, possible coma, respiratory depression, or even death

BAC, blood alcohol content.

intoxication vary with severity and can include slurred speech, nystagmus, disinhibited behavior, incoordination, unsteady gait, memory impairment, stupor, or coma.

It is important to remember that a patient's clinical presentation may not directly correlate with his/her blood alcohol content (BAC). Those with chronic alcohol abuse may show greater functionality than those who are naïve to alcohol use. Among patients who do not abuse alcohol chronically, clinical signs most often associated with particular ranges of the BAC are as follows (Table 26.1).

Alcohol Withdrawal

Alcohol withdrawal syndromes (AWSs) are demonstrated in Table 26.2 (10). Acute reduction in serum alcohol concentration leads to symptoms that begin within 6 to 8 hours, peak at 72 hours, and diminish by days 5 to 7 of abstinence (11,12). Broad withdrawal signs and symptoms include insomnia, anxiety, nausea/vomiting, tremulousness, headache, diaphoresis, palpitations, increased body temperature, tachycardia, and hypertension (11,13). Patients taking beta-blockers or alpha-2 agonists may display blunted vital signs (14,15). If the patient's withdrawal does not progress, these withdrawal symptoms may resolve within 24 to 48 hours but more commonly 5 to 7 days (16). Severe withdrawals with seizures or delirium tremens (DTs) occur in approximately 5% of patients (11,13). Further sequelae of AWSs can be seen in Figure 26.1 (17).

Figure 26.2 shows neurotransmitter changes associated with alcohol withdrawal (17). DTs typically begins 3 days after the last drink and can last for days, but symptoms may occur quicker than that, including as quick as 8 hours after the last drink (10). Mortality of DTs can be up to 4%. DTs can be predicted by several factors, including history of previous DTs, recent withdrawal seizures, history of sustained drinking, systolic blood pressure over 150 mm Hg, age over 30 years, last drink >2 days, misuse of other medications such as benzodiazepines, and current medical illness (18–20). The "Prediction of Alcohol Withdrawal Severity Scale" (PAWSS) was recently developed and validated (21) and has been implemented at various institutions (22).

Patients who are in the initial withdrawal period are oriented and goal directed. Given that alcohol is a depressant, initial withdrawal symptoms can present as the opposite of a depressant—specifically anxiety and agitation. They may also have tremor, mild tachycardia, and sensory sensitivity. The goal for this initial withdrawal is to prevent withdrawal from progressing. As such, treatment should begin to prevent with possibility of withdrawal seizures or DTs. Blood alcohol level at presentation is not predictive of withdrawal seizures or DTs.

Alcohol withdrawal treatment is classically accomplished by the use of gamma-aminobutyric acid (GABA) agonists such as benzodiazepines. Research has shown that benzodiazepines are more effective than placebo in preventing withdrawal seizures. However, they were not shown to be superior to anticonvulsants or other agents (23).

Several benzodiazepines are available for the treatment of alcohol withdrawal. There is not a consensus of which benzodiazepines are preferred. Long half-life benzodiazepines, such as chlordiazepoxide

TABLE 26.2 Alcohol Withdrawal Syndromes

Syndrome	Timeline	Characteristics
Initial withdrawal symptoms	Begins 6-8 h after last drink	• Includes tachycardia, hypertension, increased body temperature, tremulousness, anxiety, nausea/vomiting, headache, diaphoresis, and palpitations
Alcohol hallucinations	12-24 h after last drink	• 7%-8% of patients with AWS • Tactile hallucinations common, visual less likely • Auditory hallucinations possible (sometimes persecutory) • May present with tremors and other withdrawal symptoms, though some do not • Normal sensorium
Withdrawal seizures	12-48 h after last drink	• Generalized tonic-clonic, though often isolated, short in duration, short postictal period • One-third of patients with withdrawal seizures will progress to delirium tremens
Delirium tremens	Begins 3 d after the appearance of withdrawal symptoms and lasts for 1-8 d	• Rapid-onset, fluctuating disturbance of attention, and cognition plus alcohol withdrawal symptoms • Diagnosis requires autonomic instability

AWS, alcohol withdrawal syndrome.
Reprinted from Long, B., & Koyfman, A. (2017). The emergency medicine management of severe alcohol withdrawal. *American Journal of Emergency Medicine, 35*(7), 1005–1011. Copyright © 2017 Elsevier. With permission.

or diazepam, have typically been used as they tend to relieve withdrawal signs and symptoms more consistently than benzodiazepines with a shorter half-life, such as lorazepam or oxazepam. However, longer half-life benzodiazepine metabolites can also accumulate, which can then lead to oversedation or delirium. As such, the medical history of the patient must be taken into consideration prior to using a benzodiazepine. For example, in patients with a head injury or concomitant ingestions, oversedation

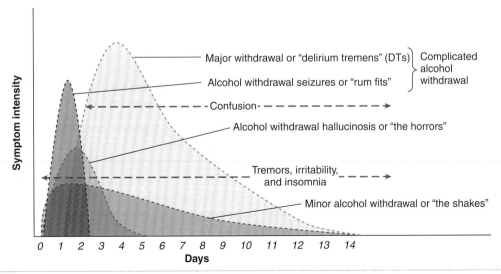

FIGURE 26.1 • Typical characteristics and timeline of unmedicated withdrawal course of alcohol dependent individuals. The timing and severity of these signs and symptoms vary by individual and level of dependency, though have a relatively predictable overall course.

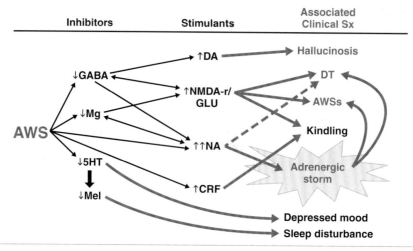

FIGURE 26.2 • Numerous neurotransmitter fluctuations are seen in the course of alcohol withdrawal. Most prominent is the decrease in inhibitors, and increase in stimulant neurotransmitters leading to the common clinical symptoms of withdrawal. AWS, alcohol withdrawal syndrome; AWSz, alcohol withdrawal seizures; CRF, corticotropin-releasing factor; DA, dopamine; DT, delirium tremens; GABA, gamma-aminobutyric acid; GLU, glutamate; Mg, magnesium; NA, noradrenaline or norepinephrine; NMDA, N-methyl-D-aspartate receptor.

would not be desirable. In patients with severe liver disease, a medication that is excreted via hepatic glucuronidation only such as oxazepam or lorazepam is preferred to one requiring hepatic oxidation and glucuronidation, such as chlordiazepoxide or diazepam.

There have been several different ways to treat alcohol withdrawal. One method is with a fixed schedule, in which the patient is giving a loading dose of a benzodiazepine and then gradually tapering doses of the next several days. It does appear that many clinicians now favor the symptoms-triggered approach, and some studies have shown that there was less need of pharmacological treatment duration and cumulative dosage of medication compared to the fixed-schedule protocol, potentially reducing costs and risk of adverse medication reactions (24,25).

The Clinical Institute Withdrawal Assessment for Alcohol—Revised is the most common accepted standard to help to facilitate the symptom-triggered approach. The scale contains 10 items that are typical in alcohol withdrawal, whose scores ranging from 0 to 67. Score over 9 indicate mild-moderate withdrawal; scores over 20 indicate severe withdrawal. Although this approach is more time consuming, patients can be rapidly stabilized without the risk of oversedation and receive

medication only when the situation requires it and not when their addiction demands it. Patients also remain alert and awake so they can speak with the provider about other options for treatment (26).

Although detoxification is typically performed in a residential or inpatient setting, it can be performed in the outpatient setting. Shaking, elevated pulse, increased blood pressure, agitation without progression to hallucinations are optimal patients to be treated as outpatients. In the outpatient setting, the patient who is undergoing withdrawal must be monitored by a person who is committed to staying with the patient throughout the detoxification process. In addition, daily physician visits are necessary until detoxification has been completed and the patient is medically stable (27).

Alternative Agents for Alcohol Withdrawal

There appears to be a subset of patients who may have benzodiazepine-resistant alcohol withdrawal (10). Benzodiazepines may also inhibit cognition, lead to delirium, increase alcohol cravings, and risk psychomotor retardation and ataxia (17).

Phenobarbital

Phenobarbital is efficacious in alcohol withdrawal management and has been shown to be an effective alternative to the standard-of-care protocol of symptom-triggered benzodiazepine therapy (28). Given that phenobarbital increases the duration of GABA-receptor opening and inhibits glutamate receptor activity, combined they oppose alcohol withdrawal effects (15). Phenobarbital has an onset of action at 5 minutes, has peaks at 20 to 30 minutes, and has an extremely long half-life of 3 to 4 days. The dosing cannot be easily titrated because of the long half-life, and unlike benzodiazepines, standardized dosing of phenobarbital for the treatment alcohol withdrawal does not exist (29). Combination therapy with benzodiazepines has also been noted to be effective (29).

Anticonvulsants

There is evidence that many of the anticonvulsants can have an effect on preventing and treating alcohol withdrawal, including carbamazepine, valproic acid, gabapentin, pregabalin, tiagabine, and vigabatrin. The mechanism by which these other agents exert their positive effects on the prevention and management of alcohol withdrawal symptoms is likely associated with their effects on glutamate and calcium channels. Nine randomized, controlled studies (n = 800) have demonstrated the effectiveness of carbamazepine in alcohol detoxification, compared with benzodiazepines; six randomized, controlled studies (n = 900 subjects) have demonstrated the effectiveness of valproic acid in alcohol detoxification when compared with benzodiazepines (17). Other agents have also shown promise, and one author notes: "anticonvulsants appear to be more effective against a larger range of withdrawal symptoms than benzodiazepines, especially among alcoholics with moderate to severe withdrawal symptoms" (30).

Alpha-2 Agonists

Alcohol withdrawal symptoms are characterized by a reduction in the inhibitory effects of GABA (disinhibition) and activation of the sympathetic nervous system (stimulation). The severity of alcohol withdrawal symptoms correlates positively with the amount of released norepinephrine. Excess norepinephrine activity may indeed drive the excess glutamate activity even further, contributing to agitation, psychosis, and even seizure activity. Given the current understanding of the effects of chronic alcohol use in the central nervous system and the effects of alcohol withdrawal symptoms in the catecholamine system, it makes sense to consider the potential use of alpha-2 agonists in the management of alcohol withdrawal symptoms. Seven double-blind, placebo-controlled trials demonstrate clonidine's utility in managing AWSs (17). When compared with benzodiazepines, subjects on clonidine experienced significantly lower mean withdrawal scores, significantly lower mean systolic blood pressure, and significantly lower mean heart rate, and subjects in the clonidine group experienced less anxiety and better cognitive recovery. In addition, clonidine provided better management of psychological symptoms (eg, anxiety, irritability, agitation) and central nervous system excitation (ie, seizures, DTs) associated with alcohol withdrawal. Animal data suggested that other alpha-2 agonists, such as guanfacine and dexmedetomidine, can be effective treatment of alcohol withdrawal (17).

Given the evidence with some of the alternative agents listed above, alcohol withdrawal protocols limiting the use of benzodiazepines are becoming more common.

BENZODIAZEPINE INTOXICATION

Oral benzodiazepines (BZDs), taken in overdose without a coingestant, rarely cause significant toxicity (31). Many patients with an isolated BZD overdose consist of central nervous system depression with normal vital signs. Many patients are able to provide an adequate history. Unfortunately, most intentional ingestions of BZDs involve a coingestant, the most common being ethanol (32).

Patients with a clinically apparent ingestion manifest slurred speech, ataxia, and altered (most commonly depressed) mental status. Respiratory compromise is uncommon with isolated oral ingestions but may be seen when patients ingest additional sedative hypnotic agents (such as ethanol) or opioids (32). The use of flumazenil is associated with a significantly increased risk of serious adverse events compared with placebo. Flumazenil should not be used routinely, and the harms and benefits should be considered carefully in every patient (33).

Benzodiazepine Withdrawal

The onset of withdrawal can vary according to the half-life of the BZD involved. Symptoms may be delayed up to 3 weeks in BZDs with long half-lives but may appear as early as 24 to 48 hours after cessation of BZDs with short half-lives. The severity and duration of withdrawal are determined by many factors, including the period of BZD use, how rapidly use was tapered (if at all), the pharmacokinetics of the particular drug, as well as possible genetic factors (33–35).

A number of medications have been used to treat BZD withdrawal, but none has been found to be as effective as BZDs. Beta-blockers, antipsychotics, selective serotonin reuptake inhibitors, and antihistamines have all been shown to be inferior to standard treatment. BZD withdrawal is treated with a BZD that has a prolonged clinical effect, such as diazepam, given intravenously and titrated to effect. The goal is to eliminate withdrawal symptoms without causing excessive sedation or respiratory depression (32,36,37).

OPIOIDS

Opioid use disorders have been increasing as of recent. Drug overdose is the leading cause of accidental death in the United States, with 52,404 lethal drug overdoses in 2015. Opioid addiction is driving this epidemic, with 20,101 overdose deaths related to prescription pain relievers and 12,990 overdose deaths related to heroin in 2015 (38). In fact, the director of the Centers for Disease Control and Prevention said in November 2018 that life expectancy in the United States is declining, driven by deaths from drug overdose and suicide (39). As such, providers in the ED need to have a keen awareness to recognize and treat opioid use disorders.

Opioid Intoxication

The signs of opioid intoxication vary between patients, dosing, and strength of the opiate used. In low doses or in those who use frequently, the most common symptoms may be drowsiness, mild confusion, and miosis. With larger doses, or in those with less tolerance to opiates, patients may exhibit severe confusion, stupor, or potentially fatal respiratory depression. Patients who present with opioid intoxication may be given the opioid antagonist naloxone to reverse life-threatening sedation with opioid overdose. However, clinicians need to be aware that naloxone has a half-life of about 1 hour, and with many opioids having longer half-lives, the patient after a small period of time can again lapse into life-threatening sedation.

Providers should also be aware of the interaction of comorbid benzodiazepine and opioid use. It has been well established that there are synergistic respiratory depressant effects when these benzodiazepines and opioids are combined (40), with an elevated risk of drug-related death previously observed among individuals receiving both opioids and benzodiazepines (41). Although naloxone is beneficial to reverse the effects of opioid overdose, there are no prospective human studies that asses how the co-use of benzodiazepines may alter the effectiveness of naloxone to reverse opioid overdose (42). Opioids are involved in approximately 75% of benzodiazepine overdose deaths, whereas benzodiazepines are involved in 31% of opioid overdose deaths (43). The increasing concurrent use of benzodiazepines and opioids is cited as a cause for increases in overdoses across the United States (44). One study noted that prescribing of opioids and benzodiazepines occurred across multiple locations in a large healthcare system to patients with a previous overdose, whereas another study funded by the Veterans' Administration noted that 82% of patients with an opioid overdose were subsequently prescribed opioids and 25% of those patients went on to have another overdose (45). Patients who abuse both opioids and benzodiazepines may be at higher risk for communicable diseases such as hepatitis C and human immunodeficiency virus (HIV) (42).

Of strong importance is the use of methadone. Methadone has a unique pharmacology, as it is absorbed by the stomach and is 36% to 100% (mean 75%) bioavailable, with a peak plasma concentration 2.5 to 4 hours post dose (46). Absorbed methadone quickly moves out of the blood compartment, where it can act on its target receptors, and into lipophilic tissues (alpha phase). An equilibrium of methadone concentration between the tissues and blood compartment is reached after saturation of lipophilic tissues, and the slow beta-phase of elimination begins, with a variable elimination half-life of 5 to 130 hours (average of

22 hours) (47). The risk of side effects, however, including respiratory depression, persists beyond this analgesic window (48). This author has personally taken care of a patient where the patient was abusing methadone and was suicidal with normal alertness and was admitted to an inpatient psychiatric unit, only to be found dead several hours later as a result of respiratory depression from methadone's pharmacology. Providers should also be aware that methadone can lead to QTc prolongation, potentially leading to torsades de pointes.

Opioid Withdrawal

Treating opioid use disorder is a multimodal process with interventions that occur in various healthcare settings. The ED serves as an essential transition point for opioid use disorder patients presenting with overdose, acute withdrawal, or associated medical complications (49). Motivational interviewing has been used to assist the patient in recognizing potentially harmful use, though evidence supporting the effectiveness of brief intervention in the ED setting to improve illicit drug–related outcomes is limited (3). Various nonopioid strategies have been tried to help patients with opioid withdrawal, including clonidine (50) as well as protocol of scheduled tizanidine, hydroxyzine, and gabapentin (51). However, initiating buprenorphine in the ED may decrease the acute withdrawal syndrome better than current symptom-based therapies, reduce illicit opioid use, and protect patients from opioid overdose (52–54). Although methadone and buprenorphine appear to have similar treatment success, the safety, ease of administration, and referral options of the latter may make it a better ED-based treatment (52,53). Perhaps most consequentially, initiating buprenorphine in the ED bridges patients to medication-assisted treatment, particularly if coordinated treatment follow-up is used (a "warm handoff") (55). Ideally, buprenorphine treatment initiation should not be delayed until the patient accesses a treatment program or requires an inpatient hospital admission (56). A 2015 randomized clinical trial of ED patients with opioid dependence found a significant increase in treatment engagement at 30 days for patients randomized to the brief intervention, buprenorphine-induction, and primary care

follow-up group (78%) in comparison to brief intervention and facilitated referral (45%) and referral to treatment (38%) (57). As such, many EDs are increasingly treating opioid withdrawal with buprenorphine and actively linking the ED patient with opioid use disorder to care by starting buprenorphine in the ED and referring to treatment (49). Evidence suggests that maintenance treatment with buprenorphine is more effective than detoxification (58). Of note, any prescriber can treat patients in an emergency setting with buprenorphine; a DATA 2000 waiver is only required for providers treating patients with opioid use disorders in the outpatient setting.

For patients who choose not to start on buprenorphine, emerging evidence on the effectiveness of overdose prevention education and community naloxone distributions to individuals likely to witness or experience an overdose laid the foundation for the integration of overdose prevention and naloxone distribution into EDs which provide care to particularly high-risk patient populations, including those with ED visits for nonfatal overdose (59–64). The US Surgeon General in 2018 in broadly supports clinicians to prescribe or dispense naloxone to individuals at risk of opioid overdose and their friends and family and "increase the awareness, possession and use of naloxone among at-risk populations and broader communities." (65).

COCAINE

Cocaine plays a significant role in drug-related ED visits. Data from the 2011 Drug Abuse Warning Network report showed that cocaine was involved in 505,224 of the nearly 1.3 million visits to EDs for drug misuse or abuse. This translates to more than one in three drug misuse or abuse-related ED visits (40%) that involved cocaine (66).

Cocaine has also become one of the primary drugs involved in drug-related ED deaths. According to the US Centers for Disease Control and Prevention, among the deaths attributed to drug overdose, cocaine, heroin, and opioid painkillers are the most common substances involved (67).

Cocaine increases alertness, feelings of well-being and euphoria, energy and motor activity, and feelings of competence and sexuality.

Its effects appear almost immediately after a single dose and disappear within a few minutes or an hour. Taken in small amounts, cocaine usually makes the user feel euphoric, energetic, talkative, and mentally alert, especially to the sensations of sight, sound, and touch. It can also temporarily decrease the need for food and sleep. A common pharmacokinetic-based issue is the increased risk when cocaine is taken in combination with alcohol. In most users, it produces more euphoria and possesses a longer duration of action than cocaine. Data suggest that it may be more cardiotoxic than cocaine and is associated with a greater risk of sudden death than with cocaine alone (68).

The short-term physiologic effects of cocaine use include constricted blood vessels and dilated pupils and increased body temperature, heart rate, and blood pressure. Large amounts of cocaine may intensify the user's high but can also lead to bizarre, erratic, and violent behavior. Some cocaine users report feelings of restlessness, irritability, anxiety, panic, and paranoia. Users may also experience tremors, vertigo, and muscle twitches (69).

The signs and symptoms of cocaine overdose are related to the psychological and stimulant effects of the drug. The use of cocaine causes tachyarrhythmia and a marked elevation of blood pressure, which can be life-threatening. This increase in blood pressure can lead to death from respiratory failure, stroke, cerebral hemorrhage, or heart failure. Cocaine also leads to increased body temperature, because the stimulation and increased muscular activity cause greater heat production. Heat loss is inhibited by the intense vasoconstriction. Cocaine-induced hyperthermia may cause muscle cell destruction and myoglobinuria, resulting in renal failure. The classic signs are hypertension, tachycardia, and tachypnea. This occurs with agitation, confusion, irritability, sweating, and hyperthermia. Sometimes seizures may occur.

Cocaine overdose can also present as a myocardial infarction with chest pain. This is thought to result from "spasm" of the coronary arteries that feed the heart muscle or from insufficient supply of blood flow to meet the needs of the stimulated heart muscle. Unfortunately, sudden death may also be the initial presentation to the ED; this is due to a lethal heart rhythm precipitated by cocaine consumption. It is important to avoid beta-blockers.

Cocaine overdose is treated as a medical emergency owing to the risk of cardiac toxicity. Physical cooling (ice, cold blankets, etc.) and acetaminophen may be used to treat hyperthermia, while specific treatments are then developed for any further complications. Sedation with agents such as diazepam is recommended for the agitation, irritability, seizures, and hyperexcitable state. This measure also helps to control the rapid heart rate and elevated blood pressure. Antipsychotics have also been used to help with agitation and psychosis (70).

Cocaine Withdrawal

Withdrawal symptoms are characterized by symptoms and signs that appear over a period of a few hours to several days after the cessation or reduction in heavy or prolonged use of cocaine. It consists of dysphoric mood and two or more of the following: fatigue, vivid and unpleasant dreams, insomnia or hypersomnia, increased appetite, and either psychomotor agitation or retardation. Cocaine craving and anhedonia are also present. Cocaine withdrawal peaks in 2 to 4 days with symptoms such as lowering of mood, fatigue, and general malaise lasting for several weeks.

Withdrawal from cocaine may not be as unstable as withdrawal from alcohol. However, withdrawal from any chronic substance abuse is very serious. There is a risk of suicide or overdose. Symptoms usually disappear over time. Individuals may benefit from anxiolytics and antidepressants. Almost one-half of all people who are addicted to cocaine also have a mental disorder (71). These conditions should be suspected and treated. When cocaine use disorder is diagnosed and treated, relapse rates are reduced dramatically.

MARIJUANA AND CANNABINOIDS

The physiologic effects of cannabinoid ingestion include dry mouth, red eyes, lowering of blood pressure, fine shakes or tremors, decreased body temperature, and decreases in muscle strength and balance. Respiratory effects include acute dilation of the bronchial tubes, decreased bronchial diameter, and worsening of breathing problems. Cardiac effects include increased heart rate and an increased cardiac workload, which may be associated with heart attacks. Urinary effects include increased urinary frequency. Gastrointestinal effects include decreased nausea/vomiting. (67).

The effects of cannabis on mood are variable. Mood effects include altered consciousness, mild euphoria, increased giddiness, increased and then decreased social interaction, and a decrease in feeling of anxiety or stress. However, some people report increased feeling of anxiety, depression, and panic symptoms with use of cannabis. Animal studies have shown that cannabis has a double-edge effect on mood, improving depressive symptoms at lower dosages and increasing depressive symptoms at higher dosages (71). A meta-analysis reviewing effects of cannabis and depression showed that heavy cannabis use increases the risk of patients developing depressive symptoms (72).

A meta-analysis of 267 studies showed that cannabis use is associated with increased anxiety (73). Cannabis-induced psychotic symptoms are of concern in the ED setting. Acute intoxication has been associated with increased suspiciousness, paranoia, derealization, lack of insight, and also increased anxiety. At very high doses, cannabis has been known to cause increased hallucinations and paranoid delusions. Some patients have also reported increased severe anxiety including increased panic symptoms during acute intoxication. Some patients experience increased aggressiveness with cannabis intoxication, although there are patients who report reduced aggression. During acute intoxication, the main concerns include cardiac risk factors associated with intoxication including arrhythmia (74).

Treatment should focus on managing presenting symptoms. If patients are agitated, benzodiazepines should be used to manage symptoms. If there are psychotic symptoms present, antipsychotics should be used to treat presenting symptoms. Charcoal has been reported to be helpful depending on the amount ingested (75). Intravenous fluid supplementation may also be needed.

Synthetic cannabinoids, colloquially referred to as "K2," "Spice," or "fake marijuana," are a class of recently developed designer drugs that contain chemical analogs of the psychoactive component of marijuana: tetrahydrocannabinol (THC) (76). The analogs of THC found in synthetic cannabinoid products act as full agonists at the same CB1 receptor, increasing the inhibition of GABA neurotransmission and therefore the severity of the psychoactive symptoms (77,78). Many synthetic cannabinoids have since become schedule I controlled substances. However, new synthetic derivatives are constantly created to avoid regulation and are rebranded and redistributed across the United States (78).

The most common symptoms with which patients present include tachycardia, agitation, diaphoresis, confusion, emesis, anxiety, headache, and dizziness (76,78). In more severe cases, patients may be in an almost semicatatonic state, unresponsive to verbal or painful stimuli with other physical signs and symptoms such as bradycardia, hypotension, renal failure, or severe secondary trauma. In most cases, the treatment for synthetic cannabinoid intoxication is supportive. Tachycardia should be treated with benzodiazepines and IV fluids, and an electrocardiogram should be performed to rule out myocardial ischemia and dysrhythmia. Benzodiazepines, such as lorazepam, starting with 2 to 4 mg and titrated to effect, can be used to treat agitation, catatonia, and anxiety (78). Patients presenting with psychosis and more severe psychological symptoms should be closely monitored and may be treated with antipsychotics if deemed necessary.

METHAMPHETMINE

Methamphetamine is a highly addictive methylated derivate of amphetamine (79). It is available in three main forms of increasing purity: powdered "speed," a yellow paste "base," and crystalline "ice" (80). Methamphetamine potentiates the release and blocks the reuptake of catecholamines, stimulating the sympathetic and central nervous systems (81). Acute poisoning is associated with a sympathomimetic toxidrome, which can vary from mild psychomotor agitation to severe toxicity with hyperthermic crisis, myocardial ischemia, arrhythmia, and intracerebral hemorrhage (79). Chronic use is associated with dependence, mental health conditions, including anxiety, depression, and psychosis, and societal dysfunction (82).

Crystal methamphetamine can induce psychotic symptoms in up to 40% of users (83,84). These commonly include auditory and tactile hallucinations, ideas of reference, and persecutory delusions. It may also precipitate or exacerbate a more enduring psychotic disorder in susceptible individuals. Methamphetamine use can also lead to symptoms of anxiety and mood disorders. Users can present in a highly agitated and aggressive state to EDs, often requiring immediate interventions (83).

During the acute intoxication, it may be difficult to take the medical history from the person affected. Therefore, information from a third party and consideration of the social environment of the patient are important for making a diagnosis. The possibility of methamphetamine intoxication should be considered in every patient presenting with diaphoresis, hyperthermia, hypertonia, tachycardia, severe agitation, or psychosis. Initially, the amount and type of substance (or substances) involved are mostly unknown. Hence, it is difficult to predict the clinical course. The management of any sympathoadrenergic syndrome including methamphetamine intoxication follows a syndrome-oriented approach. Monitoring the autonomic nervous system and psychopathological symptoms is crucial. A positive result from a qualitative urine test increases the probability of methamphetamine intoxication. However, a negative test cannot rule out life-threatening methamphetamine intoxication (85).

According to clinical experience, a quiet, protective space and talking down the patient are crucial. In the case of methamphetamine intoxication with severe agitation, aggressiveness, or psychotic symptoms requiring pharmacological treatment, benzodiazepines should be given as first-line medication. Fast-acting benzodiazepines are the first choice in the case of severe agitation, threatening or manifesting aggressive behavior toward the patient himself/herself or others, or psychotic symptoms. Sedation should not be so deep that the patient becomes unconscious. In most cases, no other medication apart from benzodiazepines is needed (85). In the case of methamphetamine intoxication, an additional medication with an antipsychotic may be considered if the administration of benzodiazepines is not sufficient.

In the case of hallucinations and delusions, it may be appropriate to administer an add-on antipsychotic medication. Based on clinical experience, second-generation antipsychotics such as olanzapine are the first choice. First-generation antipsychotics, such as butyrophenones (haloperidol), may be an alternative choice; however, they have a high risk for acute side effects (in particular acute dystonia) (85).

Once there is no further intake of methamphetamine, the ingested methamphetamine has been excreted and normal sleep patterns have been reestablished; psychotic symptoms from methamphetamine intoxication mostly ease within hours or 1 to 2 days. The need for continuation of antipsychotic medication should be reviewed continuously during the course of treatment of methamphetamine intoxication and at the latest after 3 days (85,86).

In regards to methamphetamine withdrawal, according to clinical experience, the need for treatment in methamphetamine-dependent users is similar to heroin and cocaine addicts. Withdrawal symptoms include craving, exhaustion, cognitive impairments, sleep disorders, irritability, agitation, depressive-anxious moods, and sometimes even suicidal ideation. Withdrawal symptoms may be very heavy for at least 1 week and somewhat milder for at least another 2 weeks. There is no evidence-based medication for the treatment of methamphetamine-related withdrawal symptoms and craving (85,87).

MDMA (ECSTASY)

MDMA (3,4-methylenedioxymethamphetamine) has stimulant and hallucinogenic properties, and intoxication typically results in elevated mood, empathy, and increased energy. Formulations contain varying and unknown quantities of MDMA and may contain other drugs, including amphetamines, ketamine, dextromethorphan, acetaminophen, and caffeine (88).

MDMA can independently cause serotonin syndrome, although the risk is higher if multiple drugs associated with serotonin syndrome are ingested, including amphetamines, cocaine, antidepressants, and opioids. Serotonin syndrome is characterized by altered mental status, increased muscle tone, clonus, hyperreflexia, and hyperthermia. Management of severe cases may include sedation, mechanical ventilation, rapid cooling, and pharmacologic paralysis (88,89).

Withdrawal syndrome from chronic MDMA use is related to serotonin depletion. Symptoms, including depression and fatigue, typically occur the day following use and can last up to 5 days (90).

CATHINONES

Cathinone derivatives (ie, bath salts) augment presynaptic concentrations of dopamine, norepinephrine, and serotonin by stimulating their release and antagonizing monoamine reuptake (91–93). Clinically, the effects of synthetic cathinones (bath salts) are similar to other stimulants with euphoria, increased attention, sexual arousal, tachycardia, and hypertension (92–94). After nasal insufflation and oral ingestion, effects are felt within 10 to 20 minutes and 15 to 45 minutes, respectively, and last 1 to 4 hours (94). There is a spectrum of associated toxicities reported from synthetic cathinone use. Psychiatric manifestations account for a large portion of individuals seeking medical care and include mild agitation to severe psychosis. Anxiety, paranoia, and suicidal ideation have also been reported. Additional effects include seizure, coma, tachycardia, hypertension, hyperthermia, shortness of breath, chest pain, acute kidney injury, blurred vision, rhabdomyolysis, hyponatremia, respiratory failure, and serotonin syndrome among others. Treatment of acute toxicity targets controlling agitation with benzodiazepines being the agents of choice (94,95). In controlling agitation, benzodiazepines may mitigate other toxicities such as hypertension and hyperthermia. The benzodiazepines often need frequent redosing to achieve adequate sedative effect, in which patients may ultimately require higher than normal doses (94). In rare cases where patients cannot be controlled with benzodiazepines alone, other sedatives such as propofol, barbiturates, and antipsychotics have been used (94,96–98). Severe ingestions can lead to serotonin syndrome, which has been effectively managed using benzodiazepines and cyproheptadine (99). Clinicians should also keep in mind other substances may be contributing to toxic effects. Vigilance for other coingestions is important, because polysubstance use with synthetic cathinones is particularly common. Repeated cathinone use, like methamphetamine, has shown to decrease dopaminergic transport, putting users at increased risk of parkinsonismlike symptoms and other neuropsychiatric disorders (100,101).

PIPERAZINES

Piperazine derivatives are rapidly becoming a popular class of designer drugs and are unique in the fact that they are entirely synthetic (102). They produce stimulant and hallucinogeniclike effects manifesting in euphoria, increased energy, and socialization (102–104). "Molly" is one of the more popular drugs in this class. Studies have evaluated the pharmacology of synthetic piperazines, finding them to centrally stimulate dopamine, serotonin, and norepinephrine release, as well as inhibit their reuptake (102,103,105). Effects are similar to amphetamine but 10 times weaker (102,103). At low doses, piperazines produce stimulant effects, whereas higher doses often result in hallucinations (106). Hypertension, tachycardia, euphoria, increased sociability, and feelings of self-confidence are experienced after use (107,108). Common neuropsychiatric effects include anxiety, confusion, paranoia, short temper, and auditory hallucinations (109). Symptoms are consistent with a sympathomimetic toxicity identified in acutely intoxicated patients. The toxidrome may include hyperthermia, diaphoresis, mydriasis, and tremors as well (110). Prolongation of the QT interval has also been reported (111).

Diagnosis and management is determined by the history obtained and clinical presentation. The sympathomimetic toxidrome associated with piperazine toxicity is managed in much the same way as the cathinones. General supportive measures should be initiated along with electrocardiogram and electrolyte monitoring (111,112). Antipsychotics are not recommended for severe agitation as they may impede the natural thermoregulation, cause extrapyramidal side effects, and induce hypotension or arrhythmias (113).

OTHER HALLUCINOGENS

25I-NBOMe is a designer hallucinogen with high affinity for or potency at 5HT-2a receptor, leading to its hallucinogenic properties. It additionally acts as an agonist on α-adrenergic receptors, causing sympathomimetic effects. It is available in preparations such as a vapor, intravenous, pill, and blotter. Duration of its effects may last 3 to 13 hours, whereas its toxicity may last for days. Intoxication with 25I-NBOMe resembles that of lysergic acid diethylamide (LSD) and psilocybin (114).

Intoxication of phencyclidine (PCP) may have other effects from classical hallucinogens. PCP was formerly used as an anesthetic before its popularity as a street drug. In differentiating this from other hallucinogens, PCP intoxication may produce nystagmus, hypesthesia, hyperacusis, or even coma with significant amounts of ingestion. Adrenergic symptoms occur in intoxication with PCP as well as other hallucinogens; however, the latter may involve other physical signs such as pupillary dilation, vision disturbance, diaphoresis, and tremors. Significant behavioral changes are noticed with intoxication and the signs and symptoms of intoxication are not secondary to another cause (114,115).

It is important to note that several other hallucinogens are gaining popularity. These hallucinogens fall into the category of "New World" tryptamine hallucinogens, and their use originated with the indigenous peoples of the Americas. In these communities the psychedelic plants are used for shamanic or ethnomedical practices (116). Although there are over 100 plants used for these purposes, the most likely to be used widely are Psilocybe mushrooms ("magic mushrooms") and Ayahuasca. Psilocybe mushrooms are consumed orally and historically have been used recreationally and explored for medical purposes, rather than for religious purpose (117). Ayahuasca is often used in shamanic training and is consumed as a beverage by both shamans and their patients. Although Ayahuasca has gained popularity in general culture, it was and is an important part of religious practices and under specific religious protectios is allowed to be consumed legally within the United States.

Some users of hallucinogens may experience other or persistent neuropsychiatric sequelae after episodes of ingestion. Hallucinogen-persisting perception disorder (HPPD) is a syndrome in which users will have continued perceptual symptoms that occurred during intoxication, and these symptoms lead to significant distress or impairment. Others may develop psychiatric disorders such as mood disturbance, anxiety, or psychosis, secondary to their hallucinogen use. In these instances, there are no other medical or psychiatric conditions that would better account for the symptoms (114).

Behavioral and supportive interventions are often best for patients intoxicated with hallucinogens, as noted in Table 26.3 (114). However, pharmacologic approaches for agitation and anxiety include use of benzodiazepines and use of haloperidol if benzodiazepines are not sufficient.

TABLE 26.3 Behavioral and Supportive Interventions for Intoxicated Patients

Reality testing: the "Talkdown"	Describes this as guiding the patient through his/her experience and using simple statements to aid in reality testing. Stating the patient's name or even labeling objects in the environment may provide reassurance.
Observation	A clinician or staff person should remain with the patient until the patient has "come down" from his/her "trip."
Environment	Creating a low stimulus environment—although too little stimulation might exacerbate the patient's distressed state.
Support	Offering emotional support and constant monitoring are also helpful for management.
Acuity	Hospitalization for psychotic or mood symptoms persisting longer than 24 h.

Reprinted from Hardaway, R., Schweitzer, J., & Suzuki, J. (2016). Hallucinogen use disorders. *Child and Adolescent Psychiatric Clinics of North America*, 25(3), 489–496. Copyright © 2016 Elsevier. With permission.

Given the α-2 antagonist properties and potential to lower the seizure threshold, use of some antipsychotics (eg, chlorpromazine) should be carefully considered. It is recommended to also remain cognizant of the patient's underlying medical comorbidities and presentation with medication management (118). In addition, agents may have a paradoxic effect or worsen HPPD symptoms (119,120).

MANAGEMENT OF THE ADDICTION

Screening, brief intervention, and referral to treatment (SBIRT) for substance use offer opportunities for early detection, motivational enhancement, and targeted encouragement to seek substance use treatment, when indicated. The hospital ED is an appealing setting for SBIRT, because these patients may have higher rates of substance use than community samples (121–123).

Motivational interviewing is a method for enhancing intrinsic motivation in order to change behavior. The principles of brief motivational interviewing (BMI) are (1) asking for permission to discuss alcohol use, (2) providing feedback on current drinking and consequences, (3) assessing readiness to change, and (4) providing options to help with behavioral changes and assisting in obtaining appointments or placements if desired (124). A recent Cochrane review concluded that motivational interviewing–focused interventions for adult substance users are efficacious, but it could not differentiate efficacy based on substance (125). BMI combined with booster sessions delivered following an ED visit have the unknown potential to help solidify the effects of SBIRT (126).

Certified peer recovery specialists, also known as "recovery coaches," provide experiential, nonclinical support to people living with SUD who are seeking recovery assistance. Peer recovery specialists have lived experience with addiction and recovery, allowing for guidance that may not be typically found in medical settings (127,128). Peer support groups typically exist as a component to addiction recovery programs and are found to be correlated to either a reduction in substance use (129) or increased addiction treatment adherence (130). The deployment of Peer Recovery Specialists in targeted settings, like that of EDs and in high-burden neighborhoods, to prevent future overdose is novel and widely viewed as an important tool to address the overdose epidemic (131). A recent study of an ED-based motivational brief intervention, delivered by a therapist and guided by computer, appeared to reduce drug use among adults seeking ED care compared with enhanced usual care (132).

Many hospitals are implementing pathways to enhance availability for maintenance treatments such as buprenorphine/naloxone for those who seek ED care. This is the result of a process referred to as "screening, treatment initiation, and referral" (STIR) (133).

DEALING WITH HIGH UTILIZERS

Many patients with SUDs frequent psychiatric EDs. Part of this is the failure of the medical system to provide good longitudinal follow-up, housing, and social services. This can lead to a lot of countertransference among the staff who are working with the patient. There may be the feeling of betrayal as well as the feeling if treatment is actually beneficial. Many have family or personal histories with substance abuse experiences that, on the one hand, may motivate them to work with this population and make them especially sensitive to the needs of substance abuse patients but, on the other, may impede their work if attendant countertransference issues are not adequately understood. The providers should seek supervision from other members of the team who can help to identify behavior that is influenced by countertransference, as making the unconscious conscious is the first step toward resolution of destructive countertransference (134).

SUMMARY

A large majority of patients (up to 60%) (135) presenting to PESs have a SUD, whether primary or part of a dual diagnosis with a mood or psychotic disorder. Effectively treating these patients can lead to significant reduction in morbidity and a concomitant improvement in psychosocial functioning, and as such, PESs can be the portal to recovery.

REFERENCES

1. Zealberg, J. J., & Brady, K. T. (1999). Substance abuse and emergency psychiatry. *Psychiatric Clinics of North America, 22*(4), 803–817.

2. The DAWN report. *Highlights of the 2010 Drug Abuse Warning Network (DAWN) findings on drug-related emergency department visits.* Retrieved from https://www.samhsa.gov/data/sites/default/files/DAWN096/DAWN096/SR096EDHighlights2010.htm.

3. Hawk, K., & D'Onofrio, G. (2018). Emergency department screening and interventions for substance use disorders. *Addiction Science & Clinical Practice, 13*(1), 18.

4. Substance Abuse and Mental Health Services Administration. (2017). *Key substance use and mental health indicators in the United States: Results from the 2016 National Survey on Drug Use and Health* (HHS Publication No. SMA 17-5044, NSDUH Series H-52). Rockville, MD: Center for Behavioral Health Statistics and Quality, Substance Abuse and Mental Health Services Administration.

5. Di Florio, A., Craddock, N., & van den Bree, M. (2014). Alcohol misuse in bipolar disorder. A systematic review and meta-analysis of comorbidity rates. *European Psychiatry, 29*(3), 117–124.

6. Nesvåg, R., Knudsen, G. P., Bakken, I. J., Høye, A., Ystrom, E., Surén, P., Reneflot, A., Stoltenberg, C., & Reichborn-Kjennerud, T. (2015). Substance use disorders in schizophrenia, bipolar disorder, and depressive illness: A registry-based study. *Social Psychiatry and Psychiatric Epidemiology, 50*(8), 1267–1276.

7. Mullins, P. M., Mazer-Amirshahi, M., & Pines, J. M. (2017). Alcohol-related visits to US emergency departments, 2001–2011. *Alcohol, 52*(1), 119–125.

8. Cherpitel, C. J. (1989). Breath analysis and self-reports as measures of alcohol-related emergency room admissions. *Journal of Studies on Alcohol, 50*(2), 155.

9. Pepa, P. A., Lee, K. C., Huynh, H. E., & Wilson, M. P. (2017). Safety of risperidone for acute agitation and alcohol intoxication in emergency department patients. *The Journal of Emergency Medicine, 53*(4), 530–535.

10. Long, B., & Koyfman, A. (2017). The emergency medicine management of severe alcohol withdrawal. *American Journal of Emergency Medicine, 35*(7), 1005–1011.

11. Kosten, T. R., & O'Connor, P. G. (2003). Management of drug and alcohol withdrawal. *The New England Journal of Medicine, 348*(18), 1786–1795.

12. Mainerova, B., Prasko, J., & Latalova, K. (2015). Alcohol withdrawal delirium – Diagnosis, course and treatment. *Biomedical Papers of the Medical Faculty of Palacký University, Olomouc, Czech Republic, 157*, 1–9.

13. American Psychiatric Association. (2013). *Diagnostic and statistical manual of mental disorders* (5th ed.). Washington, DC: American Psychiatric Publishing.

14. Schuckit, M. A. (2014). Recognition and management of withdrawal delirium (delirium tremens). *The New England Journal of Medicine, 371*(22), 2109–2113.

15. Schmidt, K. J., Doshi, M. R., Holzhausen, J. M., Natavio, A., Cadiz, M., & Winegardner, J. E. (2016). Treatment of severe alcohol withdrawal. *Annals of Pharmacotherapy, 50*(5), 389–401.

16. Etherington, J. M. (1996). Emergency management of acute alcohol problems: Part 1: Uncomplicated withdrawal. *Canadian Family Physician, 42*, 2186–2190.

17. Maldonado, J. R. (2017). Novel algorithms for the prophylaxis and management of alcohol withdrawal syndromes—beyond benzodiazepines. *Critical Care Clinics, 33*(3), 559–599.

18. Ferguson, J. A., Suelzer, C. J., Eckert, G. J., Zhou, X. H., & Dittus, R. S. (1996). Risk factors for delirium tremens development. *Journal of General Internal Medicine, 11*(7), 410.

19. Cushman, P., Jr. (1987). Delirium tremens. Update on an old disorder. *Postgraduate Medicine, 82*(5), 117.

20. Schuckit, M. A., Tipp, J. E., Reich, T., Hesselbrock, V. M., & Bucholz, K. K. (1995). The histories of withdrawal. Convulsions and delirium tremens in 1648 alcohol dependent subjects. *Addiction, 90*(10), 1335.

21. Maldonado, J. R., Sher, Y., Ashouri, J. F., Hills-Evans, K., Swendsen, H., Lolak, S., & Miller, A. C. (2014). The "prediction of alcohol withdrawal severity scale" (PAWSS): Systematic literature review and pilot study of a new scale for the prediction of complicated alcohol withdrawal syndrome. *Alcohol, 48*(4), 375–390.

22. Leung, J. G., Rakocevic, D. B., Allen, N. D., Handler, E. M., Perossa, B. A., Borreggine, K. L., Stark, A. L., Betcher, H. K., Hosker, D. K., Minton, B. A., Braus, B. R., Dierkhising, R. A., & Philbrick, K. L. (2018). Use of a gabapentin protocol for the management of alcohol withdrawal: A preliminary experience expanding from the consultation-liaison psychiatry service. *Psychosomatics, 59*(5), 496–505.

23. Schaefer, T. J., & Hafner, J. W. (2013). Are benzodiazepines effective for alcohol withdrawal? *Annals of Emergency Medicine, 62*, 34–35.

24. Skinner, R. T. (2014). Symptom-triggered vs. fixed-dosing management of alcohol withdrawal syndrome. *Medsurg Nursing, 23*(5), 307–315, 329.

25. Müller, U. J., Schuermann, F., Dobrowolny, H., Frodl, T., Bogerts, B., Mohr, S., & Steiner, J. (2016). Assessment of pharmacological treatment quality: Comparison of symptom-triggered vs. fixed-schedule alcohol withdrawal in practice. *Pharmacopsychiatry, 49*(5), 199–203.

26. Sullivan, J. T., Sykora, K., Schneiderman, J., Naranjo, C. A., & Sellers, E. M. (1989). Assessment of alcohol withdrawal: The revised clinical institute withdrawal assessment for alcohol scale (CIWA-Ar). *British Journal of Addiction, 84*(11), 1353–1357.

27. Prater, C. D., Miller, K. E., & Zylstra, R. G. (1999). Outpatient detoxification of the addicted or alcoholic patient. *American Family Physician, 60*(4), 1175–1183.

28. Tidwell, W. P., Thomas, T. L., Pouliot, J. D., Canonico, A. E., & Webber, A. J. (2018). Treatment of alcohol withdrawal syndrome: Phenobarbital vs CIWA-Ar protocol. *American Journal of Critical Care, 27*(6), 454–460.

29. Nelson, A. C., Kaucher, K. A., Sankoff, J., Mintzer, D., Taub, J., & Kehoe, J. (2018). Incorporating phenobarbital into your symptom-based benzodiazepine alcohol withdrawal protocol in the emergency department. *American Journal of Emergency Medicine, 36*(11), 2120–2212.

30. Ait-Daoud, N., Malcolm, R. J., & Johnson, B. A. (2006). An overview of medications for the treatment of alcohol withdrawal and alcohol dependence with an emphasis on the use of older and newer anticonvulsants. *Addictive Behaviors, 31*, 1628–1649.

31. Höjer, J., Baehrendtz, S., & Gustafsson, L. (1989). Benzodiazepine poisoning: Experience of 702 admissions to an intensive care unit during a 14-year period. *Journal of Internal Medicine, 226*(2), 117.

32. Greller, H., & Gupta, A. (2018). Benzodiazepine poisoning and withdrawal. In Grayzel, J., (Ed.), *UpToDate*. Waltham, MA: UpToDate Inc. Retrieved April 25, 2019, from https://www.uptodate.com.

33. Penninga, E. I., Graudal, N., Ladekarl, M. B., & Jürgens, G. (2016). Adverse events associated with flumazenil treatment for the management of suspected benzodiazepine intoxication – A systematic review with meta-analyses of randomised trials. *Basic & Clinical Pharmacology & Toxicology, 118*(1), 37–44.

34. Hood, H. M., Metten, P., Crabbe, J. C., & Buck, K. J. (2006). Fine mapping of a sedative-hypnotic drug withdrawal locus on mouse chromosome 11. *Genes, Brain and Behavior, 5*(1), 1.

35. Authier, N., Balayssac, D., Sautereau, M., Zangarelli, A., Courty, P., Somogyi, A. A., Vennat, B., Llorca, P. M., & Eschalier, A. (2009). Benzodiazepine dependence: Focus on withdrawal syndrome. *Annales Pharmaceutiques Françaises, 67*(6), 408.

36. Lader, M., Tylee, A., & Donoghue, J. (2009). Withdrawing benzodiazepines in primary care. *CNS Drugs, 23*(1), 19.

37. Parr, J. M., Kavanagh, D. J., Cahill, L., Mitchell, G., & McD Young, R. (2009). Effectiveness of current treatment approaches for benzodiazepine discontinuation: A meta-analysis. *Addiction, 104*(1), 13–24.

38. Rudd, R. A., Seth, P., David, F., & Scholl, L. (2016). Increases in drug and opioid-involved overdose deaths — United States, 2010–2015. *Morbidity and Mortality Weekly Report, 65*, 1445–1452.

39. *CDC Director's media statement on U.S. life expectancy*. Retrieved November 30, 2018, from https://www.cdc.gov/media/releases/2018/s1129-US-life-expectancy.html.

40. White, J. M., & Irvine, R. J. (1999). Mechanisms of fatal opioid overdose. *Addiction, 94*(7), 961–972.

41. Gomes, T., Mamdani, M. M., Dhalla, I. A., Paterson, J. M., & Juurlink, D. N. (2011). Opioid dose and drug-related mortality in patients with nonmalignant pain. *Archives of Internal Medicine, 171*(7), 686–691.

42. Jones, J. D., Mogali, S., & Comer, S. D. (2012). Polydrug abuse: A review of opioid and benzodiazepine combination use. *Drug and Alcohol Dependence, 125*(1–2), 8–18.

43. Jones, C., & McAninch, J. (2015). Emergency department visits and overdose deaths from combined use of opioids and benzodiazepines. *American Journal of Preventive Medicine, 49*, 493–501.

44. Griggs, C., Wyatt, S., Wally, M. K., Runyon, M., Hsu, J. R., Seymour, R. B., Beuhler, M., Bosse, M. J., Fogg, R., Gibbs, M., Haas, E., Jarrett, S., Leas, D., Saha, A., Schiro, S., Watling, B., & PRIMUM Group. (2019). Prescribing of opioids and benzodiazepines among patients with history of overdose. *Journal of Addiction Medicine, 13*(5), 396–402.

45. Boyle, J., Clement, C., Atherton, A., & Stock, C. (2017). A retrospective chart review of opioid prescribing following nonfatal overdose at a Veterans Affairs hospital. *Mental Health Clinician, 7*, 276–281.

46. Eap, C. B., Buclin, T., & Baumann, P. (2002). Interindividual variability of the clinical pharmacokinetics of methadone: Implications for the treatment of opioid dependence. *Clinical Pharmacokinetics, 41*, 1153–1193.

47. Barbosa Neto, J. O., Garcia, M. A., & Garcia, J. B. (2015). Revisiting methadone: Pharmacokinetics, pharmacodynamics and clinical indication. *Revista Dor, 16*, 60–66.

48. Sunilkumar, M. M., & Lockman, K. (2018). Practical pharmacology of methadone: A long-acting opioid. *Indian Journal of Palliative Care, 24*(Suppl. 1), S10–S14.

49. Love, J. S., Perrone, J., & Nelson, L. S. (2018). Should buprenorphine be administered to patients with opioid withdrawal in the emergency department? *Annals of Emergency Medicine, 72*(1), 26–28.

50. Fresquez-Chavez, K. R., & Fogger, S. (2015). Reduction of opiate withdrawal symptoms with use of clonidine in a county jail. *Journal of Correctional Health Care, 21*(1), 27–34.

51. Koch, J., Ward, S., & Thomas, C. J. (2018). Implementation and results of a symptom-triggered opioid withdrawal protocol at a Veterans Affairs medical center. *Mental Health Clinician, 7*(6), 282–286.

52. Sordo, L., Barrio, G., Bravo, M. J., et al. (2017). Mortality risk during and after opioid substitution treatment: Systematic review and meta-analysis of cohort studies. *BMJ, 357*, j1550.

53. Garcia-Portilla, M. P., Bobes-Bascaran, M. T., Bascaran, M. T., et al. (2014). Long term outcomes of pharmacological treatments for opioid dependence: Does methadone still lead the pack? *British Journal of Clinical Pharmacology, 77*, 272–284.

54. Mattick, R. P., Breen, C., Kimber, J., et al. (2014). Buprenorphine maintenance versus placebo or methadone maintenance for opioid dependence. *The Cochrane Database of Systematic Reviews*, (2), CD002207.

55. D'Onofrio, G., Chawarski, M. C., O'Connor, P. G., Pantalon, M. V., Busch, S. H., Owens, P. H., Hawk, K., Bernstein, S. L., & Fiellin, D. A. (2017). Emergency department–initiated buprenorphine for opioid dependence with continuation in primary care: Outcomes during and after intervention. *Journal of General Internal Medicine, 32*(6), 660–666.

56. Sigmon, S. C., Schwartz, R. P., & Higgins, S. T. (2017). Buprenorphine for persons on waiting lists for treatment for opioid dependence. *The New England Journal of Medicine, 376*, 1000–1001.

57. D'Onofrio, G., O'Connor, P. G., Pantalon, M. V., Chawarski, M. C., Busch, S. H., Owens, P. H., Bernstein, S. L., & Fiellin, D. A. (2015). Emergency department-initiated buprenorphine/naloxone treatment for opioid dependence: A randomized clinical trial. *JAMA, 313*(16), 1636–1644.

58. Kakko, J., Svanborg, K. D., Kreek, M. J., & Heilig, M. (2003). 1-year retention and social function after buprenorphine-assisted relapse prevention treatment for heroin dependence in Sweden: A randomised, placebo-controlled trial. *Lancet, 361*(9358), 662–668.

59. Walley, A. Y., Xuan, Z., Hackman, H. H., et al. (2013). Opioid overdose rates and implementation of overdose education and nasal naloxone distribution in Massachusetts: Interrupted time series analysis. *BMJ, 346*, f174.

60. McDonald, R., & Strang, J. (2016). Are take-home naloxone programmes effective? Systematic review utilizing application of the Bradford Hill criteria. *Addiction, 111*(7), 1177–1187.

61. Lagu, T., Anderson, B. J., & Stein, M. (2006). Overdoses among friends: Drug users are willing to administer naloxone to others. *Journal of Substance Abuse Treatment, 30*(2), 129–133.

62. Hawk, K. F., Vaca, F. E., & D'Onofrio, G. (2015). Reducing fatal opioid overdose: Prevention, treatment and harm reduction strategies. *Yale Journal of Biology and Medicine, 88*(3), 235.

63. Wheeler, E., Jones, T. S., Gilbert, M. K., & Davidson, P. J. (2015). Opioid overdose prevention programs providing naloxone to laypersons—United States, 2014. *Morbidity and Mortality Weekly Report, 64*(23), 631–635.

64. Seal, K. H., Thawley, R., Gee, L., et al. (2005). Naloxone distribution and cardiopulmonary resuscitation training for injection drug users to prevent heroin overdose death: A pilot intervention study. *Journal of Urban Health, 82*(2), 303–311.

65. Adams, J. M. (2018). Increasing naloxone awareness and use. *JAMA, 319*(20), 2073.

66. National Institute on Drug Abuse (NIDA). (2016). *Cocaine*. Retrieved December 2, 2018, from https://www.drugabuse.gov/publications/research-reports/cocaine.

67. Akerele, E., & Olupona, T. (2017). Drugs of abuse. *Psychiatric Clinics of North America, 40*(3), 501–517.

68. Jatlow, P., McCance, E. F., Bradberry, C. W., Elsworth, J. D., Taylor, J. R., & Roth, R. H. (1996). Alcohol plus cocaine: The whole is more than the sum of its parts. *Therapeutic Drug Monitoring, 18*(4), 460–464.

69. Akerele, E., & Nahar, N. (2016). Cocaine. In Mack, A. H., Brady, K. T., & Frances, R. J. (Eds.), *Clinical textbook of addictive disorders* (pp. 220–238). New York, NY: Guilford Publications.

70. Roncero, C., Ros-Cucurull, E., Palma-Álvarez, R. F., Abad, A. C., Fadeuilhe, C., Casas, M., & Grau-López, L. (2017). Inhaled loxapine for agitation in intoxicated patients: A case series. *Clinical Neuropharmacology, 40*(6), 281–285.

71. Falck, R. S., Wang, J., Siegal, H. A., & Carlson, R. G. (2004). The prevalence of psychiatric disorder among a community sample of crack cocaine users: An exploratory study with practical implications. *The Journal of Nervous and Mental Disease, 192*(7), 503–507.

72. Bambico, F. R., Katz, N., Debonnel, G., & Gobbi, G. (2007). Cannabinoids elicit antidepressant-like behavior and activate serotonergic neurons through the medial prefrontal cortex. *The Journal of Neuroscience, 27*(43), 11700–11711.

73. Lev-Ran, S., Roerecke, M., Le Foll, B., George, T. P., McKenzie, K., & Rehm, J. (2014). The association between cannabis use and depression: A systematic review and meta-analysis of longitudinal studies. *Psychological Medicine, 44*(4), 797–810.

74. Kedzior, K. K., & Laeber, L. T. (2014). A positive association between anxiety disorders and cannabis use or cannabis use disorders in the general population - A meta-analysis of 31 studies. *BMC Psychiatry, 14*, 136.

75. Campbell, C. T., Phillips, M. S., & Manasco, K. (2017). Cannabinoids in pediatrics. *The Journal of Pediatric Pharmacology and Therapeutics, 22*(3), 176–185.

76. Pourmand, A., Mazer-Amirshahi, M., Chistov, S., Li, A., & Park, M. (2018). Designer drugs: Review and implications for emergency management. *Human & Experimental Toxicology, 37*(1), 94–101.

77. Cass, D. K., Flores-Barrera, E., & Thomases, D. R. (2014). CB1 cannabinoid receptor stimulation during adolescence impairs the maturation of GABA function in the adult rat prefrontal cortex. *Molecular Psychiatry, 19*(5), 536.

78. Gurney, S. M., Scott, K. S., & Kacinko, S. L. (2014). Pharmacology, toxicology, and adverse effects of synthetic cannabinoid drugs. *Forensic Science Review, 26*(1), 53–78.

79. Schep, L. J., Slaughter, R. J., & Beasley, D. M. (2010). The clinical toxicology of metamfetamine. *Clinical Toxicology, 48*, 675–694.

80. Jones, R., Woods, C., & Usher, K. (2018). Rates and features of methamphetamine-related presentations to emergency departments: An integrative literature review. *Journal of Clinical Nursing, 27*, 2569–2582.

81. Gray, S. D., Fatovich, D. M., McCoubrie, D., & Daly, F. F. (2007). Amphetamine-related presentations to an inner-city tertiary emergency department: A prospective evaluation. *Medical Journal of Australia, 186*, 336–339.

82. Isoardi, K. Z., Ayles, S. F., Harris, K., Finch, C. J., & Page, C. B. (2019). Methamphetamine presentations to an emergency department: Management and complications. *Emergency Medicine Australasia, 31*(4), 593–599.

83. Unadkat, A., Subasinghe, S., Harvey, R. J., & Castle, D. J. (2019). Methamphetamine use in patients presenting to emergency departments and psychiatric inpatient facilities: What are the service implications? *Australasian Psychiatry, 27*(1), 14–17.

84. Glasner-Edwards, S., & Mooney, L. (2014). Methamphetamine psychosis: Epidemiology and management. *CNS Drugs, 28*, 1115–1126.

85. Wodarz, N., Krampe-Scheidler, A., Christ, M., Fleischmann, H., Looser, W., Schoett, K., Vilsmeier, F., Bothe, L., Schaefer, C., & Gouzoulis-Mayfrank, E. (2017). Evidence-based guidelines for the pharmacological management of acute methamphetamine-related disorders and toxicity. *Pharmacopsychiatry, 50*(3), 87–95.

86. Jenner, J., Spain, D., et al. (2006). *Management of patients with psychostimulant toxicity: Guidelines for emergency departments.* Canberra: Australian Government Department of Health and Ageing.

87. McGregor, C., Srisurapanont, M., Jittiwutikarn, J., et al. (2005). The nature, time course and severity of methamphetamine withdrawal. *Addiction, 100*, 1320–1329.

88. Armenian, P., Mamantov, T. M., Tsutaoka, B. T., Gerona, R. R., Silman, E. F., Wu, A. H., & Olson, K. R. (2013). Multiple MDMA (ecstasy) overdoses at a rave event: A case series. *Journal of Intensive Care Medicine, 28*(4), 252–258.

89. Davies, O., Batajoo-Shrestha, B., Sosa-Popoteur, J., & Olibrice, M. (2014). Full recovery after severe serotonin syndrome, severe rhabdomyolysis, multi-organ failure and disseminated intravascular coagulopathy from MDMA. *Heart & Lung, 43*(2), 117–119.

90. Donroe, J. H., & Tetrault, J. M. (2017). Substance use, intoxication, and withdrawal in the critical care setting. *Critical Care Clinics, 33*(3), 543–558.

91. Kersten, B. P., & McLaughlin, M. E. (2015). Toxicology and management of novel psychoactive drugs. *Journal of Pharmacy Practice, 28*(1), 50–65.

92. Simmler, L. D., Buser, T. A., & Schramm, Y. (2013). Pharmacological characterization of designer cathinones in vitro. *British Journal of Pharmacology, 168*(2), 458–470.

93. Prosser, J. M., & Nelson, L. S. (2012). The toxicology of bath salts: A review of synthetic cathinones. *Journal of Medical Toxicology, 8*(1), 33–42.

94. Warrick, B. J., Hill, M., Hekman, K., et al. (2013). A 9-state analysis of designer stimulant, "bath salt," hospital visits reported to poison control centers. *Annals of Emergency Medicine, 62*(3), 244–251.

95. Levine, M., Levitan, R., & Skolnik, A. (2013). Compartment syndrome after bath salts. *Annals of Emergency Medicine, 61*(4), 480–483.

96. Zawilska, J. B., & Wojcieszak, J. (2013). Designer cathinones—An emerging class of novel recreational drugs. *Forensic Science International, 231*(1–3), 42–53.

97. Coppola, M., & Mondola, R. (2012). Synthetic cathinones: Chemistry, pharmacology and toxicology of a new class of designer drugs of abuse marketed as "bath salts" or "plant food". *Toxicology Letters, 211*(2), 144–149.

98. Spiller, H. A., Ryan, M. L., & Weston, R. G. (2011). Clinical experience with and analytical confirmation of "bath salts" and "legal highs" (synthetic cathinones) in the United States. *Clinical Toxicology, 49*(6), 499–505.

99. Mugele, J., Nanagas, K. A., & Tormoehlen, L. M. (2012). Serotonin syndrome associated with MDPV use: A case report. *Annals of Emergency Medicine, 60*(1), 100–102.

100. McCann, U. D., Wong, D. F., & Yokoi, F. (1998). Reduced striatal dopamine transporter density in abstinent methamphetamine and methcathinone users: Evidence from positron emission tomography studies with [^{11}C]WIN-35,428. *The Journal of Neuroscience, 18*(20), 8417–8422.

101. Stepens, A., Logina, I., & Liguts, V. (2008). A parkinsonian syndrome in methcathinone users and the role of manganese. *The New England Journal of Medicine, 358*(10), 1009–1017.

102. Elliott, S. (2011). Current awareness of piperazines: Pharmacology and toxicology. *Drug Testing and Analysis, 3*(7–8), 430–438.

103. Mauer, H. H., Kraemer, T., & Springer, D. (2004). Chemistry, pharmacology, toxicology and hepatic metabolism of designer drugs of the amphetamine (ecstasy), piperazine, and pyrrolidinophenone types. *Therapeutic Drug Monitoring, 26*, 127–131.

104. Kalant, H. (2001). The pharmacology and toxicology of "ecstasy" (MDMA) and related drugs. *CMAJ, 165*(7), 917–928.

105. Fong, M. H., Garattini, S., & Caccia, S. (1982). 1-*m*-Chlorophenylpiperazine is an active metabolite common to the psychotropic drugs trazodone, etoperidone and mepiprazole. *Journal of Pharmacy and Pharmacology, 34*(10), 674–675.

106. Rosenbaum, C. D., Carreiro, S. P., & Babu, K. M. (2012). Here today, gone tomorrow... and back again? A review of herbal marijuana alternatives (K2, Spice), synthetic cathinones (bath salts), kratom, *Salvia divinorum*, methoxetamine, and piperazines. *Journal of Medical Toxicology, 8*(1), 15–32.

107. Lin, J. C., Bangs, N., & Lee, H. (2009). Determining the subjective and physiological effects of BZP on human females. *Psychopharmacology, 207*(3), 439–446.

108. Lin, J. C., Jan, R. K., & Lee, H. (2011). Determining the subjective and physiological effects of BZP combined with TFMPP in human males. *Psychopharmacology, 214*(3), 761–768.

109. Wilkins, C., Sweetsur, P., & Girling, M. (2008). Patterns of benzylpiperazine/trifluoromethylphenylpiperazine party pill use and adverse effects in a population sample of New Zealand. *Drug and Alcohol Review, 27*(6), 633–639.

110. Nicholson, T. C. (2006). Prevalence of use, epidemiology and toxicity of 'herbal party pills' among those presenting to the emergency department. *Emergency Medicine Australasia, 18*(2), 180–184.

111. Gee, P., Richardson, S., & Woltersdorf, W. (2005). Toxic effects of BZP-based herbal party pills in humans: A prospective study in Christchurch, New Zealand. *The New Zealand Medical Journal, 118*(1227), 1–10.

112. Durham, M. (2011). Ivory wave: The next mephedrone? *Emergency Medicine Journal, 28*(12), 1059–1060.

113. Arbo, M. D., Bastos, M. L., & Carmo, H. F. (2012). Piperazine compounds as drugs of abuse. *Drug and Alcohol Dependence, 122*(3), 174–185.

114. Hardaway, R., Schweitzer, J., & Suzuki, J. (2016). Hallucinogen use disorders. *Child and Adolescent Psychiatric Clinics of North America, 25*(3), 489–496.

115. American Psychiatric Association. (2013). *Diagnostic criteria from DSM-5.* Washington, DC: American Psychiatric Publishing.

116. McKenna, D., & Riba, J. (2018). New World tryptamine hallucinogens and the neuroscience of ayahuasca. In Halberstadt, A. L., Vollenweider, F. X., & Nichols, D. E. (Eds.), *Behavioral neurobiology of psychedelic drugs. Current topics in behavioral neurosciences* (Vol. 36, pp. 283–311). Berlin/Heidelberg: Springer.

117. Daniel, J., & Haberman, M. (2018). Clinical potential of psilocybin as a treatment for mental health conditions. *Mental Health Clinician, 7*(1), 24–28.

118. Tacke, U., & Ebert, M. H. (2005). Hallucinogens and phencyclidine. In Kranzler, H. R., & Ciraulo, D. A. (Eds.), *Clinical manual of addiction psychopharmacology* (pp. 211–241). Washington, DC: American Psychiatric Publishing.

119. Morehead, D. B. (1997). Exacerbation of hallucinogen-persisting perception disorder with risperidone. *Journal of Clinical Psychopharmacology, 17*(4), 327–328.

120. Strassman, R. J. (1984). Adverse reactions for psychedelic drugs: A review of the literature. *The Journal of Nervous and Mental Disease, 172*(10), 577–595.

121. Cherpitel, C. J., Bond, J., Ye, Y., Borges, G., MacDonald, S., Stockwell, T., Giesbrecht, N., & Cremonte, M. (2003). Alcohol-related injury in the ER: A cross-national meta-analysis from the Emergency Room Collaborative Alcohol Analysis Project (ERCAAP). *Journal of Studies on Alcohol, 64*, 641–649.

122. Fuda, K. K., & Immekus, R. (2006). Frequent users of Massachusetts emergency departments: A statewide analysis. *Annals of Emergency Medicine, 48*, 9–16.

123. Blow, F. C., Walton, M. A., Bohnert, A. S. B., Ignacio, R. V., Chermack, S., Cunningham, R. M., Booth, B. M., Ilgen, M., & Barry, K. L. (2017). A randomized controlled trial of brief interventions to reduce drug use among adults in a low-income urban emergency department: The HealthiER You study. *Addiction, 112*(8), 1395–1405.

124. D'Onofrio, G., & Degutis, L. C. (2002). Preventive care in the emergency department: Screening and brief intervention for alcohol problems in the emergency department: A systematic review. *Academic Emergency Medicine, 9*(6), 627–638.

125. Smedslund, G., Berg, R. C., Hammerstrøm, K. T., Steiro, A., Leiknes, K. A., Dahl, H. M., & Karlsen, K. (2011). Motivational interviewing for substance abuse [review]. *The Cochrane Library*, 1–128.

126. Longabaugh, R., Woolard, R. E., Nirenberg, T. D., Minugh, A. P., Becker, B., Clifford, P. R., Carty, K., Licsw, Sparadeo, F., & Gogineni, A. (2001). Evaluating the effects of a brief motivational intervention for injured drinkers in the emergency department. *Journal of Studies on Alcohol, 62*, 806–816.

127. Bassuk, E. L., Hanson, J., Greene, R. N., Richard, M., & Laudet, A. (2016). Peer-delivered recovery support services for addictions in the United States: A systematic review. *Journal of Substance Abuse Treatment, 63*, 1–9.

128. Reif, S., Braude, L., Lyman, D. R., Dougherty, R. H., Daniels, A. S., Ghose, S. S., Salim, O., & Delphin-Rittmon, M. E. (2014). Peer recovery support for individuals with substance use disorders: Assessing the evidence. *Psychiatric Services, 65*(7), 853–861.

129. Tracy, K., Burton, M., Miescher, A., Galanter, M., Babuscio, T., Frankforter, T., Nich, C., & Rounsaville, B. (2012). Mentorship for alcohol problems (MAP): A peer to peer modular intervention for outpatients. *Alcohol and Alcoholism, 47*(1), 42–47.

130. Huselid, R. F., Self, E. A., & Gutierres, S. E. (1991). Predictors of successful completion of a halfway-house program for chemically-dependent women. *American Journal of Drug and Alcohol Abuse, 17*(1), 89–101.

131. Formica, S. W., Apsler, R., Wilkins, L., Ruiz, S., Reilly, B., & Walley, A. Y. (2018). Post opioid overdose outreach by public health and public safety agencies: Exploration of emerging programs in Massachusetts. *International Journal of Drug Policy, 54*, 43–50.

132. Waye, K. M., Goyer, J., Dettor, D., Mahoney, L., Samuels, E. A., Yedinak, J. L., & Marshall, B. D. L. (2019). Implementing peer recovery services for overdose prevention in Rhode Island: An examination of two outreach-based approaches. *Addictive Behaviors, 89*, 85–91.

133. Bernstein, S. L., & D'Onofrio, G. (2017). Screening, treatment initiation, and referral for substance use disorders. *Addiction Science & Clinical Practice, 12*(1), 18.

134. Vannicelli, M. (2001). Leader dilemmas and countertransference considerations in group psychotherapy with substance abusers. *International Journal of Group Psychotherapy, 51*(1), 43–62.

135. Simpson, S. A., Joesch, J. M., West, I. I., & Pasic, J. (2014). Risk for physical restraint or seclusion in the psychiatric emergency service (PES). *General Hospital Psychiatry, 36*(1), 113–118.

27

Loss and Trauma

Janet S. Richmond

The views and opinions expressed are those of the author and do not necessarily reflect the official policy or position of the Veterans Health Administration.

Trauma and loss are intrinsic to the emergency department (ED). They represent either the aftermath of a catastrophic event or an event that may occur within the ED itself. Loss may be through death, but it may also be loss of one's sense of safety, security, and the belief in a "just world" (1,2).

Other losses are those of the spirit such as the loss of an ideal or a life's dream. The ED experience itself can be traumatic, reminding the patient of past traumas and losses, or it may be the setting where devastating news is delivered. This chapter will focus on both normative and traumatic loss and how acute and chronic states may present in the ED. As secondary or vicarious trauma is an occupational hazard for ED staff, it will also be discussed.

NORMAL GRIEF AND MOURNING

Grief is the circumscribed set of emotions that occur after notification of the death and in the following 2 to 4 weeks. Bereavement, the process of grieving, takes place over the months to a year after the death depending on religious and cultural norms. Grief elicits a series of predictable and painful emotions. Initially, the mourner may appear to be in shock or in actual denial, referring to the deceased as though they are still alive. The griever may be crying and inconsolable or angry and hostile, especially if they believe that negligence prompted the death. Resolution of grief can either lead to the deterioration of the person's psychological baseline or promote psychic growth (3,4). Case 27.1 exemplifies the complexities of normal grief reactions.

As the news of the death is absorbed, the numbed disbelief and shock are punctuated by acutely painful feelings of despair and emptiness, a deep pining and yearning for the deceased, and feelings of anger and rage. There may be a transient sense of worthlessness or a wish to die to join the deceased. Crying spells, anxiety, feelings of abandonment, and guilt over actions taken—or not taken—may occur. Somatic symptoms may occur with sensations of tightening in the throat, a choking sensation, and empty feelings in the abdomen whenever the deceased is mentioned (4-6). Sleep and appetite may be disturbed. It is useful to let the person know that intense emotions are normal and wash over the bereaved suddenly without warning and leave just as suddenly. Some bereaved people believe that they are "going crazy" from the intensity and suddenness of feelings; others believe that the lull between these intense emotional waves indicates that they are not properly mourning the deceased or are not giving proper honor to the magnitude of the loss. In those cases, people may have difficulty reintegrating into routine life, believing that any enjoyment is inappropriate.

Misperceptions and transient hallucinations may occur (4,6). The bereaved person may believe that they see the deceased or can hear the deceased's voice. They may mistake strangers on the street for the deceased. This is called "searching behavior" and while normative, these phenomena add to a person's belief that they are out of control.

There is also maddening indifference that the person encounters: while the mourner's world has completely changed, society functions as always without stopping to acknowledge the enormity of the loss. Cultural mourning rituals can help acknowledge this profound event.

Grief is not a medical illness, and bereavement is a normal response to loss (4,6,7). Thus, most bereaved persons do not come to the attention of clinicians. When these patients do present to the ED, psychoeducation helps the mourner predict the course of the bereavement and the vicissitudes of emotions it brings. Some people do not know how to mourn and need to learn how to do so. These people may have very limited or no experience with it or have had difficulty in the past. Thus, let the mourner know that there is no prescribed way to grieve, and that honoring one's dead does not mean stopping one's own life. As social supports are crucial to effective mourning, inquire about their supports. Some mourners find bereavement support groups comforting. Evaluate the mourner's resiliency prior to the death and their success at dealing with prior losses.

The bereaved need to tell their story, and the emergency service may be the place where people go for that. In Case 27.1, the patient began telling a complex, heartfelt story with little prompting.

Allow the patient to talk about the deceased and allow the emotions to be expressed. This can model for the patient that their feelings are not dangerous, can be contained, and do not lead to loss of control. When cultural and religious differences interfere with the expression and management of grief, consultation with chaplains can be very helpful, especially when they are a part of the ED team.

The role of medication for symptoms of grief is controversial. Many mourners report insomnia. Nonpharmacologic treatments such as education regarding sleep hygiene and cognitive behavioral interventions are recommended. The use of benzodiazepines is not advised because as in posttraumatic stress disorder (PTSD), they may interfere with learning and memory consolidation (8). The literature on the prescribing of medication is mainly among the elderly bereaved who have lost a spouse (9). There are no clear recommendations other than the possibility of selective serotonin

 CASE 27.1

Ms. Jones is a 45-year-old female who presents to the ED with a chief complaint of painful wrist after falling on ice. During her physical examination which was completely negative except for a sprained wrist, she stated that her husband had died 8 months ago in a fatal motor vehicle accident. The physician expressed sympathy and asked how she was handling the loss. The patient opened up unexpectedly. She stated that the first several weeks were "horrible." She was stunned and shocked when she heard the news. "I couldn't breathe when the hospital called me on the telephone." He died 2 hours after she and their two children arrived in the ED. The patient stated that initially she had had immense difficulty functioning. Family and friends brought food, her primary care physician prescribed zolpidem, and she had wrenching crying spells. "I felt disoriented and numb, and then suddenly I'd have a spasm of the most intense wrenching (emotional) pain I have ever experienced. I cried to the point of gasping for air. I tried to be stoic for my girls, but at the funeral, I collapsed in tears, I could hardly walk. I wanted to be buried with him. I went in and out of this kind of state.

When I went grocery shopping, I thought I saw my husband in the aisle in front of me, and I would run to that person, then was embarrassed when the stranger turned around and looked confused as to why I was calling them by the Frank's name. I still visualize his hands, and I imagine him holding me. Nights are hard. The children have returned to school and their activities. We talk about their Dad, but they're not always interested in talking. I understand, I guess at that age that's normal." She noted that initially she could only visualize her husband as he lay dying in the ED hospital stretcher, but more and more remembered him in different settings when he was well. Initially she could not look at pictures of him, but now she had a favorite picture of him with her and their two daughters sailing. She was able to "lose herself and be back on that boat," which gave her great comfort. She had a "rocky start" going back to work—"I couldn't get behind the wheel" but had a friend offer to drive with her a few times and she stopped feeling phobic about driving. "I'll never stop loving him; they say I'll be able to open my heart up to new people and new relationships, but I can't imagine that."

reuptake inhibitors (SSRIs) (10), but these agents are often impractical in the ED because of the need for follow-up. This author has noted anecdotal evidence that for temporary treatment of anxiety or insomnia, some ED clinicians are using limited dosages of hydroxyzine in place of benzodiazepines. Some clinicians prescribe limited supplies of benzodiazepines or soporifics such as eszopiclone, temazepam, zolpidem, or lorazepam, but there are no formal recommendations for the use of these agents. If they are used, a careful evaluation for a personal or family history of substance abuse is essential, as is educating the patient on the risks for addiction. The patient should be advised that this is a limited prescription and cautioned that the ED will not refill the prescription. If the patient continues to be symptomatic, they should follow up with their primary care physician who can arrange a psychiatric referral if necessary. This should all be written in the patient's discharge plan.

The ultimate goal of bereavement is to grieve the loss of the existing relationship and reestablish a new and different relationship with the loved one (4). Death does not have to end the relationship, but it does change it. Framing this for the patient is comforting and healing.

As seen with Ms. Jones, even uncomplicated acute grief causes significant disruption in all spheres of the person's life. Normal grief renders gut-wrenching pain. Withstanding that pain is the hallmark of uncomplicated grief. The goal of uncomplicated grief is not to avoid such feelings, but to garner the ability to tolerate them, return to normal functioning, and integrate the loss in a new and comforting direction. People need to know that intense feelings are normal, so that they are not blindsided by the intensity of feeling. They also need to know that these feelings are self-limited and part of the human condition. When these feelings are not self-limited and the mourner cannot integrate them into their psyche, then abnormal grief is present.

If a grieving person is seen in the ED, the provider's goal is to differentiate between normal grief and abnormal grief or other psychiatric pathology such as major depression. Normal grief calls for a supportive role, allowing painful emotions to be expressed, and psychoeducation on the grieving process. No referral for psychiatric care should be given.

As with all psychiatric presentations, mourners should also be evaluated for other psychiatric illness such as major depressive disorder, psychotic disorders, substance abuse, suicidal (11) or homicidal preoccupation, traumatic grief, or PTSD that may complicate their presentation and require referral for specialized psychiatric care. Abnormal grief may take several forms; identifying the exact one is not the goal of the ED but understanding how different types of grief may present helps the clinician distinguish between a normal versus abnormal response to the loss. Intense emotions, as described in the case above, are not an indicator of abnormal grief. For an instrument to determine impaired grief, Shear offers the Brief Grief Questionnaire (6).

IMPAIRED, COMPLICATED, OR TRAUMATIC GRIEF

Dysfunctional bereavements are referred to as either complicated, prolonged, delayed, or traumatic grief, the latter considered to be a variant of PTSD (4,5,7,12). Traumatic grief is more likely when there is a sudden, unplanned, particularly grotesque, or stigmatized death.

Table 27.1 summarizes the differences between normal and impaired/traumatic grief.

For example, if Ms. Jones from Case 27.1 reported repeated and haunting images of her dying husband and the inability to speak about him without intense pain even after 8 months, she would be experiencing symptoms of traumatic grief. If she reported decreased functioning (inability to return to work or decreased job performance) difficulty parenting, unexplained somatic symptoms, persistent insomnia, and/or social isolation, she would be suffering from complicated or prolonged grief. If she reported autonomous neurovegetative symptoms, she would be experiencing a major depressive episode. All three may be combined, making the diagnosis difficult to discern. Table 27.2 summarizes risk factors for the development of complicated grief.

Bereaved persons, especially those with complicated bereavement, have increased morbidity. The elderly, particularly those with complicated grief, are at higher risk for mortality, including suicide (14). The stress of both complicated and uncomplicated grief can lead to catecholamine

TABLE 27.1 Signs and Symptoms of Normal Versus Impaired/Traumatic Grief

Symptom Response	Bereavement	Impaired/Traumatic Grief
Thinking or talking about the deceased	Comforting recollections; encourages conversation about deceased	Painful, wrenching sadness, and despair Intrusive, unwanted thoughts of the deceased[a] Avoidance of thinking about the deceased[a]
Mood	Feelings of sadness or anger; pining and yearning which decrease in intensity	Horror[a], terror[a], fear, anger; persistent pining and yearning
Social functioning (work, family, friends)	Returns to normal	Prolonged impairment, social isolation, decreased activities, refusing or avoiding social gatherings such as invitations to dinner
Appetite	Returns to normal	Prolonged anorexia, weight loss, decreased taste or pleasure in eating, swallowing and gastrointestinal complaints (difficulty swallowing, nausea)
Cognition	Initial decreased attention and concentration returns to normal	Persistent attention and concentration complaints
Sleep	Initial insomnia Pleasant dreams of the deceased	Sustained impairment Grotesque or terrifying nightmares[a]
Sense of future	Future oriented	Sense of foreshortened future; belief that one cannot go on without deceased[a]
Suicidal ideation	Transient wish to join the deceased	Suicidal thoughts
Anger and guilt	Transient, nonpervasive	Persistent and may be independent of thoughts of deceased (eg, accompanying signs/symptoms of an autonomous clinical depression); these feelings onto others, eg, may be angry at medical providers for perceived medical errors or family for not caring, etc.
Relationship with the deceased	Integrates the loss and establishes a new relationship with the deceased	Clinging to the deceased in a wish to keep him alive

[a]denotes specific signs of traumatic grief.

and cortisol surges and subsequent hypertension, elevated heart rate, and changes in the immune system. The bereaved are uniquely at risk for takotsubo cardiomyopathy (broken heart syndrome) (6).

Thus, for patients who present to the ED with unexplainable physical complaints and new or worsening psychiatric symptoms, an inquiry into recent loss or trauma is indicated. Inquire about the deceased's medical issues and physical state prior to death. If there is a similarity in symptom presentation, gently ask the patient what they make of that. They may see no connection or may find relief with that revelation.

TABLE 27.2 Risk Factors for the Development of Complicated Grief

- Age and gender (females over 60 years old (6), children, and adolescents)
- A past or current history of psychiatric illnesses
- A history of multiple losses or traumas
- A loss that has occurred through traumatic or otherwise sudden, unanticipated, or societally stigmatized death (eg, suicide, murder)
- Out-of-phase deaths such as the death of a child or death of a child or adolescent's parent is considered a risk factor (6,11)
- High degree of dependency on the deceased prior to death (13)

TRAUMA

A traumatic event is a uniquely solitary experience, even when others are experiencing the same event at the same time (15-19). That existential awareness can be quite troubling. As noted above, it can shatter one's sense of safety and the belief that the world is safe and predictable. There is a lost innocence (1,19).

Psychological trauma is defined as a witnessed or experienced event or series of events involving actual or threatened death, serious injury, or a threat to the integrity of self or others (19). Table 27.3 lists potentially traumatic events.

Acute stress disorder (ASD) refers to symptoms of PTSD which are present within the first 4 months after the event, whereas PTSD occurs 4 months or more following the event. PTSD may be delayed and may present many years later when a nontraumatic life-cycle event occurs such as birth of a child or retirement or after the diagnosis of a new medical illness (25,26). Subthreshold symptoms (27) such as discreet phobias or anxiety and depression; substance abuse; and impulsivity may be the presenting behavior. This may be in combination with or without a traumatic brain injury, the latter making PTSD worse and more complicated to treat. Long-term consequences of trauma can cause impaired work and social functioning, can cause difficulty with intimacy and relationships, and contribute to a deep sense of ennui. For example, for the combat soldier, coming home can actually increase stress because of the loss of one's buddies, the mission,

TABLE 27.3 Examples of Potentially Traumatic Events

- Serious medical illness and its treatment
- Subsequent visits to the clinic or doctor after treatment (triggering event)
- Awakening during surgery (20)
- Torture
- Rape or sexual assault
- Childhood sexual/physical/verbal abuse
- Natural disasters—hurricanes, tornadoes, earthquakes, etc.
- Accidents—car or plane crash
- Combat—witnessing gruesome maiming or death, witnessing or participating in atrocities
- Humiliation (21,22)
- Moral injury (22,23)
- Physical incapacitation
- Forced loss of cultural identity (17)
- Forced assimilation (17)
- Listening about or witnessing trauma (first responders, medical professionals—secondary traumatization) (17,24)
- Terrorism
- Traumatic loss (5,7,8,11,14)

and a sense of great meaning and purpose (28). While in combat, the soldier must respond in a circumscribed and highly skilled manner which becomes maladaptive back in civilian life.

Immediately following a disaster or trauma, the victim may appear dissociated- and numbed with a "detached calm." Alternatively, they may be agitated, tremulous, tearful or edgy, suspicious, irritable, or even hostile (19).

Potential consequences of unresolved ASD/PTSD include substance abuse, comorbid psychiatric illness (depression, anxiety, and impulse disorders), and suicidal or homicidal ideation (19,25,26). Patients with PTSD also have a higher risk of medical comorbidities such as cardiovascular/arterial disease, lower gastrointestinal, dermatological and muscular skeletal disorders (29), and insulin resistance and diabetes mellitus. PTSD symptoms and exposure to traumatic events have been associated with greater use of medical services (30) and treatment nonadherence (31).

Trauma causes changes in the amygdala, hippocampus, and anterior cingulate (32). Time can distort and minutes may be experienced as hours (17,19). Therefore, memories of the event may be incomplete or distorted yet, survivors report an inability to forget and complain of persistent and at times relentless intrusive thoughts of the event (17,19). The traumatic event may be recalled in a dissociative manner. An example is that of a rape victim who remembers her rape as a spectator from the side of the bed on which she was raped (16).

Immediately following a traumatic event, the goal for the ED is to minimize stress, to prevent the development of ASD, and to allow for natural healing to proceed with the least amount of interference. As with grief, natural healing is best without medical intervention. Premature suggestions for psychiatric referral pathologize the trauma and should be avoided (33).

People who experience trauma feel isolated and reconnecting them quickly with their family and community is essential. The ED should allow relatives, friends, and other victims to be together despite logistical challenges it may cause the ED. Comfort; consolation; protection from further threat and distress; and food, shelter, and clothing should be provided (24). Allowing but not requiring the person to describe the events and the attendant emotions is helpful (1), especially when the caregiver can help the victim normalize the survivor's emotions. EDs should establish protocols for treating survivors of sexual assault and make appropriate referrals to law enforcement, including evidence collection (34). Debriefing is not recommended and can be harmful (1,24).

It is not uncommon for strong emotions to overwhelm the clinician who is working with trauma survivors. A quick assessment is necessary: is it the patient or the clinician who cannot tolerate these feelings? If the latter, pulling in another colleague to share the burden can be helpful. A rushed or otherwise inelegant withdrawal from the case communicates to the survivor that their emotions are dangerous and that they should not talk about the event. Survivors of trauma frequently conceal their experience from family, friends, and their medical providers. Self-disclosure in this case is best: "What you are describing is very painful for me to hear, but it is important that you talk about it freely. I'd like to have a colleague join us to help me steady myself, so I can be more present with you. Is that OK?" Such a statement can model for the patient the importance of self-care and the ability to self-regulate.

Inquire about the patient's usual coping style. Is the patient able to manage their daily affairs? Problem-solving interventions and helping the person regain control are useful (eg, how will the person get home from the ED).

Psychoeducation is important: let the person know that getting back to normal activities is the best antidote for trauma. Follow-up is essential; the traumatized person should not feel alone in the aftermath. As with the bereaved, hospital chaplains can be particularly helpful.

Assess for risk factors for PTSD development (Table 27.4), as well as for suicidal or homicidal ideation or intent, and psychiatric comorbidities. Determine the patient's support network. Evaluate the survivor's resiliency by inquiring how they have managed past adversity and what their support system is.

As with the bereaved, sleep may be disrupted, and as noted above, the use of sleep medication is controversial but may be necessary on a short-term basis.

TABLE 27.4 Risk Factors for the Development of Posttraumatic Stress Disorder

Patient Characteristics	Clinical/Premorbid Factors	Protective Characteristics
Age: Children and adolescents	Personal history of psychiatric illness	Strong social support
Female from 40 to 60 y of age	Family history of psychiatric illness	Cognitive flexibility
Non-Caucasian	Elevated heart rate or blood pressure (24,28,34)	"Hardiness," resilience (13,18,20,35)
Lower educational attainment	Decreased or nonelevated cortisol levels (24,35,36)	Ability to self-regulate emotions (13,18,21,26)
Lower socioeconomic status	Pending litigation or disability	Ability to maintain independence
	Horrific/intrusive memories	Ability to return to routine quickly (18)
	Shame or humiliation related to the trauma	Good coping skills, hope for the future, self-confidence (18)
	Premature "meaning-making" (2,18,37,38)	Ability to retain the belief that life is safe (16)
	Psychic numbing (30,31)	Ability to avoid giving excessive meaning to the event (16)
	Peritrauma dissociative states (2,18,30,35,36,39,40)	Extent to which patient's own skills/resources to help the community recover (16)

Another goal of the ED is the help the patient self-regulate. Farchi (36) has established protocols for immediate first aid interventions for the acutely traumatized person in order to address both agitation and "catatonic" presentations. For the immobilized person, he recommends vigorous attempts to make contact. For example, calling the person's name repeatedly and actively moving them out of their frozen state are some techniques. For the agitated patient, he recommends grounding techniques and movement which will decrease autonomic hyperarousal such as pacing with the patient and guiding the patient into a slower pace. Such techniques are similar to those used to verbally de-escalate agitated patients (35,37). As memory consolidation theory suggests Iyadurai et.al. (38) have used virtual reality in the ED through the use of the videogame Tetrus to assist with memory consolidation as there appears to be a "time window of several hours post trauma during which memory is malleable and vulnerable to disruption." Although this intervention has some promise, it is not yet ready for ED use.

For patients who are several days or weeks post trauma, assess whether the survivor has been able to resume daily activities and has been able to reestablish psychological equilibrium and return to pretrauma functioning. Offer reassurance, emphasize coping strategies, and normalize the emotions. Educate the patient about normal psychological responses to trauma. When spiritual issues or crises are identified, appropriate referral to a clergyperson or chaplain is indicated. If the patient appears to be having difficulty reintegrating into their daily routine, has persistent sleep difficulty, comorbidities of anxiety, depression, and suicidal thoughts, a referral for psychiatric treatment is indicated.

To date, there are no clear biochemical markers to predict ASD or PTSD and no pharmacological intervention known to prevent it. Pitman et. al. (32) summarize the various mechanisms studied thus far. Among them are dysregulation in catecholamine reactivity, genetic factors, neuropeptide Y, inflammation, serotonin, the NMDA (N-methyl-ᴅ-aspartate) receptor, DHEA (dehydroepiandrosterone), the HPA (hypothalamic-pituitary-adrenal axis, specifically glucocorticoids/cortisol levels which counter-intuitively remain static or may even decrease), and glutamate (24,32).

There are currently no recognized medications which prevent the development of ASD or PTSD. Research has been done using hydrocortisone administration shortly after exposure and morphine. Since amnesia appears to prevent the onset of PTSD symptoms (33), morphine's amnestic properties may account for its effectiveness. These are preliminary studies and these drugs should not be used in the emergency setting as prophylaxis or treatment. Trials of propranolol, escitalopram, temazepam, gabapentin, and divalproex were ineffective in preventing the development of PTSD (34).

POSTTRAUMATIC STRESS DISORDER

As noted above, posttraumatic stress symptoms can be quiescent or persistent and may come to the attention of emergency psychiatry clinicians during crisis times even years after the initial trauma—anniversaries of trauma, new-onset physical illness, retirement, or other acute situations that render the person symbolically as vulnerable as they were during the original trauma (19,25,26). Some patients may not have insight into how their past trauma connects to their current emotional state, making it challenging for the clinician to tease out what is happening. These cases illustrate common presentations of PTSD in the ED:

The clinician should be careful to avoid attributing patients' symptoms or behavior to other disorders such as psychosis, an impulse control disorder, or willful, histrionic behavior. For example, in Case 27.2, rather than immediately involving police authorities, identifying the precipitant to the threats helped not only defuse the situation so that there was no longer danger to the doctor, but the patient felt listened to and understood, enhancing doctor-patient relationship. In the third case, bizarre, histrionic behavior can startle the clinician and make him wary of the patient. Understanding helps reequilibrate the situation. In Case 27.3, an innocuous question led to the revelation of important history which facilitated the understanding as to why the patient was suddenly feeling suicidal after years of what had appeared to be good functioning. and in Case 27.4 an extreme reaction to a sensitive test is explained by past trauma.

The patient may be reluctant to disclose the nature of the trauma either because of the perceived shame and fear of being humiliated or because of distrust of the medical profession. Such patients may be vague about why they have come to the ED or may be defensive and angry. Others may complain of anxiety, depression, irritability, and a "short fuse." Others may identify intrusive memories of an event or dissociative states. Others may feel suicidal or have homicidal ideation. Still others may complain of marital or work problems.

As with all ED patients, eliciting the patient's request in addition to the chief complaint is essential. Verbal de-escalation techniques should be employed (37). If patients' symptoms are so severe as to render them dysfunctional, or if they are suicidal or homicidal, psychiatric hospitalization may be required. Gentle exploration of feelings of guilt, shame, humiliation, and spiritual

 CASE 27.2

A 65-year-old man was referred to the psychiatric ED by his urologist after the patient threatened to kill the doctor during an appointment where he received a diagnosis of prostate cancer. The patient had been healthy all his life. After careful evaluation in the ED, it became clear that this medical diagnosis had been experienced as a narcissistic injury to the patient, who had been traumatized years earlier by an uncle who had sexually molested him between the ages of 9 and 12 over a 2-year period. The current diagnosis of prostatic cancer had triggered (unexplained) panic and rage in the patient.

CASE 27.3

A 28-year-old man came to the ED complaining of symptoms of a clinical depression with suicidal ideation. Upon learning that the patient was a veteran, the clinician asked about his military experience at which point the patient broke down into tears stating that he had recently met the wife of his best buddy who had been killed by an IED (improvised explosive device) while driving a Humvee. The patient had been sitting in the front seat next to him. He was wracked with guilt for not having spotted the land mine. Since that meeting with the buddy's widow, the patient had not been able to stop thinking about the event with intrusive memories and nightmares of the buddy's blood and tissues splashing onto him. Themes of survivor guilt and moral injury surfaced for the first time since his military discharge 5 years earlier.

CASE 27.4

A 45-year-old female came to the ED because of abnormal vaginal bleeding. She agreed to and appeared to understand the need for an endometrial biopsy. She was instructed about the procedure and what to expect. During the procedure, as the uterus contracted around the tenaculum, the patient let out a series of sudden and involuntary blood curdling screams. She was diaphoretic, tremulous, and hyperventilating. She was also and profusely apologetic. The equally startled clinician was also shaken by the patient's extreme response. The patient was able to verbalize that she had been sexually molested by a relative as a child and then remembered that she had had similar reaction about 15 years earlier when undergoing the same procedure for an infertility workup. She recalled that at the time her husband had told her that he had been able to hear her scream "all the way out in the waiting room," and that he had become alarmed.

or religious crises is important, and appropriate referral is often helpful for the patient.

The ED clinician should be prepared to provide psychoeducation on PTSD and teach the patient about possible treatment options. Regarding new pharmacologic treatments for (chronic) PTSD in the outpatient setting, current research cites the potential for intranasal oxytocin to reduce intrusive thoughts and mood dysregulation, particularly anxiety and irritability. Corticotropin releasing factor (ACTH, adrenocorticotropin hormone), substance P, and neuropeptide Y (NPY), as well as D-cycloserine have been studied. Baclofen was noted to be effective with an even more robust response in combination with citalopram (26). Ketamine and ganaxolone may have beneficial effects. There are preliminary findings that cannabinoids and NMDA may be effective (24). Once again however, none of these agents are accepted treatments for PTSD and have no place in the ED.

Among the more conventional therapies for the treatment of PTSD, SSRIs, SNRIs, tricyclic antidepressants, MAOIs, bupropion, and the anticonvulsant mood stabilizers (except for divalproex) have had some but not widespread positive effect. Methylphenidate may be effective in PTSD patients who also have traumatic brain syndrome. Prazosin has been shown to be helpful for nightmares. In some cases, mirtazapine and trazodone have also been used for nightmares (24). Trials of propranolol, escitalopram, temazepam, and gabapentin and divalproex were ineffective (28). The National Center for PTSD recommends against second-generation antipsychotics (34).

Benzodiazepines may produce a "paradoxical increase in fear-driven behavior and PTSD symptoms" and should generally be avoided for even short-term treatment of PTSD (26).

If the ED begins a psychopharmacologic treatment regimen, then close follow-up and monitoring plus referral is crucial. Because of these concerns, prescribing from the ED might not be the best option and rapid referral may be the preferred option.

VICARIOUS OR SECONDARY TRAUMATIZATION: A PERSONAL REFLECTION

After 15 years of working with veterans, I traveled to Washington, DC, coincidentally on the same weekend as the unveiling of the Women's Vietnam Memorial. The statue portrays three nurses in the jungle in various positions reflecting their futile attempts to save a seriously wounded soldier. None have medical equipment. One sits on her knees, head bent, perhaps in prayer and with shoulders hung in defeat. Another looks toward the sky perhaps searching for a rescue chopper or divine guidance, her arm resting on the shoulder of the third nurse who has the wounded soldier draped over her lap and arms, looking intently into his face with a strength and resolve. Visitors had strewn red roses over the sculpture of that third nurse. I, too, was drawn to her. I studied her face, her arms, and her eyes and suddenly began weeping and sobbing, choking as I tried to suppress the tears. A middle-aged woman who had been standing on a low wall surveying the crowd came down, put her arms around me, and rocked me. She became my comforting nurse as I continued to cry. Finally, I thanked her and moved on through the memorial. I wondered if she had given herself the job of comforting those who came to visit the memorial and thought how brave and noble she was.

I returned to work at my VA hospital 2 days later and without warning, saw a picture of the statue on one of the hallway walls. I froze and began to tear up. I couldn't understand what was happening to me, but I sensed that I had identified with the nurse's sense of strength in the face of hopelessness and the helplessness of the other two nurses. I also realized that it was the sense of hopelessness and everlasting pain reflected in the other nurses that I identified with. I was feeling the weight of caring for a very troubled and traumatized patient population. I sought out my Chief who kindly and attentively listened to me and then pointed out the obvious—"You've been (vicariously) traumatized a bit after all these years."

For 6 months, I could not go by that picture without having a physiologic reaction of some sort. Now, as I look back after another 15 years of treating veterans, I understand the healing power of "being there." Traumatized people believe that their suffering is for naught. However, I have learned that to bear witness to traumatized peoples' suffering is my gift of healing to them. It also allows them to see meaning in their suffering, and I have become stronger in my capacity both to listen to them and care for myself. Their suffering also has a ripple effect: I take their story, incorporate it into my understanding, bring that empathy not only to that veteran, but to those who come after him. I approach my work now feeling reinvigorated and humbled. I am also forever indebted to my Chief for his attentive kindness, his nonjudgmental attitude, and his unwavering respect and regard for me.

Emergency psychiatry work is intoxicatingly rewarding, ennobling, and satisfying for those of us who make it our life's work (19). However, like soldiers, firefighters, or police officers, the many hours of downtime and then sudden, unpredictable spurts of great intensity can render even the hardiest emergency clinician vulnerable to vicarious traumatization. The ED is itself a traumatic place where overwhelming and traumatic news of a severe illness, the need for life-threatening treatments, or death are communicated routinely. The sheer number of traumatic events that the average emergency clinician witnesses or hears about is staggering. Secondary traumatization is an occupational hazard of this work, and the clinician must know that this can occur.

It is also referred to in the literature as compassion fatigue and vicarious traumatization. Although called by different names, there is no debate that the phenomenon does exist (39) and that it can affect even the most senior clinician (18) by virtue of overexposure to patients' traumatic stories and presentations.

With the current concern about physician burnout, it is important to point out that secondary traumatization may be unrelated to burnout. From this author's perspective, one way to distinguish it is that burnout refers to an overall dysfunction in the workplace which results in cynicism, disillusionment, anger, and irritability, whereas vicarious traumatization may include a sense of failure, social isolation, and at times dissociation or intrusive thoughts of traumatic events that patients have shared with the clinician or that they have witnessed. In other words, burnout refers to the person's inability to tolerate the often relentless and unreasonable demands of patients and/or the organization, whereas secondary traumatization refers solely to the impact overexposure to traumatic events has upon the clinician.

Signs of secondary traumatization are overidentification with the patient either through distancing, numbing, excessive or punitive limit setting, or what may superficially appear to be a lack of empathy (shutting down). Elwood (40) opines that the experience of "low-level" symptoms of secondary trauma is normal, common, likely transient and does not reach a level of clinical impairment.

Risk factors for the development of secondary traumatization include both the degree of intensity and frequency of exposure to others' traumatic losses, exposure to children's trauma, and the lack of variation in clinical practice beyond treating trauma patients and survivors (18). Clinicians with a past personal or family history of trauma, those who minimize their own personal or family needs, and those "addicted" to the adrenaline rush of the ED are also at risk. New clinicians and those without awareness of the possibility of secondary traumatization are at risk (18).

Remedies for the prevention and management of secondary trauma include a consistent work-life balance, strong social supports both within and outside the clinician's place of work, plenty of rest, nourishment, exercise, working collaboratively with others rather than in isolation, and cultivating relationships with colleagues with whom the clinician can share their own stories. The individual clinician needs to know when to take a break and when they are being overexposed. One way of recognizing this is when one goes on "automatic pilot" or feels that one "has to" treat the patient because no one else can and that rest can come later (17). Also essential are supervisors who create an environment of physical and emotional safety, who encourage and expect their staff to discuss issues and who help them keep a sense of meaning in the face of tragedy. Organizations need to respect staff and allow for

a mix of various kinds of clinical work and other activities such as built-in teaching, administration, or a less intense shift or two. Flexible schedules allow for a good work-home balance, so that clinicians can be present for family and friends. Some clinicians will require professional care and may need referral to mental health professionals. This should be done with care and sensitivity.

Brom (17) recommends that once a year every trauma clinician take stock by asking: "Why do I do this work, why am I continuing to work in the trauma field, and what do I need to continue to do this work?"

REFERENCES

1. Gray, M. L. B., & Papa, T. (2006). Crisis debriefing: What helps, and what may not? *Current Psychiatry, 5*, 17–29.
2. Mancini, A. D., Prati, G., & Bonanno, G. A. (2011). Do shattered worldviews lead to complicated grief? Prospective and longitudinal analyses. *Journal of Social and Clinical Psychology, 30*(2), 184–215.
3. Maciejewski, P. K., Zhang, B., Block, S. D., & Prigerson, H. G. (2007). An empirical examination of the stage theory of grief. *JAMA, 297*(7), 716–723.
4. Zisook, S., & Shear, K. (2009). Grief and bereavement: What psychiatrists need to know. *World Psychiatry, 8*(2), 67–74.
5. Zisook, S., Simon, N. M., Reynolds, C. F., III, Pies, R., Lebowitz, B., Young, I. T., Madowitz, J., & Shear, M. K. (2010). Bereavement, complicated grief, and DSM: Part 2: Complicated grief. *The Journal of Clinical Psychiatry, 71*(8), 1097–1098.
6. Shear, M. K. (2015). Clinical practice. Complicated grief. *The New England Journal of Medicine, 372*(2), 153–160.
7. Zisook, S., Iglewicz, A., Avanzino, J., Maglione, J., Glorioso, D., Zetumer, S., et al. (2014). Bereavement: Course, consequences, and care. *Current Psychiatry Reports, 16*(10), 482.
8. Simon, N. M. (2013). Treating complicated grief. *JAMA, 310*(4), 416–423.
9. Shear, M. K., Muldberg, S., & Periyakoil, V. (2017). Supporting patients who are bereaved. *BMJ, 358*, j2854.
10. Bui, E., Nadal-Vicens, M., & Simon, N. M. (2012). Pharmacological approaches to the treatment of complicated grief: Rationale and a brief review of the literature. *Dialogues in Clinical Neuroscience, 14*(2), 149–157.

11. Boelen, P. A., Van den Bout, J., & De Keijser, J. (2003). Traumatic grief as a disorder distinct from bereavement-related depression and anxiety: A replication study with bereaved mental health care patients. *American Journal of Psychiatry, 160*(7), 1339–1341.

12. Zisook, S., Pies, R., & Corruble, E. (2012). When is grief a disease? *The Lancet, 379*(9826), 1590.

13. Piper, W. E., Ogrodniczuk, J. S., Joyce, A. S., McCallum, M., Weideman, R., & Azim, H. F. (2001). Ambivalence and other relationship predictors of grief in psychiatric outpatients. *The Journal of Nervous and Mental Disease, 189*(11), 781–787.

14. Shear, M. K., Ghesquiere, A., & Glickman, K. (2013). Bereavement and complicated grief. *Current Psychiatry Reports, 15*(11), 406.

15. Vanderkolk, B. (1996). The complexity of adaptation to trauma. In Vanderkolk, B., McFarlane, A. C., & Weisaeth, L. (Eds.), *Traumatic stress: The effects of overwhelming experiences on mind, body, and society* (pp. 183–205). New York, NY: Guilford.

16. Herman, J. (1997). *Trauma and recovery.* New York, NY: Basic Books.

17. Brom, D., Agassi, G., Pat-Horenczyk, R., & Baum, N. (2010). *Trauma & resilience: Theory & practice from the Israeli experience.* International Course. Rothberg International School of the Hebrew University of Jerusalem I. Jerusalem: Israel Center for the Treatment of Psychotrauma.

18. Brom, D., & Kleber, R. (2008). Resilience as the capacity for processing traumatic experiences. In Brom, D., Pat-Horenczyk, R., & Ford, J. (Eds.), *Treating traumatized children: Risk, resilience and recovery.* London: Routledge.

19. Richmond, J. S. (2013). Trauma and loss in the emergency setting. In Zun, L. S., Chepenik, L., & Mallory, M. N. S. (Eds.), *Behavioral emergencies for the emergency physician* (pp. 235–243). New York, NY: Cambridge University Press.

20. Osterman, J. E., Hooper, J., Heran, W. J., Keane, T. M., & van der Kolk, B. A. (2001). Awareness under anesthesia and the development of posttraumatic stress disorder. *General Hospital Psychiatry, 23*(4), 198–204.

21. Moore, A., Ben-Meir, E., Golan-Shapira, D., & Farchi, M. (2013). Rape: A trauma of paralyzing dehumanization. *Journal of Aggression, Maltreatment and Trauma, 22*(10), 1051–1069.

22. Lazare, A. (1987). Shame and humiliation in the medical encounter. *Archives of Internal Medicine, 147*(9), 1653–1658.

23. Litz, B. T., Stein, N., Delaney, E., Lebowitz, L., Nash, W. P., Silva, C., et al. (2009). Moral injury and moral repair in war veterans: A preliminary model and intervention strategy. *Clinical Psychology Review, 29*(8), 695–706.

24. U.S. Department of Veterans Affairs. PTSD: National Center for PTSD. Retrieved September 25, 2019, from https://www.ptsd.va.gov/PTSD/professional/index.asp.

25. Richmond, J. S., & Beck, J. C. (1986). Posttraumatic stress disorder in a World War II veteran. *American Journal of Psychiatry, 143*(11), 1485–1486.

26. Shalev, A., Liberzon, I., & Marmar, C. (2017). Post-traumatic stress disorder. *The New England Journal of Medicine, 376*(25), 2459–2469.

27. Marshall, R. D., Olfson, M., Hellman, F., Blanco, C., Guardino, M., & Struening, E. L. (2001). Comorbidity, impairment, and suicidality in subthreshold PTSD. *American Journal of Psychiatry, 158*(9), 1467–1473.

28. Richmond, J. S. (in press). Mental health issues in veterans. In Zun, L., et al. (Eds.), *Behavioral emergencies for the healthcare professional.* Dog Ear Publishers.

29. Vaccarino, V., Goldberg, J., Magruder, K. M., Forsberg, C. W., Friedman, M. J., Litz, B. T., et al. (2014). Posttraumatic stress disorder and incidence of type-2 diabetes: A prospective twin study. *Journal of Psychiatric Research, 56,* 158–164.

30. Stein, M. B., McQuaid, J. R., Pedrelli, P., Lenox, R., & McCahill, M. E. (2000). Posttraumatic stress disorder in the primary care medical setting. *General Hospital Psychiatry, 22*(4), 261–269.

31. Shemesh, E., Rudnick, A., Kaluski, E., Milovanov, O., Salah, A., Alon, D., et al. (2001). A prospective study of posttraumatic stress symptoms and nonadherence in survivors of a myocardial infarction (MI). *General Hospital Psychiatry, 23*(4), 215–222.

32. Pitman, R. K., Rasmusson, A. M., Koenen, K. C., Shin, L. M., Orr, S. P., Gilbertson, M. W., et al. (2012). Biological studies of post-traumatic stress disorder. *Nature Reviews Neuroscience, 13*(11), 769–787.

33. Zohar, J., Sonnino, R., Juven-Wetzler, A., & Cohen, H. (2009). Can posttraumatic stress disorder be prevented? *CNS Spectrums, 14*(1 Suppl. 1), 44–51.

34. Linden, J. A. (2011). Clinical practice. Care of the adult patient after sexual assault. *The New England Journal of Medicine, 365*(9), 834–841.

35. Berlin, J. S. (2017). Collaborative de-escalation. In Zeller, S. L., Nordstrom, K., & Wilson, M. P. (Eds.), *The diagnosis and management of agitation* (pp. 144–155). Cambridge, UK: Cambridge University Press.

36. Farchi, M. (2011). From a helpless victim to a coping survivor: Innovative mental health intervention methods during emergencies and disasters. *Prehospital and Disaster Medicine*, 26(Suppl. 1), S3.

37. Richmond, J. S., Berlin, J. S., Fishkind, A. B., Holloman, G. H., Jr., Zeller, S. L., Wilson, M. P., et al. (2012). Verbal de-escalation of the agitated patient: Consensus statement of the American Association for Emergency Psychiatry Project BETA De-escalation Workgroup. *The Western Journal of Emergency Medicine, 13*(1), 17–25.

38. Iyadurai, L., Blackwell, S. E., Meiser-Stedman, R., Watson, P. C., Bonsall, M. B., Geddes, J. R., et al. (2018). Preventing intrusive memories after trauma via a brief intervention involving Tetris computer game play in the emergency department: A proof-of-concept randomized controlled trial. *Molecular Psychiatry, 23*(3), 674–682.

39. Figley, C. R. (Ed.), (1995). *COMPASSION FATIGUE: Coping with secondary traumatic stress disorder in those who treat the traumatized*. New York: Routledge, Taylor & Francis.

40. Elwood, L. S., Mott, J., Lohr, J. M., & Galovski, T. E. (2011). Secondary trauma symptoms in clinicians: A critical review of the construct, specificity, and implications for trauma-focused treatment. *Clinical Psychology Review, 31*(1), 25–36.

28

Personality Disorders

Victor Hong, Priyanka P. Reddy, Shami Entenman

Among patients who receive psychiatric emergency care, those with personality disorders are high utilizers, visit recurrently, and present unique challenges for assessment, treatment, and disposition (1-4). Whether the primary diagnosis or a comorbidity, a personality disorder significantly influences presenting symptoms and often complicates crisis management. A patient with narcissistic personality disorder may present with increased depressive symptoms secondary to a perceived injury to their ego, whereas the trigger for heightened depression in a patient with borderline personality disorder (BPD) may be feelings of abandonment. In both instances, the emergency clinician must address the depressive symptoms, with a broader lens to the underlying personality structure. This chapter offers techniques and approaches emergency clinicians can utilize to more skillfully address presenting problems while managing personality disorder–related issues. The chapter focuses on the most prevalent personality disorder in psychiatric emergency settings: BPD (5).

THE PERSONALITY DISORDERS

Personality traits are enduring patterns of perceiving, relating to, and thinking about others and oneself that are exhibited in a wide range of social and personal contexts (6). A personality disorder is characterized by "an enduring pattern of inner experience and behavior that deviates markedly from the expectations of the individual's culture" and is manifested in at least two of the following areas: cognition, affectivity, interpersonal functioning, or impulse control (6). The diagnosis of a personality disorder requires an evaluation of the person's long-term patterns of functioning, and the particular personality features must be evident by adolescence or early adulthood (6). Table 28.1 briefly describes the personality disorders, how they might present in the emergency department

(ED), and proposed approaches. Understanding the patient's perspective and unique way of interacting with the world will assist the emergency clinician regardless of the presenting complaints.

BORDERLINE PERSONALITY DISORDER

Patients with BPD are high utilizers of psychiatric emergency services, with recurrent visits being a hallmark (4). Emotion dysregulation is a frequent presenting symptom of the BPD patient in crisis and often interferes with their ability to rationally process information. Such dysregulation can trigger desperate, impulsive acts, often involving self-harm or suicidal behaviors. Treating a dysregulated patient may engender dysregulation in ED staff (10), adding fuel to the fire in an often chaotic environment. Excessive countertransference can impair rational, objective evaluation and hinder sound treatment decision-making.

It is important to recognize that given the core characteristic of interpersonal hypersensitivity in those with BPD, interpersonal conflicts often trigger emotion dysregulation and prompt ED visits (11). Relationship stressors may contribute to depression, anxiety, substance use, dissociation, self-injurious behaviors, and/or suicidal ideation or acts for those with BPD. Notably, the patient may present with vague complaints, such as anxiety or depression, while avoiding, or failing, to recognize the interpersonal triggers in play. The emergency provider is well-served to focus the discussion on interpersonal factors as doing so can illuminate details of their support system, assist the patient's development of insight, and can inform the provider's safety risk assessment. If interpersonal conflict is understood to trigger self-injury or suicidality, then focusing on the inciting incident can expedite the evaluation by getting to the heart of why they are in crisis (2). Over time, particularly if the patient is

TABLE 28.1 Personality Disorders: Presenting Features and Clinical Approaches in the Emergency Department

Personality Disorder	Characteristic Behaviors	Presenting Features	Approach to the Patient
Cluster A: Odd/eccentric			
Schizoid	"Detachment from social relation-ships, restricted range of emotional expression"	Social disconnection often leaves them few supports in the community.	Recognize that the patient is likely not comfortable talking to strangers and may not have cho-sen to come to the ED. Assess acute safety risk: suicide and homicide risk. Obtain corroborating history from others who may know the patient's history or details of the acute situation. Consider medications for psycho-sis/anxiety/agitation (low-dose atypical antipsychotics, benzodi-azepines) (7-9). Refer to social service agencies for increased support and if addi-tional issues such as housing are problematic.
Schizotypal	"Discomfort in close relationships, cog-nitive or perceptual distortions, eccentric-ities of behavior"	Usually presents with disorganized thoughts/behaviors, eccentricity or bizarre behavior, magical thinking, delusions, or other psychotic symptoms.	
Paranoid	"Distrust and sus-piciousness of others such that their motives are interpreted as malevolent"	Paranoid beliefs and distrust make for dif-ficult encounters and vague histories.	
Cluster B: Erratic/dramatic			
Borderline	"Marked impulsivity, unstable interper-sonal relationships, self-image, and affect"	Interpersonal conflicts are common, likely with difficulty in regu-lating emotions.	Assess for acute changes that ele-vate suicide risk above baseline. Verbal de-escalation techniques, shows of support and validation are preferred over medications. Be aware of one's own excessive emotional reactions so as not to influence the evaluation. Probe for recent interpersonal stressors which may have trig-gered the present crisis.
Histrionic	"Excessive emotion-ality and attention seeking"	Overly dramatic behavior makes determining facts difficult.	Assess suicide/homicide risk apart from affect. Differentiate excitement and drama from other psychiatric dis-orders such as bipolar disorder or a primary psychotic disorder.
Narcissistic	"Grandiosity, need for admiration, and a lack of empathy"	May present with suicidal ideation or suicide attempts. May also exhibit rage or assaultive behavior.	Uncover possible interpersonal situation or other trigger (nar-cissistic injury) that may have brought on acute crisis. Focus on suicide/homicide risk and other acute issues as opposed to addressing longer-term issues related to narcissism.

TABLE 28.1 Personality Disorders: Presenting Features and Clinical Approaches in the Emergency Department   (Continued)

Personality Disorder	Characteristic Behaviors	Presenting Features	Approach to the Patient
Antisocial	"Disregard for, and violation of, the rights of others"	Often brought in by police or others to assess reasons for criminal or aggressive behavior. Issues of secondary gain (avoiding incarceration, needing housing, etc.) may be relevant.	Rule out other psychiatric disorders and organic medical factors as primary cause of behavior. Assess suicide/homicide risk given high incidence of violence. If assault has occurred or patient is unkempt and/or intoxicated, evaluate medical status. May use antipsychotics or benzodiazepines for agitation. Work closely with law enforcement, consider "duty to warn" in cases of elevated risk of violence.
Cluster C: Anxious/fearful			
Avoidant	"Social inhibition, feelings of inadequacy, and hypersensitivity to negative evaluation"	Complaints are usually related to anxiety and behavior conducted in an effort to reduce the anxiety. Can have severe and prolonged panic/anxiety states. May have dissociative experiences.	Support and calm reassurance can be helpful. Emphasize that physical symptoms are neither life-threatening nor permanent. If safe for discharge, refer for cognitive behavioral therapy.
Dependent	"Excessive need to be taken care of that leads to submissive and clinging behavior and fears of separation"		
Obsessive-compulsive	"Preoccupation with orderliness, perfectionism, and control"		

a recurrent visitor to the ED, connecting their stressors to their symptoms and behaviors can gradually improve their self-awareness and reveal opportunities to mitigate future decompensation.

COMORBIDITIES

Patients with personality disorders frequently present with comorbid psychiatric disorders including primary mood or substance use disorders, which can confound the presentation of personality pathology and vice versa (12). The clinician should not assume that just because a person has a comorbid personality disorder diagnosis, the

ED presentation is all due to personality pathology. At the same time, it is important to recognize that no matter the chief complaint, it is likely the personality traits will indeed influence the presentation and evaluation. Some comorbidities, such as concurrent major depression or substance use, can elevate acute safety risk in those with personality disorders (13).

TREATMENT APPROACH

In the ED, where safe and efficient evaluation and disposition are prized, rapid development of a therapeutic alliance is ideal. For BPD in particular, guidelines of how best to engage with an individual are useful, with Good Psychiatric Management (GPM) being a notable example (14). If the clinician adopts an active and engaged approach, they may quickly build rapport by demonstrating trustworthiness, compassion, and interest in the patient. Incorporating direct but empathetic responses can help the patient feel validated, foster the therapeutic alliance, and repair fluctuating disruptions. Common, negative staff reactions (such as fear, hostility, and emotional detachment) to patients with personality disorders, particularly those with BPD, may challenge providers' abilities to engage productively. In turn, manifestations of these negative attitudes can cause the patient to withdraw or act out, making the assessment much more difficult. To effectively engage and rationally treat patients with personality disorders, clinicians must maintain insight into their own moods, thoughts, and behaviors. Potential iatrogenic actions toward patients with BPD are described in Table 28.2.

If patients resist meaningful dialogue with providers, clinicians should explicitly underscore that without the patient's authentic participation and provision of crucial information, the

evaluation cannot be completed. The clinician can advertise that they are not a "mind reader" and indeed require the patient's active participation to make the most appropriate treatment decision.

MANAGEMENT OF SAFETY RISK

Across all diagnoses seen in the ED, safety assessment is critical, but it is especially nuanced with patients with personality disorders. This issue is complex when managing individuals with BPD, for whom chronic suicidality and acute safety risks are constant concerns, above and beyond the other personality disorders (15,16). BPD is, after all, the only psychiatric diagnosis in which recurrent suicidal behavior is one of the diagnostic criteria (6). Safety concerns are at the center of most emergency psychiatric evaluations with this patient group. A helpful model for assessing safety in BPD involves distinguishing between acute versus chronic risks (17).

At baseline, a BPD patient's chronic level of suicide risk is elevated above the general population, yet this fact should rarely be used as the basis for treatment decisions in the emergency setting. Chronic suicidal thoughts may indicate

TABLE 28.2 How to Avoid Pitfalls When Managing Borderline Personality Disorder in the Emergency Department

Poor Management	Potential Etiologies and Consequences	Good Management
Negative staff attitudes and behaviors	Excessive countertransference reactions leading to worse outcomes and ineffective evaluations	Recognition that patients are doing "the best they can," have brain-based deficits, and that an engaged, optimistic approach can expedite the evaluation
Excessive prescribing of medications	Inadequate verbal de-escalation, limited provider or patient distress tolerance leading to overreliance on medications, adverse side effects	Validation of the patient's distress and offering verbal support and calming techniques; de-emphasizing the role of medications in the treatment of BPD
Suboptimal safety risk assessments	Difficulty distinguishing acute versus chronic risk factors, poor communication with collateral informants, reaction to fears of liability leading to unnecessary hospitalizations or dismissing clear warning signs of suicide	Emphasize acute changes in presentation over chronic behaviors, thoroughly assess social support system and follow-up care, discuss with colleagues and supervision to make a team decision, utilize safety planning and follow-up contacts

the patient has an overwhelmed coping system, which habitually defaults in crisis to a "solution of suicide" rather than a problem-solving process (18). In contrast, an acute exacerbation of risk can be related to substance use, discharge from structured treatments, major depression, negative life events, or delayed family support (13,19-21).

A question that might further elucidate acute versus chronic risk is to ask "When was the last time you were *not* having suicidal thoughts?" Often the patient reports that they have had these thoughts regularly since adolescence or early adulthood. Although this information does not diminish the intensity of the situation, it does provide a context in which the evaluating clinician can proceed. A provider may ask what pushed them into their acute crisis, and if there are ways that they have handled intense, painful emotions in the past. This line of questioning may help the patient consider alternatives to suicide as well as possible triggers for the crisis. Patients may deny any discrete triggers to their acute distress, either because they lack insight into them or because they are reluctant to participate in this dialogue. In this case, a detailed chain analysis can help to lay bare the events, emotions, and behaviors precipitating the ED visit (22). Again, given the interpersonal hypersensitivity inherent to most patients with BPD, one can assume that an interpersonal trigger may be involved (23).

The detailed safety assessment is not the time to up the ante by challenging the patient to prove they are suicidal. Rather, it is an opportunity to validate their suffering, recognize they are overwhelmed, and communicate that you are taking them seriously, even if the patient has presented numerous times in the past with similar complaints. Providers should recall that patients can quickly sense their disinterest and dismissiveness, and when they do, the resultant increase in feelings of abandonment and hopelessness is likely to interfere with the evaluation.

Patients with chronic suicidality may be frequent visitors to the ED and therefore clinicians may be known to them. This familiarity can be useful if the clinician consistently focuses on the outpatient setting, serving to bolster the ongoing treatment. Patients may eventually realize that they are utilizing emergency visits and inpatient hospitalizations to avoid coping with affect and distress. The emergency clinician must also focus on interpreting what the words "I am suicidal" actually means. Does this mean that the patient wants to die and intends to carry out a plan of suicide or that they are distressed, lonely, and feeling abandoned? These differences are crucial in deciding the optimal disposition. If they are engaged in outpatient treatment, questions can be asked about that treatment, what it entails, their commitment to it, and their follow-through with recommendations, coping skills, and strategies. For those receiving dialectical behavioral therapy (DBT), the emergency clinician can ask what previously beneficial skills the patient has utilized when in distress or crisis.

Although inpatient hospitalization has traditionally been employed to manage patients with BPD in acute crisis, this is no longer considered standard practice. Hospitalizations, while still playing a role for acute suicidality above and beyond the BPD patient's chronic risk level, are equivocally effective in reducing overall risk. Some have even argued that recurrent hospitalizations are damaging to the overall course of BPD (24). If inpatient hospitalization is considered, the goal should be a short, structured admission, focused on coping skill development and buoying of social supports (25).

Given the concerns for liability in managing chronically high-risk individuals, the importance of collecting information from others (such as family, romantic partners, friends, outpatient providers) should be underscored. As with all situations in which there are safety concerns, collateral informants can and should be contacted even in cases when the patient protests their involvement. Speaking with others in the patient's life can provide more context for the patient's presentation, contribute significantly to the safety risk assessment, assist in safety planning, and offer providers additional resources for close follow-up upon discharge. Utilizing the team approach (gathering opinions from colleagues and supervisors) in crafting a disposition plan is also of paramount importance in complex cases, as this not only "spreads out the worry" but also serves as a risk management tool.

Discharge may be a reasonable option if in the emergency setting the patient's emotional dysregulation can be improved, the availability of lethal means can be mitigated, supports can be increased, follow-up care can be arranged, and the determination can be made that the crisis has either passed or at least that the patient can tolerate it safely. Follow-up phone calls and engaging the patient in safety planning are essential interventions to reducing suicide risk post discharge (26,27).

In individuals with personality disorders, risk of harming others may be addressed by a somewhat similar framework in that the history of violence along with acute behavioral warning signs are the building blocks of assessment. The clinician must be aware of the increased risk of violent behavior in those with personality disorders compared to the general population (28). When threats are credible and associated with elevated risk, interventions such as medications or inpatient hospitalization for a potential contributing mental illness are indicated. In addition, in these instances, it is important to contact law enforcement and to issue a *Tarasoff* notification, in which the clinician informs the threatened individuals of the risk (29). Other factors to consider include the presence of agitation and substance use, as these increase an individual's risk to be violent (30,31). As with a suicide risk assessment, consultation with colleagues and supervisors about a patient's potential danger to others is an important risk management tool.

MEDICATION MANAGEMENT

There are no US Food and Drug Administration–approved medications specifically for the treatment of any personality disorder, as no medications have been shown as consistently or significantly effective. That notwithstanding, many patients with personality disorders are prescribed various psychopharmacologic medications for long-term symptoms and also frequently receive medication to address acute anxiety and agitation in the ED (5,32). Antipsychotics are often prescribed for schizotypal personality disorder and antisocial personality disorders; selective serotonin reuptake inhibitors (SSRIs) are sometimes prescribed for avoidant personality disorder and obsessive compulsive personality disorder, and

polypharmacy is very common in treating BPD (33,34). Certainly, in the ED, antipsychotics and benzodiazepines are often prescribed to mitigate intense anxiety or agitation (5).

It is important to recall that unless a patient's behavior poses imminent danger to themselves or others or their anxiety precludes the provision of a thorough evaluation, verbal de-escalation techniques are preferred (35). Not only can medications have adverse side effects, but they can also establish or reaffirm expectations that medications are the solutions to their problems. In addition, if medications succeed in temporarily reducing intense emotions, this may reinforce the appropriateness of utilizing the ED for symptom relief or as a regular coping mechanism. It is unlikely that changes to a patient's home medication regimen will be useful in stabilizing the acute crisis, and therefore modifications to standing regimens should not be made without consulting the patient's outpatient provider, who should have a better grasp of the patient's medication history (2). In general, in the ED and beyond, the role of medications for treating personality disorders should be de-emphasized, and for BPD in particular, psychotherapy should be promoted as the treatment of choice.

EVALUATION OF SUPPORT NETWORK

For patients with personality disorders and certainly those with BPD, a critical aspect of assessment, management, and treatment of patients in the ED is incorporating their support network, which can be comprised of family, friends, and providers. These individuals can provide vital collateral information, help to problem solve, and engage in safety planning. Although the ED setting and the underlying BPD personality constructs may make including members of the patient's support network challenging, it is nevertheless important to make a concerted effort. These individuals may be key to creating a plan that diverts from an inpatient hospitalization. If attempts to engage supports reveal that the support system is limited or unreliable, then the likelihood is higher that a hospitalization will be necessary for acute, short-term stabilization.

Family involvement in the emergency setting also provides a valuable opportunity to engage family members in psychoeducation. The purpose of this is to not only address their own fears or confusion but also to connect them with resources and information so they can become more meaningfully supportive of their loved ones. In BPD, family and loved ones can be crucial partners in the patient's treatment and should know the basics about the diagnosis, typical symptoms, thoughts, and behaviors, prognosis, and effective treatments (36,37). In addition, they can be provided guidelines of how best to interact with the patient, which can decrease their stress and burden and help them avoid behaviors and missteps which may complicate treatment (38).

DIAGNOSTIC EVALUATION AND PSYCHOEDUCATION

A personality disorder diagnosis requires information about the patient's history and behaviors over an extended period of time. Given that an emergency visit is a brief and limited view of the patient's symptoms and behaviors, it has long been considered prudent to avoid diagnosing a personality disorder during a one-time ED visit. Furthermore, when in acute crisis, an individual's level of functioning, ability to control emotions and behaviors, and interpersonal style may not accurately represent their baseline. That said, in cases when adequate collateral information has been gathered, there is an abundance of information from the medical records and past visits, and the symptoms are clear, it behooves the emergency clinician to honestly offer a professional opinion about potential diagnoses in play. This is particularly important with BPD, as initiating discussion about the diagnosis and providing psychoeducation can be useful in establishing appropriate expectations, identifying helpful resources, and improving the patient's level of insight (39). In many cases, patients experience a sense of relief when they learn about a diagnosis that fits their symptoms, for which there are evidence-based treatments, and that can have a good prognosis. It is important to recall that owing to BPD's frequency of comorbidities, and the heterogeneity and complexity of presentation, misdiagnosis and

therefore inappropriate foci of treatment is common (40). The emergency visit can be reframed as an opportunity for clarification and perhaps optimization of treatment.

Psychoeducation can provide patients with BPD a context for their emotions and behaviors. Presenting BPD as a genetically based brain disorder, with specific vulnerabilities such as emotion dysregulation and interpersonal hypersensitivity, is helpful in reshaping the patient's view of their mental health problems. Psychoeducation is also important in guiding patients toward effective, evidence-based treatments (interventions with a psychosocial focus such as DBT or GPM) rather than toward less validated treatments such as medication management.

DISPOSITION MANAGEMENT

The frequent comorbidities associated with personality disorders and the significant safety concerns involved frequently make an appropriate disposition challenging (41,42). Generally, the role of the emergency clinician is to manage the short-term crisis and decide whether to hospitalize or refer to a partial hospital or outpatient treatment. If the patient is a recurrent visitor to the ED, staff should pursue ongoing collaboration with outpatient providers and, when they are in the ED, can assist the patient in deepening insight and more effectively managing their moods and behaviors.

Given the focus on safety in the emergency setting, there are several guidelines to follow when deciding to discharge. As with all patients with an elevated risk of suicide, engaging the individual in active safety planning is key (26). It is also recommended to follow-up with the patient post discharge, which is a cost-effective and evidence-based way to optimize safety (27,43). When interpersonal issues are a notable factor to a patient's distress, this sort of follow-up can indicate authentic care and clinical compassion and reinforce that helping resources and institutions exist to help maintain their safety in times of crisis. As those who are referred to outpatient treatment actually follow up at a low rate, outreach from ED staff after a crisis may also be a useful tool to encourage follow-through with recommendations (44).

CONCLUSION

In conclusion, the presence of comorbidities, diagnostic complexity, significant interpersonal difficulties, and safety issues is central to the challenge of managing personality disorders in the emergency setting. With an underlying knowledge of the ways in which the different personality disorders manifest, and an understanding of how to avoid common pitfalls, emergency clinicians can optimize care for these individuals without causing iatrogenic harm.

REFERENCES

1. Penfold, S., Groll, D., Mauer-Vakil, D., et al. (2016). A retrospective analysis of personality disorder presentations in a Canadian university-affiliated hospital's emergency department. *BJPsych Open, 2*, 394–399.
2. Hong, V. (2016). Borderline personality disorder in the emergency department: Good psychiatric management. *Harvard Review of Psychiatry, 24*(5), 357–366.
3. Chaput, Y. J., & Lebel, M. J. (2007). Demographic and clinical profiles of patients who make multiple visits to psychiatric emergency services. *Psychiatric Services, 58*, 335–341.
4. Pasic, J., Russo, J., & Roy-Byrne, P. (2005). High utilizers of psychiatric emergency services. *Psychiatric Services, 56*, 678–684.
5. Pascual, J. C., Córcoles, D., Castaño, J., et al. (2007). Hospitalization and pharmacotherapy for borderline personality disorder in a psychiatric emergency service. *Psychiatric Services, 58*, 1199–1204.
6. American Psychiatric Association. (2013). *Diagnostic and statistical manual of mental disorders (DSM-5)*. Washington, DC: American Psychiatric Association.
7. Goldberg, S. C., Schulz, S. C., Schulz, P. M., et al. (1986). Borderline and schizotypal personality disorders treated with low-dose thiothixene vs placebo. *Archives of General Psychiatry, 43*, 680–686.
8. Soloff, P. H. (1990). What's new in personality disorders? An update on pharmacologic treatment. *Journal of Personality Disorders, 4*, 233–243.
9. Koenigsberg, H. W., Reynolds, D., Goodman, M., et al. (2003). Risperidone in the treatment of schizotypal personality disorder. *The Journal of Clinical Psychiatry, 64*, 628–634.
10. Gabbard, G. O., & Wilkinson, S. M. (1994). *Management of countertransference with borderline patients*. Washington, DC: American Psychiatric Press.
11. Gunderson, J. G. (1984). *Borderline personality disorder*. Washington, DC: American Psychiatric Press.
12. Zanarini, M. C., Frankenburg, F. R., Dubo, E. D., et al. (1998). Axis I comorbidity of borderline personality disorder. *American Journal of Psychiatry, 155*, 1733–1739.
13. Kelly, T. M., Soloff, P. H., Lynch, K. G., et al. (2000). Recent life events, social adjustment, and suicide attempts in patients with major depression and borderline personality disorder. *Journal of Personality Disorders, 14*, 316–326.
14. Gunderson, J. G., & Links, P. (2014). *Handbook of good psychiatric management for borderline personality disorder*. Washington, DC: American Psychiatric Publishing.
15. Elisei, S., Verdolini, N., & Anastasi, S. (2012). Suicidal attempts among emergency department patients: One-year of clinical experience. *Psychiatria Danubina, 24*(Suppl. 1), S140–S142.
16. Oldham, J. M. (2006). Borderline personality disorder and suicidality. *American Journal of Psychiatry, 163*, 20–26.
17. Sansone, R. A. (2004). Chronic suicidality and borderline personality. *Journal of Personality Disorders, 18*(3), 215–225.
18. Putnam, K., & Silk, K. R. (2005). Emotion dysregulation and the development of borderline personality disorder. *Development and Psychopathology, 17*, 899–925.
19. Links, P. S., Eynan, R., Heisel, M. J., et al. (2007). Affective instability and suicidal ideation and behavior in patients with borderline personality disorder. *Journal of Personality Disorders, 21*, 72–86.
20. Soloff, P. H., Fabio, A., Kelly, T. M., et al. (2005). High-lethality status in patients with borderline personality disorder. *Journal of Personality Disorders, 19*, 386–399.
21. Yen, S., Shea, M. T., Sanislow, C. A., et al. (2004). Borderline personality disorder criteria associated with prospectively observed suicidal behavior. *American Journal of Psychiatry, 161*, 1296–1298.
22. Rizvi, S. L., & Ritschel, L. A. (2014). Mastering the art of chain analysis in dialectical behavior therapy. *Cognitive and Behavioral Practice, 21*, 335–349.
23. Gunderson, J. G., & Lyons-Ruth, K. (2008). BPD's interpersonal hypersensitivity phenotype: A gene-environment-developmental model. *Journal of Personality Disorders, 22*, 22–41.
24. Paris, J. (2004). Is hospitalization useful for suicidal patients with borderline personality disorder? *Journal of Personality Disorders, 18*, 240–247.

25. Silk, K. R., Eisner, W., Allport, C., et al. (1994). Focused time-limited inpatient treatment of borderline personality disorder. *Journal of Personality Disorders, 8*, 268–278.

26. Stanley, B., Brown, G. K., Brenner, L. A., et al. (2018). Comparison of the safety planning intervention with follow-up vs usual care of suicidal patients treated in the emergency department. *JAMA Psychiatry, 75*, 894–900.

27. National Action Alliance for Suicide Prevention: Transforming Health Systems Initiative Work Group. (2018). *Recommended standard care for people with suicide risk: Making health care suicide safe*. Washington, DC: Education Development Center, Inc.

28. Yu, R., Geddes, J. R., & Fazel, S. (2012). Personality disorders, violence, and antisocial behavior: A systematic review and meta-regression analysis. *Journal of Personality Disorders, 26*, 775–792.

29. Felthous, A. R. (2006). Warning a potential victim of a person's dangerousness: Clinician's duty or victim's right? *Journal of the American Academy of Psychiatry and the Law, 34*, 338–348.

30. Witt, K., van Dorn, R., & Fazel, S. (2013). Risk factors for violence in psychosis: Systematic review and meta-regression analysis of 110 studies. *PLOS One, 8*, e55942.

31. Soyka, M. (2000). Substance misuse, psychiatric disorder and violent and disturbed behaviour. *British Journal of Psychiatry, 176*, 345–350.

32. Zanarini, M. C., Frankenburg, F. R., Hennen, J., et al. (2004). Mental health service utilization by borderline personality disorder patients and axis II comparison subjects followed prospectively for 6 years. *Journal of Clinical Psychiatry, 65*, 28–36.

33. Ripoll, L. H., Triebwasser, J., & Siever, L. J. (2011). Evidence-based pharmacotherapy for personality disorders. *The International Journal of Neuropsychopharmacology, 14*, 1257–1288.

34. Zanarini, M. C., Frankenburg, F. R., Bradford Reich, D., et al. (2015). Rates of psychotropic medication use reported by borderline patients and axis II comparison subjects over 16 years of prospective follow-up. *Journal of Clinical Psychopharmacology, 35*, 63–67.

35. Richmond, J. S., Berlin, J. S., Fishkind, A. B., et al. (2012). Verbal de-escalation of the agitated patient: Consensus statement of the American Association for Emergency Psychiatry Project BETA De-escalation Workgroup. *The Western Journal of Emergency Medicine, 13*, 17–25.

36. Hoffman, P. D., & Fruzzetti, A. E. (2007). Advances in interventions for families with a relative with a personality disorder diagnosis. *Current Psychiatry Reports, 9*, 68–73.

37. Hoffman, P. D., Fruzzetti, A. E., Buteau, E., et al. (2005). Family connections: A program for relatives of persons with borderline personality disorder. *Family Process, 44*, 217–225.

38. Gunderson, J. G., & Berkowitz, C. (2016). *Family connections: Borderline personality disorder family guidelines*. Retrieved from http://www.borderlinepersonalitydisorder.com/family-connections/familyguidelines/.

39. Zanarini, M. C., Conkey, L. C., Temes, C. M., et al. (2018). Randomized controlled trial of web-based psychoeducation for women with borderline personality disorder. *The Journal of Clinical Psychiatry, 79*(3).

40. Ruggero, C. J., Zimmerman, M., Chelminski, I., et al. (2010). Borderline personality disorder and the misdiagnosis of bipolar disorder. *Journal of Psychiatric Research, 44*, 405–408.

41. Links, P., Ansari, J., Fazalullasha, F., & Shah, R. (2012). The relationship of personality disorders and Axis I clinical disorders. In Widiger, T. (Ed.), *Oxford handbook of personality disorders* (pp. 237–259). New York, NY: Oxford University Press.

42. Lenzenweger, M. F., Lane, M. C., Loranger, A. W., et al. (2007). DSM-IV personality disorders in the National Comorbidity Survey Replication. *Biological Psychiatry, 62*, 553–564.

43. Denchev, P., Pearson, J. L., Allen, M. H., et al. (2018). Modeling the cost-effectiveness of the interventions to reduce suicide risk among hospital emergency department patients. *Psychiatric Services, 69*, 23–31. doi:10.1176/appi.ps.201600351.

44. Klinkenberg, W. D., & Calsyn, R. J. (1999). Predictors of receiving aftercare 1, 3, and 18 months after a psychiatric emergency room visit. *Psychiatric Quarterly, 70*, 39–51.

29

Somatic Symptom and Related Disorders

Julia C. Cromwell, Lucy A. Hutner, Theodore A. Stern

Somatic symptom disorder (SSD) and related disorders all have in common the presence of somatic complaints that are accompanied by significant distress and impairment (1). Symptoms can be quite disabling; many individuals with somatic symptoms have lower overall functioning than do patients with chronic medical illnesses (2,3). Patients who somatize account for up to one-third of all cases seen in the outpatient setting (4) and roughly one-third (36%) of all cases of psychiatric disability (5). They also have higher case complexity scores and double the medical care utilization (and cost) of their nonsomatizing counterparts (6,7). The etiology of SSD and related disorders is multifactorial, including biological, psychological, and social factors (8-14), and there is increasing interest in cognitive-behavioral explanations based on maladaptive illness thoughts and behaviors (15). Discussion in the literature is ongoing regarding the terminology of these disorders (eg, the use of terms such as medically unexplained symptoms, functional symptoms, and somatization), with substantial changes made to their classification in the *Diagnostic and Statistical Manual of Mental Disorders, 5th Ed. (DSM-5)* (1,9,16).

Psychiatrists are likely to encounter patients with somatic complaints in the emergency department (ED). Such presentations are common (eg, 60%-80% of Americans experience a somatic symptom in any given week) (17), they comprise physical symptoms that typically mandate a medical evaluation, and somatization is often associated with psychiatric illness (most often depression and anxiety) (3,13,14,18-21). SSD can be difficult to evaluate and manage in the time-limited setting of the ED, thus misdiagnoses are possible. However, since the 1970s studies have found misdiagnosis of conversion or hysteria symptoms to be consistently low at 4%

(22-24). In the ED, treatment is focused on ruling out life-threatening causes of symptoms, encouraging a treatment alliance with a primary care provider (PCP) and promoting improvement in daily functioning.

PRESENTING CLINICAL FEATURES

Somatic symptom and related disorders are now included in the DSM-5, with SSD being a new classification that reflects elements of the previously defined somatization disorder, undifferentiated somatoform disorder, pain disorder, and hypochondriasis with somatic symptoms (16). Individuals with SSD have at least one somatic symptom causing significant distress or disruption of daily quality of life. They have excessive behaviors, thoughts, and feelings related to their somatic symptom(s), including excessive time and energy devoted to managing their symptoms, excessive worry about their symptoms, and excessive thinking about the potential seriousness of their symptoms. This symptomatic state typically lasts more than 6 months and may have pain as a predominant feature (previously this was referred to as pain disorder). The severity of one's preoccupation with his or her symptoms can be rated as mild, moderate, or severe (16). The importance of medically unexplained symptoms has been de-emphasized in the current criteria for SSD. Instead, the diagnostic focus is on the dysfunction and functional limitation caused by the amplification of the experience of having the somatic symptom(s) (17).

The case vignette below illustrates a presentation of SSD, with Mr. A endorsing multiple somatic complaints, leading to severe distress and overutilization of the ED to address his symptoms (Case 29.1). The somatic symptoms may

CASE 29.1

Mr. A, a 35-year-old man, presented repeatedly to the ED reporting a "diffusely positive" review of systems and severe anxiety that his symptoms were not being treated effectively. The ED staff said they were no longer sure "how much of this was psychological," but they were concerned about missing an obscure etiology of his symptoms. A review of the medical record revealed multiple visits for headache, *abdominal pain, and vague somatic complaints over the preceding years; no obvious physical cause had ever been identified. The ED psychiatrist recommended proceeding with an appropriate medical evaluation in the ED and establishing consistent follow-up with the patient's PCP, who could consider a referral to a cognitive-behavioral therapist or outpatient provider if the patient was amenable.*

---

be associated with an underlying medical illness, but the presence of excessive thoughts, feelings, or behaviors regarding the symptoms is essential for the diagnosis. The prevalence of SSD is estimated to be around 5% to 7% and is associated with female gender, low socioeconomic status, neuroticism, fewer years of education, older age, social stress, and comorbid psychiatric illness. Reinforcing social factors, such as obtaining illness benefits, may also contribute to the disorder (16,25-27). Unlike Mr. A, some patients with SSD will have only one somatic complaint (typically pain).

Roughly 75% of patients who would have been diagnosed with hypochondriasis in the past are now considered to have SSD (16). Hypochondriasis was the term used to describe patients who were preoccupied with the belief that they had a serious medical illness, despite repeated evaluations and reassurances to the contrary (28). Such individuals misattribute trivial symptoms to serious causes and intensely fear disease; thus, they are preoccupied by bodily symptoms. However, about 25% of those who met criteria for hypochondriasis did not have somatic complaints yet continued to excessively worry

about their health. These patients are now classified under the term illness anxiety disorder, with both "care-seeking" and "care-avoidant" subtypes (16).

Ms. B meets criteria for conversion disorder (also known as functional neurological symptom disorder), because of having at least one symptom of abnormal motor or sensory function incompatible with physical examination and incompatible with any recognized neurological cause (Case 29.2). Patients with conversion disorder present with acute physical symptoms, which may be imposed on a known medical illness (such as psychogenic nonepileptic seizures in the setting of a known seizure disorder). Other symptoms may include paralysis, tremor, sensory loss, speech symptoms (eg, slurred speech), or a gait abnormality, some of which have specific signs (eg, an entrainable tremor or positive Hoover sign) suggesting conversion disorder (29). Symptoms may appear, and resolve, abruptly; other patients have persistent symptoms that last longer than 6 months. Functional brain imaging studies have implicated the anterior cingulate gyrus, orbitofrontal cortex, striatum, thalamus, and the primary sensorimotor cortex in the disorder (30).

CASE 29.2

Concerned parents brought their 19-year-old daughter, Ms. B, into the ED in a wheelchair. They reported that her left leg suddenly became weak 2 hours earlier, causing an inability to walk. When asked when her symptoms started, Ms. B stated that it may have *been soon after her parents announced they were getting a divorce. There was adequate strength in the limb and her imaging results were normal; nevertheless, Ms. B still insisted that her leg was immobile.*

CASE 29.3

Mr. C, 56-year-old man, presented to the ED numerous times for evaluation of skin abscesses. The abscesses, which grew multiple bacteria, responded well to basic medical treatment. After his fifth presentation, the ED resident, puzzled by the unclear etiology *of the symptoms, called the patient's PCP for collateral and was informed that Mr. C had a history of injecting fecal matter under his skin. No obvious external reward was found for this repeated behavior. Psychiatry was consulted to help manage the situation.*

Although the disorder is often associated with psychological distress and trauma, identifying a clear precipitating stressor is no longer required for diagnosis (nor is excluding feigning) (16).

Mr. C's behaviors are consistent with factitious disorder (Case 29.3). Factitious disorder occurs when a patient falsifies symptoms or induces injury to present himself or herself as ill. Although the patient is intentionally deceiving others, there is no clear secondary gain perpetuating the behavior (if obvious external reward is found, the patient would be diagnosed with malingering instead). Factitious symptoms can be physical (eg, injecting oneself with warfarin) or psychological (eg, reporting suicidal ideation after a divorce, when it was later found out that the patient was never married). If the false symptoms are induced in another person (eg, someone's child or elderly parent), the creator of the symptoms is diagnosed with factitious disorder imposed on another (16).

EVALUATION

History

The ED psychiatrist must attempt to gather a complete history from the patient, focusing on the presenting somatic complaint(s). A medical team may have already asked about medical symptoms (including their pattern, quality, frequency, duration, and severity). The ED psychiatrist can add to the history by attempting to redress physical complaints with an ear tuned to the underlying affect, such as symptoms that arise suddenly after a personal loss. The ED psychiatrist should then conduct a full psychiatric interview to help clarify the underlying diagnosis, evaluate for comorbid psychiatric disorders, and assess for psychosocial factors contributing to the symptoms. The assessment should include a history of psychiatric symptoms (including their timing, severity, frequency, nature, and precipitants) and any known relationship to the current physical symptoms. The psychiatric consultant should also perform a psychiatric review of systems, covering symptoms from the affective, behavioral, and psychotic realms (and ruling out thoughts of suicide or homicide). Obtaining a history of substance abuse is crucial, as is that of any past trauma. Finally, a psychiatric history (eg, of suicide attempts, hospitalizations, medication trials, and current treaters) should be gathered.

Examination

The mental status examination (MSE) is a detailed observation of a patient's behavior, speech, language, mood, affect, and cognition. The MSE can be helpful in making a diagnosis of SSD. For example, a patient with extreme anxiety and persistent rumination about the seriousness of his or her symptoms is more likely to have SSD than is a patient with a neutral affect and no evidence of preoccupation with his or her physical complaints. Attention to vital signs (eg, that suggest substance intoxication or withdrawal), neurologic signs (such as facial asymmetry), cardiac abnormalities, and gastrointestinal signs (such as stigmata of liver disease) may suggest the need for further medical evaluation. Among the most important physical findings are those that indicate frontal lobe dysfunction, because the frontal lobes govern executive function—including decision-making, planning, and inhibition of behavior. Tests that assess the status of the frontal lobes (by assessing the presence of frontal release signs and performing go-no-go tests) are brief and easily performed, whereas documentation of a memory screening test such as the Montreal Cognitive Assessment may be helpful to clarify the patient's baseline cognitive functioning (31).

Differential Diagnosis

The key to creating a differential diagnosis for patients with somatic complaints is to think broadly, with consideration of medical, social, and psychological contributions. SSD is no longer a diagnosis of exclusion, and if a patient meets criteria for SSD and another psychiatric or medical disorder, the patient should be diagnosed with both disorders. For instance, patients with functional somatic syndromes, such as systemic exertion intolerance disease, fibromyalgia, and chronic Lyme disease, often exhibit maladaptive illness thoughts and behaviors that meet diagnostic criteria for SSD (15).

An extensive differential of other psychiatric disorders involving somatic complaints should also be considered as possible primary diagnoses (eg, SSD should not be diagnosed if somatic preoccupation only occurs during depressive episodes). Affective disorders (such as major depressive disorder [MDD] or persistent depressive disorder), anxiety disorders (such as panic disorder or generalized anxiety disorder), obsessive-compulsive disorders (such as body dysmorphic disorder), and primary psychotic disorders (such as delusional disorder or schizophrenia) can all include somatic complaints. In fact, about 75% of patients with MDD or panic disorder initially present to their PCP with somatic symptoms (17). Thus, an alternative psychiatric disorder such as MDD is a more common reason for somatic complaints than is SSD.

Another important consideration is a substance use disorder, which commonly produces physical complaints (such as fatigue, headache, insomnia, and appetite change). Patients with dissociative disorders (such as dissociative identity disorder), characterized by disruption in consciousness, identity, perception, or memory (16), can provide an inconsistent or vague history that may not correlate with objective findings. A personality disorder is also on the differential, such as exaggeration of somatic symptoms by a patient with histrionic personality disorder, or intense fixation on somatic symptoms in a patient with paranoid personality disorder (17). Finally, it is important to remember that cultural components of psychiatric presentations are often somatic (32); a diagnosis of SSD fits less well, in general, in cultures that have a more unified view of mind and body (9). Also, the cultural background of the physician matters. If the physician's cultural background has less focus on the interconnectedness of the body and mind, somatic symptoms may be interpreted differently and SSD underdiagnosed.

MANAGEMENT

Criteria for Hospitalization

A patient with suspected SSD or a related disorder may be medically or psychiatrically hospitalized for a variety of reasons. First, patients with factitiously produced medical illnesses, such as hypoglycemia or sepsis, may require medical hospitalization for acute treatment. There may be a need for further inpatient medical evaluation that would be difficult to achieve in the ED (eg, performance of a colonoscopy or another diagnostic procedure in the setting of persistent abdominal pain). Psychiatric hospitalization may also be warranted when a comorbid psychiatric disorder causes concern for a patient's safety because of imminent risk of suicide, homicide, or an inability to care for self because of mental illness. Finally, a medical or psychiatric hospitalization should be considered when a patient's symptoms are severe enough to significantly limit activities of daily living (such as a stated inability to ambulate). If a hospital stay is offered, the focus should be on a time-limited process that emphasizes creating a treatment plan for functional recovery in the outpatient setting. A short hospitalization also provides an opportunity to consult additional services to help in treatment planning, including social work or case management consults to address clear social factors contributing to repeated ED presentations, neurology consults for patients with conversion disorder, physical therapy and occupational therapy consults for disposition planning, and neuropsychological testing to aid in diagnosis.

Treatment Within the Emergency Setting

A general approach to treating SSD in the ED includes evaluating for medical causes of symptoms, focusing on building a treatment alliance, and referring to outpatient follow-up for further management. It is important to emphasize that limit setting and avoidance of prolonged ED stays are key management tools for SSD and related disorders, given the iatrogenic risks with unnecessary procedures and invasive evaluations as well as the tendency of long ED and hospital stays to induce emotional regression in certain patients. Thus, a patient may be safely diverted from the ED if an acute life-threatening medical illness has been reasonably excluded and the patient is able to follow-up with outpatient appointments provided. For patients with an extensive history of ED visits, more detailed management plans developed in conjunction with the patient's outpatient providers can be made easily accessible place in the medical record (8).

Evaluation of Medical Causes

Ruling out a medical cause for somatic symptoms is no longer central to the diagnosis of SSD; instead, the patient's excessive emotional and behavioral focus on the symptoms, regardless of their cause, is the main criteria for diagnosis. In general, somatic symptom and related disorders do not represent medical emergencies requiring acute treatment in the ED, but they can mimic serious medical emergencies that do need to be addressed imminently. Thus, life-threatening emergencies (eg, myocardial infarction, pulmonary embolism) should be ruled out in any patient presenting to the ED with concerning medical symptoms. Beyond this general rule, deciding whether it is safe to avoid or defer a complete medical workup of symptoms when SSD is high on the differential is challenging. The extent of the medical workup is typically decided on a case-by-case basis. The ED team should make this decision, with the ED psychiatrist aiding in clarifying the diagnosis via gathering further psychosocial history and collateral or helping with management and treatment planning.

Although it may be tempting to dismiss medical complaints from patients with SSD, one must remember that occult disease can (on occasion) be detected among those who repeatedly seek examinations and treatment. Alternatively, if a life-threatening emergency is excluded, rather than dismissing the patient's concerns, one should take the time to consider nonemergent causes for somatic complaints that could be effectively treated in the outpatient setting (eg, acid reflux in a patient repeatedly presenting with acute chest pain) (8). If the diagnosis is still unclear and one is considering low-probability conditions, one should recall that each procedure carries its own risks (including iatrogenic anxiety from false-positive or inconclusive results). Thus, one needs to balance a thorough investigation of a complaint with the potential risk of testing itself. This is especially true for patients with illness anxiety, in which the physician's reassurance about a negative result is unlikely to produce a sense of relief.

For patients with factitious disorder, knowing the etiology of their physical symptoms minimizes unnecessary diagnostic testing during repeated ED visits. Particularly for those patients who refuse to discuss their behaviors or accept psychiatric care, it is essential to communicate the diagnosis with the patient's PCP and other local EDs (in part by adding the diagnosis to the patient's medical record).

Alliance Building

Throughout the medical evaluation, the physician should aim for an effective therapeutic alliance with patients by validating their suffering via focusing on the impact (rather than the etiology) of their somatic complaints (eg, avoiding telling patients that, based on lab results, nothing is "seriously" wrong with them) (15). Many patients with SSD or conversion disorder do not believe that their physical symptoms are related to psychological or social distress (26), thus abruptly highlighting the connection among biologic, psychological, and social factors in their presentation before creating a therapeutic alliance may backfire. In general, the ED team should reinforce the fact that a patient's somatic symptoms can improve, even if their origin is unclear. In the ED, this is best done by either collaborating with a patient's existing PCP or referring the patient to a new PCP, who can see the patient for time-limited, regular outpatient appointments (17). This can decrease a possible unconscious need of patients to present as "sick" to receive medical attention (15) and can help to facilitate further referrals to outpatient care (eg, physical therapy, psychiatry). Finally, the persistence of the patients' complaints can lead to feelings of boredom, hostility, and derision on the part of the physician, who may feel that such patients waste his or her time or use up hospital (and societal) resources. Physicians should learn to recognize possible negative countertransference reactions to patients with SSD and counter them by remaining cognizant of patients' underlying suffering.

If a patient has factitious disorder, direct confrontation of deceitful actions while in the ED should typically be avoided, as the patient may feel stigmatized or humiliated and may start accessing care at a different ED instead of changing behaviors. However, for some patients, confrontation of maladaptive behaviors in a supportive manner and offering psychiatric care could be beneficial.

Psychopharmacologic and Psychotherapeutic Options

Psychopharmacologic management may be helpful. For example, a patient with MDD and concurrent pain may benefit from dual-acting agents, such as tricyclic antidepressants (eg, amitriptyline) or serotonin and norepinephrine reuptake inhibitors (SNRIs) (eg, duloxetine) (33). Additionally, antidepressant therapy in general has been shown to be useful both in the treatment of medically unexplained symptoms and functional somatic symptoms (34). The psychiatrist should avoid prescribing these agents in the ED and should instead refer to a colleague who can prescribe and monitor their use and effects in the outpatient setting. It is a good idea to avoid polypharmacy in those with SSD because they may become preoccupied with medication side effects (and have lesser susceptibility to placebo benefits). Additionally, narcotics should be avoided so that additional problems (eg, dependence, diversion, and the need for further presentations for secondary gain) do not develop.

Therapy treatments, such as short-term dynamic psychotherapy or CBT, can help reduce psychological distress, depression, and catastrophic thinking and can limit excessive use of medical care (35,36). Other therapeutic techniques may include graded exercise, physical therapy (specifically for conversion disorder), biofeedback, and mindfulness (15). Although psychotherapeutic treatments beyond psychoeducation or brief supportive therapy are unlikely to be feasible in the ED, building a therapeutic alliance may help a patient more easily accept any type of mental health referral.

REFERENCES

1. Dimsdale, J. E., Creed, F., Escobar, J., et al. (2013). Somatic symptom disorder: An important change in DSM. *Journal of Psychosomatic Research, 75*, 223–228.
2. Smith, G. R., Monson, R. A., & Ray, D. C. (1986). Patients with multiple unexplained symptoms: Their characteristics, functional health, and health care utilization. *Archives of Internal Medicine, 146*, 69–72.
3. Kroenke, K., Spitzer, R. L., Williams, J. B. W., et al. (1994). Physical symptoms in primary care: Predictors of psychiatric disorders and functional impairment. *Archives of Family Medicine, 3*, 774–779.
4. Bass, C., & Sharpe, M. (2003). Medically unexplained symptoms in patients attending medical outpatient clinics. In Weatherall, D. A., Ledingham, J. G., & Warrell, D. A. (Eds.), *Oxford textbook of medicine* (4th ed., pp. 1296–1303). Oxford, UK: Oxford University Press.
5. Nejad, S. H., & Alpay, M. (2018). Pain. In Stern, T. A., Herman, J. B., & Rubin, D. H. (Eds.), *Massachusetts General Hospital psychiatry update and board preparation* (4th ed., pp. 455–467). Boston, MA: MGH Psychiatry Academy Publishing.
6. Van Eck van der Sluijs, J. F., de Veroege, L., van Manen, A. S., et al. (2017). Complexity assessed by the INTERMED in patients with somatic symptom disorder visiting a specialized outpatient mental health care setting: A cross-sectional study. *Psychosomatics, 58*, 331–342.
7. Barsky, A. J., Orav, J., & Bates, D. W. (2005). Somatization increases medical utilization and costs independent of psychiatric and medical comorbidity. *Archives of General Psychiatry, 62*, 903–910.
8. Stephenson, D. T., & Price, J. R. (2006). Medically unexplained symptoms in emergency medicine. *Emergency Medicine Journal, 23*, 595–600.
9. Mayou, R., Kirmayer, L. J., Simon, G., et al. (2005). Somatoform disorders: Time for a new approach in DSM-V. *American Journal of Psychiatry, 162*(5), 847–855.
10. Newman, M. G., Clayton, L., Zuellig, A., et al. (2000). The relationship of childhood sexual abuse and depression with somatic symptoms and medical utilization. *Psychologie Médicale, 30*(5), 1063–1077.
11. Drossman, D. A., Leserman, J., Nachman, G., et al. (1990). Sexual and physical abuse in women with functional or organic gastrointestinal disorders. *Annals of Internal Medicine, 113*(11), 828–833.

12. Marsden, C. D. (1986). Hysteria—A neurologist's view. *Psychologie Médicale, 16,* 277–288.

13. Hamilton, J., Campos, R., & Creed, F. (1996). Anxiety, depression, and management of medically unexplained symptoms in medical clinics. *Journal of the Royal College of Physicians of London, 30,* 18–20.

14. Brown, F. W., Golding, J. M., & Smith, R. (1990). Psychiatric comorbidity in primary care somatization disorder. *Psychosomatic Medicine, 52,* 445–451.

15. Kontos, N. (2018). Somatic symptom and related disorders. In Stern, T. A., Herman, J. B., & Rubin, D. H. (Eds.), *Massachusetts General Hospital psychiatry update and board preparation* (4th ed., pp. 227–231). Boston, MA: MGH Psychiatry Academy Publishing.

16. American Psychiatric Association. (2013). *Diagnostic and statistical manual of mental disorders* (5th ed.). Washington, DC: American Psychiatric Association.

17. Kontos, N., Beach, S. R., Smith, F. A., et al. (2018). Psychosomatic conditions: Somatic symptom and related disorders, functional somatic syndromes, and deception syndromes. In Stern, T. A., Freudenreich, O., Smith, F. A., et al. (Eds.), *Massachusetts General Hospital handbook of general hospital psychiatry* (7th ed., pp. 161–176). Edinburgh: Elsevier.

18. Russo, J., Katon, W., Sullivan, M., et al. (1994). Severity of somatization and its relationship to psychiatric disorders and personality. *Psychosomatics, 35,* 546–556.

19. Kroenke, K., Jackson, J. L., & Chamberlin, J. (1997). Depressive and anxiety disorders in patients presenting with physical complaints: Clinical predictors and outcome. *American Journal of Medicine, 103,* 339–347.

20. Simon, G. E., Von Korff, M., Piccinelli, M., et al. (1999). An international study of the relation between somatic symptoms and depression. *The New England Journal of Medicine, 341,* 1329–1335.

21. Simon, G. E., & Von Korff, M. (1991). Somatization and psychiatric disorder in the NIMH epidemiologic catchment area study. *American Journal of Psychiatry, 148,* 1494–1500.

22. Stern, T. A. (1988). Malingering, factitious illness, and somatization. In Hyman, S. E. (Ed.), *Manual of psychiatric emergencies* (2nd ed., pp. 217–225). Boston, MA: Little, Brown and Company.

23. Hurwitz, T. (2004). Somatization and conversion disorder. *The Canadian Journal of Psychiatry, 49,* 172–178.

24. Stone, J., Smyth, R., Carson, A., et al. (2005). Systematic review of misdiagnosis of conversion symptoms and "hysteria." *BMJ, 331*(7523), 989.

25. Barsky, A. J., Peekna, H. M., & Borus, J. F. (2001). Somatic symptom reporting in women and men. *Journal of General Internal Medicine, 16,* 266–275.

26. Kroenke, K., & Spitzer, R. L. (1998). Gender difference in the reporting of physical and somatoform symptoms. *Psychosomatic Medicine, 60,* 150–155.

27. Hernandez, J., & Kellner, R. (1992). Hypochondriacal concerns and attitudes toward illness in males and females. *International Journal of Psychiatry in Medicine, 22,* 251–263.

28. American Psychiatric Association. (1994). *Diagnostic and statistical manual of mental disorders* (4th ed.). Washington, DC: American Psychiatric Association.

29. McKee, K., Glass, S., Adams, C., et al. (2018). The inpatient assessment and management of motor functional neurological disorders: An interdisciplinary perspective. *Psychosomatics, 59,* 358–368.

30. Ghaffar, O., Staines, W. R., & Feinstein, A. (2006). Unexplained neurologic symptoms: An fMRI study of sensory conversion disorder. *Neurology, 67,* 2036–2038.

31. Nasreddine, Z. S., Phillips, N. A., Bédirian, V., Charbonneau, S., et al. (2005). The Montreal Cognitive Assessment, MoCA: A brief screening tool for mild cognitive impairment. *Journal of the American Geriatrics Society, 53*(4), 695–699.

32. Goldberg, D. P., & Bridges, K. (1988). Somatic presentations of psychiatric illness in primary care settings. *Journal of Psychosomatic Research, 32*(2), 137–144.

33. Dharmshaktu, P., Tayal, V., & Kalra, B. S. (2012). Efficacy of antidepressants as analgesics: A review. *The Journal of Clinical Pharmacology, 52*(1), 6–17.

34. Barsky, A. J., & Borus, J. F. (1999). Functional somatic syndromes. *Annals of Internal Medicine, 130,* 910–921.

35. Chavooshi, B., Saberi, M., Tavallaie, S. A., et al. (2017). Psychotherapy for medically unexplained pain: A randomized clinical trial comparing intensive short-term dynamic psychotherapy and cognitive-behavioral therapy. *Psychosomatics, 58,* 506–519.

36. Sharpe, M., Peveler, R., & Mayou, R. (1992). The psychological treatment of patients with functional somatic symptoms: A practical guide. *Journal of Psychosomatic Research, 36,* 515–529.

30

Malingering and Deception

Scott A. Simpson

INTRODUCTION

Malingering is the intentional fabrication of symptoms in order to gain material advantage or avoid undesired responsibility. In clinical practice, malingering is likely common and certainly challenging to identify. This chapter describes the phenomenon and epidemiology of malingering and provides a framework for assessing and managing malingering patients in the emergency department (ED).

DEFINING MALINGERING

Although malingering exhibits many varied phenotypes, certain common elements differentiate malingering from other psychiatric illnesses. For one, malingering requires that the patient's actions be intentional and conscious. Unconscious behaviors are more typical of other psychiatric illnesses such as somatic symptom disorders. Historical theories describing malingering included consideration of psychodynamic and unconscious motivations underlying these behaviors; however, these theories are no longer relevant to clinical practice.

Malingering also requires that the patient produce or hide symptoms that are not caused by illness. These symptoms may vary in quality and intensity. Some patients exhibit partial malingering by exaggerating extant symptoms. Other patients demonstrate pure malingering by fabricating entirely new symptoms. In emergency psychiatry, most malingering involves the reporting of symptoms including suicidality, hallucinations, or pain. Some patients may confer actual physical injury—for example, swallowing items, self-harming, or administering medications. It is also possible to manipulate laboratory tests to suggest the presence of disease where there is none (1). Most malingering involves the production of symptoms, and this chapter focuses on the

identification of malingering in those instances. However, malingering patients also dissimulate or intentionally obscure symptoms for external motivation (2).

Finally, malingering requires that the behaviors be motivated by the patient's desire to acquire some material gain through these actions. The goal of malingering is often described as secondary gain. Secondary gain includes the acquisition of some external benefit or aversion of responsibility. Common examples in the ED are shelter, disability payments, or avoidance of work or legal consequences. Secondary gain is differentiated from primary gain in that the latter refers to a typically unconscious need that must be fulfilled from being ill (3). This primary need is instilled through the patient's past experiences of trauma or interpersonal relationships. The intentional production of symptoms for primary gain is factitious disorder. Being ill in order to consciously elicit the material benefits of attention or caregiving is considered secondary gain and is malingering.

Table 30.1 enumerates the intrinsic elements of malingering. The Diagnostic and Statistical Manual, Fifth Edition (DSM-5) does not consider malingering a psychiatric illness (4). Rather, malingering is considered a condition with significant implications for clinical care. The DSM-5 explicitly notes that malingering for substance of abuse is considered malingering (eg, reporting pain to obtain opioids).

EPIDEMIOLOGY

It is difficult to define the prevalence of a condition whose core feature is deception. Patients are rarely motivated to report the presence of malingering—although they certainly will on occasion. Studies have attempted to ascertain the frequency of malingering through descriptions of fraud claims, clinicians' suspicions, patients' self-report, and neuropsychological testing.

TABLE 30.1 Essential Elements of Malingering

- Purposeful and conscious behavior
- Presence of somatic or psychiatric symptoms
- Motivation for secondary gain (for example, substances of abuse, housing, legal or financial benefit, abrogation of legal claims)

Regardless of methodology, it is clear that malingering is common across all clinical settings. In one study specific to the ED, clinicians suspected more than 10% of patients to be fabricating symptoms (5). Malingering appears even more common among disability claimants (6), inmates (7,8), and even outpatient psychotherapy patients (9). Malingering costs health systems in the United States tens of billions of dollars annually (10,11). The idea of formalized screening for malingering in the ED has been suggested; however, no available approach has yet proven plausible or valid (12). ED screening would be particularly difficult, given the variety of patient demographics, clinical acuity, and logistical challenges of this care environment.

IDENTIFICATION IN CLINICAL PRACTICE

Relative to its significant costs and prevalence, many clinicians receive little education around the identification and management of malingering. This discrepancy likely reflects concerns over the pejorative connotations of the term and the rightful fear of dismissing actual, even life-threatening illness as malingering (13). The idea of patients' intentionally feigning illness is also difficult to reconcile with concepts of trauma-informed and patient-centered care predominant in contemporary medicine. But notwithstanding a patient's deceptive behaviors, it remains possible and important for clinicians to build an effective therapeutic alliance with these patients and provide them effective, compassionate care. The first step in building that alliance and providing appropriate care is identifying the presence of malingering.

There is no gold standard for the diagnosis of malingering: it is ultimately impossible to know if a patient is malingering. Much research on detecting malingering has occurred in specialized forensic settings. These settings are quite different than the ED; however, there are common contextual and clinical clues that should raise the provider's suspicion for malingering. Medical and psychiatric evaluations in forensic settings (eg, for court proceedings or disability determinations) are more likely to be associated with malingered symptoms (4). Although EDs do not appear to be among the practice settings with a particularly high rate of malingering, the clear presence of secondary benefits from the patient's presentation should raise the clinician's concern, for instance, consider the patient who is adamant about sheltering in the ED or receiving controlled substances.

Malingering symptoms are often highly inconsistent—inconsistent with known pathology, other present symptoms, and the degree of observed impairment. Indeed, the variability and atypicality of malingered symptoms are in some ways the hallmark of the malingered presentation. Malingering patients often report symptoms that are inconsistent with known presentations of the purported underlying illness. In psychiatric illness, for example, patients with schizophrenia often describe auditory hallucinations that are intermittent, spoken by identifiable individuals, and ameliorated by coping skills; a patient malingering such hallucinations may be unable to describe coping skills or the identity of the voice (14). Discriminating such symptomatic nuances requires both the clinician to be familiar with the primary illness and also the malingerer to be poorly informed. Moreover, clearly some patients with true illness will exhibit atypical symptoms. It is the quality—not quantity—of reported symptoms that are most suspicious for malingering (15).

A careful history of malingering patients' symptoms often elicits further inconsistencies. The timing and quality of symptoms often vary from one visit and clinician to the next. The degree of impairment conferred by these symptoms is also often inconsistent (16,17). For example, a patient may report severe hallucinations for which hospitalization is requested, yet there is no overt evidence of distress in the ED. Or a patient may report severe pain without evidence of functional limitation. Obtaining a record of such inconsistencies requires a thorough chart review of the patient's prior presentations including at other facilities and a review of the patient's ED course with other staff. The presence of such inconsistencies is suspicious—albeit not conclusive—for malingering.

Several bedside and laboratory tests may be applicable in differentiating malingered illness. Physical, laboratory, and radiologic findings discordant with the reported illness are naturally concerning. So is the overt presence of instruments used in malingering: for instance, the discovery of hidden needles or medications in the patient's belongings requires discussion and consideration of occult symptom falsification. The laboratory presence of surreptitiously administered medications and drugs is also of concern. Certain neurological tests have been evaluated in the detection of functional illness and malingering, but there is debate as to these tests' reliability. These tests include the Hoover sign to test functional leg paresis (18), the presence of Waddell signs associated with nonorganic lower back pain (19), and isometric strength testing to assess for maximal effort (20).

Neuropsychological testing is frequently employed in forensic and psychological testing for the detection of malingering. These tests typically require trained administrators and utilize several strategies to elucidate inconsistencies in patients' response styles. Strategies include the use of misleading face validity (ie, the test appears harder than it actually is, and malingerers score poorly) and atypical symptom endorsement. Some tests have promise for application in the ED though have not been specifically validated in this setting. The Rey 15-item test evaluates a patient's effort and memory and can be administered at the bedside in about a minute (21). Another test is the longer Miller Forensic Assessment of Symptoms Test which requires 10 minutes and use of specific testing materials by a trained operator (12,22). These tests are different from polygraph ("lie-detector") tests that use a combination of carefully constructed questioning and physiological testing.

Polygraphy is used in law enforcement and not applicable for clinical practice (23,24).

Most patients who are not malingering are cooperative with the clinician's evaluation including even invasive interview questions and laboratory tests. And most patients appreciate a discussion of treatment options available to them. In contrast, malingering should be suspected in patients who are uncooperative with treatment planning and adamant about particular treatments. Malingering patients often request only specific treatments (opioids, hospitalization) and become irritable at the suggestion of alternative options (25). Conditional threats may be made ("If you don't admit me, then you'll be sorry!") (26). Patients may hinder attempts at obtaining a history of present illness through excessively vague language or refusals to allow clinicians to obtain collateral information (16,27).

Yet ultimately each of these clues is only an imperfect indicator of malingering. The accumulation of many risk factors (summarized in Table 30.2) should raise the clinician's suspicion for falsified symptoms and be considered in the approach to the patient's management.

PATHOPHYSIOLOGY

Having reviewed characteristics of the malingered presentation, it is worthwhile to consider why patients may exaggerate or entirely fabricate symptoms. Certainly, malingering patients are seeking overt gain. But why must patients resort to lying to their healthcare clinicians?

Psychological models have attempted to describe malingering as the result of unconscious motivations, but these models were discarded when they did not correlate well with the trajectory of patients' clinical course—in particular, these models could not account for why malingering ceased when the secondary gain was removed (28). Subsequent formulations, particularly older editions of the DSM, focused on the predatory nature of malingering and its association with antisocial personality disorder. These formulations correlated with neurological evidence such as abnormalities of neurotransmissions in human and animal models of aggression (29,30). Yet they again did not account for changes in behavior over time or inform a clinical approach.

TABLE 30.2 Clinical Presentations Suspicious for Malingering

Element	Example
Inconsistency in history	A patient reports he has no history of substance abuse, but he was seen for an opioid overdose in the same emergency department (ED) last month. Or, a patient reports severe pain and an inability to walk but nonchalantly roams the ED when thought to be unobserved.
Atypical symptoms and presentation	A patient who purports to have schizophrenia describes overly indulgent, bizarre, and well-formed visual hallucinations.
Absence of objective impairment	The above psychotic patient does not appear distressed by these symptoms—or to react to them in any way.
Clear objective evidence of surreptitious behavior	Drug paraphernalia is found in a patient's hospital room.
Presence or absence of objective laboratory evidence	A patient reports overdosing on lithium but has a negative lithium serum level. Or, a patient denies a substance use history but has objective stigmata of injection drug use.
Forensic setting	The patient comes to the ED from a local jail.
Presence of antisocial personality disorder	The patient has a long history of prison time including for assault, forgery, and larceny; old notes suggest the patient has a history of conduct disorder as an adolescent.
Uncooperative in treatment planning	The patient refuses to talk with the behavioral health consultant about coping skills to manage anxiety and instead continually requests benzodiazepines.
Evidence from bedside neuropsychological testing	The patient has a low score on a Rey 15-item test.
Clear evidence of secondary gain	The patient was kicked out of a friend's home and is now homeless.

A more sensible and helpful formulation of malingering is an adaptational model that posits that the patient's decision to malinger is the choice that poses the greatest possible reward with the least possible risk (28). This model is both sensible and helpful in clinical practice. Patients with substantial, imminent needs and no other way to meet those needs are more likely to malinger. And if the costs of malingering are low, as they are in the ED, then malingering behaviors are more likely. This formulation is consistent with evidence that malingering appears more likely when the potential external reward is greater (8,31). The presence of an adversarial relationship with providers only escalates the potential for somebody to resort to malingering to have their needs met. Figure 30.1 illustrates the risk of malingering in terms of this model.

The adaptational model is agnostic as to the presence of psychiatric illness. Social conventions often dissuade many patients from lying and falsifying illness to their clinicians. These conventions are often disregarded by patients with antisocial personality disorder or unfamiliar to patients with serious mental illness. More often, the use of malingering reflects the patient's inability to meet their needs through other means. For example, a patient with a substance use disorder cannot achieve sobriety or obtain treatment and so malingers for substances to relieve withdrawal. Or a patient with severe trauma-associated anxiety struggles to spend the night in a busy shelter and so malingers for the safety of the ED. Formulating malingering as the best option available to the patient at the time of presentation

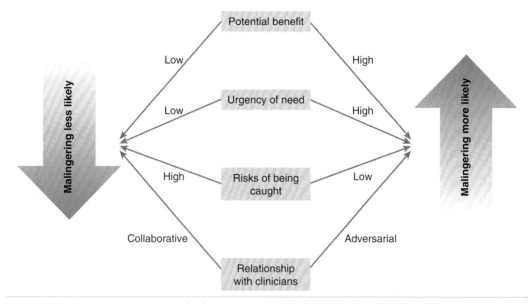

FIGURE 30.1 • Application of the adaptational model in assessing the likelihood of malingering.

averts the need to apply a psychiatric diagnosis and guides the clinician in a compassionate, practical approach to managing these behaviors.

MANAGEMENT

Having suspected and identified malingering, the next—and for many clinicians the most challenging—step in managing malingering is being aware of one's own emotional reaction to the malingering patient. It is not uncommon or unreasonable for the clinician to respond with frustration, annoyance, anger, or hostility toward the malingering patient (32). Rare is the provider who went into health care without idealizing the value of a trusting, productive clinician-patient relationship. By malingering, the patient jeopardizes that alliance and clinicians' trust.

The implications of such negative countertransference reactions are profound. Most concerning is the possibility that clinicians miss signs and symptoms suggestive of genuine illness. Indeed, over time much illness thought to be malingering or functional has proven to be previously undiscovered neurological illness (33), and medically unexplained symptoms remain common (34,35). The clinician may make demeaning statements about the patient to other staff—"oh, he's just faking"—or even directly to the patient

(36). Such behavior is an abdication of clinical leadership and diminishes the healthcare team's ability to compassionately care for not only malingerers but also for other patients. In addition, a workplace in which patients are spoken of negatively invites similar behavior toward colleagues and escalates the risk of burnout (37).

That said, it is appropriate to acknowledge one's own countertransference and model its professional management among the team. Sharing with a colleague that this patient "sometimes makes me feel angry" can normalize strong countertransference reactions among the team; a strong clinical leader can follow this statement with a demonstrable rededication to excluding serious illness and helping the patient connect with appropriate resources on ED discharge. Channeling the energy of strong negative reactions into positive, productive interventions on the patient's behalf represents mature coping by the clinician as well as a strategy more likely to reduce the risk of recurrent malingering.

Recalling that malingering arises from the patient's seeking to optimize the likelihood of a positive, desired outcome, the clinician must identify the patient's goals (eg, shelter) and reframe the conversation around those goals. What is the patient's necessary need at this time? And why can the patient not otherwise acquire these goals? Perhaps the patient has a comorbid illness that has made it difficult to navigate the shelter system or workplace environment (38). In legal settings, many inmates have a history of abuse that profoundly affects their interpersonal functioning and decision-making.

Having identified the patient's goal, the clinician should feel confident in setting firm limits around what is permissible in achieving that goal. The clinician need not excuse or be complicit in the patient's decision to lie. The goal of the ED encounter is to stabilize emergent symptoms and facilitate the patient's next stage of treatment. For example, if hospitalization or a work excuse is not indicated, the clinician ought to be forthright and unambiguous in saying so. The goal is not to confront the patient with evidence of malingering; doing so is not helpful (39). Rather, the goal is to remove any temptation on the patient's part to further feign symptoms to achieve something unobtainable. When clear limits are set, malingering patients often begin discussing alternative options (eg, how to access a shelter if they cannot be hospitalized) or simply discontinue the relationship by leaving the ED. Clearly the former is preferable even if the latter may sometimes be unavoidable.

Documentation is a critical facet of managing malingering. Appropriate documentation serves to reveal the clinician's decision-making including in the application of interventions or testing. Strong documentation aids future clinicians in discovering and managing malingering. Thus, documentation should include a thorough history including acknowledgment of collateral information from outside hospitals and observations collected from nurses, technicians, and other staff. For particularly challenging cases, performing and documenting a brief consultation with a peer colleague may improve assessment and treatment planning while reducing legal liability (40).

Documentation of the assessment should include a frank enumeration of which symptoms are suspected to be malingered, to what degree the symptoms are exaggerated, and what evidence suggests malingering. Evidence of malingering may be a listing of the above risk factors, such as the comorbid presence of antisocial personality disorder, highly atypical symptoms, or the absence of corroborating laboratory evidence. When supported, a frank diagnosis of malingering is appropriate to document (41). Unambiguous documentation aids future clinicians seeking to make a correct diagnosis, avoid iatrogenic harm from unnecessary tests and treatments, and responsibly use finite healthcare resources. Clinicians nevertheless must consider that malingering patients may re-present with genuine symptoms and deserve care regardless of their history.

The final aspect of the assessment should include identification of any factors that may have required the patient to resort to malingering and how any such comorbid illness will be managed. For example, if the patient's incipient opioid withdrawal led them to feign pain for opioid medications, what steps are being taken to ameliorate withdrawal and assist the patient in connecting to treatment? Documentation should include reference to any management undertaken in the ED, follow-up instructions, and return precautions. In emergency psychiatry, many feigned symptoms still merit follow-up similar to actual illness. A patient who exaggerates suicidal ideation would nonetheless benefit from best practices for mitigating suicide risk including lethal means restriction, familiarity with crisis resources, a written safety plan, and close psychiatric follow-up. Table 30.3 summarizes essential considerations for documentation.

TABLE 30.3 Elements of Documentation When Malingering is Suspected

- Clear description of history including incorporation of multiple sources
- Identification of which symptoms are malingered
- Enumeration of aspects of the presentation that raise suspicion for malingering
- Identification of the patient's secondary gain
- Diagnosis and treatment plan for comorbid conditions
- Description of treatments and resources offered to the patient and their reaction
- Follow-up plan and return precautions
- Suicide and violence risk assessment for psychiatric presentations

CONCLUSION

No clinical evidence supports a particular comprehensive approach to malingering. Historically there has been a mismatch between the frequency of malingering in clinical settings and the training practitioners receive to identify and manage this presentation. The result of this lack of education and research is many health professionals' propensity to view malingering patients negatively and experience frustration in managing their treatment. However, most malingering patients are choosing to feign symptoms as the most expeditious choice available to them. That this choice is perceived as their best choice speaks to an underlying deficit and distress that itself require attention and possibly treatment. The choice to malinger does not obviate the very real needs of our patients—housing, money, medication, or attention. Our obligation as clinical leaders among our community and hospitals requires a thoughtful and compassionate approach toward even these most frustrating of patient encounters.

REFERENCES

1. Wallach, J. (1994). Laboratory diagnosis of factitious disorders. *Archives of Internal Medicine, 154*(15), 1690–1696.
2. Caruso, K. A., Benedek, D. M., Auble, P. M., & Bernet, W. (2003). Concealment of psychopathology in forensic evaluations: A pilot study of intentional and uninsightful dissimulators. *Journal of the American Academy of Psychiatry and the Law, 31*(4), 444–450.
3. Barsky, A. J., & Klerman, G. L. (1983). Overview: Hypochondriasis, bodily complaints, and somatic styles. *American Journal of Psychiatry, 140*(3), 273–283.
4. American Psychiatric Association. (2013). *Diagnostic and statistical manual of mental disorders: DSM-5.* Arlington, VA: American Psychiatric Association.
5. Yates, B. D., Nordquist, C. R., & Schultz-Ross, R. A. (1996). Feigned psychiatric symptoms in the emergency room. *Psychiatric Services, 47*(9), 998–1000.
6. Mittenberg, W., Patton, C., Canyock, E. M., & Condit, D. C. (2002). Base rates of malingering and symptom exaggeration. *Journal of Clinical and Experimental Neuropsychology, 24*(8), 1094–1102.
7. Pollock, P. H., Quigley, B., Worley, K. O., & Bashford, C. (1997). Feigned mental disorder in prisoners referred to forensic mental health services. *Journal of Psychiatric and Mental Health Nursing, 4*(1), 9–15.
8. McDermott, B. E., Dualan, I. V., & Scott, C. L. (2013). Malingering in the correctional system: Does incentive affect prevalence? *International Journal of Law and Psychiatry, 36*(3–4), 287–292.
9. van Egmond, J., & Kummeling, I. (2002). A blind spot for secondary gain affecting therapy outcomes. *European Psychiatry, 17*(1), 46–54.
10. Frueh, B. C., Grubaugh, A. L., Elhai, J. D., & Buckley, T. C. (2007). US Department of Veterans Affairs disability policies for posttraumatic stress disorder: Administrative trends and implications for treatment, rehabilitation, and research. *American Journal of Public Health, 97*(12), 2143–2145.
11. Chafetz, M., & Underhill, J. (2013). Estimated costs of malingered disability. *Archives of Clinical Neuropsychology, 28*(7), 633–639.
12. Zubera, A., Raza, M., Holaday, E., & Aggarwal, R. (2015). Screening for malingering in the emergency department. *Academic Psychiatry, 39*(2), 233–234.
13. Weiss, K. J., & Van Dell, L. (2017). Liability for diagnosing malingering. *Journal of the American Academy of Psychiatry and the Law, 45*(3), 339–347.
14. Mason, A. M., Cardell, R., & Armstrong, M. (2014). Malingering psychosis: Guidelines for assessment and management. *Perspectives in Psychiatric Care, 50*(1), 51–57.
15. Taylor, S., Frueh, B. C., & Asmundson, G. J. (2007). Detection and management of malingering in people presenting for treatment of posttraumatic stress disorder: Methods, obstacles, and recommendations. *Journal of Anxiety Disorders, 21*(1), 22–41.
16. American Psychiatric Association. (2000). *Diagnostic and statistical manual of mental disorders: DSM-IV-TR* (4th ed.). Washington, DC: American Psychiatric Association.
17. Ali, S., Jabeen, S., & Alam, F. (2015). Multimodal approach to identifying malingered posttraumatic stress disorder: A review. *Innovations in Clinical Neuroscience, 12*(1–2), 12–20.
18. Mehndiratta, M. M., Kumar, M., Nayak, R., Garg, H., & Pandey, S. (2014). Hoover's sign: Clinical relevance in neurology. *Journal of Postgraduate Medicine, 60*(3), 297–299.

19. Fishbain, D. A., Cutler, R. B., Rosomoff, H. L., & Rosomoff, R. S. (2004). Is there a relationship between nonorganic physical findings (Waddell signs) and secondary gain/malingering? *The Clinical Journal of Pain, 20*(6), 399–408.

20. Fishbain, D. A., Cutler, R., Rosomoff, H. L., & Rosomoff, R. S. (1999). Chronic pain disability exaggeration/malingering and submaximal effort research. *The Clinical Journal of Pain, 15*(4), 244–274.

21. Reznek, L. (2005). The Rey 15-item memory test for malingering: A meta-analysis. *Brain Injury, 19*(7), 539–543.

22. Ahmadi, K., Lashani, Z., Afzali, M. H., Tavalaie, S. A., & Mirzaee, J. (2013). Malingering and PTSD: Detecting malingering and war related PTSD by Miller Forensic Assessment of Symptoms Test (M-FAST). *BMC Psychiatry, 13,* 154.

23. MacNeill, A. L., & Bradley, M. T. (2016). Temperature effects on polygraph detection of concealed information. *Psychophysiology, 53*(2), 143–150.

24. Li, G., & Hu, Z. (2014). An exploratory study of using polygraph to detect deception in patients with traumatic brain injury. *Neuroreport, 25*(12), 943–947.

25. Brady, M. C., Scher, L. M., & Newman, W. (2013). "I just saw Big Bird. He was 100 feet tall!" Malingering in the emergency room. *Current Psychiatry, 12*(10), 33–40.

26. Reccoppa, L. (2010). Mentally ill or malingering? 3 clues cast doubt. *Current Psychiatry, 8*(12), 110.

27. Lebourgeois, H. W., III. (2007). Malingering: Key points in assessment. *Psychiatric Times, 24*(5), 21.

28. Rogers, R. (1990). Development of a new classificatory model of malingering. *The Bulletin of the American Academy of Psychiatry and the Law, 18*(3), 323–333.

29. Siegel, A., & Victoroff, J. (2009). Understanding human aggression: New insights from neuroscience. *International Journal of Law and Psychiatry, 32*(4), 209–215.

30. Miczek, K. A., Fish, E. W., De Bold, J. F., & De Almeida, R. M. (2002). Social and neural determinants of aggressive behavior: Pharmacotherapeutic targets at serotonin, dopamine and gamma-aminobutyric acid systems. *Psychopharmacology, 163*(3–4), 434–458.

31. Greve, K. W., Ord, J. S., Bianchini, K. J., & Curtis, K. L. (2009). Prevalence of malingering in patients with chronic pain referred for psychologic evaluation in a medico-legal context. *Archives of Physical Medicine and Rehabilitation, 90*(7), 1117–1126.

32. Ekstrom, L. W. (2012). Liars, medicine, and compassion. *The Journal of Medicine and Philosophy, 37*(2), 159–180.

33. Stone, J., Smyth, R., Carson, A., et al. (2005). Systematic review of misdiagnosis of conversion symptoms and "hysteria". *BMJ, 331*(7523), 989.

34. Katon, W. J., & Walker, E. A. (1998). Medically unexplained symptoms in primary care. *The Journal of Clinical Psychiatry, 59*(Suppl. 20), 15–21.

35. Swanson, L. M., Hamilton, J. C., & Feldman, M. D. (2010). Physician-based estimates of medically unexplained symptoms: A comparison of four case definitions. *Family Practice, 27*(5), 487–493.

36. Malone, R. D., & Lange, C. L. (2007). A clinical approach to the malingering patient. *The Journal of the American Academy of Psychoanalysis and Dynamic Psychiatry, 35*(1), 13–21.

37. Garcia, H. A., McGeary, C. A., Finley, E. P., McGeary, D. D., Ketchum, N. S., & Peterson, A. L. (2016). The influence of trauma and patient characteristics on provider burnout in VA post-traumatic stress disorder specialty programmes. *Psychology and Psychotherapy, 89*(1), 66–81.

38. Brennaman, L. (2012). Crisis emergencies for individuals with severe, persistent mental illnesses: A situation-specific theory. *Archives of Psychiatric Nursing, 26*(4), 251–260.

39. Adetunji, B. A., Basil, B., Mathews, M., Williams, A., Osinowo, T., & Oladinni, O. (2006). Detection and management of malingering in a clinical setting. *Primary Psychiatry, 13*(1), 61–69.

40. Clayton, S., & Bongar, B. (1994). The use of consultation in psychological practice: Ethical, legal, and clinical considerations. *Ethics & Behavior, 4*(1), 43–57.

41. Kontos, N., Taylor, J. B., & Beach, S. R. (2018). The therapeutic discharge II: An approach to documentation in the setting of feigned suicidal ideation. *General Hospital Psychiatry, 51,* 30–35.

31

Suicide

Gregory L. Iannuzzi, Leigh J. Ruth, Ryan C. Wagoner, Glenn W. Currier

EPIDEMIOLOGY

Suicide is the 10th leading cause of death in the United States, and the second leading cause of death in individuals 10- to 35-year-old, with rates increasing in nearly all states (1). In 2016, nearly 45,000 Americans of age 10 or older died by suicide (1). According to the Centers for Disease Control and Prevention (1), from 1999 to 2016 percentage increases in suicide rates ranged from 6% to 57% and 25 states had suicide rate increases of more than 30%. This problem is not unique to the United States—suicide is the 15th leading cause of death globally, with an estimated 800,000 deaths per year (2). Moreover, for each completed suicide, there are estimated to be an additional 25 suicide attempts (3).

The lifetime prevalence for attempting suicide is 4.6% (4). Men are more than 3.5 times as likely to die by suicide than women, with non-Hispanic American Indian/Alaska Native and non-Hispanic White population groups at highest risk (1). Other population groups disproportionately impacted by suicide include middle-aged adults, whose rates increased 35% from 2000 to 2015, with steep increases seen among both males (29%) and females (53%) aged 35 to 64 years (1). Veterans and other military personnel (whose suicide rate nearly doubled from 2003 to 2008), as well as sexual minority youth, have also seen significant increases in suicide (1). The vast majority of completed suicides utilize firearms, suffocation, and poisoning (3).

It is no surprise that, regardless of chief complaint (CC), nearly 10% of *all* patients who present to an emergency department (ED) have been found to have suicidal ideation or behaviors (5-7). There are 420,000 ED visits for suicide attempts and self-harm each year, and this represents a doubling of ED presentations compared to a decade earlier (8). Approximately 40% of people who die by suicide have presented to the ED in the prior year, and nearly 40% of these presentations were for nonlethal self-injury (9). Thus, the ED may represent a unique opportunity to intervene during a crisis and connect patients to outpatient care (10).

This chapter will discuss basic considerations for the clinician evaluating patients in the emergency setting who may have an elevated risk for suicide. There is no gold standard for evaluating suicide risk, and this chapter is not intended to serve as one. Rather, the authors hope that by sampling a variety of suicide assessment tools, this chapter may serve as a practical companion to the clinician in the emergency setting.

A FIVE-STEP SUICIDE ASSESSMENT

There are numerous standardized suicide risk assessment instruments available in the current literature, but no single suicide risk assessment instrument stands out as superior. Loosely based on the Columbia-Suicide Severity Rating Scale (C-SSRS), (11) we will discuss a five-step suicide assessment that can potentially be integrated into the clinician's routine evaluation:

1. Explore the chief complaint
2. Identify suicidal behavior
3. Evaluate risk and protective factors
4. Obtain collateral information
5. Document your decision

Step 1: Explore the Chief Complaint

Although gathering the patient's chief complaint (CC) and exploring the history of the present illness (HPI) is second nature to the seasoned clinician for general complaints, eliciting this information in the context of suicide may be unfamiliar to clinicians outside of mental health. When clarifying what the patient means when they voice suicidal ideation, consider the questions listed below (Table 31.1).

TABLE 31.1 Explore the Chief Complaint

HPI Element	Sample Questions to Elicit
Modifying factors and context	"What makes your suicidal thoughts more intense? Less intense?" "What stressors are occurring in your life that make your suicidal thoughts worse?" "What are some things that are important to you and keep you from acting on thoughts of suicide?"
Quality	"Do you wish that you were dead? Do you have a desire to end your life?" "Have you thought of ways to harm yourself? Do you have a plan?" "How close have you come to acting on your plan? Have you done anything to prepare, such as writing letters to loved ones, making arrangements for your death, seeking access to lethal means such as stockpiling medications or obtaining a weapon?" "Did you attempt suicide before coming to the hospital?"
Severity	"How strongly do you feel that you may harm yourself here in the ED? If admitted to the hospital? If discharged?"
Duration and timing	"When did you start feeling suicidal?" "Have your thoughts of suicide changed since they began?" "Are your suicidal thoughts increasing or decreasing in intensity? Do they come and go?" "Is there a trigger that makes your suicidal thoughts worse?"
Associated symptoms	"Do you think things can get better?" "Do you feel like a burden to people who care about you?" "Do you feel isolated or alone?" "What does the future hold for you?"

ED, emergency department; HPI, history of present illness.

Having clarified what the patient means when they voice concern for suicide and having explored some of the circumstances resulting in these disruptive thoughts, the clinician screens for other factors that may contribute to suicidality using their review of systems (or symptoms) (ROS). In addition to their usual ROS, the ED clinician may explore psychiatric symptoms relevant to the patient's presentation, such as depression, anxiety, mania, psychosis, derogatory auditory hallucinations, command auditory hallucinations to harm self or others, obsessions, compulsions, and sleep disturbances. These symptoms often indicate the presence of a primary psychiatric disorder, which increases risk for suicide.

A thorough evaluation of the CC, HPI, and ROS provides a foundation of information about the patient's current suicidal thoughts. This database could now be compared to a semistandardized continuum of increasing severity such as described in the C-SSRS, which uses five different levels of intensity to stratify suicidal thoughts

(Table 31.2). It is important to note that not all stages in the continuum proposed are always evident prior to a suicide attempt (12).

Step 2: Identify Suicidal Behavior

Having completed the evaluation of the patient's suicidal thoughts, the next step is to determine whether the patient has demonstrated suicidal behavior. Suicidal behavior consists of any action taken by the patient toward the goal of ending their life, such as seeking means and writing notes to loved ones. Similar to suicidal thoughts, suicidal behaviors can be loosely organized on a continuum similar to the C-SSRS (Table 31.3).

Step 3: Evaluate Risk and Protective Factors

After assessing current suicidal thoughts and suicidal behavior, the clinician's next step is to gather historical information about the patient's relationship with suicide and self-harm. This complements the standard assessment of past

TABLE 31.2 The Spectrum of Suicidal Ideation (SI)

Level of SI	Sample Questions to Elicit
Wish to be dead	"Do you view death as a means to relieve suffering?" "Do you wish you would go to sleep and not wake up?" "What purpose does death serve for you?" "Do you have a desire for death?"
Nonspecific active suicidal thoughts	"Do you want to do something to end your life or accelerate your death?"
Active suicidal ideation with any methods (not plan) without intent to act	"Have you thought about what you might do if you were to end your life?"
Active suicidal ideation with some intent to act, without specific plan	"How likely do you think you are to act on these thoughts or plan?"
Active suicidal ideation with specific plan and intent	"What's holding you back from completing this specific plan?"

medical history (PMH), social history (SH), and family history (FH). There are several important pieces of information that a clinician may consider adding to their typical assessment in order to elicit risk factors for suicide and protective factors against suicide (Table 31.4).

Step 4: Obtain Collateral Information

Unfortunately, patients who are at highest risk for suicide and have decided to end their life often do not view the evaluating physician as their ally (13) and therefore may intentionally withhold and minimize information during an evaluation. Consider the accuracy of their history and whether consulting with a close friend or family member is warranted to gather further information. Be suspicious when a patient declines to give you permission to speak with a collateral contact. If they agree, verify the relationship between the patient and the named individual. The ideal collateral contact is someone with whom the patient has regular and recent contact, and that the patient confides in when they are in crisis such

TABLE 31.3 The Spectrum of Suicidal Behavior

Level of Behavior	Sample Questions to Elicit
Nonlethal self-injury	"What did you think could happen when you did this behavior? Did you believe that by doing this behavior, you might die?"
Preparatory acts or behavior	"How far did you get in carrying out your plan? Did you begin stockpiling medications? Have you sought out the means to harm yourself? Did you write any notes to loved ones? Have you given away any possessions?"
Aborted attempt	"What stopped you from carrying through with your plan?"
Interrupted attempt	"Would you have continued with your plan if you were not interrupted?"
Actual attempt (nonfatal)	"How do you feel about having survived?" "Are you thinking about attempting suicide again?"
Suicide	Death

TABLE 31.4 Exploring the past medical history (PMH), social history (SH), family history (FH)

PMH	"Have you ever attempted suicide in the past?" "Have you ever done something to harm yourself without intending to end your life, such as cutting or burning yourself?" "Have you ever received a psychiatric diagnosis like depression, anxiety, bipolar, schizophrenia, OCD, or PTSD?" "Have you ever been hospitalized for psychiatric reasons?" "Do you take any psychiatric medications?" "Do you have chronic pain?" "Have you ever had a traumatic brain injury?"
Medications	Evaluate for high-risk medications and medications that are especially lethal in overdose such as benzodiazepines, opioids, sedative hypnotics, tricyclic antidepressants, and mood stabilizers such as lithium.
Social history	Income: "What is your source of income? Are you working? Is your income appropriate to meet your needs, or are finances a significant stressor for you? Housing: "Where do you live? Do you feel safe there and able to take care of your needs? Are you or have you recently been homeless?" Relationships: "Are you married? Divorced? How do you identify your sexuality? Do you identify as LGBTQ? How do you view your role in your children's life?" Religion: "Do you identify as religious? How does your religion view suicide? Is this enough to prevent you from attempting suicide?" Substance abuse: "Do you use any illegal drugs or prescription drugs that are not prescribed to you? Alcohol? Tobacco?" Trauma and abuse: "Do you have a history of trauma? Have you ever experienced verbal, psychological, physical, or sexual abuse?" Military: "Have you ever served in the military? Do you struggle with memories or guilt from your time in the service?" Access to firearms: "Do you own a firearm? How is it stored? What prevents access to the gun and ammunition?"
Family history	"Does anyone in your family struggle with mental health problems?" "Has anyone in your family ever died by suicide?" "Does anyone in your family use drugs or alcohol?"

OCD, obsessive-compulsive disorder; PTSD, posttraumatic stress disorder.

as a close family member, friend, or roommate. When speaking with the collateral contact, your job is to verify the information provided to you by the patient. If the collateral contact contradicts some or much of the patient's history or if the collateral contact is not familiar enough with the patient to comment on such sensitive information, be concerned that the patient may be attempting to manipulate your clinical decision-making. In situations where collateral is not immediately available, it may be prudent to keep the patient in a supervised setting until collateral can be obtained, if the clinician determines that this is necessary.

Step 5: Document Your Decision-Making

After assessing the patient's suicidal thoughts, suicidal behavior, risk factors, protective factors, and collateral information, it is time to make a decision about how to treat the patient. This decision is rarely easy, but tends to be simpler when both patient and clinician agree on a treatment plan, either for hospitalization or for close outpatient follow-up. When the patient and clinician disagree, decision-making becomes difficult. This typically occurs when patients decline voluntary hospitalization and the clinician feels it is necessary to take legal action to hospitalize the patient against their will. Local laws governing involuntary commitment vary by state, so it is important for clinicians to become familiar and abide by local statutes. A commonly used criterion for involuntary commitment is, "based on your assessment, does the patient represent an imminent danger to themselves or others?"

Clinicians are limited in their ability to predict future behavior, and "foreseeability" is commonly debated in malpractice lawsuits against clinicians whose patients ultimately attempt or die by suicide. Unfortunately, there is no way for clinicians to predict with adequate sensitivity and specificity what an individual patient may do once they leave the ED. Instead, physicians must consider if the risk of suicide was so high at the time of evaluation that it was foreseeable the patient would harm themselves. A common formulation in malpractice cases such as these is, "was the risk so great that any reasonably prudent practitioner would have foreseen that the patient was going to attempt suicide if not hospitalized?"

The risk of a patient leaving the ED and attempting/completing suicide is a major fear for many clinicians. From a legal perspective, this fear may be at least partially justified, as post-suicide lawsuits account for the largest number of malpractice lawsuits against psychiatrists (14). However, even when these lawsuits occur, clinicians overwhelmingly prevail in these cases (15).

When considering the risk of liability in suicide risk assessments, there are some key factors that can guide a clinician in navigating this area. The first is that the clinician should provide evaluation and treatment that meets the "standard of care." Physicians are not expected to be perfect but must maintain an appropriate level of skill comparable to other physicians in their field. Appropriate documentation can play a major role in establishing that a physician met the standard of care in a particular case, especially if the clinician documents the rationale behind the important decisions they made.

The second is to understand the limitations of both the assessment and treatment options available. Errors of fact, which are based on the collection of information, are different than errors of judgment, which are based on the way a physician synthesizes the information and makes a decision (16). Courts are often more forgiving of errors in judgment, as errors in fact are usually the result of not gathering sufficient information.

This suggests that clinicians should consider gathering information in a suicidal patient from multiple sources, as suggested previously in this chapter. Treatment options may also guide liability, particularly in the area of involuntary commitment. Familiarity with the involuntary commitment laws in your state may help to guide exactly what you are able to do in a situation where a suicidal patient may not want inpatient treatment, as clinical judgment should still fall within the confines of what is legally permissible.

The third factor to consider in the area of liability is to focus on serving the best interests of the patient. Although multiple competing factors influence a clinician's decision about how to treat a suicidal patient such as staffing issues, caseload volume, and insurance considerations, the primary focus of decision-making should be how to best protect and meet the needs of the patient. With that mindset, a clinician is far more likely to land within the standard of care by focusing on their role as a physician helping the sick.

SUICIDE RISK ASSESSMENT

The suicide risk assessment is a formal accounting of an individual's risk factors for suicide and protective factors against suicide. These factors have been elicited using the above interview, and clearly summarizing them in the assessment can clarify the management plan for the treating physician. A sample suicide risk assessment is listed below (Table 31.5).

Risk and protective factors can be categorized as modifiable and nonmodifiable. Modifiable risk factors such as current suicidal thoughts, intoxication and substance use, access to lethal means, poor social support and housing, and poorly controlled psychiatric symptoms contribute to the clinician's understanding of their foreseeable acute risk for self-harm. The patient who has numerous modifiable risk factors during an ED presentation may require hospitalization to resolve these risks. Protective factors such as strong religious beliefs that suicide is immoral and feelings of obligation toward children and family members strengthen a patient's resolve against suicide. These may also be modifiable and, when reduced or attenuated, the patient may benefit from hospitalization. Nonmodifiable risk factors such as previous suicide attempts, recent self-injury, a

TABLE 31.5 Sample Suicide Risk Assessment

Risk Factors	
Age/ethnicity/gender	
Current SI	Y/N
Previous attempt	Y/N
Uncontrolled psychiatric symptoms	Y/N
Impulsive behavior	Y/N
Self-injurious behavior	Y/N
Recent substance use	Y/N
Active intoxication	Y/N
Access to lethal means	Y/N
Homelessness	Y/N
Family history of suicide	Y/N
Protective Factors	
Religious preclusion	Y/N
Obligation toward family	Y/N
Social support	Y/N
Identifies reasons for living	Y/N
Chronic risk for suicide	Low, moderate, high
Acute risk for suicide	Elevated or at baseline

history of impulsive behavior, FH of completed suicide, and personal history of trauma and abuse all help establish the patient's chronic risk for suicide. A patient may have a chronically elevated risk for suicide based on history, but their modifiable risk and protective factors are controlled and the patient may be appropriate for continued outpatient treatment. Taking inventory of a patient's risk and protective factors helps the clinician determine if their acute risk is consistent with their chronic risk or if exacerbation of acute stressors raises their acute risk for suicide above baseline. Acutely elevated suicide risk typically results in hospitalization.

MANAGEMENT AND DISPOSITION IN THE EMERGENCY DEPARTMENT

Identifying which patients in the ED are at greatest risk for suicide can be difficult. Occult suicidality may be present in nearly 10% of all ED patients (5-7). One proposed solution to detect these individuals is to implement universal screening, which has been shown to feasibly identify more individuals with suicidal thoughts and behaviors (17) without overwhelming available resources (18). There exist a variety of suicide screening tools including the C-SSRS which served as an outline for our earlier discussion, ED-Safe, the Suicide Assessment Five-step Evaluation and Triage (SAFE-T), the Convergent Functional Information for Suicidality (CFI-S), the Beck Scale for Suicide Ideation (BSSI), the Patient Safety Screener (PSS-2 and PSS-3), and others (19). No single screen has emerged as superior, and screening alone does not significantly affect future suicidal behavior, rather it is the intervention that follows that may reduce future suicidal behavior (20-23).

As patients with suicidal ideation are often identified prior to evaluation by a physician, EDs may consider implementing universal precautions to minimize potential harm to patients and staff while the patient awaits evaluation by the physician. Depending on your facility and the specific needs of the patient, an increased level of observation may be necessary, including use of a one-to-one sitter, video observation, or other means to monitor the patient more closely. Removing potential hazards from the patient examination room, such as sharp objects, unnecessary medical equipment, and searching the patient's belongings should also be considered.

When it is time for the clinician to evaluate the patient, preparation sets the stage for a successful interview. The ED can be a chaotic environment to elicit intimate details about a person's struggle with thoughts of self-harm. Thus, controlling the setting may help establish the therapeutic relationship necessary to unearth this information. The examination room should be quiet and removed from the tumult of the main emergency setting. Some EDs have a separate area for patients with mental health concerns that have been cleared medically. Ideally, the patient's evaluation room should provide equal access to the exit for both parties. Consider asking family and friends who have accompanied the patient to leave the room for the duration of the evaluation. While conducting the evaluation, the clinician may elicit more useful information with an interview style that is compassionate, yet indifferent. The patient is likely to provide emotional testimony, and indifference may prevent the patient from over- or underendorsing their symptoms based on the clinician's reaction to hearing the history. Patients are also more likely to reveal sensitive information to the empathetic yet indifferent clinician.

After completing the evaluation, the treating clinician can decide on the appropriate patient disposition. Inpatient psychiatric settings are typically limited in the ability to provide medical services. Patients who have attempted suicide and/or performed self-injury may require initial medical hospitalization to treat health conditions resulting from their attempt (i.e., surgical disposition for tissue wounds, medical disposition for overdose or poisoning). Patients who can be medically cleared in the ED yet remain at acutely elevated risk for suicide may be hospitalized with psychiatry, either on a voluntary or involuntary status. Be sure to abide by local laws and regulations when pursuing inpatient treatment.

Psychiatric hospitalization serves several purposes such as limiting the patient's access to means to harm themselves, providing an increased level of patient observation and temporary removal from the stressful environment in which their suicide risk became elevated.

Outpatient levels of care may be considered, including partial hospitalization programs (PHPs), intensive outpatient programs (IOPs), and close outpatient follow-up with the patient's mental health clinician. PHP and IOP typically offer a structured daily routine and increased frequency of contact with mental health professionals than is available in the general outpatient setting. Consult with local resources to learn which services are available in your area. These programs may serve as alternatives to hospitalization, depending on the level of care provided and the clinician's evaluation of the patient. Close outpatient follow-up will place the patient back with their usual outpatient mental health provider, who may choose to schedule more frequent visits in the period following the ED visit. Patients who do not have a provider may be referred to local resources. For some patients, integration of these resources into a personalized safety plan may help the patient identify early warning signs and behavior as well as coping strategies to help patients reduce their suicidal thoughts (23). More personally relevant safety plans may predict lower likelihood of suicidal behavior (24), and internet-based suicide safety plan interventions are being studied (25). Safety plans can also incorporate involvement from family members and limiting access to lethal means, such as storing firearms with a family member or changing how firearms are stored in the home to reduce the patient's ability to act impulsively.

CONCLUSION AND FUTURE CONSIDERATIONS

Current management of acutely suicidal patients presenting to the ED often take a disposition-based rather than treatment-based approach. There is a need to shift this paradigm and provide patients with a standardized, evidence-based, algorithm-driven care similar to that which is offered to patients with medical complaints (26). Emerging evidence suggests that interventions performed in the ED and during the acute period following discharge may decrease suicidal behavior during this immediate period (20,27,28). There is growing evidence for acute pharmacologic interventions in the ED, such as ketamine and buprenorphine, that may reduce suicidality. Ketamine may reduce suicidal ideation in the short term, with serial administrations providing additional improvement (29). Buprenorphine may also reduce suicidal ideation both in patients with (30) and without (31) comorbid opioid dependence. However, these interventions have not yet become the standard of care. Future treatment of suicidal patients may involve ED administration of agents such as these.

In conclusion, the ED serves as an important point of contact for many individuals to access medical care, particularly patients with suicidal thoughts and self-harming behaviors. We hope that the topics outlined in this chapter provide a useful framework to guide emergency mental health clinicians through the evaluation of these patients, and we encourage clinicians to innovate emergency mental health services in the ever-changing landscape of healthcare delivery.

REFERENCES

1. Stone, D. M., Simon, T. R., Fowler, K. A., et al. (2018). Vital signs: Trends in state suicide rates – United States, 1999–2016 and circumstances contributing to suicide – 27 states, 2015. *Morbidity and Mortality Weekly Report, 67*(22), 617–624.

2. World Health Organization. (2018, Updated). *Suicide.* Retrieved November 23, 2018, from http://www.who.int/news-room/fact-sheets/detail/suicide.

3. American Foundation for Suicide Prevention. (2016, Updated). *Suicide statistics.* Retrieved from https://afsp.org/about-suicide/suicide-statistics/.

4. Kessler, R. C., Borges, G., & Walters, E. E. (1999). Prevalence of and risk factors for lifetime suicide attempts in the National Comorbidity Survey. *Archives of General Psychiatry, 56*(7), 617–626.

5. Claassen, C. A., & Larkin, G. L. (2005). Occult suicidality in an emergency department population. *British Journal of Psychiatry, 186,* 352–353.

6. Ilgen, M. A., Walton, M. A., Cunningham, R. M., et al. (2009). Recent suicidal ideation among patients in an inner city emergency department. *Suicide and Life-Threatening Behavior, 39*(5), 508–517.

7. Boudreaux, E. D., Clark, S., & Camargo, C. A., Jr. (2008). Mood disorder screening among adult emergency department patients: A multicenter study of prevalence, associations and interest in treatment. *General Hospital Psychiatry, 30*(1), 4–13.

8. Ting, S. A., Sullivan, A. F., Boudreaux, E. D., Miller, I., & Camargo, C. A., Jr. (2012). Trends in US emergency department visits for attempted suicide and self-inflicted injury, 1993–2008. *General Hospital Psychiatry, 34*(5), 557–565.

9. Gairin, I., House, A., & Owens, D. (2003). Attendance at the accident and emergency department in the year before suicide: Retrospective study. *British Journal of Psychiatry, 183,* 28–33.

10. D'Onofrio, G., Jauch, E., Jagoda, A., et al. (2010). NIH roundtable on opportunities to advance research on neurologic and psychiatric emergencies. *Annals of Emergency Medicine, 56*(5), 551–564.

11. The Columbia Lighthouse Project. (2016, Updated). *Columbia-suicide severity rating scale.* Retrieved November 23, 2018, from http://cssrs.columbia.edu/.

12. Baca-Garcia, E., Perez-Rodriguez, M. M., Oquendo, M. A., Keyes, K. M., Hasin, D. S., Grant, B. F., & Blanco, C. (2011). Estimating risk for suicide attempt: Are we asking the right questions? Passive suicidal ideation as a marker for suicidal behavior. *Journal of Affective Disorders, 134*(1–3), 327–332.

13. Resnick, P. (2002). Recognizing that the suicidal patient views you as an "adversary." *Current Psychiatry, 1*(1), 8.

14. Packman, W. L., Pennuto, T. O., Bongar, B., & Orthwein, J. (2004). Legal issues of professional negligence in suicide cases. *Behavioral Sciences & the Law, 22*(5), 697–713.

15. Baerger, D. R. (2001). Risk management with the suicidal patient: Lessons from case law. *Professional Psychology: Research and Practice, 32*(4), 359–366.

16. Resnick, P. J. (2017). *Suicide risk assessment and malpractice prevention.* Presented at U.S. Psychiatric and Mental Health Congress, New Orleans, LA, September 16–19, 2017.

17. Boudreaux, E. D., Camargo, C. A., Jr., Arias, S. A., et al. (2016). Improving suicide risk screening and detection in the emergency department. *American Journal of Preventive Medicine, 50*(4), 445–453.

18. Roaten, K., Johnson, C., Genzel, R., Khan, F., & North, C. S. (2018). Development and implementation of a universal suicide risk screening program in a safety-net hospital system. *The Joint Commission Journal on Quality and Patient Safety, 44*(1), 4–11.

19. Lotito, M., & Cook, E. (2015). A review of suicide risk assessment instruments and approaches. *Mental Health Clinician, 5*(5), 216–223.

20. Miller, I. W., Camargo, C. A., Arias, S. A., et al. (2017). Suicide prevention in an emergency department population: The ED-SAFE study. *JAMA Psychiatry, 74*(6), 563–570.

21. Chang, B. P., & Tan, T. M. (2015). Suicide screening tools and their association with near-term adverse events in the ED. *The American Journal of Emergency Medicine, 33*(11), 1680–1683.

22. Betz, M. E., Wintersteen, M., Boudreaux, E. D., et al. (2016). Reducing suicide risk: Challenges and opportunities in the emergency department. *Annals of Emergency Medicine, 68*(6), 758–765.

23. Boudreaux, E. D., Miller, I., Goldstein, A. B., et al. (2013). The Emergency Department Safety Assessment and Follow-up Evaluation (ED-SAFE): Method and design considerations. *Contemporary Clinical Trials, 36*(1), 14–24.

24. Green, J. D., Kearns, J. C., Rosen, R. C., Keane, T. M., & Marx, B. P. (2018). Evaluating the effectiveness of safety plans for military veterans: Do safety plans tailored to veteran characteristics decrease suicide risk? *Behavior Therapy, 49*(6), 931–938.

25. Klein, J. P., Hauer, A., Berger, T., Fassbinder, E., Schweiger, U., & Jacob, G. (2018). Protocol for the REVISIT-BPD trial, a randomized controlled trial testing the effectiveness of an internet-based self-management intervention in the treatment of borderline personality disorder (BPD). *Front Psychiatry, 9*, 439.

26. Bridge, J. A., Horowitz, L. M., & Campo, J. V. (2017). ED-SAFE—Can suicide risk screening and brief intervention initiated in the emergency department save lives? *JAMA Psychiatry, 74*(6), 555–556.

27. Fleischmann, A., Bertolote, J. M., Wasserman, D., et al. (2008). Effectiveness of brief intervention and contact for suicide attempters: A randomized controlled trial in five countries. *Bulletin of the World Health Organization, 86*(9), 703–709.

28. Vaiva, G., Vaiva, G., Ducrocq, F., et al. (2006). Effect of telephone contact on further suicide attempts in patients discharged from an emergency department: Randomised controlled study. *BMJ, 332*(7552), 1241–1245.

29. Wilkinson, S. T., Ballard, E. D., Bloch, M. H., et al. (2018). The effect of a single dose of intravenous ketamine on suicidal ideation: A systematic review and individual participant data meta-analysis. *American Journal of Psychiatry, 175*(2), 150–158.

30. Ahmadi, J., Jahromi, M. S., & Ehsaei, Z. (2018). The effectiveness of different singly administered high doses of buprenorphine in reducing suicidal ideation in acutely depressed people with co-morbid opiate dependence: A randomized, double-blind, clinical trial. *Trials, 19*(1), 9.

31. Yovell, Y., Bar, G., Mashiah, M., et al. (2016). Ultra-low-dose buprenorphine as a time-limited treatment for severe suicidal ideation: A randomized controlled trial. *American Journal of Psychiatry, 173*(5), 491–498.

32

Violence: Violence Risk as a Psychiatric Emergency

John S. Rozel

Evaluation of violence risk is a critical aspect of every evaluation in the psychiatric emergency service (PES). Violence is a frequent chief complaint, a frequent risk, and must be assessed for even when not identified as a presenting concern. How ironic, then, it is to note that psychiatric illness is actually only a small contributor to violent behavior.

Effective psychiatric evaluation in the emergency setting requires a broad perspective: careful diagnostic skill to identify pertinent diagnoses and the capacity to identify the historical, social, and psychological factors which often play an even greater role than the illness itself. Whether ascribed to the biopsychosocial approach or the recovery model, effective evaluation and management of psychiatric risk requires significantly more than mere diagnostic acumen.

Added to this is the challenge of effective engagement of friends and family of psychiatric patients in the evaluation. Engaging friends and family as collateral informants and collaborating allies in the care of the patient is important in emergency evaluation. Violence by people with psychiatric illness is more often targeted toward immediate family, friends, or other caregivers than toward strangers (1). The notion of a person with severe mental illness posing a serious threat to a stranger is extremely low but may still play a role in public perception (2,3).

Although specific scales and measures may be of limited use for violence risk management, especially in the PES setting, some simple mnemonic devices may be helpful to promote consistent clinical approaches. A simple approach is to adhere to the ABCs of violence risk management (see Table 31.1) (5).

No single chapter can encompass all of violence risk management in the emergency setting.

This chapter will focus on essential rubrics to guide evaluation, cognitive issues in decision-making, special considerations on risk factors, and legal considerations including criminal justice interventions. A second chapter in this volume will address the evaluation and management of threats in the context of concerns of mass shootings, active attacks, and high magnitude attacks.

SIX ESSENTIAL MAXIMS OF VIOLENCE

There are six essential maxims about the relationship between violence and psychiatric illness that must be understood to effectively manage risk in clinical settings. They are summarized in Table 31.2 and discussed in detail below.

First, most violence is not due to mental illness or people with mental illness. Our best estimates are that less than 10% of the violence that occurs in our society is attributable to psychiatric illness and perhaps as little as 3% to severe mental illness (6-8). Mental illness plays a similarly small role in firearm violence (9,10).

Second, most people with mental illness are not violent. Violence rates for people with and without severe mental illness are similar, although in both populations with substance use increases the risk (11,12).

Third, people with mental illness are more likely to be a victim of violence than to be a perpetrator of violence (6,13). Severe mental illness is associated with a fivefold increased risk of being murdered and a greater than 20-fold increased risk of being a victim of sexual assault. Notably, recent and severe victimization may increase risk of imminent violence in people with mental illness and many people with mental illness are at risk for both victimization and perpetration

TABLE 31.1 The ABCs of Violence Risk Management

Assess violence risk through interview and a review of relevant history
Behaviorally manage immediate risk with de-escalation, medication, or physical interventions(4)
Conceptualize the patient's dynamic and static risk and protective factors
Document formulation and plan
Execute a clinical plan
Follow up to assure plan followed and appropriate modifications are made
Get help through consultation on challenging cases

(14,15). Notably, recent violent victimization may be one of our strongest predictors for imminent violence in people with mental illness (16).

Fourth, there is definitely an intersection between psychiatric illness and violence and it is critical for PES clinicians to recognize and manage that risk. Certain subgroups of people with mental illness—especially those with active symptoms and comorbid substance use—may be at elevated risk for violence (17). It is essential that people at risk for violence due to their psychiatric illness be correctly identified and properly linked to appropriate clinical interventions to decrease their risk.

Fifth, even when risk for violence is not driven by psychiatric illness, PES professionals should not miss opportunities to reduce risk. Many of the major acute and chronic risk factors for violence are psychosocial factors, similar to what is often seen in people with severe and chronic mental illness, and which may be better addressed by crisis models of care or the resources more readily available to the social workers of the PES than the medical ED (18). This holds true for patients with and without psychiatric illness. Even in people with psychiatric illness, violence is not necessarily the product of the mental illness (19).

Sixth, and finally, many of the most robust risk factors for violence are similar for people with and without psychiatric illness.

MODELS OF VIOLENCE

It is beyond the scope of this chapter to enumerate and discuss all of the models of violence however some essential and useful models warrant recognition—and qualification. Different modes of violence may have different social purposes, biological causes and states, and amenability to intervention. An intervention well-tailored to violence caused by reactive fear may have little use for violence intended to coerce or control others. Violence is not intrinsically pathological and may serve an important function in some settings, possibly even socially condoned or celebrated; soldiers, special weapons and tactics (SWAT) officers, and even the proverbial good person with a gun may engage in violence that is neither pathological nor driven by psychopathology.

Often in clinical settings, we discuss categories of proactive/instrumental/predatory violence versus reactive/affective violence. The models, well discussed in the literature, imply that

TABLE 31.2 The Six Maxims of Violence

1. Most violence is not due to mental illness.
2. Most people with mental illness are not violent.
3. People with mental illness are more likely to be a victim of violence than a perpetrator.
4. There is an intersection and it is critical for PES professionals to effectively identify and manage risk.
5. Even when risk for violence is not driven by psychiatric illness, PES professionals should not miss opportunities to reduce risk.
6. Most of the more robust risk factors for violence are valid whether or not a person has mental illness.

behavior-driven overt and conscious goals may be less amenable to acute psychiatric care than aggression driven by affective reactivity (20,21). This is a useful schema and should be considered in emergency psychiatric settings: the person who became aggressive when overwhelmed by the symptoms of schizophrenia or posttraumatic stress disorder (PTSD) may well be a better candidate for psychiatric intervention than the person who was aggressive while robbing a bank. There is growing neurobiological evidence to support these phenotypes (22).

Perhaps more clinically useful is a less well-vetted but broader schema known as the quadripartite model (23,24). This model, renamed more simply, the Four Rs, consists of: Rage, Revenge, Reward, and Recreation (25). These categories have either high or low impulsivity (impulsive v. controlled) and high or low affect (aversive v. appetitive). The Four Rs are summarized in Table 31.3 below.

Models may be of limited use in clinical work for a number of reasons. Not all violent behaviors will fall into specific categories, either cutting across domains or merely being difficult to classify. Often, while an individual has a preferred mode of aggression, they may also engage in more than one type of violence. The schema do provide useful reminders for the role of intent, impulsivity, and emotion in violent behavior.

THE AVAILABILITY HEURISTIC AND THE BASE RATE FALLACY

Thinking in an emergency situation is challenging, especially when one is expected to manipulate and juxtapose rare and common risks. A broad understanding of human thinking, heuristics, and cognitive errors in risk-related decision-making can be extremely helpful for clinicians working in the PES (26,27). Two essential concepts are the availability heuristic and the base rate fallacy (28,29).

The availability heuristic suggests that we are more likely to classify an event into a category if we have been exposed to other recent members of that category (30). Put simply, if we have seen a lot of violent patients recently, one is likely to classify the next patient as being at risk for violence, regardless of the actual risk of the patient. In a context like the PES (or other acute psychiatric settings), this bias is especially pernicious. Legal constraints (such as limiting involuntary interventions to people who are imminently dangerous) and clinical constraints (such as limiting payment for inpatient care to people who are imminently dangerous) create a violence-rich environment in the PES and acute inpatient unit.

The base rate fallacy (or base rate neglect) means that when people apply a general rule about frequency (the base rate) to a specific case with additional case-specific information, the base rate data are ignored. This is especially true if the case-specific information includes social stereotype information (31). Put together, this means that clinicians who frequently see people who are violent and have psychiatric illness are more likely to overestimate violence risk in future evaluations of people with psychiatric illness.

STRUCTURED CLINICAL JUDGMENT AND VIOLENCE RISK

There are, broadly, three approaches to violence risk evaluation: clinical, structured clinical judgment, and actuarial. A clinical assessment is essentially a basic interview: the clinician talks to the patient, reviews the record, and comes to a formulation of risk. An actuarial approach is a highly systematic, psychometric approach using standardized clinical tools which have been normed to specific populations. Structured clinical judgment is a hybrid approach. Often in PES settings, a clinical or structured clinical judgment approach is best, but it is important to understand all three approaches.

TABLE 31.3 The Four Rs of Violence

	Appetitive	Aversive
Impulsive	Recreation	Rage
Controlled	Reward	Revenge

Most research suggests that, when applied to the proper population, the psychometric or actuarial approach yields superior results to clinical assessment alone (32-34). And, there is no shortage of psychometric tools assessing violence risk (35,36). Unfortunately actuarial and psychometric tools are only effective when applied to homogeneous populations. Deviations based on language preference, age, gender, psychiatric history or severity, criminal history, intoxication, or other factors as well as lack of information about developmental or behavioral history all significantly degrade the accuracy and utility of actuarial tools. Further, the tools take considerable time to administer and interpret. One would consider it, given that the typical PES boasts neither a homogeneous patient population nor ready access to extensive historical data nor ample time for such explorations.

Even the structured professional judgment (SPJ) approach—as a looser approach to actuarial assessment—has limitations. SPJ prompts clinicians to look at a specific number of risk and protective factors and to integrate them with their own judgment to formulate risk (37). Again, although there are many available instruments, training and implementation take time and none will be useful across the broad array of people presenting to the PES (38,39).

Operationally, a raw score from a psychometric tool suggesting a degree of risk is of relatively little value in the PES. First, that score describes the nomothetic risk for people with similar characteristics and does not necessarily translate accurately or precisely to the idiographic risk of the individual of concern. Second, numerous factors can impact the reliability of those scores (40). In fact, simply asking a person how likely they are to engage in violence, is nearly as effective as many of the most well-respected violence assessment tools (41). Finally, a risk score, no matter how accurate, does not necessarily give clear direction for next steps to mitigate risk.

DYNAMISM AND VIOLENCE RISK MANAGEMENT

Focus on dynamic risk and protective factors may be the single most useful strategy to understand and reduce violence risk. Prediction of violence is challenging and often impossible to do with any degree of accuracy. Management of violence risk is an adaptable approach that provides an actionable plan to contain violence risk. To do so effectively, clinicians must consider not only risk and protective factors but also static and dynamic factors. Static factors are those which change little or not at all; dynamic factors are those which can change significantly based on environmental or individual processes as well as by clinical intervention. Although static factors should not be ignored, a clinical plan to disrupt dynamic risk factors and to monitor or reinforce dynamic protective factors is essential (42). See Table 31.4 below.

These categories may have some ambiguity or overlap depending on the context. Use of marijuana may be an effective coping strategy for some people at risk for violence, but it may be a significant risk factor for people with underlying schizophrenia to engage in violence (43). Similarly, not all risk or protective factors are of equal weight: violent video game use is likely only

TABLE 31.4 Risk Factors

	Static	Dynamic
Risk	Unchanging factors which increase risk (eg, history of violent victimization or child abuse, history of violence, low IQ, TBI)	Changeable factors which increase risk (eg, active psychiatric symptoms, intoxication, unstable relationships)
Protective	Unchanging factors which decrease risk (eg, older age, female gender)	Changeable factors which decrease risk (eg, stable relationships, employment)

TBI, traumatic brain injury

a weak risk factor (and may serve as a protective factor for some) whereas a history of attempting to strangle a partner is an extreme risk factor (44,45).

Shifting clinical thinking from yes/no or high/low assessments of likelihood to if/then thinking can be an important way to more effectively manage violence risk in clinical settings including the PES (46).

IMMINENT RISK FACTORS

Generally, static risk factors contribute to chronic and long-term risk whereas dynamic risk factors contribute to short term risk. Inevitably in the work of emergency psychiatry, patients will be recognized as having significant and long-term risk for violence. Most acute psychiatric interventions—that is, inpatient admission and medication management—are best suited for the acute and imminent risk factors. Chronic risk for violence may not be reduced by inpatient admission, and, for some patients, acute risk may be increased by admission.

Patients with schizophrenia and recurrent psychosis are often at elevated risk for violence. It is important to note that the acute risk is modulated by only a few select aspects of the illness. Current or recent positive symptoms (hallucinations or delusions), treatment resistance or lack of access to treatment, and comorbid substance use appear to be the most robust risk factors among these patients according to a number of meta-analyses (2,47-49). Notably, it is active and recent symptoms more so than this diagnosis itself which drives risk (50). Persecutory ideation and delusional content may be of additional concern even if only present as a trait (51,52).

Drug and alcohol use—especially frequent or current intoxication—are powerful risk factors for violence in people with and without psychiatric illness (11). Alcohol use is strongly associated with violence risk (53,54). The effect is robust and may even be demonstrated by geographic proximity to liquor stores in some communities (55). There are varying data on other illicit substances and violence largely because of the confounding role of the criminal activity that is often necessary to procure an ongoing supply of illicit substances which can be difficult to separate from the direct neuropsychiatric effects of those substances (54). Current, recent, and frequent intoxication is the operant risk factor although clearly underlying substance use disorder will predispose many to those states (56).

As noted above, recent violent victimization has long been seen as a significant risk factor for violence. Recent and severe violence carry greater risk than remote or milder violence. The effect of recent victimization is seen in people with and without psychiatric illness, but the effect appears most pronounced in those with severe psychiatric illness. Even so, prior victimization in and of itself is not a sufficient risk factor for future violence. In one recent meta-analysis, current alcohol use, recent violence, and recent victimization were the most robust predictors of short-term violence risk in people with psychiatric illness (57).

MAGNITUDE AMPLIFIERS

Three factors warranting additional consideration in violence risk management include firearm access, military veteran status, and psychopathy or antisocial personality. Although they all serve, to a degree, as risk factors for violence, it is worth noting that they have a greater effect on the magnitude of potential violence.

Firearm Access

Compared to other developed countries, Americans actually have a relatively low rate of interpersonal violence. It is access to firearms which drives the extremely high rates of lethal violence (58). There are an estimated 393 million firearms in US civilian hands (59). Estimates for ownership by home range from 30% to 44% (60,61). Access to a firearm makes the severity of violence significantly higher including elevated risk of impulsive violence, domestic violence, and suicide (62). Access to firearms should always be explored and temporary removal or safer storage advised.

Antisocial and Psychopathic Personality

Psychopathy is a rare personality disorder, often seen as an intersection between antisocial and narcissistic personality disorder (63). Exploitation, manipulativeness, and sadism are common and concerning features (64). Psychopathy is neither necessary nor sufficient as a risk factor for violence, however when present is often associated with repeated severe violence; this is true for both impulsive aggression (rage and recreation) and planful aggression (revenge and reward) (65). Although there are few direct treatments for antisocial or psychopathic personality, management of comorbid illnesses (eg, depression, substance use) may be helpful. A patient likely should not be admitted for violence risk when the risk is solely attributable to personality disorder; however, neither should a patient with psychopathy be excluded from admission if they would otherwise meet admission criteria and benefit from care for other comorbidities.

Veteran Status

Most veterans, even those with combat experience in recent engagements, do not have PTSD. However, of those who do—and especially when also using alcohol—violence frequency may be increased (66). However, any veteran, provided they have completed basic training, has had explicit and specific training in how to kill other people that is well beyond what most civilians experience (67). This means that although the risk of violence in veterans in general is low, their capacity for higher magnitude violence is greater than in people without military training. Added to this, veterans may have higher rates of gun ownership, pain, and substance use adding to their risk (68-70). Getting a detailed history of military experience can be broadly helpful in clinical assessment and specifically useful in evaluating violence risk (71).

LEGAL CONCERNS

There are numerous legal concerns encountered in the clinical evaluation and care for potentially violent patients in the PES. Any and all legal issues are best reviewed with hospital legal advisors, and most PES teams find they are well served by a close and collegial working relationship with those attorneys. Arguably, the PES encounters complex legal questions at a rate and intensity seldom seen in other areas of clinical care. Nothing in this chapter is intended or offered as legal advice. Four key issues are duties to third parties, involuntary commitment, red flag laws, and malpractice liability.

Duties to Third Parties

Duties to protect or warn third parties of potential violence from a patient vary highly between states, but most states have enacted some type of duty, usually tethered directly or otherwise to the original Tarasoff decision (72). States have varying standards about whether there is an affirmative duty, in what situations it may apply, and how it may be discharged. Some states impose no duty at all. Some states impose a duty only for specific, imminent, and severe violence toward a known target; others modify one or more of these attributes: the duration of imminence, the severity of violence, the specificity of the threat, or the identifiability of the victim. There are some broad listings of duties cataloged across jurisdictions (73,74). The Health Insurance Portability and Accountability Act of 1996 (HIPAA) provides permission to warn insofar as such warning is congruent with one's professional ethics and the standards of the local jurisdiction. To wit: clinicians do not need to fear HIPAA repercussions for warning (75). Ultimately, each state determines its own standard, by statute or case law, and these standards evolve over time. The PES is usually fully capable of admitting a patient at risk, in theory defusing any imminent risk such that conundrum of locating and warning a victim is usually moot, barring the rare elopement.

Commitment

Involuntary inpatient commitment is a special power given to psychiatric professionals and few others in our society. The three general categories of involuntary admission recognized by most states are suicide risk, inability to care for self, and violence risk. Specific involuntary commitment criteria and procedures will vary significantly by state (76). Commitment, voluntary or involuntary, may be a useful intervention to prevent violence over the short term by placing the patient in a more contained setting and allowing for rapid and intense psychiatric management of symptoms. It should be a surprise to no one that inpatient units have high rates of violence: commitment is one of several steps needed to mitigate risk.

Red Flag Laws

More states are looking at the use of red flag laws (also known as gun violence restraining orders or extreme risk protection orders) as a tool to prevent intentional violence in people with and without psychiatric illness. They have demonstrated benefit in preventing suicide in some studies, but there is inadequate data so far to reach conclusions about efficacy for violence prevention (77,78). It is hoped that such laws may allow affirmative removal of firearms from people with significant violence risk but not significant psychiatric illness (79).

Malpractice Liability

Medical malpractice risk in psychiatry is low compared to other specialties; however one could reasonably argue that the emergency setting increases risk (80,81). Again, standards will vary highly by state but generally, a provider will need to be found in dereliction of duty to a patient or third party, leading directly to harm. Reassuringly, many of the same interpersonal strategies that are effective in de-escalating aggression are also effective in mitigating risk after adverse outcomes through thoughtful interaction with the patient or impacted parties (82).

There are a number of other legal concerns as well which are beyond the scope of this chapter including staff safety and employee rights, premises security and liability, insider threat issues, and others. Criminal charges against patients may be a consideration in some situations and this will be discussed later.

INTERVENTIONS

Not all violence risk requires immediate admission. In fact, some violence risk may escalate with admission. The intrusiveness or restrictiveness of a given intervention must be balanced against the plausible clinical benefit in general and against the prevailing legal and ethical standards. Although beginning with less intrusive, autonomy promoting interventions (eg, psychotherapy) may be ethically ideal in general, the imminence and severity of risk can easily override and justify more intrusive interventions. Thus, motivational interviewing is not the ideal intervention to interrupt an attack on a fellow healthcare worker.

In clinical settings, common interventions to reduce violence risk may include referral for outpatient treatment, increased level of care, addition or modification of medications, and involuntary admission. Seclusion, restraint, or involuntary medication may be needed in certain acute circumstances. The spectrum of interventions for imminent violence in the emergency setting is summarized in Table 31.5.

There will also be circumstances where violence risk is identified, criteria for involuntary commitment are not met, and the patient is unwilling to agree to further care. In such circumstances, passive monitoring may be all that is possible: crafting a thoughtful note for the day's encounter and awaiting a re-presentation to the PES. When possible, engaging with primary supports or family can be extremely helpful in such a situation: prompting them to monitor for evidence of decompensation, worsening symptoms,

TABLE 31.5 Spectrum of Interventions in Emergency Settings

Passive monitoring
Active monitoring (including evaluation, reevaluation)
Problem solving and cognitive interventions (with potential assailant, with others)
Voluntary medication
Distraction
Redirection
Direction/explicit guidance on appropriate behaviors (and notification of consequences)
Restriction (to one section of a unit or away from a high-risk area)
Confinement (to seclusion room or locked inpatient unit)
Manual or mechanical restraint
Involuntary medication

increasing substance use, increased agitation, or threats. Mere awareness is not enough. Families and friends will also need to know how to reach appropriate crisis or law enforcement sources and may benefit from linkage to support groups such as the Parent to Parent program from the National Alliance on Mental Illness.

CRIMINAL JUSTICE INTERVENTION

Outside of psychiatric settings, threats or acts of violence are often given other descriptors: misdemeanors and felonies. There is often significant reticence in healthcare settings to consider or seek criminal charges against patients, especially for psychiatric patients. It comes perilously close to compromising the physician-patient relationship. It raises questions of agency and responsibility. And, at a fundamental level, it can be inconsistent with the concepts of beneficence and nonmaleficence inherent in modern medical ethics (83).

It would seem reasonable that, in a PES setting, we begin with the assumption that threats and violent behavior are the product of a psychiatric or medical cause (84,85). That is, at first approximation, behavioral emergencies should be seen as a medical concern not a criminal justice concern. However as discussed throughout this chapter, much of violence is unrelated to psychiatric illness. There are circumstances where, in the course of psychiatric evaluation, it is determined that recent or threatened violence is not the substantial product of psychiatric illness. That is, whether or not the patient has psychiatric illnesses, the illness is not the driving force behind the violence risk.

Additionally, in a subset of those cases, it may be felt that inpatient admission is not only not beneficial but may be harmful as well. If we accept that our clinical goal is to reduce risk for the patient and others, then our general principles of medical ethics may permit consideration of legal interventions in lieu of clinical interventions. Often, PES teams will not stand in the way of ongoing criminal prosecution of an act such as when a patient is criminally arrested and brought through the medical ED or PES for clearance prior to booking at the jail. On occasion, PES clinicians may support or even encourage family or others criminally victimized by a patient to pursue

charges. PES professionals may see family repeatedly bringing a loved one to the PES for what is essentially criminal behavior; it is difficult enough to accept that a loved one may have mental illness; it can be more difficult to accept that they are criminal as well. Such discussions are challenging but may be justified by the value of harm reduction: we are helping out patient's family or supports decrease their risk of future violence by helping them choose a potentially more effective intervention for the violent behavior of concern. It is still incredibly difficult to contemplate initiating criminal charges against a loved one.

There may also be circumstances where criminal charges are considered or pressed for a patient's conduct in the clinical setting (86). This may be for solid clinical reasons reached after careful deliberation and review of the records. It may be for the simple reason that no staff member relinquished their right to seek criminal charges against a person by virtue of their employment. That said, most reasonable clinicians will quickly note the difference between an elderly patient with dementia who, startled and confused, grabs the arm of a staff member providing a sponge bath and a younger patient who, angry and entitled, grabs the arm of a staff member declining to give them a prescription for a controlled substance.

Such interventions should be rare and considered as an intervention of last resort, used when there is a documented history of the failure of those clinical interventions for similar behavior, reasonable clinical confidence that the behavior is not driven by psychiatric issues amenable to traditional psychiatric interventions, and, preferably, after a patient has been expressly told that future criminal acts may lead to charges (87). It has been noted that criminal justice system may be less responsive than hoped to such charges (potentially further positively reinforcing the criminal behavior) (88). Proactive development of policies in coordination with regional law enforcement may be helpful (89).

Many psychiatric patients may encounter the criminal justice system despite being better served by the psychiatric system as their behavior is driven by psychiatric factors more than criminogenic factors (90,91). Whenever logistically possible and clinically appropriate, diversion of patients out of the criminal justice system into the mental health system is desirable. However, some people with mental illness also have high degrees of criminality. Increasingly, it is seen that for such rare individuals, neglect of either category of risk can be dangerous. Thus, even for people with significant psychiatric illness, sometimes criminal interventions may be appropriate when there is a reasonable degree of confidence that their violent behavior is substantially unrelated to their psychiatric illness (92).

CONCLUSION

Clinicians must use a broad biopsychosocial approach to violence risk assessment. Myopic focus on symptoms and diagnoses limits clinicians' abilities to recognize the fullness of the risk and protective factors impacting a patient's life and risk. By including a broader, recovery-oriented, and biopsychosocial approach, clinicians are better able to identify the risk factors linked to elevated violence risk including personal and social history, acute and chronic stressors, the role of substances, and the presence and stability of supports and family. Thoughtful evaluation and management of dynamic risk factors can not only help with identifying those at risk of violence but also help reduce this risk in people with and without psychiatric illness.

REFERENCES

1. Monahan, J., Steadman, H. J., Silver, E., Appelbaum, P. S., Robbins, P. C., Mulvey, E. P., et al. (2001). *Rethinking risk assessment: The MacArthur study of mental disorder and violence.* New York, NY: Oxford University Press.
2. Nielssen, O., Bourget, D., Laajasalo, T., Liem, M., Labelle, A., Hakkanen-Nyholm, H., et al. (2011). Homicide of strangers by people with a psychotic illness. *Schizophrenia Bulletin, 37*(3), 572–579.
3. McGinty, E. E., Kennedy-Hendricks, A., Choksy, S., & Barry, C. L. (2016). Trends in news media coverage of mental illness in the United States: 1995–2014. *Health Affairs, 35*(6), 1121–1129.
4. Holloman, G., & Zeller, S. (2012). Overview of Project BETA: Best practices in evaluation and treatment of agitation. *The Western Journal of Emergency Medicine, 13*(1), 1–2.
5. Rozel, J. S., Jain, A., Mulvey, E. P., & Roth, L. H. (2017). Psychiatric assessment of violence. In Sturmey, P. (Ed.), *The Wiley handbook of violence and aggression* (pp. 697–709). Chichester: John Wiley & Sons.
6. Choe, J. Y., Teplin, L. A., & Abram, K. M. (2008). Perpetration of violence, violent victimization, and severe mental illness: Balancing public health concerns. *Psychiatric Services, 59*(2), 153–164.
7. Beeber, L. S. (2018). Disentangling mental illness and violence. *Journal of the American Psychiatric Nurses Association, 24*(4), 360–362.
8. Ahonen, L., Loeber, R., & Brent, D. A. (2017). The association between serious mental health problems and violence: Some common assumptions and misconceptions. *Trauma, Violence, & Abuse, 20*(5), 613–625.
9. Anacker, L., & Pinals, D. A. (2018). In the crosshairs: Examining firearms, violence, and mental illness. *Psychiatric Annals, 48*(9), 416–420.
10. Rozel, J. S., & Mulvey, E. P. (2017). The link between mental illness and gun violence: Implications for social policy. *Annual Review of Clinical Psychology, 13*(1), 445–469.
11. Steadman, H. J., Mulvey, E. P., Monahan, J., Robbins, P. C., Appelbaum, P. S., Grisso, T., et al. (1998). Violence by people discharged from acute psychiatric inpatient facilities and by others in the same neighborhoods. *Archives of General Psychiatry, 55*(5), 393–401.
12. Rueve, M. E., & Welton, R. S. (2008). Violence and mental illness. *Psychiatry, 5*(5), 34–48.
13. Bhavsar, V., & Bhugra, D. (2018). Violence towards people with mental illness: Assessment, risk factors, and management. *Psychiatry and Clinical Neurosciences, 72*, 811–820.
14. Desmarais, S. L., Van Dorn, R. A., Johnson, K. L., Grimm, K. J., Douglas, K. S., & Swartz, M. S. (2014). Community violence perpetration and victimization among adults with mental illnesses. *American Journal of Public Health, 104*(12), 2342–2349.
15. Monahan, J., Vesselinov, R., Robbins, P. C., & Appelbaum, P. S. (2017). Violence to others, violent self-victimization, and violent victimization by others among persons with a mental illness. *Psychiatric Services, 68*(5), 516–519.
16. Hiday, V. A., Swanson, J. W., Swartz, M. S., Borum, R., & Wagner, H. R. (2001). Victimization: A link between mental illness and violence? *International Journal of Law and Psychiatry, 24*(6), 559–572.

17. Swanson, J. W. (2008). Preventing the unpredicted: Managing violence risk in mental health care. *Psychiatric Services, 59*(2), 191–193.

18. Bernstein, R. (2009). *Practice guidelines: Core elements in responding to mental health crises* (Report No.: SMA-09-4427). Bethesda, MD: US Department of Health and Human Services, Substance Abuse and Mental Health Services Administration.

19. Peterson, J. K., Skeem, J., Kennealy, P., Bray, B., & Zvonkovic, A. (2014). How often and how consistently do symptoms directly precede criminal behavior among offenders with mental illness? *Law and Human Behavior, 38*(5), 439–449.

20. Meloy, J. R. (2006). Empirical basis and forensic application of affective and predatory violence. *Australian and New Zealand Journal of Psychiatry, 40*(6–7), 539–547.

21. McEllistrem, J. E. (2004). Affective and predatory violence: A bimodal classification system of human aggression and violence. *Aggression and Violent Behavior, 10*(1), 1–30.

22. Stahl, S. M. (2014). Deconstructing violence as a medical syndrome: Mapping psychotic, impulsive, and predatory subtypes to malfunctioning brain circuits. *CNS Spectrums, 19*(5), 357–365.

23. Howard, R. (2011). The quest for excitement: A missing link between personality disorder and violence? *The Journal of Forensic Psychiatry & Psychology, 22*, 692–705.

24. Runions, K. C. (2013). Toward a conceptual model of motive and self-control in cyber-aggression: Rage, revenge, reward, and recreation. *Journal of Youth and Adolescence, 42*(5), 751–771.

25. Runions, K. C., Salmivalli, C., Shaw, T., Burns, S., & Cross, D. (2018). Beyond the reactive-proactive dichotomy: Rage, revenge, reward, and recreational aggression predict early high school bully and bully/victim status. *Aggressive Behavior, 44*(5), 501–511.

26. Kahneman, D. (2013). *Thinking, fast and slow*. New York, NY: Farrar, Straus and Giroux.

27. Fischhoff, B., & Kadvany, J. D. (2011). *Risk: A very short introduction*. Oxford, NY: Oxford University Press.

28. Tversky, A., & Kahneman, D. (1974). Judgment under uncertainty: Heuristics and biases. *Science, 185*(4157), 1124–1131.

29. Saposnik, G., Redelmeier, D., Ruff, C. C., & Tobler, P. N. (2016). Cognitive biases associated with medical decisions: A systematic review. *BMC Medical Informatics and Decision Making, 16*(1), 138.

30. Tversky, A., & Kahneman, D. (1973). Availability: A heuristic for judging frequency and probability. *Cognitive Psychology, 5*(2), 207–232.

31. Locksley, A., Hepburn, C., & Ortiz, V. (1982). Social stereotypes and judgments of individuals: An instance of the base-rate fallacy. *Journal of Experimental Social Psychology, 18*(1), 23–42.

32. Gardner, W., Lidz, C. W., Mulvey, E. P., & Shaw, E. C. (1996). Clinical versus actuarial predictions of violence of patients with mental illnesses. *Journal of Consulting and Clinical Psychology, 64*(3), 602–609.

33. Hart, S. D., Michie, C., & Cooke, D. J. (2007). Precision of actuarial risk assessment instruments. *British Journal of Psychiatry, 190*(49), s60–s65.

34. Smee, J. E., & Bowers, T. G. (2008). A comparative test of clinical judgment versus actuarial prediction of future violence. *Journal of Police and Criminal Psychology, 23*(1), 1–7.

35. Singh, J. P., Grann, M., & Fazel, S. (2011). A comparative study of violence risk assessment tools: A systematic review and metaregression analysis of 68 studies involving 25,980 participants. *Clinical Psychology Review, 31*(3), 499–513.

36. Fazel, S., Singh, J. P., Doll, H., & Grann, M. (2012). Use of risk assessment instruments to predict violence and antisocial behaviour in 73 samples involving 24 827 people: Systematic review and meta-analysis. *BMJ, 345*(2), e4692.

37. Doyle, M., & Dolan, M. (2002). Violence risk assessment: Combining actuarial and clinical information to structure clinical judgements for the formulation and management of risk. *Journal of Psychiatric and Mental Health Nursing, 9*(6), 649–657.

38. Singh, J. P., Fazel, S., Gueorguieva, R., & Buchanan, A. (2014). Rates of violence in patients classified as high risk by structured risk assessment instruments. *British Journal of Psychiatry, 204*(3), 180–187.

39. Abidin, Z., Davoren, M., Naughton, L., Gibbons, O., Nulty, A., & Kennedy, H. G. (2013). Susceptibility (risk and protective) factors for in-patient violence and self-harm: Prospective study of structured professional judgement instruments START and SAPROF, DUNDRUM-3 and DUNDRUM-4 in forensic mental health services. *BMC Psychiatry, 13*(1), 197.

40. Lidz, C. W., Mulvey, E. P., & Gardner, W. (1993). The accuracy of predictions of violence to others. *JAMA, 269*(8), 1007–1011.

41. Skeem, J. L., Manchak, S. M., Lidz, C. W., & Mulvey, E. P. (2013). The utility of patients' self-perceptions of violence risk: Consider asking the person who may know best. *Psychiatric Services, 64*(5), 410–415.

42. Douglas, K. S., & Skeem, J. L. (2005). Violence risk assessment: Getting specific about being dynamic. *Psychology, Public Policy, and Law, 11*(3), 347–383.

43. Arseneault, L., Moffitt, T. E., Caspi, A., Taylor, P. J., & Silva, P. A. (2000). Mental disorders and violence in a total birth cohort: Results from the Dunedin study. *Archives of General Psychiatry, 57*(10), 979–986.

44. Ferguson, C. J. (2015). Do angry birds make for angry children? A meta-analysis of video game influences on children's and adolescents' aggression, mental health, prosocial behavior, and academic performance. *Perspectives on Psychological Science, 10*(5), 646–666.

45. Strack, G. B., McClane, G. E., & Hawley, D. (2001). A review of 300 attempted strangulation cases. Part I: Criminal legal issues. *The Journal of Emergency Medicine, 21*(3), 303–309.

46. Mulvey, E. P., & Lidz, C. W. (1995). Conditional prediction: A model for research on dangerousness to others in a new era. *International Journal of Law and Psychiatry, 18*(2), 129–143.

47. Fazel, S., Langström, N., Hjern, A., Grann, M., & Lichtenstein, P. (2009). Schizophrenia, substance abuse, and violent crime. *JAMA, 301*(19), 2016–2023.

48. Witt, K., van Dorn, R., & Fazel, S. (2013). Risk factors for violence in psychosis: Systematic review and meta-regression analysis of 110 studies. *PLOS One, 8*(2), e55942.

49. Skeem, J., Kennealy, P., Monahan, J., Peterson, J., & Appelbaum, P. (2016). Psychosis uncommonly and inconsistently precedes violence among high-risk individuals. *Clinical Psychological Science, 4*(1), 40–49.

50. Skeem, J. L., Schubert, C., Odgers, C., Mulvey, E. P., Gardner, W., & Lidz, C. (2006). Psychiatric symptoms and community violence among high-risk patients: A test of the relationship at the weekly level. *Journal of Consulting and Clinical Psychology, 74*(5), 967–979.

51. Coid, J. W., Ullrich, S., Bebbington, P., Fazel, S., & Keers, R. (2016). Paranoid ideation and violence: Meta-analysis of individual subject data of 7 population surveys. *Schizophrenia Bulletin, 42*(4), 907–915.

52. Knoll, J. L., & Meloy, J. R. (2014). Mass murder and the violent paranoid spectrum. *Psychiatric Annals, 44*(5), 236–243.

53. Elbogen, E. B., & Johnson, S. C. (2009). The intricate link between violence and mental disorder: Results from the National Epidemiologic Survey on Alcohol and Related Conditions. *Archives of General Psychiatry, 66*(2), 152–161.

54. McGinty, E. E., Choksy, S., & Wintemute, G. J. (2016). The relationship between controlled substances and violence. *Epidemiologic Reviews, 38*(1), 5–31.

55. Burgason, K. A., Drawve, G., Brown, T. C., & Eassey, J. (2017). Close only counts in alcohol and violence: Controlling violence near late-night alcohol establishments using a routine activities approach. *Journal of Criminal Justice, 50*, 62–68.

56. Mulvey, E. P., Odgers, C., Skeem, J., Gardner, W., Schubert, C., & Lidz, C. (2006). Substance use and community violence: A test of the relation at the daily level. *Journal of Consulting and Clinical Psychology, 74*(4), 743–754.

57. Johnson, K. L., Desmarais, S. L., Grimm, K. J., Tueller, S. J., Swartz, M. S., & Van Dorn, R. A. (2016). Proximal risk factors for short-term community violence among adults with mental illnesses. *Psychiatric Services, 67*(7), 771–778.

58. Grinshteyn, E., & Hemenway, D. (2016). Violent death rates: The US compared with other high-income OECD countries, 2010. *American Journal of Medicine, 129*(3), 266–273.

59. Karp, A. (2018). *Estimating global civilian-held firearms numbers* (Report No.: 9). Geneva: Small Arms Survey. Retrieved June 19, 2018, from http://www.smallarmssurvey.org/fileadmin/docs/T-Briefing-Papers/SAS-BP-Civilian-Firearms-Numbers.pdf.

60. Pew Research Center. (2017). *The demographics of gun ownership in the U.S.* Retrieved November 25, 2018, from http://www.pewsocialtrends.org/2017/06/22/the-demographics-of-gun-ownership/.

61. *Guns | Gallup historical trends*. Retrieved November 25, 2018, from https://news.gallup.com/poll/1645/guns.aspx.

62. Moyer, M. W. (2017, October). Journey to gunland: More firearms do not keep people safe, hard numbers show. Why do so many Americans believe the opposite? *Scientific American*, 54–63.

63. Cleckley, H. M. (1976). *The mask of sanity: An attempt to clarify some issues about the so-called psychopathic personality* (5th ed.). St. Louis, MO: Mosby.

64. Paulhus, D. L. (2014). Toward a taxonomy of dark personalities. *Current Directions in Psychological Science, 23*(6), 421–426.

65. Camp, J. P., Skeem, J. L., Barchard, K., Lilienfeld, S. O., & Poythress, N. G. (2013). Psychopathic predators? Getting specific about the relation between psychopathy and violence. *Journal of Consulting and Clinical Psychology, 81*(3), 467–480.

66. Elbogen, E. B., Johnson, S. C., Wagner, H. R., Sullivan, C., Taft, C. T., & Beckham, J. C. (2014). Violent behaviour and post-traumatic stress disorder in US Iraq and Afghanistan veterans. *British Journal of Psychiatry, 204*(5), 368–375.

67. Grossman, D. (2009). *On killing: The psychological cost of learning to kill in war and society* (Rev. ed.). New York, NY: Little, Brown and Co.

68. Cleveland, E. C., Azrael, D., Simonetti, J. A., & Miller, M. (2017). Firearm ownership among American veterans: Findings from the 2015 National Firearm Survey. *Injury Epidemiology, 4*, 33.

69. Elbogen, E. B., Wagner, H. R., Kimbrel, N. A., Brancu, M., Naylor, J., Graziano, R., et al. (2017). Risk factors for concurrent suicidal ideation and violent impulses in military veterans. *Psychological Assessment, 30*, 425–435.

70. Tripp, J. C., McDevitt-Murphy, M. E., & Henschel, A. V. (2016). Firing a weapon and killing in combat are associated with suicidal ideation in OEF/OIF veterans. *Psychological Trauma: Theory, Research, Practice, and Policy, 8*(5), 626–633.

71. Morrison, J., & Boehnlein, J. (2007). Our favorite tips for interviewing veterans. *Psychiatric Clinics of North America, 30*(2), 269–273.

72. Buckner, F., & Firestone, M. (2000). Where the public peril begins: 25 years after Tarasoff. *Journal of Legal Medicine, 21*(2), 187–222.

73. Werth, J. L., Welfel, E. R., & Benjamin, G. A. H. (Eds.). (2009). *The duty to protect: Ethical, legal, and professional considerations for mental health professionals*. Washington, DC: American Psychological Association.

74. Widgery, A., & Winterfield, A. (2013). Mental health professionals' duty to warn. *NCSL Legisbrief, 21*(1), 2.

75. Rodriguez, L. (2013). *Message to our nation's health care providers*. Retrieved from http://www.hhs.gov/ocr/office/lettertonationhcp.pdf.

76. Pinals, D. A., & Mossman, D. (2012). *Evaluation for civil commitment. Best Practices in Forensic Mental Health Assessment*. New York, NY: Oxford University Press.

77. Swanson, J. W., Norko, M. A., Lin, H.-J., Alanis-Hirsch, K., Frisman, L. K., Baranoski, M. V., et al. (2017). Implementation and effectiveness of Connecticut's risk-based gun removal law: Does it prevent suicides. *Law & Contemporary Problems, 80*, 179.

78. RAND Corporation. (2018). *The science of gun policy: A critical synthesis of research evidence on the effects of gun policies in the United States*. Santa Monica, CA: RAND.

79. Kapoor, R., Benedek, E., Bonnie, R. J., Gandhi, T., Gold, L. H., Judd, S., et al. (2018). *Resource document on risk-based gun removal laws*. Washington, DC: American Psychiatric Association. Retrieved from https://www.psychiatry.org/File%20Library/Psychiatrists/Directories/Library-and-Archive/resource_documents/2018-Resource-Document-on-Risk-Based-Gun-Removal-Laws.pdf.

80. Schaffer, A. C., Jena, A. B., Seabury, S. A., Singh, H., Chalasani, V., & Kachalia, A. (2017). Rates and characteristics of paid malpractice claims among US physicians by specialty, 1992-2014. *JAMA Internal Medicine, 177*(5), 710–718.

81. Jena, A. B., Seabury, S., Lakdawalla, D., & Chandra, A. (2011). Malpractice risk according to physician specialty. *The New England Journal of Medicine, 365*(7), 629–636.

82. Rozel, J. S. (2018). Difficult relationships: Patients, providers, and systems. *Current Emergency and Hospital Medicine Reports, 6*(1), 1–7.

83. Beauchamp, T. L., & Childress, J. F. (2013). *Principles of biomedical ethics* (7th ed.). New York, NY: Oxford University Press.

84. Nordstrom, K., Zun, L., Wilson, M., Stiebel, V., Ng, A., Bregman, B., et al. (2012). Medical evaluation and triage of the agitated patient: Consensus statement of the American Association for Emergency Psychiatry Project BETA Medical Evaluation Workgroup. *The Western Journal of Emergency Medicine, 13*(1), 3–10.

85. Stowell, K., Florence, P., Harman, H., & Glick, R. (2012). Psychiatric evaluation of the agitated patient: Consensus statement of the American Association for Emergency Psychiatry Project BETA Psychiatric Evaluation Workgroup. *The Western Journal of Emergency Medicine, 13*(1), 11–16.

86. Flogen, S., Waddell, A., Russell, B., Luczak, S., Garmaise, C., & Mangla, K. (2015). Pursuing criminal charges against patients who are reported as having assaulted healthcare professionals: Considerations. *Healthcare Quarterly, 18*(2), 25–30.

87. Clark, C. R., McInerney, B. A., & Brown, I. (2012). The prosecution of psychiatric inpatients: Overcoming the barriers. *The Journal of Forensic Psychiatry & Psychology, 23*(3), 371–381.

88. Hoge, S. K., & Gutheil, T. G. (1987). The prosecution of psychiatric patients for assaults on staff: A preliminary empirical study. *Hospital and Community Psychiatry, 38*(1), 44–49.

89. Gupta, S., Akyuz, E. U., Flint, J., & Baldwin, T. (2018). Violence and aggression in psychiatric settings: Reporting to the police. *BJPsych Advances, 24*(3), 146–151.

90. Munetz, M. R., & Griffin, P. A. (2006). Use of the Sequential Intercept Model as an approach to decriminalization of people with serious mental illness. *Psychiatric Services, 57*(4), 544–549.

91. Griffin, P. A. (Ed.). (2015). *The sequential intercept model and criminal justice: Promoting community alternatives for individuals with serious mental illness.* Oxford, NY: Oxford University Press.

92. Skeem, J. L., Winter, E., Kennealy, P. J., Louden, J. E., & Tatar, J. R. (2014). Offenders with mental illness have criminogenic needs, too: Toward recidivism reduction. *Law and Human Behavior, 38*(3), 212–224.

33

Violence: Managing Major Threats

John S. Rozel

Threat management is a multidisciplinary approach to preventing targeted violence, including mass shootings. It consists of deliberate and planned collaboration across different disciplines (eg, law enforcement and investigation) to prevent targeted violence from occurring. Unlike traditional psychiatric approaches, threat management looks beyond the scope of diagnoses and symptoms to look at criminogenic and contextual factors. The field, now built on over 25 years of research, both complements and informs our own work in clinical care of behavioral emergencies (1,2). For both threat management and emergency psychiatry, all threats must be taken seriously.

TARGETED VIOLENCE

Targeted violence encompasses all attacks that are contemplated, planned, and/or enacted toward a specific individual or group and is neither spontaneous or random. Targeted violence includes most homicides, as well as mass shootings, vehicle attacks, bombings, arson, and other attacks intended to injure large numbers of people. Most targeted violence homicides in the United States happen within small groups or dyads—a bar fight, domestic violence, a drug deal gone bad—and by definition are intentionally directed to a specific target, chosen by who they are or their membership in a class. Contrary to popular perceptions, the US homicide rate has decreased significantly over the past 30 years (3,4). There has been an uptick in homicides in 2015 to 2016 that is specifically attributable to firearms and which is not reflected in homicides by other means such as stabbing or strangulation (5).

Mass shootings or attacks account for only about 1% of all homicides but also appear to be occurring with increased frequency (9-12). Mass shootings can be defined in a number of different ways leading to confusion about the varying interpretations of different data sets (6-8). Mass shootings also appear to be distinctly more common in the United States than in other economically developed nations (83,84).

Collectively, this grouping is called targeted violence. Threat management is a specialized approach to managing targeted violence that can be extremely useful to psychiatric emergency service (PES) professionals. Its models, techniques, and tools are informative whether the target is one or many and even when there is no specific target at all.

THE PATHWAY TO VIOLENCE

The conceptualization of a pathway to violence is central to threat management. This model describes how persons of concern rarely, if ever, snap; rather, they follow a pathway beginning with grievance, transitioning to thoughts of violence and contemplation of a target, evolving to preparation and, ultimately, to attack. This pathway to violence often takes days, weeks, or even years which provide an extended window of opportunity for identification, investigation, and intervention (13-15). This model is summarized in Figure 33.1.

Conceptually, grievance is the first step on the pathway to violence. As risk factors accumulate and protective factors weaken, fixation intensifies and people progress up the stairway toward an attack. The goal is to disrupt and

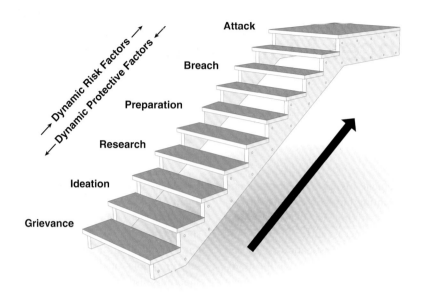

FIGURE 33.1 • Pathway to violence (15). (From Calhoun, F. S., & Weston, S. W. (2003). Contemporary threat management: a practical guide for identifying, assessing, and managing individuals of violent intent (p. 280). San Diego, CA: Specialized Training Services. [A practical guide series.] With permission.)

divert a person before they reach the attack stage. People at highest risk may be those who are already at or near the top of the staircase or who seem to be moving upwards more quickly. Threat management embraces using either criminal justice or mental health interventions as needed because each given person of concern transits the pathway in a unique and distinct manner. Careful clinical judgment is always essential for no model can truly countenance the subtleties of all human behavior. What follows are brief descriptions of each stage based primarily upon the Calhoun and Weston version of the pathway to violence (15).

Grievance

Grievance, in the context of threat management, is the idea that one has been wronged and treated unjustly by another, an organization, or the world writ large. All people encounter frustrating situations by circumstance or the acts of others; most let the frustrations effervesce away. Some people ruminate on these slights, be they real or imagined. They let the feelings fester and grow and, increasingly, to become a central part of their self-perception. In a psychiatric interview, this is a person who readily identifies how their problems or adverse experiences are attributable to a person or parties. Persistent rumination itself may be harmful to the individual in other psychological ways (16). The clinician should be especially wary of the person who readily catalogs the numerous slights and offenses of their lives (so called "grievance collectors") and those who, often through characterological pathology, seek repeatedly to create situations where they can claim injustices against themselves ("grievance creators.")

Ideation

Ideation is the pivot from "I've been harmed by others" to "I will harm them back." It is the beginning of the progression toward an attack. It may be marked by increased empathy with others who engage in violence and shifting from a viewpoint of passive victimization to embracing a proactive position that, by harming others, the person of concern can somehow address the injustices they have suffered. Although persons of concern may be cognizant of the fact that the world may view their actions as immoral or illegal, they often perceive themselves as the one who is just. Increased fixation on how the target or the world deserves the intended harm becomes more common. Themes of entitlement are common and perhaps a predisposing risk factor as well. Fantasies about being an avenging, righteous warrior whose actions will be remembered by others become more common (17). It should be noted that homicidal ideation and violent fantasies are not uncommon and, in and of themselves, not necessarily concerning. The therapeutic space is often used as a safe way to express those urges so as not to act on them; the critical nuance is when they evolve from fantasy to intent (18).

Research and Preparation

At this stage, the person of concern moves beyond simple contemplation of an act of violence to planning and exploration of how they might attack their target. It may include the development of an operational plan or merely readiness to act when the opportunity arises by carrying a weapon. It can include surveillance, reconnaissance, or probing the security of the target. It may be accompanied by increased fixation on and fantasies about how they will be perceived during or after their attack. This phase may include acquisition and practice with weapons, costuming and dress, and interest in how their message will be conveyed and portrayed (19). Often, this may include communications which become leakage through varying social media or interpersonal connections (20).

Breach

Breach is the pivot from the preparation to dangerous action. It may include "walk throughs" or rehearsals, probes of security such as bringing a weapon to a setting where they know they should not have one, or a verbal altercation or threat toward their intended target. Actions to strengthen commitment toward the final act are common including sabotage of their own personal resources and protective factors; examples include dropping out of treatment, distancing themselves from personal relationships, and even destroying their own home or apartment. Some assailants may escalate substance use, knowing it will disinhibit them while others may shift to abstinence to increase their focus and dexterity. It can also include cruelty to animals as a form of practice or fixating into commitment, such as killing the family dog before killing the family itself (21).

Attack

This is the final stage and is the act or attempt to physically injure the target. Successful attacks, especially when consequences (natural, logical, or legal) do not occur, may reinforce aggressive behavior in the person of concern. A history of violence is one of the best predictors of future violence. It is not uncommon to see persistently violent offenders who, following an initial successful attack, demonstrate increasing magnitude and decreasing thresholds to attack again when slighted.

Many clinicians may see immediate parallels between the pathway to violence and the stages of change (22). Grievance is similar to precontemplation. Ideation and research are similar to contemplation. Planning and breach correlate to determination or commitment. And, of course, action corresponds to attack. The correlation of the models invites the use of motivational interviewing methodology in interview, assessment, and development of strategies for the person of concern to change their behavioral pathway. Just as substance users are often ambivalent about their use, ambivalence can be common in potential assailants up to the moment of attack. Motivational interviewing techniques and strategy may be helpful by creating an alliance with the person of concern, building understanding through exploration and empathy, and ultimately helping the individual move toward changing their behaviors. Some possible interview questions are provided in Table 33.1.

THE CASE FOR THE ROLE OF EMERGENCY PSYCHIATRY

In most cases, psychiatric illness has little to do with gun violence or with mass shootings (23,24). Examined purely statistically, the rates of mental illness among perpetrators of violence is lower than the rate of mental illness in the general population. Nonetheless, after many high-profile events, there is often an immediate ascription of blame to mental illness from pundits and policy makers (25,26). In American adults, the prevalence of a prior diagnosis of mental illness is 25% and the lifetime prevalence approaches 55% (27). In comparison, a study from the FBI Behavioral Analysis Unit looked closely at recent mass shooting offenders and identified psychiatric illness in only 25% of offenders (28). A long-term study looking at a century of data on mass murderers found a rate of 25% for mental illness

TABLE 33.1 Interview Questions to Explore Progress Along the Pathway to Violence

Grievance	Who has wronged you in your life? What experiences have you had where others have wronged you? What makes it difficult to forgive people who have wronged you?
Ideation	You have described a number of ways others have hurt you; what can you do to set things right? Do you ever want to hurt people they way you have been hurt? What fantasies do you have about harming others?
Research and preparation	How would you attack this person (when, where, how)? What has kept you from attacking this person so far? What would be the most effective way to take care of the person who wronged you?
Breach	What is the closest you have gotten to attacking them? What has kept you from attacking them so far? What is your "go-ahead" condition to attack them?

as well (29). And, notably, although psychotic illnesses play a substantial role in general violence risk, they accounted for only a minority of these active assailants in both studies. Some studies, have found lower rates of mental illness in mass shooting offenders: only 17% in school shooters, only 11% in other shooters, and one study found that only 4.7% of mass shooters in public locations had a psychiatric history severe enough to disqualify them from legally acquiring a firearm (ie, involuntary commitment, found incompetent to stand trial, or not guilty be reason of insanity) (30,31,32).

Although it is rarely stated explicitly, the implication is that if psychiatric services were better, somehow the person at risk would have been identified and helped (or hospitalized—not that they are mutually exclusive) prior to the attack. Thus, one could argue, emergency psychiatry is the linchpin: if, as suggested, these offenders were seriously mentally ill, then certainly if they had only been brought to a PES in time and been treated or admitted, then such tragedies would not occur. Emergency psychiatry is involved in the discussion about mass shootings because we were invited. It is an issue squarely in the lane of emergency health professionals. No studies have ever suggested that people with mental illness never engage in such violence and so the role of emergency psychiatry is to identify and stabilize those at risk.

In response to the debate, the American Association for Emergency Psychiatry (AAEP) issued a position statement about the role of mental illness in violence and mass shootings (33). It recognizes both that the role of mental illness in violence and mass violence is often exaggerated and that psychiatrists and emergency psychiatrists have an important role to play both in the evaluation and care of people at risk and in the ongoing public dialogue about appropriate public policy remedies for this issue. Anchored to the mission of promoting evidence-based and compassionate care for people with behavioral emergencies, it endeavors to mitigate stigma and risk alike through application of science and collaboration with other stakeholders. And, by including the idea of collaboration across disciplines, the AAEP position statement is compatible with and complements threat management. The core recommendations of the position statement are summarized in Table 33.2.

PSYCHIATRIC ILLNESS AND THE PATHWAY TO VIOLENCE

In threat management, a mental illness is relevant in as much as it either facilitates a person of concern's progression up the pathway to violence or slows down that progression. It is always an assessment based on the individual, their experience of the illness, and within the context of

TABLE 33.2 Recommendations From the American Association for Emergency Psychiatry (33)

1. All threats of violence must be taken seriously and receive a psychiatric evaluation within the capacity of the facility.
2. Optimal use of emergency and general psychiatric services will not eliminate community violence or mass shootings because of the limited role psychiatric illness plays in such events; however, when such cases do arise and are clinically identified, every reasonable clinical intervention should be considered.
3. Recognizing that violence is often multifactorial, consultation and collaboration amongst professionals (including health care and law enforcement) should be used to support multidisciplinary assessment and intervention including accessible psychiatric treatment.
4. Emergency department and PES decision-making should reflect clinically appropriate, ethical, and legal practices.
5. Care of violent and threatening patients is challenging and PES and ED programs should provide staff wellness resources to support optimal team performance.
6. The science of violence and firearm injury prevention is an actively developing science. Clinicians should consider violence an essential element of continuing education and the AAEP will prioritize relevant education and training for the membership.
7. Understanding concerns about media-related contagion, communications by healthcare providers or hospital spokespersons relating to such events should adhere when possible to best practices (www.reportingonmassshootings.org) including avoiding glamorizing the assailant or attack, using behavioral health experts to explain the science, and explaining that violence and mass shootings are complex with multiple causes.

AAEP, American Association for Emergency Psychiatry; ED, emergency department; PES, psychiatric emergency service.

other risk and protective factors. Extrapolating population-level, nomothetic research to understand individual level and idiographic behavior is challenging and fraught with inaccuracy and risk (34). Mental illness is relatively uncommon in people who engage in violence, including severe violence (35,36). There is no psychiatric illness or symptom which, in and of itself, necessary or sufficient as a risk factor for targeted violence. When psychiatric illness is present in a person at risk for violence, early identification, appropriate treatment, and careful follow-up can be essential to reducing the risk of attack or necessity for criminal justice involvement.

Perhaps it will turn out in future studies that the risk for engaging in mass violence intersects not with severe mental illness but with moderate mental illness. That is, the broad and severe impairment that typifies severe mental illness may be substantially incompatible with the capacity to plan and carry out a complex plan of attack. There are some disorders which may be seen more frequently in state or trait in individuals who engage or attempt to engage in planned and intentional violence which warrant additional discussion.

Psychopathy

Psychopathy, as an intersection of antisocial and narcissistic personality, is often seen as an important risk factor for violence in general and targeted violence in particular (37,38). As with all risk factors, it is neither necessary nor sufficient in and of itself. However, the presence of psychopathy in a person who is contemplating targeted violence or otherwise at risk for violence may be at risk for greater magnitude or severity due to the lack of moral inhibitions against violence (39). Although oft debated, psychopathy is not currently recognized as a psychiatric disorder in the Diagnostic and Statistical Manual of Mental Disorders (DSM).

Psychosis and Paranoia

Major psychotic disorders, especially schizophrenia and bipolar I, are often associated with violence especially earlier in the course of illness, with comorbid substance use, when resistant to treatment and when acutely symptomatic (40-42). Recent data have suggested that mental illness is uncommon in people who engage in mass shootings, and psychotic illnesses in particular are uncommon within that subset (28). There is also a frequent pattern of suspiciousness, mistrust, and alienation that is seen in people who engage in planned violence and which seems to suggest, at least, the trait of psychosis and persecutory and paranoid ideology (43).

Autism Spectrum

Several high-profile active shooters have been identified as having autism spectrum features. In general, autism is not significantly linked to violence, especially once attention-deficit/hyperactivity disorder (ADHD) and conduct disorder are controlled for (44,45). However, it has been suggested that features of autism, including persistence and planning, limited emotional reciprocity, and elevated risk of being psychologically abused or bullied by others (none of which are the exclusive domain of autism), may facilitate planned violence in some people already otherwise predisposed to engage in more extreme violence (46,47). Notably, although most experienced mental health professionals can readily discern autism spectrum from schizophrenia or antisocial personality and psychopathy, professionals in other disciplines may confuse the symptoms and the diagnoses. This may undermine the success of a threat management intervention plan constructed without the input of a mental health professional who can recognize the differences and help adapt the plan accordingly (48).

LEAKAGE AND THREATS

A threat is when a person of concern expresses intent to harm the target in a way that the target is aware of the danger; leakage is when that information is directed to or through a third party (49). Leakage and threats are a sensitive but nonspecific risk factor for engaging in serious violence; studies often identify leakage or threats in 80% or more of serious attacks including mass shootings and school attacks (28,31,50,51). Threatening behavior as a cause for admission is also a strong risk factor for inpatient violence (52). Numerous

PES evaluations occur because a person has leaked or threatened a desire to harm others.

After a highly publicized event such as a mass shooting, PESs often receive an influx of people flagged as potential risks for similar acts. The initial response of many clinicians is exasperation and a sense that others are overreacting. Indeed, people are more likely to categorize a person as being at risk if they have just been thinking about a highly risky event (53,54). Apophenia—a tendency to see threatening patterns in behavior which are not actually present is a known reaction to fear and stress (55,56). However, clustering of mass shootings does occur after highly publicized events so there likely is an increased probability of encountering a person at risk for engaging in a major attack amid the flurry of other referrals (57-59). Although it may be frustrating to be seeing an increased number of persons who may or may not have made a bona fide threat, it is important to evaluate each threat and each threatener carefully. Threats and leakage are a sensitive but not a specific risk factor for future violence.

Consider four basic categories of the potential threats and threateners seen in the PES, especially after highly publicized violent events: pseudothreateners, hoaxers, hotheads, and bona fide threats.

Pseudothreatening Outliers

This category includes people with no intent to threaten or harm but behavior is awkward, intimidating, or disruptive enough to provoke anxiety in others. These may be people with autism spectrum disorders or schizotypy, people with an unexpectedly loud or disruptive tone or merely people who are engaging in benign activities who are misperceived because of stereotype or prejudice (60). Although PES clinicians should in no way pathologize a target of stereotype or stigma, some of these persons may show developmental or personality features, communication disorders, or other issues that, if not previously identified, may benefit from clinical intervention or support.

Hoaxers and Trolls

The concept of instrumental or sadistic threats is well understood and, while possibly exacerbated in an era of social media and electronic communication, has been present for some time. These threats are often anonymous but are occasionally traced back to the perpetrator. They are made without any intent to actually harm the target physically but merely to intimidate that person or disrupt operations of a facility (eg, anonymous bomb threats to a school). Clinicians may identify conduct disorder or personality disorder in these persons; treating comorbid mood or substance use disorders may decrease their risk for future antagonistic behavior as will, of course, natural consequences for criminal conduct.

Hotheads

This category impulsively makes menacing or threatening statements when upset or angry without sustained (or any) intent to carry out attack. Intermittent explosive disorder, other impulse control disorders, mania, or substance use may be identified and may benefit from targeted treatment including education on coping skills.

Bona Fide Threats

This is the most concerning category: a person contemplating or moving toward an attack with real intent to harm others. This category may or may not have treatable psychopathology, but, if and when present, such illness should be treated aggressively.

ALL THREATS MUST BE TAKEN SERIOUSLY

Conceptually, the premise that all threats must be investigated and all threateners evaluated for clinical needs is cardinal. As discussed above, threats and a history of violence are critical risk factors to consider in the evaluation of violence; threats

and leakage are a highly sensitive risk factor for future violence. Additionally, acute stressors and losses including romantic or personal relationships, employment and financial security, medical illness, and housing have all been associated with risk of violence in people with and without mental illness and across the spectrum of violence types (28,31,46,61,62). Substance use and intoxication has been widely recognized as a potent risk factor for violence and also is significant both for people with and without other mental illness (63-66). People who perceive the world as an inherently dangerous or threatening place automatically believe neutral actions of others are intentionally harmful or demeaning to them, or have other features of a hostile attribution bias have significant risk for violence (67,68). Similarly, external attributional style including an inability to take personal responsibility and blaming others for their own shortcomings or failures is at elevated risk for violence—and this may come out in the aforementioned paranoid or persecutory delusional pattern (69,70). Finally, suicidality and hopelessness may also be a risk factor for violent behavior (as the opposite is true as well); notably, many mass shooters either kill themselves or expect to be killed in their attacks (71,72). Consider the mnemonic in Table 33.3 as a useful tool.

ATTACKS, TARGETS, AND AGGRESSORS

Targeted violence is a complex, dynamic problem, both in the colloquial and the scientific sense of those terms. Effective interventions themselves will also need to be complex and nuanced—and to move beyond the traditional concept of merely

TABLE 33.3 All THREATS Must Be Taken Seriously

T	**Threats** and leakage about violence toward others
H	**History** of violence toward others, especially the identified target
R	**Recent stressors** or losses (financial, relationship, medical, employment, housing)
E	**Ethanol** or other drug abuse
A	**Agitated or annoyed** easily (hostile attributional style)
T	**Takes no responsibility** for actions (external attributional style)
S	**Suicidal** or hopeless

disrupting or stopping the attack through admission (or arrest) of the person of concern or warning of the target.

Security professionals often discuss the idea of hardening the target: this is a concept which extends the traditional idea of warning and adds some degree of counseling or provision of resources to potential targets. If the target is an organization, especially one with its own security resources, this could take the form of adding security professionals, surveillance for threats, countersurveillance to disrupt or block stalking or pursuit, or simply relocation of the target from the zone of danger (eg, paid leave). As clinical professionals, PES providers may also consider helping the target, especially if the target is an individual person. Although law enforcement colleagues may be able to provide essential counseling in situational awareness or even self-defense training to a potential target, attending to the psychological needs of the individual or linkage to appropriate victim advocacy services may be helpful as well. Targets of workplace threats or violence can be linked to Employee Assistance Programs; the impact of threats or violence can be significant, and Critical Incident Stress Management or similar interventions for impacted individuals or teams should be considered.

Although our role as clinicians is often focused on the person of concern (ie, identifying and treating contributing psychiatric illnesses), this concept of aiding the aggressor to decrease their risk may not be identified as a priority by others involved in threat management. It should not be neglected as doing so may both decrease the risk of harm to the current (or future) targets but can also improve the quality of life and well-being of the person of concern.

COLLABORATION: AD HOC AND INTENTIONAL

Psychiatry, acting alone, will often struggle to fully and effectively evaluate a threat. In part, this is due to many risk factors extending beyond mere diagnosis and symptoms. In part, this is due to many elements of data relevant to assessment often being unavailable to evaluating clinicians in a PES. Input from collateral and coordination with law enforcement is often necessary

to mitigate violence risk. This is not to say that PES clinicians should be routinely involving law enforcement, but rather to suggest that such collaboration and coordination of efforts may be ethical, legal, and even clinically optimal for the person of concern. This may be a particular concern when assessment and treatment as usual are expected to yield foreseeably unsatisfactory results.

Threat management, as a multidisciplinary approach to an interdisciplinary problem, integrates subject matter and operational expertise to identify effective strategies and tactics to disrupt attacks before they happen. Categories of interventions include blocking the attack, hardening the target and altering target behavior, and intervening with the person of concern (73). Threat management draws expertise and evidence from behavioral sciences, law enforcement, law and risk management, intelligence, operational security, and other fields; it uses an investigative and preventive mindset to derail attacks before they occur (74). Arguably, with expertise in violent behavior management and legal aspects relating to commitment and duties to third parties, emergency psychiatrists and emergency medicine physicians can be especially effective team members.

Collaboration may occur ad hoc when a person of concern is identified by law enforcement and brought to a PES for evaluation or the PES team identifies a person of concern and reaches out to law enforcement for collaboration. Ideally, established teams exist on an ongoing basis, working closely together through actual cases and role plays, with explicitly defined roles and processes (75). Of course, many ongoing teams begin when the same professionals find themselves working through similar cases repeatedly and opt to shift from a reactive to a proactive stance (76).

The Health Insurance Portability and Accountability Act of 1996 Privacy (HIPAA) regulations specifically permit sharing of information to prevent intentional and severe violence when doing so is within the ethical standards of the professional or the applicable jurisdictional laws (77,78). Jurisdictional and professional standards vary and evolve over time; the prudent practitioner would be well served in attending to their nuances (79,80). Resources providing guidance in the ethical and legal sharing of information with law enforcement are worth careful consideration by clinicians and hospital counsel alike (81,82). Although HIPAA is oft criticized for being confusing and difficult to implement, clinicians and legal advisors should reframe their legal and ethical analysis to identification of opportunities where even limited disclosure may be possible and helpful. Even when HIPAA or other factors prevent sharing of direct information with law enforcement, a professional may still be able to offer opinions to threat management teams about what behavioral factors may or may not be relevant to a case under review.

CONCLUSION

Violence risk is one of the most common and concerning chief complaints in the PES. Our clinical evaluations can benefit from integrating threat management principles into our direct work and by developing collaborative threat management processes through ad hoc cooperation or the development of formal and informal teams. Although only a minority of violence is attributable to psychiatric illness, psychiatric emergency professionals have valuable expertise nurtured from their experience with high-risk patients, familiarity with legal issues including commitment and duties to third parties, and through their comfort working with complex cases and relationships. Although media coverage may falsely portray mass violence as psychiatric issue, the increasing frequency of mass violence is also creating a growing need for effective collaboration between emergency psychiatry and other threat management professionals.

REFERENCES

1. Meloy, J. R. (2015). Threat assessment: Scholars, operators, our past, our future. *Journal of Threat Assessment and Management, 2*(3–4), 231–242.
2. Calhoun, F. S., & Weston, S. W. (2015). Perspectives on threat management. *Journal of Threat Assessment and Management, 2*(3–4), 258–267.
3. Criminal Justice Information Services Division. (2018). *2017, Crime in the US: Expanded offense*. FBI. Retrieved December 9, 2018, https://ucr.fbi.gov/crime-in-the-u.s/2017/crime-in-the-u.s.-2017/topic-pages/expanded-offense.
4. Pew Research Center. (2013, May). *Gun homicide rate down 49% since 1993 peak; Public unaware. Pace of decline slows in past decade*. Washington, DC: Pew Research Center. Retrieved May 6, 2015, from http://www.pewsocialtrends.org/files/2013/05/firearms_final_05-2013.pdf.
5. Pifer, H., & Minino, A. (2018). QuickStats: Number of homicides committed, by the three most common methods – United States, 2010–2016. *Morbidity and Mortality Weekly Report, 67*(29), 806.
6. DeSilver, D. (2014). *Why timely, reliable data on mass killings is hard to find*. Washington, DC: Pew Research Center. Retrieved March 11, 2015, from http://www.pewresearch.org/fact-tank/2014/06/17/why-timely-reliable-data-on-mass-killings-is-hard-to-find/.
7. Huff-Corzine, L., McCutcheon, J. C., Corzine, J., Jarvis, J. P., Tetzlaff-Bemiller, M. J., Weller, M., et al. (2014). Shooting for accuracy: Comparing data sources on mass murder. *Homicide Studies, 18*(1), 105–124.
8. Duwe, G. A. (2005). Circle of distortion: The social construction of mass murder in the United States. *Western Criminology Review, 6*(1), 59–78.
9. Follman, M., Aronsen, G., Pan, D., & Caldwell, M. *US mass shootings, 1982–2012: Data from Mother Jones' investigation*. Mother Jones. Retrieved March 11, 2015, from http://www.motherjones.com/politics/2012/12/mass-shootings-mother-jones-full-data.
10. Schweit, K. W. (2016). *Active shooter incidents in the United States in 2014 and 2015*. Washington, DC: Federal Bureau of Investigation, US Department of Justice. Retrieved July 16, 2016, from https://www.fbi.gov/about-us/office-of-partner-engagement/active-shooter-incidents/a-study-of-active-shooter-incidents-in-the-u.s.-2000-2013.
11. Blair, J. P., & Schweit, K. W. (2014). *A study of active shooter incidents in the United States between 2000 and 2013*. Washington, DC: Texas State University and Federal Bureau of Investigation. Retrieved September 24, 2014, from http://www.fbi.gov/news/stories/2014/september/fbi-releases-study-on-active-shooter-incidents/pdfs/a-study-of-active-shooter-incidents-in-the-u.s.-between-2000-and-2013?utm_campaign=email-Immediate&utm_content=359251.
12. Lin, P.-I., Fei, L., Barzman, D., & Hossain, M. (2018). What have we learned from the time trend of mass shootings in the U.S.? *PLOS One, 13*(10), e0204722.

13. Fein, R. A., & Vossekuil, B. (1999). Assassination in the United States: An operational study of recent assassins, attackers, and near-lethal approaches. *Journal of Forensic Sciences, 44*(2), 321–333.

14. Borum, R., Fein, R., Vossekuil, B., & Berglund, J. (1999). Threat assessment: Defining an approach to assessing risk for targeted violence. *Behavioral Sciences & the Law, 17*(3), 323.

15. Calhoun, F. S., & Weston, S. W. (2003). *Contemporary threat management: A practical guide for identifying, assessing, and managing individuals of violent intent. A practical guide series.* San Diego, CA: Specialized Training Services.

16. Poon, K.-T., & Wong, W.-Y. (2018). Stuck on the train of ruminative thoughts: The effect of aggressive fantasy on subjective well-being. *Journal of Interpersonal Violence.* doi:10.1177/0886260518812796.

17. Knoll, J. L. (2010). The "pseudocommando" mass murderer: Part I, The psychology of revenge and obliteration. *Journal of the American Academy of Psychiatry and the Law, 38*(1), 87–94.

18. Smith, C. E., Fischer, K. W., & Watson, M. W. (2009). Toward a refined view of aggressive fantasy as a risk factor for aggression: Interaction effects involving cognitive and situational variables. *Aggressive Behavior, 35*(4), 313–323.

19. Knoll, J. L. (2010). The "pseudocommando" mass murderer: Part II, The language of revenge. *Journal of the American Academy of Psychiatry and the Law, 38*(2), 263–272.

20. Lankford, A., & Madfis, E. (2018). Don't name them, don't show them, but report everything else: A pragmatic proposal for denying mass killers the attention they seek and deterring future offenders. *American Behavioral Scientist, 62*(2), 260–279.

21. Arluke, A., Lankford, A., & Madfis, E. (2018). Harming animals and massacring humans: Characteristics of public mass and active shooters who abused animals. *Behavioral Sciences & the Law, 36*, 739–751.

22. Prochaska, J. O., & Velicer, W. F. (1997). The transtheoretical model of health behavior change. *American Journal of Health Promotion, 12*(1), 38–48.

23. Knoll, J. L., & Annas, G. D. (2016). Mass shootings and mental illness. In Gold, L. H., & Simon, R. I. (Eds.), *Gun violence and mental illness* (1st ed., pp. 81–104). Arlington, VA: American Psychiatric Association Publishing.

24. Rozel, J. S., & Mulvey, E. P. (2017). The link between mental illness and gun violence: Implications for social policy. *Annual Review of Clinical Psychology, 13*(1), 445–469.

25. Huetteman, E., & Pérez-Peña, R. (2015, December 1). Paul Ryan pushes changes in mental health care after Colorado shooting. *The New York Times.* Retrieved December 2, 2015, from http://www.nytimes.com/2015/12/02/us/obama-repeats-call-for-stricter-gun-laws-after-colorado-shooting.html.

26. Trump, D. J. (2018). *So many signs that the Florida shooter was mentally disturbed, even expelled from school for bad and erratic behavior. Neighbors and classmates knew he was a big problem. Must always report such instances to authorities, again and again!.* @realDonaldTrump. Retrieved November 26, 2018, from https://twitter.com/realDonaldTrump/status/964110212885106689.

27. Kessler, R. C., Berglund, P., Demler, O., Jin, R., Merikangas, K. R., & Walters, E. E. (2005). Lifetime prevalence and age-of-onset distributions of DSM-IV disorders in the National Comorbidity Survey Replication. *Archives of General Psychiatry, 62*(6), 593–602.

28. Silver, J., Simons, A., & Craun, S. (2018, June). *A study of the pre-attack behaviors of active shooters in the United States between 2000 and 2013.* Washington, DC: Federal Bureau of Investigation, US Department of Justice. Retrieved from https://www.fbi.gov/file-repository/pre-attack-behaviors-of-active-shooters-in-us-2000-2013.pdf/view.

29. Stone, M. H. (2015). Mass murder, mental illness, and men. *Violence and Gender, 2*(1), 51–86.

30. *Analysis of recent mass shootings* (2015, August). Everytown for Gun Safety. Retrieved December 16, 2015, from http://everytownresearch.org/documents/2015/09/analysis-mass-shootings.pdf.

31. Vossekuil, B., Fein, R. A., Reddy, M., Borum, R., & Modzeleski, W. (2002). *The final report and findings of the Safe School Initiative: Implications for the prevention of school attacks in the United States* (p. 63). Washington, DC: U.S. Department of Education, Office of Elementary and Secondary Education, Safe and Drug-Free Schools Program and U.S. Secret Service, National Threat Assessment Center. Retrieved March 11, 2015, from https://www.secretservice.gov/data/protection/ntac/ssi_final_report.pdf.

32. Silver, J., Fisher, W., & Horgan, J. (2018). Public mass murderers and federal mental health background checks for firearm purchases. *Law & Policy, 40*(2), 133–147.

33. American Association for Emergency Psychiatry. (2018). *AAEP position statement: Evaluation of persons of concern in relation to violence, mass shootings and mental illness.* Retrieved November 26, 2018, from https://www.emergencypsychiatry.org/position-statements.

34. Swanson, J. W. (2011). Explaining rare acts of violence: The limits of evidence from population research. *Psychiatric Services, 62*(11), 1369–1371.

35. Steadman, H. J., Mulvey, E. P., Monahan, J., Robbins, P. C., Appelbaum, P. S., Grisso, T., et al. (1998). Violence by people discharged from acute psychiatric inpatient facilities and by others in the same neighborhoods. *Archives of General Psychiatry, 55*(5), 393–401.

36. Choe, J. Y., Teplin, L. A., & Abram, K. M. (2008). Perpetration of violence, violent victimization, and severe mental illness: Balancing public health concerns. *Psychiatric Services, 59*(2), 153–164.

37. Brazil, I. A. (2015). Considering new insights into antisociality and psychopathy. *The Lancet Psychiatry, 2*(2), 115–116.

38. Marcus, D. K., Preszler, J., & Zeigler-Hill, V. (2018). A network of dark personality traits: What lies at the heart of darkness? *Journal of Research in Personality, 73*, 56–62.

39. Cardinale, E. M., & Marsh, A. A. (2015). Impact of psychopathy on moral judgments about causing fear and physical harm. *PLOS One, 10*(5), e0125708.

40. Swanson, J. W., Van Dorn, R. A., Swartz, M. S., Smith, A., Elbogen, E. B., & Monahan, J. (2008). Alternative pathways to violence in persons with schizophrenia: The role of childhood antisocial behavior problems. *Law and Human Behavior, 32*(3), 228–240.

41. Skeem, J., Kennealy, P., Monahan, J., Peterson, J., & Appelbaum, P. (2016). Psychosis uncommonly and inconsistently precedes violence among high-risk individuals. *Clinical Psychological Science, 4*(1), 40–49.

42. Large, M. M., & Nielssen, O. (2011). Violence in first-episode psychosis: A systematic review and meta-analysis. *Schizophrenia Research, 125*(2–3), 209–220.

43. Knoll, J. L., & Meloy, J. R. (2014). Mass murder and the violent paranoid spectrum. *Psychiatric Annals, 44*(5), 236–243.

44. Im, D. S. (2016). Template to perpetrate: An update on violence in autism spectrum disorder. *Harvard Review of Psychiatry, 24*(1), 14–35.

45. Heeramun, R., Magnusson, C., Gumpert, C. H., Granath, S., Lundberg, M., Dalman, C., & Rai, D. (2017). Autism and convictions for violent crimes: Population-based cohort study in Sweden. *Journal of the American Academy of Child & Adolescent Psychiatry*, 56(6), 491–497.e2.

46. Allely, C. S., Minnis, H., Thompson, L., Wilson, P., & Gillberg, C. (2014). Neurodevelopmental and psychosocial risk factors in serial killers and mass murderers. *Aggression and Violent Behavior, 19*(3), 288–301.

47. Allely, C. S., Wilson, P., Minnis, H., Thompson, L., Yaksic, E., & Gillberg, C. (2017). Violence is rare in autism: When it does occur, is it sometimes extreme? *The Journal of Psychology, 151*(1), 49–68.

48. White, S. G., Meloy, J. R., Mohandie, K., & Kienlen, K. (2017). Autism spectrum disorder and violence: Threat assessment issues. *Journal of Threat Assessment and Management, 4*(3), 144–163.

49. Meloy, J. R., & O'Toole, M. E. (2011). The concept of leakage in threat assessment. *Behavioral Sciences & the Law, 29*(4), 513–527.

50. Silver, J., Horgan, J., & Gill, P. (2018). Foreshadowing targeted violence: Assessing leakage of intent by public mass murderers. *Aggression and Violent Behavior*, 38, 94–100.

51. Gill, P., Silver, J., Horgan, J., & Corner, E. (2017). Shooting alone: The pre-attack experiences and behaviors of U.S. solo mass murderers. *Journal of Forensic Sciences*, 62(3), 710–714.

52. McNiel, D. E., & Binder, R. L. (1989). Relationship between preadmission threats and later violent behavior by acute psychiatric inpatients. *Psychiatric Services, 40*(6), 605–608.

53. Tversky, A., & Kahneman, D. (1973). Availability: A heuristic for judging frequency and probability. *Cognitive Psychology, 5*(2), 207–232.

54. Ropeik, D. (2010). *How risky is it really? Why our fears don't always match the facts*. New York, NY: McGraw-Hill.

55. Kahneman, D. (2013). *Thinking, fast and slow*. New York, NY: Farrar, Straus and Giroux.

56. Schneier, B. *Living in code yellow*. Fusion. Retrieved September 24, 2015, from http://fusion.net/story/200747/living-in-code-yellow/.

57. Langman, P. (2018). Different types of role model influence and fame seeking among mass killers and copycat offenders. *American Behavioral Scientist, 62*(2), 210–228.

58. King, D. M., & Jacobson, S. H. (2017). Random acts of violence? Examining probabilistic independence of the temporal distribution of mass killing events in the United States. *Violence & Victims, 32*(6), 1014–1023.

59. Towers, S., Gomez-Lievano, A., Khan, M., Mubayi, A., & Castillo-Chavez, C. (2015). Contagion in mass killings and school shootings. *PLOS One, 10*(7), e0117259.

60. Victor, D. (2018, May 11). When white people call the police on black people. *The New York Times*, A19.

61. Abo-Zena, D. M. M. (2017). Exploring the interconnected trauma of personal, social, and structural stressors: Making "sense" of senseless violence. *The Journal of Psychology, 151*(1), 5–20.

62. Johnson, K. L., Desmarais, S. L., Grimm, K. J., Tueller, S. J., Swartz, M. S., & Van Dorn, R. A. (2016). Proximal risk factors for short-term community violence among adults with mental illnesses. *Psychiatric Services, 67*(7), 771–778.

63. Swartz, M. S., Swanson, J. W., Hiday, V. A., Borum, R., Wagner, H. R., & Burns, B. J. (1998). Violence and severe mental illness: The effects of substance abuse and nonadherence to medication. *American Journal of Psychiatry, 155*, 226–231.

64. Pickard, H., & Fazel, S. (2013). Substance abuse as a risk factor for violence in mental illness: Some implications for forensic psychiatric practice and clinical ethics. *Current Opinion in Psychiatry, 26*(4), 349–354.

65. Mulvey, E. P., Odgers, C., Skeem, J., Gardner, W., Schubert, C., & Lidz, C. (2006). Substance use and community violence: A test of the relation at the daily level. *Journal of Consulting and Clinical Psychology, 74*(4), 743–754.

66. McGinty, E. E., Choksy, S., & Wintemute, G. J. (2016). The relationship between controlled substances and violence. *Epidemiologic Reviews, 38*(1), 5–31.

67. Dodge, K. A. (2006). Translational science in action: Hostile attributional style and the development of aggressive behavior problems. *Development and Psychopathology, 18*(3), 791–814.

68. Castro, B. O. D., Veerman, J. W., Koops, W., Bosch, J. D., & Monshouwer, H. J. (2002). Hostile attribution of intent and aggressive behavior: A meta-analysis. *Child Development, 73*(3), 916–934.

69. Zimbardo, P. G. (2004). A situationist perspective on the psychology of evil: Understanding how good people are transformed into perpetrators. In Miller, A. (Ed.), *The social psychology of good and evil: Understand our capacity for kindness and cruelty* (pp. 21–50). New York, NY: Guilford Press.

70. Kaney, S., & Bentall, R. P. (1989). Persecutory delusions and attributional style. *British Journal of Medical Psychology, 62*(2), 191–198.

71. Hagan, C. R., Podlogar, M. C., & Joiner, T. E. (2015). Murder-suicide: Bridging the gap between mass murder, amok, and suicide. *Journal of Aggression, Conflict and Peace Research, 7*(3), 179.

72. Warren, L. J., Mullen, P. E., & Ogloff, J. R. P. (2011). A clinical study of those who utter threats to kill. *Behavioral Sciences & the Law, 29*(2), 141–154.

73. Behavioral Analysis Unit. (2016). *Making prevention a reality: Identifying, assessing, and managing the threat of targeted attacks*. Washington, DC: Federal Bureau of Investigation, US Department of Justice. Retrieved February 27, 2017, from https://www.fbi.gov/file-repository/making-prevention-a-reality.pdf.

74. Simons, A., & Meloy, J. R. (2017). Foundations of threat assessment and management. In Van Hasselt, V. B., & Bourke, M. L. (Eds.), *Handbook of behavioral criminology* (pp. 627–644). Cham: Springer International Publishing. Retrieved from http://drreidmeloy.com/wp-content/uploads/2017/12/2017_FoundationsOfThreat.pdf.

75. Hughes, A. M., Gregory, M. E., Joseph, D. L., Sonesh, S. C., Marlow, S. L., Lacerenza, C. N., et al. (2016). Saving lives: A meta-analysis of team training in healthcare. *Journal of Applied Psychology, 101*(9), 1266–1304.

76. Edmondson, A. C. (2012). Teamwork on the fly. *Harvard Business Review, 90*(4), 72–80.

77. Department of Health and Human Services. (2016). Health Insurance Portability and Accountability Act (HIPAA) privacy rule and the National Instant Criminal Background Check System (NICS) 45 CFR Part 164. *Federal Register, 81*(3), 382–396.

78. Rodriguez, L. (2013). *Message to our nation's health care providers*. Retrieved January 15, 2013, from https://www.hhs.gov/sites/default/files/ocr/office/lettertonationhcp.pdf.

79. Werth, J. L., Welfel, E. R., & Benjamin, G. A. H. (Eds.), (2009). *The duty to protect: Ethical, legal, and professional considerations for mental health professionals*. Washington, DC: American Psychological Association.

80. Widgery, A., & Winterfield, A. (2013). Mental health professionals' duty to warn. *National Council of State Legislatures Legisbrief, 21*(1), 2.

81. Castro, J. (2015). Piercing the privacy veil: Towards a saner balancing of privacy and health in cases of severe mental illness. *Hastings Law Journal, 66*, 1769.

82. Petrila, J., & Fader-Towe, H. (2010). *Information sharing in criminal justice - Mental health collaborations: Working with HIPAA and other privacy laws*. New York, NY: Council of State Governments Justice Center. Retrieved June 4, 2017, from https://www.bja.gov/Publications/CSG_CJMH_Info_Sharing.pdf.

83. Lankford, A. (2016). Public mass shooters and firearms: A cross-national study of 171 countries. *Violence and Victims, 31*(2), 187–199.

84. Schildkraut, J., & Elsass, H. J. (2016). *Mass shootings: Media, myths, and realities. Crime, media, and popular culture*. Santa Barbara, CA: Praeger.

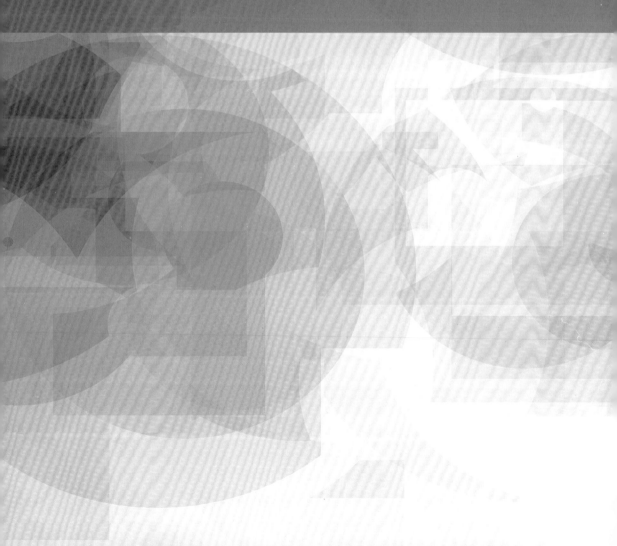

PART V

Special Populations

Section Editor: Victor Hong

34

The Psychiatric Emergency Care of Children and Adolescents

Bernard Biermann, Jennifer G. Votta

According to the Annual Report on Health Care for Children and Youth in the United States, emergency department (ED) visits for pediatric mental health conditions increased by 21% between 2006 and 2011, with a 34% increase in ED visits for substance use disorders and 71% increase in visits for impulse control disorders (1). More recent data presented at the American Academy of Pediatrics (2) showed an increase in the rates of mental health visits, from 50.4 to 78.5 per 100,000 children in 2012 and 2016, respectively. In the psychiatric emergency services (PESs) at the University of Michigan, while the number of total patient visits increased 29% from 5,003 in FY 2010 to 6,433 in FY 2018, the number of visits by patients aged 17 years and younger increased from 1,377 to 2,269 over the same period, an increase of 65% (3).

In one study, more than half of youth requiring ED care for mental health had not previously sought such care in other settings (4). Almost as many patients with psychiatric concerns (up to 45%) are repeat visitors to the ED (5). With wait times for outpatient child psychiatry appointments as long as 10 weeks (6), EDs often become the default location for patients to receive care. Owing to EMTALA requirements, the ED is essentially the only setting that mandates some level of evaluation and crisis stabilization.

Across the country, EDs at only 25% of academic medical centers and 8% of community hospitals have a child psychiatrist available to evaluate youths (7). Many PESs serve mainly adult patients. Such settings are not optimal as the environments might be overly stimulating and frightening to youth and families. EDs are often faced with "boarding" of patients awaiting admission or stabilization (up to 34% of patients in one study) (8). Patients with a diagnosis of autism, cognitive impairment or developmental delay, or a medical illness requiring intensive nursing care pose unique challenges. Emergency physicians and psychiatrists caring for youth in emergency settings face a daunting task.

MODELS OF CARE

Settings specifically designed with pediatric psychiatric patients in mind and with multidisciplinary staffing have shown reduced use of security and restraint and decreased length of stay (9). Such models, described by Mroczkowski et al (10), include designated, safely designed psychiatric space within the confines of a larger general pediatric ED or "flexible" ED space for both medical and psychiatric use. A more optimal setting, such as the specialized Children's Comprehensive Psychiatric Emergency Program at Bellevue hospital in New York, is staffed 24 hours a day, 7 days a week by psychiatrists and child psychiatric nurses and has a few brief (up to 72 hours) stabilization beds and an interim crisis clinic. Children's Hospital of Philadelphia has developed a clinical pathway for patients with autism spectrum disorder who present with agitation or aggression and has a 12-bed medical behavioral unit, costaffed by pediatrics and psychiatry.

In some communities, urgent care models have the potential for averting ED visits and admissions. Sunderji et al (11) highlight findings of urgent care clinics showing improvements in symptom severity and distress, subjective well-being, and satisfaction with care along with decreased wait times for post ED ambulatory care. Alternatively, mobile crisis teams attempt to bring trained staff to homes and into the community to decrease utilization of hospital emergency services and more rapidly deliver care.

In various remote areas, telepsychiatry has emerged as a viable, cost-effective mechanism for delivering care. Studies indicate that it is generally acceptable to patients and families that patient outcomes are similar to face-to-face interactions (12-14). The use of telepsychiatry requires equipment with secure connections, replication of face-to-face interviews, and a team who are able to access services in cases where transfer for admission is needed.

GENERAL CONSIDERATIONS IN THE ASSESSMENT OF CHILDREN AND ADOLESCENTS

Medical Evaluation

An important part of the psychiatric emergency assessment is evaluating for an underlying medical etiology. The approach to medical clearance varies by institution, as there are no specific standards for routine screening (15,16). General guidelines suggest pursuing focused medical workup based on the history and physical examination (17,18). Many pediatric psychiatric hospitals require medical clearance through a set of routine laboratory work, commonly including toxicology screening, complete blood count, comprehensive metabolic panel (including BUN and liver function tests), thyroid function tests, pregnancy test, and electrocardiogram (19-21). Additional testing should be guided by the history and physical examination, such as pursuing head imaging for a patient with recent head trauma.

A physical examination and comprehensive review of systems are important for all pediatric patients, as there are many medical illnesses that can cause or worsen psychiatric symptoms (22). Suspicion for an underlying medical etiology should rise in the setting of acute onset of new symptoms, sudden change in behavior, age under 12 years, vital sign abnormalities, abnormalities on physical or neurological examination, impaired attention or memory, nonauditory hallucinations (visual, tactile, olfactory), disorientation, fluctuating mental status, evidence of trauma or head injury, recent change in medications, or the presence of seizures (18-20). One of the most common medical illnesses masquerading as an acute psychiatric disorder is delirium (20,23). A more comprehensive medical workup is warranted if there is any concern for delirium, as there is a marked increase in mortality if the underlying cause of delirium goes untreated (18,24). Other medical issues that can present with psychiatric symptoms are detailed in Table 34.1, though this is not a comprehensive list.

Clinicians should also include a detailed medication history as part of the assessment. Inquiring about recent changes in medication, both prescribed and over-the-counter, is of high importance, as there are many medication side effects that need to be taken into consideration. Recently starting an antidepressant can result in activation syndrome, or abruptly stopping an antidepressant could result in discontinuation syndrome, both of which can present with symptoms of irritability, aggression, altered mood, and/or psychotic symptoms (25-27). Though rare, initiation of an antidepressant in someone under the age of 25 years has been associated with spontaneous reporting of suicidal thoughts (28). The two most acute medical issues associated with psychotropic medications are neuroleptic malignant syndrome (NMS) and serotonin syndrome. NMS is potentially lethal and presents as altered mental status, autonomic instability, hyperthermia, and rigidity. Treatment includes removal of the causative medication and supportive measures, sometimes with administration of dantrolene, bromocriptine, or amantadine. Serotonin syndrome involves rapid onset of altered mental status, autonomic instability, myoclonus, and hyperreflexia, with the latter two symptoms considered highly diagnostic. Discontinuation of the precipitating agent and supportive measures are the main treatment, though sometimes cyproheptadine may be used (8,29). Keeping these syndromes in mind is especially important when assessing an adolescent with a history of depression who presents with agitation and mental status change, as the precipitating event may have been a suicide attempt by overdose.

TABLE 34.1 Psychiatric Presentations of Medical Illnesses

Psychiatric Presentation	Possible Medical Causes
Depression/suicidality	Hypothyroidism, anemia, hypoglycemia, mononucleosis, lithium toxicity, substance abuse, systemic lupus erythematous, chronic fatigue syndrome
Aggression/agitation	CNS infections (meningitis, encephalitis), intracranial bleeding, thyroid storm, Wilson's disease, lead poisoning
Psychosis	Delirium, CNS infection or lesion (meningitis, encephalitis, bleeding, tumor), sepsis, seizures, diabetic ketoacidosis, drug toxicity, pheochromocytoma, porphyria, steroid use, lipid storage disorders, velocardiofacial syndrome
Mania	Hyperthyroidism, toxic encephalopathy, temporal lobe epilepsy, Kluver-Bucy syndrome, Kleine-Levin syndrome
Anxiety	Akathisia, hyperthyroidism, hypoglycemia, cardiac arrhythmia (Wolff-Parkinson-White), caffeine consumption
Tics/obsessions/compulsions	Streptococcal (group A beta-hemolytic) throat infection, dystonia, postviral encephalitis, carbon monoxide poisoning

CNS, central nervous system.
Adapted from Rocker, J. A., & Oestreicher, J. (2018). Focused medical assessment of pediatric behavioral emergencies. *Child and Adolescent Psychiatric Clinics of North America, 27*(3), 399–411; Guerrero, A. P. (2003). General medical considerations in child and adolescent patients who present with psychiatric symptoms. *Child and Adolescent Psychiatric Clinics of North America, 12*, 613–628; and Tucci, V., Siever, K., Matorin, A., & Moukaddam, N. (2015). Down the rabbit hole: Emergency department medical clearance of patients with psychiatric or behavioral emergencies. *Emergency Medicine Clinics of North America, 33*(4), 721–737.

Role of Collateral Contacts

Collateral information is generally paramount in the evaluation of a child or adolescent and is recommended by the AACAP practice parameters (30). Both parents should be interviewed, as each may be able to offer a different perspective, especially if they are living apart. Obtaining information from the school can offer additional insights into the onset and progression of symptoms, as well as any psychosocial stressors (eg, bullying on social media). Other important sources of information can include outpatient providers, juvenile justice personnel, or clinicians (eg, court-run drug treatment program). For foster children, there are numerous people (eg, case worker, current or previous foster parent(s), biological parent(s) or sibling(s), other relatives) who can assist in the overall understanding of the child/adolescent. Appropriate consents should always be obtained when necessary.

Screening Instruments

Several instruments, requiring minimal training or commitment, are available. (31) At least three such tools have been described in the literature and have been tested for reliability and validity. The Ask Suicide-Screening Questionnaire (ASQ) has been shown to be highly sensitive with 98% accuracy for screening for and ruling out risk of suicide (32). The Columbia-Suicide Severity Rating Scale has shown predictive validity with adolescent psychiatric emergency patients (33). The HEADS—ED, (25,63) which has gained widespread use in Canada as part of clinical protocol, is designed to assist with disposition and determination of level of care (1).

Approach to the Interview

There are a few important elements to take into consideration in the assessment of a pediatric patient. First is recognizing that children are not "little adults." A primary objective in an emergency evaluation is determining whether a true emergency, where there is imminent risk of harm either to the patient or to others, is present and warrants acute inpatient psychiatric hospitalization (34). Making this determination often requires taking into consideration social and environmental factors that may not be considered when assessing an adult. Second, psychiatric illness frequently does not present in a traditional manner in a child or adolescent because of their developmental status, especially if a developmental disorder or cognitive impairment is present (30). Therefore, the interview of a child or adolescent needs to be handled in a more comprehensive manner, rather than the problem-focused nature in which adult psychiatric patients are evaluated in an emergency setting. Third is remembering that a child is part of several systems (eg, family, school) and therefore a system-based approach, as opposed to individual, is necessary. Therefore, collateral information is extremely important and is discussed in more detail in a separate section in this chapter. A suggested outline for specific areas to focus on in the interview can be found in Table 34.2.

There often will be multiple people to interview. For children under the age of 12 years, a good general rule of thumb is to interview the parents first separately from the child (34). Sometimes the parents will not be able to provide full details, especially if the inciting incident occurred in a different setting such as school. In those instances, the clinician should consider reaching out to the school next, saving the interview with the child for last. For an adolescent over the age of 12 years, the recommendation is to interview them first, as this can help give them a sense of agency and make them feel like they are being listened to and taken seriously. With a child under the age of 12 years, start the interview with the parent in the room, but for an adolescent over the age of 12 years, minimal time should be spent interviewing them with a parent present, as this may lead to them minimizing symptoms, self-harm, substance use, and sexual activity (34).

Taking into consideration a patient's developmental level is extremely important for effectively interviewing a child or adolescent. The type of language used, as well as certain nonverbal communication cues, can have a major impact on how much or how little a child/adolescent will engage. For example, when asking about substance use or progression of symptoms, a better clinical picture is built by using more direct language ("how many days a week do you smoke") as opposed to more open language ("how often do you smoke"). In a situation where the patient is being extremely uncooperative, suggested techniques include being fully transparent about the process and potential outcomes as well as joining with the patient to encourage their involvement in their treatment (eg, "I understand how difficult your current situation is to be in. Let's work together to figure out how we can make things better for you.") (34).

Of note, the clinician should be mindful of the language used over the course of the evaluation and when discussing diagnosis or treatment/disposition with both the patient and the parents, as negative or punitive words can have a long-lasting effect on how the parent views the child or how the child views themselves (35).

Working With Families

In the ED, working with a child or adolescent's caregivers is a critical part of the evaluation and treatment plan as ultimately the decision for how to proceed with treatment rests with the patient's parent/guardian. Given that children are part of family systems, brief family assessments are especially important for guiding disposition and safety planning, especially if the decision is made to discharge the patient home. At times, a child or adolescent will present to the ED in the midst of an interpersonal crisis or conflict with their parents, which may necessitate an initial period of separation to help facilitate information gathering. Once reunited, members of the treatment team can model appropriate interactions with the child, especially in regards to communication and limit setting. Additionally, ED staff, can provide reassurance, psychoeducation, and guidance for parents, who are often frightened and feel unsure about their ability to adequately ensure their child's safety. If the decision is made to discharge the patient home, parents should be actively involved in safety planning, including supervision, suicide means restriction, and knowing when to return to the ED, contact emergency

TABLE 34.2 Components of a Child/Adolescent Psychiatric Assessment in the Emergency Setting

Chief complaint	What prompted presentation right now, who is labeling this an emergency (eg, parents, school), does the child/adolescent know why they are here
Identification	Demographics (eg, age, sex, gender identity), grade level and school status (truancy or attendance issues), previous diagnoses
History of present illness	Specific symptoms, onset and progression of symptoms, impact of symptoms on patient and family, current stressors
Psychiatric history	Current or previous treatment, specific type of treatment (psychotherapy, medication, day program), effectiveness of treatment, history of suicidal ideation/suicide attempts/self-injury, past hospitalizations/ED visits, history of trauma (physical, sexual, emotional or witnessed)
Medical history	Chronic medical or neurological issues, recent illness, history of seizures or head trauma, current or recent medications
Developmental history	Intrauterine complications or exposure to drugs/alcohol, weeks gestation at time of delivery, postnatal complications, temperament as infant/toddler, any delays in milestones (motor, cognitive, speech/language)
Family history	Family history of mental illness, suicide attempts or completions, treatment used in other family members
Social history	Living arrangement, relationship with family members, peer relationships, social media usage, hobbies, sexual activity, risk-taking behavior, level of supervision at home
Educational history	Current grade level, type of classes (regular or special education), any accommodations (IEP), current/recent/past academic performance, any changes in academic performance, issues with school avoidance
Substance use	What substances, age of first use, pattern of use/changes in frequency, use alone or with friends
Legal history	Involvement of social services (CPS), current case worker or probation officer; if parents are divorced who has legal custody, or if parental rights have been terminated who is designated legal guardian

CPS, Child Protective Services; IEP, Individualized Education Program.

personnel, or their child's therapist or physician. Sometimes this will be a family's first interaction with a mental health professional, thus presenting an opportunity to provide parents with psychoeducation as well as resources for families (eg, NAMI, Al Anon, Autism Alliance, CHADD). For more information on working with families, see Chapter 17.

Trauma-Informed Care

The importance and implementation of trauma-informed care are rapidly growing, as there is increased recognition about the prevalence of trauma in childhood, symptoms of which may mimic other psychiatric disorders such as attention-deficit/hyperactivity disorder (ADHD), bipolar disorder, or psychosis. Approximately 60% of children experienced a traumatic event within the past year (36) and two-thirds of the population experienced one or more traumatic events in childhood (37). Children in the foster care system are three times more likely to suffer physical abuse and two to three times more likely to be the victim of sexual abuse (35). Furthermore, the experience of being in an emergency department can be traumatic for children and adolescents (38).

A child or adolescent with a trauma history may be triggered by witnessing a violent patient or having someone touch them for a physical examination. Even for a child/adolescent without an overt trauma history, the process of being evaluated and admitted to a psychiatric hospital can be a traumatic experience for both the patient and the family.

Trauma-informed care is a model in which healthcare professionals take an approach to all patients, akin to other universal precautions, that aims to prevent or minimize emotional trauma. Past trauma is not always disclosed right away and all patients are at risk of experiencing emotional trauma during the course of acute medical or psychiatric treatment (35,39). The underlying components of trauma-informed care are outlined in Table 34.3. Clinicians taking a trauma-informed approach has a strong understanding of how trauma can be experienced in the medical setting and how symptoms of both prior or current trauma can manifest, thus guiding care and treatment. Goals include reducing the negative impact of potentially traumatic events in the medical setting and recognizing and addressing signs/symptoms of both preexisting trauma reactions and newly manifesting trauma reactions from medical care (39-41).

The Center for Pediatric Traumatic Stress created HealthCareToolBox.org, which is a website where healthcare professionals as well as patients and families can find numerous resources for learning about and coping with trauma in the medical setting (42).

Disposition

One of the main goals of emergency assessment and planning is determining an appropriate disposition based upon safety, risk of further decompensation, and environment of care. In general, patients who continue to endorse a desire to die, remain agitated or hopeless, cannot meaningfully engage in safety planning, do not have an adequate support system, or who cannot be adequately monitored or receive follow up are in need of admission. Highly lethal suicide attempts with clear expectation of death generally warrant hospital admission. Other factors include impulsivity, substance abuse, and significant anger (8). Patients with a first episode of psychosis or with active symptoms of psychosis should also likely be admitted (43). The symptoms and diagnoses that typically warrant inpatient psychiatric admission are outlined in Table 34.4.

Once a pediatric patient has undergone a complete psychiatric evaluation in the emergency department, disposition planning can begin. The first step is determining whether or not acute psychiatric treatment is needed. It is important to note that insurance parameters and limitations in bed availability may result in delayed admission and the child/adolescent having to "board" in the ED, where direct treatment options are limited. In these situations, clinicians are encouraged to consider whether there are any possible interventions to reduce delay in treatment (eg, starting an antipsychotic for an acutely manic patient). There are instances where a pediatric patient will

---

TABLE 34.3 Approach to Trauma-Informed Care

- Understanding the prevalence and impact of trauma
- Recognizing how patients and families may experience and be affected by trauma
- Incorporating knowledge about trauma into the provision of medical care
  - Strong rapport building
  - Transparency about evaluation and treatment decisions
  - Careful approach to assessing for a history of trauma
- Preventing new trauma or retraumatization

Adapted from Marsac, M. L., Kassam-Adams, N., Hildenbrand, A. K., Nicholls, E., Winston, F. K., Leff, S. S., & Fein, J. (2016). Implementing a trauma-informed approach in pediatric health care networks. *JAMA Pediatrics, 170*(1), 70–77 and Heppell, P. J., & Rao, S. (2018). Social services and behavioral emergencies: Trauma-informed evaluation, diagnosis, and disposition. *Child and Adolescent Psychiatric Clinics of North America, 27*(3), 455–465.

TABLE 34.4 Presenting Concerns That Warrant Inpatient Psychiatric Hospitalization

- Suicide attempt (after medical clearance)
- Active suicidal ideation with plan, intent, and/or means
- Agitation/aggression that cannot be stabilized and is not due to a medical issue
- Danger to others due to homicidal thoughts or violent outbursts
- Psychotic symptoms without clear medical cause
- Manic symptoms without clear medical cause
- Catatonia
- Evidence of imminent suicide risk despite denial of suicidal ideation
  - Feeling hopeless, trapped, or without a sense of purpose
  - Giving away possessions
  - Dramatic mood changes
  - Reckless behavior or uncontrolled rage
  - Withdrawal from family and friends

be admitted to a general medical service with the psychiatry consultation/liaison service advising treatment, though this clinical scenario is far from ideal and should only be pursued if there are no options available for inpatient psychiatric hospitalization.

For patients who do not require acute inpatient admission, disposition planning is more extensive as there are more variables to consider such as level of care for follow-up. Outpatient options range from lower intensity treatment (eg, referral to outpatient mental health services) to higher intensity treatment (eg, partial hospitalization or day treatment programs). Other potential disposition plans include substance abuse rehabilitation, referral for specific counseling (eg, substance abuse, disordered eating), respite care or emergency foster care placement, or returning to follow-up with existing services.

Safety Planning

Another important aspect of disposition planning with a patient who is not being hospitalized is developing a safety plan to be followed upon leaving the emergency department. Although studies have shown that having a patient sign a no-suicide contract does not reduce or prevent suicide (AACAP parameters), discussing ways to improve safety at home is still valuable. The components of a safety plan are outlined in Table 34.5. For children and adolescents, arguably one of the most important aspects of safety planning is

means restriction. Many suicide attempts in children/adolescents occur impulsively (44) and with underestimated lethality (45), so reducing access to lethal means and creating barriers to quick actions are important steps in keeping the child or adolescent safe.

Child-Specific Areas of Assessment

In a review by case (46), common psychiatric diagnoses among youth seen for emergency mental health visits included depression, 23.9%; anxiety, 21.6%; disruptive behavior and ADHD, 19.8%; substance use, 14.4%; psychosis, 7.2%; bipolar disorder, 4.4%; adjustment disorder, 3.5%; and other psychiatric diagnoses, 5.0%. Content areas for evaluation of children in the psychiatric emergency setting must be tailored to the developmental age of the child or adolescent. The mental status examination must be conducted using concrete, developmentally appropriate questions. For example, when questioning a 5-year-old about having attempted to kill himself by holding his breath, suicidal intent might be ascertained by asking, "Did you think you would die if you held your breath?" Future orientation might be determined by asking, "If you had died, would you still be able to celebrate Christmas next week?" Likewise, a teen might well be able to answer questions related to day, month, and year in relationship to orientation, but it would be more developmentally appropriate to ask a younger child whether it is morning or night.

TABLE 34.5 Components of a Safety Plan

- Identify early warning signs and any triggers that may induce suicidal thoughts
- Develop coping skills to use in the face of suicidal thoughts
  - CBT skills (eg, distraction, play the tape through)
  - DBT skills (eg, mindfulness, distress tolerance)
- Outline which adults the child/adolescent can go to for support
- Provide clear instructions for when to return to the emergency department
- Means restriction
  - Remove firearms and other violent weapons from the home
  - Lock up medications and household chemicals

CBT, cognitive behavioral therapy; DBT,dialectical behavior therapy.
Reproduced with permission from Chun, T. H., Mace, S. E., & Katz, E. R. (2016). Evaluation and management of children and adolescents with acute mental health or behavioral problems. Part I: Common clinical challenges of patients with mental health and/or behavioral emergencies. *Pediatrics, 138*(3), e20161570. Copyright © 2016 by the AAP.

CLINICAL ISSUES IN PRESENTATION

Suicide and Self-Injury

Suicide remains one of the top causes of death among youth in the United States. According to the Centers for Disease Control in 2016 (47), suicide was the second leading cause of death in both the 10 to 14 years and 15 to 24 years age groups. Suicide in prepubescent children is much rarer, mostly occurring in males with disorders of impulse control, such as ADHD, rather than depression. In the 10- to 14-year-old age group, suffocation and hanging are the most common methods of suicide (56.7%), followed by firearms (36.7%). The use of firearms is the most common method of suicide (46.9%) in the 15- to 24-year-old age group, followed by suffocation and hanging (36.7%). The Youth Risk Behavior Survey, conducted by the Centers for Disease Control and Prevention (CDC), indicated that 17.2% of high school students had "seriously considered attempting suicide" in the previous 12 months. 13.6% made a specific plan to attempt suicide, 7.4% reported a suicide attempt, and 2.4% made a serious suicide attempt that required medical attention (48).

In addition to suicide, the rates of nonfatal self-inflicted self-injury requiring medical attention are highest among youth age 10 to 24 years, with adolescents aged 15 to 19 years having the highest rates. Trends in self-inflicted self-injury show a marked increase among females between 2008 and 2015, particularly in females between ages 10 and 14 years. Self-inflicted injury is one of the strongest risk factors for completed suicide (49).

Adolescent psychiatric disorder, history of previous attempts, impulsivity, a family history of suicide and psychopathology, stressful life events, substance abuse, and access to firearms have been identified as risk factors for suicide. Youth who identify as lesbian, gay, bisexual, or transsexual, are also at significantly heightened risk, with feelings of social isolation being a significant factor. Recent data demonstrated that initial suicide attempts in youth are often more likely to lead to serious injury or death. In a study by McKean et al (50), lethality rates for initial attempts in male youth were 6.2%, compared to 2.9% for subsequent attempts. For females, deaths occurred in 0.7% for initial attempts versus 0.4% for survivors of an initial attempt. This highlights the importance of initial screens, careful suicide assessment, and focus on prevention, including means restriction, particularly of firearms in youth. According to one study, a large percentage of suicide attempts are impulsive: 24% occurring within 5 minutes of making the decision, 24% between 5 and 19 minutes, 20% between 20 minutes and 1 hour. For at-risk youth, this highlights the importance of safety planning (8).

When asking about suicide, it is important to ask directly about ideation, suicide plans, intent to act, and the patients' understanding about lethality. Patient's may over- or underestimate the degree of lethality of a given method. In the face of a suicide attempt, patients should be asked about events leading up to the attempt: was it planned or impulsive, did they do anything to avoid discovery, and what was their expectation of the outcome? Patients may deny that their behavior constituted a suicide attempt or may minimize the severity of their behavior. Caregivers should thus be consulted, both individually and in the presence of the patient.

Jacobsen et al. (51) stated that assessing the suicidal intent of prepubertal children requires understanding the child's comprehension of the potential lethality of a given suicidal act, the actual medical lethality of the act, and the child's motives. The cognitive level and emotional state at the time of the interview are key to determining risk. For example, although a 5-year-old child may lack the knowledge of what may hurt them, there still may be intent to die. Psychiatrists must also assess parental recognition of the child's suicidal ideation or behavior (51).

Aggression

Children and adolescents who present for psychiatric evaluation may display aggressive behavior, either as the reason for presentation or during the course of evaluation. A review by Gerson and Malas (52) noted that 1 in 15 youth presenting for psychiatric complaints were restrained, and that the numbers were even higher for individuals with autism. Causes are multifactorial. Aggression can be a manifestation of psychiatric disorders including externalizing and internalizing disorders: ADHD, oppositional defiant disorder (ODD), conduct disorder. Aggression can also be linked to medical illness, such as delirium or intoxication, pain or discomfort, and is more common in patients with limited verbal skills, such as patients with developmental disabilities including autism. Some guiding principles for working with agitated patients: 1) Maximize safety of the patient and staff, 2) Assist the patient in managing emotions and regaining control of behavior, 3) Use least restrictive, age appropriate methods of restraint, and 4) Minimize coercive interventions (8).

Managing aggression is one of the most challenging aspects of child and adolescent emergency psychiatric care. Most guidelines suggest a stepwise management approach involving providing a safe environment, using verbal or behavioral techniques, considering pharmacologic options,

and reserving restraint or seclusion for situations where other modalities have been utilized, aggression persists, and the situation does not allow other alternatives because of threats to safety of the patient or others.

Environmental strategies include minimizing stimuli such as bright lighting and loud noises, providing adequate space for patients to walk or move about, removing dangerous objects such as medical equipment, and providing distractions and nondangerous items for self-soothing. Offering food and drink and honoring reasonable requests can be helpful. In terms of communication, speaking in a calm voice, introducing oneself, reassuring patients that they are safe, giving simple and clear directives, providing choices, reflecting emotions with thoughtful hypotheses, and utilizing empathic listening can all help patients maintain emotional control. Other interventions such as involving child life programs, coping kits, and quiet activities can serve as healthy distractions.

Medications that have been used for aggressive behaviors are outlined in Table 34.6. Although widely used, the evidence base to support demonstrated efficacy of pharmacologic agents is limited, particularly when such medications are used on a PRN basis (53). Ideally, pharmacologic management of aggression should target underlying causes, when possible, rather than simply providing sedation. Examples include stimulants or alpha agonists for ADHD or significant impulsivity, neuroleptic medications for psychosis or delirium, and benzodiazepines for severe anxiety or panic or in the case of agitated catatonia. Also, an increased or extra dose of a home medication with known tolerance can be considered. It is important to consider routes of administration (PO vs IM) as it pertains to rapidity of onset and whether patients are cooperative with medication administration. As with any medication, it is important to monitor for side effects and tolerability, including extrapyramidal side effect (EPS), dystonic reactions, sedation, or QT prolongation. Certain combinations are contraindicated, as in the case of parenteral coadministration of olanzapine and benzodiazepine.

In individuals with autism, benzodiazepines or antihistamines can exacerbate symptoms and should be used with caution. Parents can often provide useful guidance regarding what medications have

TABLE 34.6 Medications for Managing Agitation/Aggression or Hyperactivity in Children/Adolescents

Medication	Dosing	Onset of Action	Indications	Potential Side Effects
Benzodiazepines Lorazepam	0.5-2 mg po or IM	20-30 min	Acute anxiety Agitation Withdrawal Catatonia	Sedation disinhibition
Alpha-2 agonist Clonidine	0.05-0.1 mg po	30 min-1 h	Impulsivity Hyperactivity Anxiety	Hypotension Orthostasis Sedation
Antihistamines Diphenhydramine	12.5-50 mg po or IM	30 min-1 h	Agitation Acute anxiety	Sedation Paradoxical worsening
Hydroxyzine	12.5-50 mg po	30 min-1 h	Agitation Anxiety	
Antipsychotics Haloperidol	0.5-5 mg PO or IM	30 min oral 5 min IM	Acute psychosis Mania Agitation Aggression Delirium	Sedation EPS Dystonia QT prolongation
Olanzapine (do not coadminister IM with IV/IM lorazepam!)	2.5-10 mg po (Zydis) or IM	15-45 min	Acute psychosis Mania Agitation Aggression Delirium	Sedation Orthostasis
Ziprasidone	5-20 mg IM	15 min	Aggression Severe agitation	Sedation Orthostasis QT prolongation
Methylphenidate	2.5-10 mg po	30 min	Hyperactivity associated with ADHD	Mood lability Appetite suppression Tachycardia

ADHD, attention-deficit/hyperactivity disorder; EPS, extrapyramidal side effect.

been effective in the past. Other considerations for managing agitation in patients with autism include decreasing stimulation and, if possible, giving them a place to retreat and isolate. Verbal techniques such as reassurances, providing explanations, or coaxing are less likely to be effective. Also, careful consideration of medical issues including constipation, seizures, and pain such as an undetected injury, an ear infection, or dental pain is important.

Seclusion or restraint is generally considered a last resort, to be used when immediate safety (imminent threat or aggressive acting out) is at stake and other approaches have failed to curtail aggressive behaviors. When utilizing restraints, staff must follow standard procedures, comply with laws, require an order and physician assessment. Guidelines for applying restraints include having at least five staff, using sturdy materials, such as leather, attach restraints to the bedframe, use at least one female staff for female patients and elevate the head of the bed. Restraint or seclusion should be discontinued as soon as it is safe to do so. When removing restraints, the technique of removing one limb at a time is generally the recommended practice.

Psychosis

Psychosis constitutes a disorder of thinking (delusions or disorganized thought patterns) or perceptual disturbance (hallucinations), along with impairment in reality testing. Youth with true psychosis often present with a change in social or cognitive functioning, including withdrawal, declining school performance, decreased self-care such as hygiene, or bizarre behaviors. Psychotic youth might appear unusually suspicious, guarded, irritable, or hostile. Given limited insight, patients are likely to be brought in by others and may be fearful, apprehensive, or mistrusting of caregivers (54).

A workup for psychotic symptoms should be completed to rule out an underlying primary medical illness or substance intoxication, withdrawal, or overdose. Semper and McClellan (55) state that the "goal of the psychiatric assessment is to determine whether the child is actually psychotic and if so, to identify the most likely cause that is producing the clinical picture." Assessment involves a complete history and physical examination, with laboratory testing guided by the history and physical. The ED is a common entry point for patients with psychotic symptoms, with as many as one-half incidents of schizophrenia initially presenting to the ED (43). One study in Ontario, Canada, showed that between 2010 and 2013, 4,628 young people aged 16 to 24 years presented with a psychotic disorder for the first time with 72% being admitted. Of those not admitted, nearly one-half received no outpatient aftercare within 30 days and 1 in 10 had not received care within a year. Clear recommendations for timely referral to specialty mental health care have been published (43).

Semper and McClellan (55) note the complexity inherent in diagnosing pediatric psychosis. Noting that the presenting symptoms of pediatric psychosis "vary depending on the acuity and the specific nature of the disorder and other relevant features of the clinical picture including age, developmental level, and confounding comorbid psychiatric and nonpsychiatric conditions." Psychosis in children or adolescents may occur as the result of a primary psychotic illness, including schizophrenia, schizoaffective disorder, bipolar disorder, or psychotic depression. Psychosis may also occur as the result of normal, developmentally appropriate phenomena such as the presence of imaginary friends. Disorganized behaviors such as those seen in trauma, abuse, disruptive behavior disorders, and developmental delays may also be a factor.

The challenge inherent in determining whether a child is psychotic during a PES evaluation can be illustrated by looking at hallucinations as a diagnostic symptom. Edelsohn (56) describes considerations for assessing hallucinations in children and adolescents in the emergency setting. She notes that hallucinations in children can be part of normal development or be associated with nonpsychotic psychopathology, psychosocial adversity, or a physical illness. These nonpsychotic hallucinations may be differentiated from psychotic hallucinations by the absence of delusional beliefs, disturbed language production, decreased motor activity, signs of incongruous mood, bizarre behavior, and social withdrawal. The content of the hallucinations may be relevant in understanding the underlying psychopathology and issues in the child's development. Edelsohn advocates careful consideration of diagnostic labeling of psychosis based on hallucinations alone because the diagnosis tends to influence future evaluation and decision-making.

Substance Use and Intoxication

Issues related to substance use are one of the top reasons for pediatric visits to the ED for psychiatric reasons and often a factor in necessitating hospitalization. According to a national survey, among teens who presented to ED for psychiatric care between 2001 and 2010, over 10% had a diagnosis of drug abuse (57). Common substances of abuse include those most easily obtained and available: alcohol, nicotine, cannabis, inhalants, sedative hypnotics, hallucinogens, stimulants, cocaine, and opioids (58).

According to the 2018 Monitoring the Future annual survey of 8th, 10th, and 12th graders, substance use among teens remains common (59). The most recent trends show a surge in rates of "vaping" among adolescents with 21% of 12th graders reporting having done so within the previous 30 days. Although steadily declining over the previous 5 years, 8.2% of 8th graders, 18.6% of

10th graders, and 30.2% of 12th graders reported alcohol use in the previous 30 days, with 14% of 12th graders reporting at least one binge episode (five or more drinks in one sitting) within the previous 2 weeks. According to a review by Wang et al (58), early onset of substance use is associated with risks such as dependence, use of other substances, school failure, high-risk sexual behaviors, and psychiatric comorbidity. Additionally, poisonings and overdoses are a leading cause of death in adolescent populations. Data from 2015 revealed a death rate from overdose deaths in youth aged 15 to 19 years as 3.7 per 100,000, an increase from 1.6 per 100,000 in 1999 (58).

The ED offers an opportunity to screen for, evaluate, and recommend treatment for substance use disorders and associated problems related to substance use among youth. Useful screening tools are available to help identify and stratify the risks of substance use. Examples include the Alcohol Use Disorders Identification Test (AUDIT) and the "Car, Relax, Alone, Forgotten, Family/friend, Trouble" (CRAFFT) screen. These instruments question teens about risk factors including age at first use, patterns of use along with impacts, and consequences of use. The American Academy of Pediatrics recommends the Screening for Substance Use, Brief Intervention, and or Referral to Treatment (SBIRT) guidelines, which were developed by the US Substance Abuse and Mental Health Services Administration, and has been shown to be associated with reduced alcohol consumption, below risky drinking guidelines, in some youth between ages 14 and 20 years (60).

PES clinicians should also be aware of common substances of abuse and be familiar with the signs and symptoms of acute intoxication and be prepared to treat medically dangerous intoxication. Solhkhah (60) indicates that "awareness of the most likely presentations of an intoxicated child or adolescent is crucial in developing an appropriate differential diagnosis and forming an integrated and complete treatment plan." He further recommends that substance use should be considered in almost every case that presents to the ED for evaluation of psychiatric symptoms, noting that acute states of confusion or agitation have a high likelihood of being substance induced. Once identified, clinicians should be familiar with basic brief interventions, including

psychoeducation, brief motivational interviewing (64), and community resources for referral to treatment programs as well as availability of 12 step groups, such as Alcoholics Anonymous and Narcotics Anonymous.

Other Risk-Taking Behaviors

Even in the absence of psychiatric illness, children and adolescents are at risk of engaging in potentially dangerous behaviors. An awareness of these various risk factors can guide assessment and provide an opportunity for brief education for youth and families. According to the CDC, examples include behaviors that contribute to unintentional injuries and violence, sexual behaviors which result in unwanted pregnancy or STDs, drug alcohol and tobacco use, unhealthy dietary behaviors, and inadequate physical activity. Some specific areas of investigation include wearing helmets and seatbelts, riding in cars with peers who have been drinking, texting while driving, school truancy, inappropriate use of internet or social media such as sexting or risky online dating, carrying weapons, dating violence, bullying, gang involvement, use of condoms and birth control, running away, or the importance of curfews. Approaching these topics in a calm, nonjudgmental, matter-of-fact manner can encourage dialogue and adult guidance with youth who might not bring up these issues on their own.

LEGAL ISSUES

Consent to Treat

Consent for evaluation and treatment of a minor usually must come from at least one parent or legal guardian. In some instances, such as with some divorced parents, clarification of legal custody or medical decision-making is necessary. Efforts made to ascertain which parent has legal rights should be carefully documented. In a situation where parents disagree on treatment and share joint legal custody, consulting with an institutional attorney is recommended. If the parents disagree but one parent has full legal custody, that parent's choice prevails.

Regarding youth in the foster care system, often the accompanying adult does not have legal authority to make medical decisions. If the parents' rights have been terminated or temporarily held, the foster care agency becomes the legal guardian, but many times that is not the case and the biological parents are still the legal authority. In the latter situation, if the biological parents cannot be contacted or refuse to provide consent and evaluation/treatment is clinically necessary, the hospital legal team should be contacted to initiate proceedings to override the legal guardian's authority (35).

There are certain situations in which a minor can consent, without parental involvement, to mental health or substance use evaluation and treatment. Laws vary by state, so clinicians should be aware of the statutes in their particular jurisdiction. Another area of concern that varies by jurisdiction is psychiatric hospitalization of a minor, as there are certain parameters that must be followed for voluntary or involuntary admission (35,61).

Confidentiality

Patients should be advised at the start of an evaluation as to what information can be kept confidential and what information must be disclosed to parents or legal authorities. Consent from the legal guardian of a pediatric patient is required to disclose information to anyone other than the patient or legal guardian(s) and to contact anyone to obtain collateral information. However, if collateral information is deemed necessary for diagnosis, treatment, or disposition planning, information can be exchanged even without consent (35,62). All measures should be taken to protect the patient's confidentiality, and information shared with the collateral source should be limited to only what is necessary. For example, if the school is contacted to obtain collateral information, they should not need any information beyond the fact that the child or adolescent is being evaluated.

Mandatory Reporting of Child Abuse

All mental healthcare providers are mandated reporters, which means that the law requires them to report any known instances of child abuse or neglect as soon as possible upon becoming aware of the issue, with potential legal repercussions if not handled appropriately (42). Some states also mandate reporting of any suspicion or concern for possible child abuse or neglect. Other situations in

which Child Protective Services (CPS) may need to be contacted include a parent leaving a child at the emergency department or a parent refusing admission when a child absolutely requires acute medical or psychiatric treatment. The process for reporting can vary, and contacting CPS for a particular state is usually a good first step. Some institutions have specialized child protection teams who can provide guidance and expertise around these issues, as well.

REFERENCES

1. Torio, C. E., Encinosa, W., Berdahl, T., et al. (2015). Annual report on health care for children and youth in the United States: National estimates of cost, utilization and expenditures for children with mental health conditions. *Academic Pediatrics, 15*, 19–35.
2. Children's National Health System. (2018). Mental health diagnoses among US children, youth continue to rise at alarming rate. Public Release.
3. Unpublished data, University of Michigan, 2018.
4. Jabbour, M., Hawkins, J., Day, D., et al. (2018). An emergency department clinical pathway for children and youth with mental health conditions. *Child and Adolescent Psychiatric Clinics of North America, 27*, 413–425.
5. Leon, S. L., Cloutier, P., Polihronis, C., et al. (2017). Child and adolescent mental health repeat visits to the emergency department: A systematic review. *Hospital Pediatrics, 7*, 177–186.
6. Stricker, F. R., O'Neill, K. B., Merson, J., et al. (2018). Maintaining safety and improving the care of pediatric behavioral health patients in the emergency department. *Child and Adolescent Psychiatric Clinics of North America, 27*, 427–439.
7. Gerson, R., Havens, J., Marr, M., et al. (2017). Utilization patterns at a specialized Children's Comprehensive Psychiatric Emergency Program. *Psychiatric Services, 68*, 1104–1111.
8. Chun, T. H., Mace, S. E., & Katz, E. R. (2016). Evaluation and management of children and adolescents with acute mental health or behavioral problems. Part I: Common clinical challenges of patients with mental health and/or behavioral emergencies. *Pediatrics, 138*(3), e20161570.
9. Newton, A. S., Hartling, L., Soleimani, A., et al. (2017). A systematic review of management strategies for children's mental health care in the emergency department: Update on evidence and recommendations for clinical practice and research. *Emergency Medicine Journal, 34*, 376–384.

10. Mroczkowski, M. M., & Havens, J. (2018). The state of emergency child and adolescent psychiatry: Raising the bar. *Child and Adolescent Psychiatric Clinics of North America, 27,* 357–365.

11. Sunderji, N., Tan de Bibiana, J., & Stergiopoulos, V. (2015). Urgent psychiatric services: A scoping review. *Canadian Journal of Psychiatry, 60,* 393–402.

12. Roberts, N., Hu, T., Axas, N., et al. (2017). Child and adolescent emergency and urgent mental health delivery through telepsychiatry: 12-month prospective study. *Telemedicine and e-Health, 23,* 842–846.

13. Butterfield, A. (2018). Telepsychiatric evaluation and consultation in emergency care settings. *Child and Adolescent Psychiatric Clinics of North America, 27,* 467–478.

14. Thomas, J. F., Novins, D. K., & Hosokawa, P. W. (2018). The use of telepsychiatry to provide cost-efficient care during pediatric mental health emergencies. *Psychiatric Services, 69,* 161–168.

15. Reeves, R. R., Perry, C. L., & Burke, R. S. (2010). What does "medical clearance" for psychiatry really mean? *Journal of Psychosocial Nursing and Mental Health Services, 48,* 2–4.

16. Santillanes, G., Donofrio, J. J., Lam, C. N., & Claudius, I. (2014). Is medical clearance necessary for pediatric psychiatric patients? *The Journal of Emergency Medicine, 46*(6), 800–807.

17. Lukens, T. W., Wolf, S. J., Edlow, J. A., et al. (2006). Clinical policy: Critical issues in the diagnosis and management of the adult psychiatric patient in the emergency department. *Annals of Emergency Medicine, 47,* 79–99.

18. Tucci, V., Siever, K., Matorin, A., & Moukaddam, N. (2015). Down the rabbit hole: Emergency department medical clearance of patients with psychiatric or behavioral emergencies. *Emergency Medicine Clinics of North America, 33*(4), 721–737.

19. Rocker, J. A., & Oestreicher, J. (2018). Focused medical assessment of pediatric behavioral emergencies. *Child and Adolescent Psychiatric Clinics of North America, 27*(3), 399–411.

20. Baren, J. M., Mace, S. E., Hendry, P. L., et al. (2008). Children's mental health emergencies. Part 2: Emergency department evaluation and treatment of children with mental health disorders. *Pediatric Emergency Care, 24,* 485–498.

21. Williams, E. R., & Moore Shephard, S. (2000). Medical clearance of psychiatric patients. *Emergency Medicine Clinics of North America, 18*(2), 185–198.

22. Guerrero, A. P. (2003). General medical considerations in child and adolescent patients who present with psychiatric symptoms. *Child and Adolescent Psychiatric Clinics of North America, 12,* 613–628.

23. Evans, D. L. (2000). Bipolar disorder: Diagnostic challenges and treatment considerations. *The Journal of Clinical Psychiatry, 61,* 26–31.

24. Kakuma, R., du Fort, G. G., Arsenault, L., et al. (2003). Delirium in older emergency department patients discharged home: Effect on survival. *Journal of the American Geriatrics Society, 51,* 443–450.

25. Nischal, A., Tripathi, A., Nischal, A., et al. (2012). Suicide and antidepressants: What current evidence indicates. *Mens Sana Monographs, 10*(1), 33–44.

26. Goodman, W. K., Murphy, T. K., & Storch, E. A. (2007). Risk of adverse behavioral effects with pediatric use of antidepressants. *Psychopharmacology, 191*(1), 87–96.

27. Gabriel, M., & Sharma, V. (2017). Antidepressant discontinuation syndrome. *CMAJ, 189*(21), E747.

28. Brent, D. A. (2016). Antidepressants and suicidality. *Psychiatric Clinics of North America, 39*(3), 503–512.

29. Sadock, B. J., & Sadock, V. A. (Eds.). (2003). *Kaplan & Sadock's synopsis of psychiatry: Behavioral sciences/clinical psychiatry* (9th ed.). Philadelphia, PA: Lippincott Williams & Wilkins.

30. King, R. A. (1995). AACAP OFFICIAL ACTION: Practice parameters for the psychiatric assessment of children and adolescents. *Journal of the American Academy of Child and Adolescent Psychiatry, 34,* 1386–1402.

31. Newton, A. S., Soleimani, A., Kirkland, S. W., & Gokiert, R. J. (2017). A systematic review of instruments to identify mental health and substance use problems among children in the emergency department. *Academic Emergency Medicine, 24,* 552–568.

32. Horowitz, L. M., Bridge, J. A., Teach, S. J., et al. (2012). Ask suicide-screening questions (ASQ): A brief instrument for the pediatric emergency department. *Archives of Pediatrics & Adolescent Medicine, 166,* 1170–1176.

33. Gipson, P. Y., Agarwala, P., Opperman, K. J., et al. (2015). Columbia-suicide severity rating scale: Predictive validity with adolescent psychiatric emergency patients. *Pediatric Emergency Care, 31,* 88–94.

34. Goldstein, A. B., & Findling, R. L. (2006). Assessment and evaluation of child and adolescent psychiatric emergencies. *Psychiatric Times, 23*(9), 1–2.

35. Heppell, P. J., & Rao, S. (2018). Social services and behavioral emergencies: Trauma-informed evaluation, diagnosis, and disposition. *Child and Adolescent Psychiatric Clinics of North America, 27*(3), 455–465.

36. Finkelhor, D., Turner, H., Ormrod, R., & Hamby, S. L. (2009). Violence, abuse, and crime exposure in a national sample of children and youth. *Pediatrics, 124*(5), 1411–1423.

37. Felitti, V. J., Anda, R. F., Nordenberg, D., et al. (1998). Relationship of childhood abuse and household dysfunction to many of the leading causes of death in adults: The Adverse Childhood Experiences (ACE) study. *American Journal of Preventive Medicine, 14*(4), 245–258.

38. Kazak, A. E., Kassam-Adams, N., Schneider, S., Zelikovsky, N., Alderfer, M. A., & Rourke, M. (2006). An integrative model of pediatric medical traumatic stress. *Journal of Pediatric Psychology, 31*(4), 343–355.

39. Marsac, M. L., Kassam-Adams, N., Hildenbrand, A. K., Nicholls, E., Winston, F. K., Leff, S. S., & Fein, J. (2016). Implementing a trauma-informed approach in pediatric health care networks. *JAMA Pediatrics, 170*(1), 70–77.

40. Ko, S. J., Ford, J. D., Kassam-Adams, N., et al. (2008). Creating trauma-informed systems: Child welfare, education, first responders, health care, juvenile justice. *Professional Psychology: Research and Practice, 39*(4), 396–404.

41. Kassam-Adams, N., Marsac, M. L., Hildenbrand, A. K., & Winston, F. (2013). Posttraumatic stress following pediatric injury: Update on diagnosis, risk factors, and intervention. *JAMA Pediatrics, 167*(12), 1158–1165.

42. Center for Pediatric Traumatic Stress. (2009). Retrieved December 16, 2018, from www.HealthCareToolbox.org.

43. Kozloff, N., Jacob, B., Voineskos, A. N., et al. (2018). Care of youth in their first emergency presentation for psychotic disorder: A population-based retrospective cohort study. *The Journal of Clinical Psychiatry, 79*, e1–e7.

44. Simon, O. R., Swann, A. C., Powell, K. E., Potter, L. B., Kresnow, M. J., & O'Carroll, P. W. (2001). Characteristics of impulsive suicide attempts and attempters. *Suicide and Life-Threatening Behavior, 32*(Suppl. 1), 49–59.

45. Brown, G. K., Henriques, G. R., Sosdjan, D., & Beck, A. T. (2004). Suicide intent and accurate expectations of lethality: Predictors of medical lethality of suicide attempts. *Journal of Consulting and Clinical Psychology, 72*(6), 1170–1174.

46. Case, S. D., Case, B. G., Olfson, M., et al. (2011). Length of stay of pediatric mental health emergency department visits in the United States. *Journal of the American Academy of Child and Adolescent Psychiatry, 50*, 1110–1119.

47. National Center for Injury Prevention and Control, CDC using WISQARS™ *10 leading causes of death by age group, United States, 2016.*

48. Centers for Disease Control and Prevention. (2018). Youth risk behavior surveillance—United States, 2017. *Morbidity and Mortality Weekly Report, 67*(8), 1–114.

49. Mercado, M. C., Holland, K., & Leemis, R. W. (2017). Trends in emergency department visits for nonfatal self-inflicted injuries among youth aged 10-24 years in the United States, 2001–2015. *JAMA, 318*, 1931.

50. McKean, A., Pabbati, C. P., Geske, J. R., et al. (2018). Rethinking lethality in youth suicide attempts: First suicide attempt outcomes in youth ages 10-24. *Journal of the American Academy of Child and Adolescent Psychiatry, 57*, 786–791.

51. Jacobson, L. K., Rabinowitz, I., Popper, M. S., et al. (1994). Interviewing prepubertal children about suicidal ideation and behavior. *Journal of the American Academy of Child and Adolescent Psychiatry, 33*, 439–452.

52. Gerson, R., Malas, N., & Mroczkowski, M. M. (2018). Crisis in the emergency department: The evaluation and management of acute agitation in children and adolescents. *Child and Adolescent Psychiatric Clinics of North America, 27*, 367–386.

53. Baker, M., & Carlson, G. A. (2018). What do we really know about PRN use in agitated children with mental health conditions: A clinical review. *Evidence Based Mental Health, 21*, 166–170.

54. Carandang, C., Gray, C., Marval-Ospino, H., & MacPhee, S. (2012). Child and adolescent psychiatric emergencies. In Rey, J. M. (Ed.), *IACAPAP textbook of child and adolescent mental health (pp. 1–31).* Geneva: International Association for Child and Adolescent Psychiatry and Allied Professions.

55. Semper, T. F., & McClellan, J. M. (2003). The psychotic child. *Child and Adolescent Psychiatric Clinics of North America, 12*, 679–691.

56. Edelsohn, G. A. (2006). Hallucinations in children and adolescents: Considerations in the emergency setting. *American Journal of Psychiatry, 163*, 781–785.

57. Pittsenbarger, Z. E., & Mannix, R. (2013). Trends in pediatric visits to the emergency department for psychiatric illnesses. *Academic Emergency Medicine, 21*, 25–30.

58. Wang, G. S., & Hoyte, C. (2018). Common substances of abuse. *Pediatrics in Review, 39,* 403–412.

59. National Institute on Drug Abuse. *Monitoring the Future 2018 Survey Results.* Retrieved from https://www.drugabuse.gov/related-topics/trends-statistics/infographics/monitoring-future-2018-survey-results.

60. Solkhah, R. (2003). The intoxicated child. *Child and Adolescent Psychiatric Clinics of North America, 12,* 693–722.

61. Rubin, D. M., Alessandrini, E. A., Feudtner, C., et al. (2004). Placement stability and mental health costs for children in foster care. *Pediatrics, 113*(5), 1336–1341.

62. Fortunati, F. G., Jr., & Zonana, H. V. (2003). Legal considerations in the child psychiatric emergency department. *Child and Adolescent Psychiatric Clinics of North America, 12,* 745–761.

63. Cappelli, M., Gray, C., Zemek, R., et al. (2012). The HEADS-ED: A rapid mental health screening tool for pediatric patients in the emergency department. *Pediatrics, 130,* e321–e327.

64. Davis, A. K., Arterberry, B. J., & Bonar, E. E. (2018). Predictors of positive drinking outcomes among youth receiving an alcohol brief intervention in the emergency department. *Drug and Alcohol Dependence, 188,* 102–108.

35

The Psychiatric Emergency Care of the Geriatric Patient

Katherine G. Levine, Harold H. Harsch, Joseph S. Goveas

THE GERIATRIC CARE SYSTEM IN THE UNITED STATES

The medical structure that provides care to older adults in the United States can be divided into the acute care system and the long-term care (LTC) system. Medicare has provided the funding for most of the acute care and rehabilitation needs for adults older than 65 years. LTC, however, is funded primarily by the Medicaid program and private resources. In 2014, fewer than 3% of individuals older than 65 years were in skilled nursing facilities (SNFs), yet a much larger number were part of the LTC system in the United States (an estimated 1.2 vs 7.5 million) (1,2).

Emergency department (ED) physicians, both psychiatrists and nonpsychiatrists, need to understand the levels of care this system offers to appropriately accept and return individuals to these facilities. Residential settings in the LTC system include SNFs, community-based residential facilities (CBRFs), and assisted living facilities (ALFs). SNFs, commonly known as *nursing homes*, are the most familiar to physicians. They provide care to the older adult who requires at least 7 hours a week of skilled nursing care. Although often understaffed, SNFs have a registered nurse and nursing aides available 24/7. CBRFs, in some areas called as *group homes*, provide care to five or more adults unable to live independently by providing supervision and supportive services. Usually they are licensed by the state; some cater to specific populations, such as those requiring dementia care. Often different licensure levels exist, which separate CBRFs by the type of resident they can admit

(eg, ambulatory, nonambulatory, mentally capable of responding to a fire alarm or not). A nurse might be on call, but CBRFs generally use nonmedical personnel, with at least one staff member being present 24/7. The phrase *assisted living* refers to a type of residential care with four or more registered beds, at least two meals a day, help with personal care (bathing, dressing) or health-related services (medication management), and around-the-clock on-site supervision (3). In most states ALFs are licensed.

Behavioral emergencies in these facilities are always difficult but become even more so at night or over the weekends because of reduced staffing. SNFs can give as-needed medication and provide some short-term acute monitoring for a resident. CBRFs usually can give as-needed medication but rarely have the staff to provide extra monitoring for residents. Assisted living is best thought of as a nonmedical housing situation with no monitoring available.

The available support and supervision in these differing levels of care must be considered when EDs make disposition decisions. Behavioral stability is required for an ALF, while an SNF could have a resident return if he or she is somewhat better but still requires extra observation. It is frustrating for physicians when LTC facilities refuse to allow a resident to return from the ED or psychiatric emergency service (PES). However, if a facility feels that it cannot manage the older adult's behaviors, it is probably safer for the patient to not be sent back to the facility from the ED or PES. This chapter discusses the issues of geriatric behavioral assessment, acute treatment, and possible hospitalization.

EMERGENCY PSYCHIATRIC ASSESSMENT OF THE OLDER ADULT

The proportion of older adults in the United States is rising. The number of people aged 65 years and older accounted for 14.9% of the total population in 2015 and is expected to reach 20% by 2030 (4). In 2015 it was estimated that the elderly constituted 15.6% of the total ED visits (5). As the population ages, geriatric patients will become an ever-increasing portion of ED visits, and physicians need to be aware of the challenges inherent in treating this population. The goals of a geriatric psychiatric evaluation in the ED are to complete an efficient assessment, investigate for underlying medical disorders, establish a provisional diagnosis and differential diagnosis, establish the patient's cognitive and functional capacity, provide emergency treatment, and arrange an appropriate disposition in a limited time frame. Obtaining the geriatric history and assessing the mental status is a time-intensive process because older patients rarely present with a single well-defined diagnosis, rather often experience multiple, comorbid medical and neurologic illnesses, and may not be reliable historians. Although ED personnel are proficient in medical history taking and performing a physical examination, they are often not trained in recognizing common psychiatric presentations in the elderly, including psychosis, depression, suicidality, behavioral disturbances, anxiety, and alcohol or drug intoxication and withdrawal. Despite the pace of the ED, it is essential to be thorough in your information gathering and medical evaluation of geriatric patients. Careful medical evaluations are especially crucial for a free-standing PES, as life-threatening medical emergencies in geriatric patients can easily masquerade as psychiatric issues. Hasty and incomplete assessments of older adults in the medical or psychiatric ED increase the likelihood of serious adverse outcomes from erroneous disposition planning because of missed diagnoses.

The psychiatric evaluation should be modified to accommodate the needs of the geriatric psychiatric patient as outlined in Table 35.1. New-onset psychiatric symptoms in the elderly that trigger an ED visit should prompt the physician to assess for precipitating factors. Environmental and physical factors such as recent losses, relocation, changes in support networks, separations, recent changes in medications, and various medical illnesses (ranging from a urinary tract infection to a recent diagnosis of a potentially life-threatening illnesses) can be associated with the onset of an anxiety, affective, cognitive, or psychotic symptomatology in an older adult. Also, new-onset psychosis in older adults is often caused by undiagnosed dementia or acute delirium. A careful review of prescription and over-the-counter medications is essential as polypharmacy is very common in the elderly. Ideally, a review of the medicine containers and a double check between the written schedule and the pill containers should be performed. This could reveal prescription drug noncompliance or overuse. Screening for alcohol, street drug, prescription, and over-the counter drug misuse or abuse in a geriatric patient is essential in the ED or PES but is often overlooked. Therefore, when suspicion arises, a blood alcohol level and urine toxicology screen should be obtained. Suicide risk assessment is a critical part of the ED geriatric psychiatric evaluation because suicide is more frequent in the elderly population compared with their younger counterparts. Moreover, approximately three-fourths of elderly patients who commit suicide have seen a physician in the previous month, and over one-third within the week of their suicide (6).

Cognitive evaluation is mandatory for all geriatric patients presenting to the ED. A sudden decline from baseline in either cognition or functional status is highly suggestive of an acute delirium. Recognizing cognitive impairment early in the ED assessment is the key for a correct medical and psychiatric differential diagnosis as well as knowing the appropriate laboratory and imaging studies, and consultations to obtain (7,8). The most widely used cognitive screening instrument is the Folstein Mini-Mental Status Examination (MMSE). The expert consensus panel for treatment of behavioral emergencies has endorsed the MMSE as the preferred cognitive instrument in ED settings (9). The Confusion Assessment Method (CAM), a brief screening instrument that is highly sensitive and specific for delirium, can be effectively administered by nonpsychiatrically trained ED staff.

TABLE 35.1 Evaluation of the Geriatric Patient in the Emergency Department

Identifying data
Reliability of the history from the patient
Reason for ED visit
History: Present episode, including onset, duration, chronology of progression of symptoms over time, and recent environmental and physical changes
Past psychiatric history: Past psychiatric diagnoses, treatment, and hospitalizations
Medical history: Medical illnesses, history of falls, strokes, head trauma, and seizures
Medication history: List of prescription and over-the-counter medications, recent changes in medications; contact pharmacy or current physician(s) if needed to verify the prescription and rationale for use
Family history: Depression, psychosis, suicide, alcohol abuse or dependence, and dementia
Substance use history: Alcohol; prescription, over-the-counter, supplements, and illicit drugs
Physical examination: Special attention to vital signs and oxygen saturation, thorough neurologic evaluation for deficits, and stat glucose level
Mental status: Folstein Mini-Mental Status Examination, appearance, grooming, attitude, ability to relate to the interviewer, speech, mood and affect, attention, behavior/psychomotor activity, thought process and thought content abnormalities (delusions, obsessions, compulsions, suicidality, homicidality, disturbance of perception), insight and judgment
Functional assessment
Physical activities of daily living: Bathing, dressing, toileting, grooming, and ability to transfer and to feed self
Instrumental activities of daily living: Shopping; ability to use the telephone, handle finances, and operate a motor vehicle; food preparation; laundry; and responsibility for own medications
Evaluate for elder abuse: Suspect with history of multiple fractures, falls, and failure to thrive presentations, delays in seeking medical care, different histories from patient and caregiver
Interview with the significant other or caregiver
Laboratory studies: Complete blood count with differential, comprehensive metabolic panel, thyroid function, serum vitamin B_{12} and folate levels, rapid plasma reagent, urinalysis, electrocardiogram (especially prior to using antipsychotics), urine toxicology and blood alcohol levels (if substance abuse is suspected), electroencephalogram (if seizures suspected), and serum drug levels (if appropriate)
Neuroimaging (if indicated): Computerized tomographic scan of head without contrast (better tolerated) or magnetic resonance imaging scan of brain

Functional assessment will provide the physician an understanding of how much care or supervision the patient requires upon discharge from the ED. Various scales have been developed for this purpose (10).

Most geriatric assessments in the ED or PES should include interviewing the significant other or caregiver. The geriatric patient may not be a reliable historian because of cognitive and behavioral disturbances, and the collateral history will provide further insight into the patient's condition. If the significant other is the caregiver, the ED staff will need to assess for caregiver burden and his or her health and ability to care for the patient. A systematic diagnostic approach as outlined in Table 35.1 and careful differential diagnoses will facilitate appropriate dispositional planning and treatment.

ACUTE BEHAVIORAL DISTURBANCES

Psychosis

Psychosis can occur at any age, including in late life. Characterized by delusions and hallucinations, the prototypical form of psychosis is schizophrenia. In the United States, the prevalence estimate of schizophrenia is 0.1% to 0.5% in people aged 65 years and older. Importantly, the number of individuals with schizophrenia aged 55 years and older will double by 2025, or about one-fourth of all persons with schizophrenia (11,12). Most older adults with schizophrenia have early-onset psychosis (ie, diagnosed earlier in life and now living into late-life with the condition). Although the onset of schizophrenia is typically in adolescence to early adulthood, it can less frequently develop later in life. When symptoms develop in individuals older than 40 years, this is considered late-onset schizophrenia. It is estimated that about 23% of patients have late-onset schizophrenia, and approximately 3% have an onset after age 60 years. When the onset of these symptoms occurs after the age of 60 years, it is considered very-late-onset schizophrenia-like psychosis and is typically due to medical conditions, such as dementia or other neurodegenerative disorders. Late-onset schizophrenia is believed to have better a prognosis and responds to lower antipsychotic doses. (12,13).

While late-onset schizophrenia is uncommon, there are other more common causes of late-onset psychosis, which include dementia with psychotic features, geriatric mood disorders, delusional disorder, and psychotic disorders secondary to medications and delirium. The prevalence of psychotic symptoms in Alzheimer disease (AD), for instance, ranges between 30% and 50%. Risk factors for late-onset psychosis include female gender, age-related deterioration of frontal and temporal lobes, cognitive deficits, premorbid paranoid and schizoid personality traits, visual or hearing impairment, polypharmacy, and illicit substance use. Late-onset psychosis is often associated with structural brain abnormalities and can be the first clinical manifestation of a medical, neurologic, or substance-induced condition, and therefore warrants a thorough diagnostic workup (11-16). It is important for the ED or PES physician to determine whether the elderly person has early- or late-onset psychosis as this significantly informs management.

Regardless of the age at onset, psychiatric and medical examinations must be performed, and appropriate laboratory and neuroimaging studies should be part of the evaluation to rule out reversible or identifiable medical etiologies.

Agitation and Aggression

Agitation and aggression are common manifestations of medical and psychiatric illnesses in older adults and are present in approximately 60% of the hospitalized elderly. Agitation is conceptualized as excessive motor or verbal activity that can escalate to verbal or physical aggression. Examples of verbal aggression include threats, vocal outbursts, name calling, cursing, and excessive verbalizations of distress. Examples of physical aggression include throwing or breaking objects, pushing, slapping, kicking, and hitting. Agitation can be precipitated by a variety of factors including medical illnesses, medications, pain, alcohol/substance intoxication and withdrawal, environmental changes, dementia, and psychosis (15,17). Approximately 40% of elderly persons older than 70 years presenting to the ED have an alteration in mental status, and 25% are diagnosed with delirium (18). Patients with dementia are highly predisposed to develop delirium.

The most common underlying causes of agitation and aggression in the elderly are dementia, delirium, or both. Dementia often causes difficulties with problem-solving and impaired communication. In these situations, agitation may be a means of expressing anxiety, discomfort, or distress. It can present as disruptive behaviors, fidgeting, pacing, and resisting care. Sometimes agitation appears repetitive (repeating sentences, questions, words, or sounds), whereas other times the agitation presents as socially inappropriate behavior (sexual disinhibition, undressing, or voiding in inappropriate places) (19,20). In 2015, the International Psychogeriatric Association developed the following consensus defining agitation in the setting of cognitive disorders as: (1) occurring in patients with cognitive impairment or dementia syndrome; (2) exhibiting behavior consistent with emotional distress; (3) manifesting excessive motor activity, verbal aggression, or physical aggression; and (4) evidencing behaviors that cause excess disability and are not solely attributable to another disorder (psychiatric, medical, or substance-related) (21).

Aggressive behaviors, regardless of the etiology, not only increase the risk of danger to the affected person and others but also lead to increased caregiver burden, stress, and depression. The safety of the patient, caregivers, and ED personnel is a priority in management of agitation or aggression in an ED or PES setting. Although treatment of agitation in the ED often combines behavioral and pharmacologic approaches, nonpharmacologic management is recommended as the first-line approach in elderly persons presenting to the ED with agitation. Identification and correction of possible reversible causes for agitation, along with environmental, interpersonal, and medical interventions, should be considered before use of pharmacologic interventions. Involvement of families, patients, and caregivers in decision making with communication of risks, benefits, and limitations of available treatments is essential. Nonpharmacologic treatment strategies are most effective when (1) used as adjuncts to pharmacotherapy, (2) pharmacotherapy is contraindicated, or (3) agitation is secondary to environmental factors (19,22).

Show of force, an often-successful nonpharmacologic intervention for an agitated young adult, is not an effective treatment modality in the elderly. Instead, approach the agitated elderly patient slowly, provide repeated reassurance, talk slowly and in a calm tone, use simple sentences, ask simple questions, be polite, and maintain a pleasant facial expression. One may need to introduce one's self and role routinely. Avoid complex, multistep tasks, and use eye contact. If the patient is becoming increasingly agitated, back off, reapproach, and ask permission. If the patient is paranoid, do not argue or try to reason; instead, try distracting him or her. If he or she is looking for certain objects that were misplaced, offer to help find them. Adjust the physical environment to be adaptive to the geriatric patient's needs. If the patient is restless, holding his or her hands, providing soft music, a hand or back massage, or meaningful activities, and having a family member or caregiver in the room might be greatly beneficial. If redirection is ineffective, place the patient in a safe, quiet room with minimal sensory stimuli. It is worth noting that for patients with dementia, circadian rhythm abnormalities, wandering, vocalizations, and catastrophic reactions are best managed behaviorally, whereas paranoia, anger, and aggression are considered more likely to respond to antipsychotic medications. (19,20,23).

Physical restraint use in the elderly is considered an indicator of poor quality in institutional settings, and routine use of physical restraints in hospitals has been closely scrutinized by federal agencies. Increased physical restraint use in the hospitalized elderly has been associated with dementia, delirium, and prior residence in an LTC facility. In fact, individuals with cognitive impairment and ones who reside at LTC facilities comprise most geriatric psychiatric ED visits. There is no evidence to support the use of physical restraints in the agitated elderly, and their use does not decrease the risk of falls. However, there is evidence to suggest that use of mechanical restraints can increase agitation in the cognitively impaired elderly. Furthermore, severe adverse outcomes, including injuries and hip fractures, pressure ulcers, functional decline, increased risk for infections, psychological trauma, and even death from asphyxiation, have been reported in the literature (24,25). The use of physical restraints should be considered only if no other viable option is available and all less restrictive measures have failed.

Suicide

The elderly has elevated suicide rates in the United States. In 2016, the 65- to 74-year-old cohort had a suicide rate of 15.4 per 100,000 individuals, with the rate climbing to 18.2 per 100,000 in the 75- to 84-year-old cohort. The suicide rate is even higher among the old-old (defined as older than 85 years), at 19.0 per 100,000 persons (26). Several risk factors for geriatric suicide have been described in the literature. The majority of completed elderly suicides occur among white men, followed by nonwhite men, white women, and nonwhite women. Depression, alcohol use disorder (AUD), substance abuse, previous suicide attempts, firearms possession, and expressed suicidal intent have been reported as independent risk factors for completed suicides. Other mental health risk factors include depression, psychosis, and dementia. Social factors include being divorced, widowed, or living alone; low social interaction; recent life change; bereavement; family discord; and anniversary of a loss. Medical risk factors include serious physical illness, greater physical illness burden with associated functional impairment, and chronic persistent pain (27). ED or PES personnel should screen for these risk factors.

Social and cognitive perspectives can help explain suicidality in the elderly. Relationship loss and health issues are a typical experience of aging. The Interpersonal Theory of Suicide posits that social disconnection through either a thwarted sense of belonging (ie, retirement, death of peers) or a perceived sense of being a burden (ie, chronic disease, functional limitations) when combined with repeated negative and painful events can result in suicidal ideation and behaviors (28). Neuropsychological alterations associated with vulnerability to suicide in the elderly include impaired decision making, cognitive inhibition, and social problem solving (29). Cognitive testing of older adults with recent suicide attempts showed decreased performance on measures of attention, memory, and executive function compared with similarly matched peers without recent suicide attempts (30). When accounting for these social and cognitive aspects, the suicidal older adult can be best conceptualized as demonstrating a decreased ability to problem solve and inhibit negative thoughts in the setting of life stressors (loss, pain, disability), insufficient social connections, and/or perceived burdensomeness (29).

Older adults are less likely to report depressive symptoms and suicidal thoughts, are more likely to use highly lethal means, and are more likely to die on a first attempt (31). Elderly patients are secretive about suicidal intent unless directly questioned. If suicidal ideation is shared, a detailed inquiry regarding specific plans and access needs to be made. The Beck Scale for Suicidal Ideation, which is relatively easy to administer, has been effectively used in geriatric suicide prevention studies (32). Elderly patients with a high risk for suicide should be psychiatrically hospitalized, either voluntarily or involuntarily, and should be closely observed during the first 24 hours of inpatient admission.

Alcohol and Substance Abuse

AUD is commonly a lifelong illness, with an early onset and relapses/recurrences later in life. Late-onset AUD is also seen; biological factors, major life events, and other psychosocial stressors later in life could play a role. Older adults do not usually volunteer information about their alcohol intake. Although alcohol use declines with age, it continues to pose a significant public health concern.

At-risk or problem drinking is defined as drinking at a level that either has resulted in adverse medical, psychological, or social consequences or substantially increases the likelihood of such problems, but does not meet the criteria for alcohol dependence, and is highly prevalent among older adults, especially in health care settings (33,34). In elderly primary care patients, 10% to 15% of the patients were found to screen positive for at-risk or problem drinking (35,36). AUD is even more prevalent in hospitalized older patients: close to 30% hospitalized on medical floors and about 50% on inpatient psychiatric units have AUD (33). Interestingly, 29% to 49% of veterans in nursing homes had a lifetime diagnosis of alcohol dependence, with about 10% to 18% meeting criteria for abuse or dependence within 1 year of admission (37,38). Despite its common occurrence, AUD in the elderly are frequently overlooked by the ED or PES providers.

Aging-related pharmacokinetic and pharmacodynamic changes increase the risk of complications from alcohol in the elderly. Older adults are more sensitive to the detrimental effects of alcohol and have higher levels than their younger counterparts for the same amount consumed. Alcohol intoxication could therefore occur at lower serum levels in the elderly, and withdrawal symptoms may be more severe, of longer duration, and more difficult to treat in this age group than in younger patients (39). Sleep disturbances and central nervous system complications from alcohol, such as Wernicke-Korsakoff syndrome and dementia, can occur. AUD could also complicate management of comorbid chronic diseases in the elderly. Older adults with AUD may present to the ED with various complaints, including dehydration, infections, recurrent falls, gait abnormalities, malnutrition and lack of self-care, head trauma, hypoglycemia, myopathy, gastrointestinal bleeding, hypothermia, delirium, and worsening or new onset of cognitive or psychiatric disorders.

Appropriate screening for late-life problem drinking and AUD can be performed using widely available, validated screening instruments such as the CAGE questionnaire and the Short Michigan Alcohol Screening Test—Geriatric Version (40,41). Appropriate dispositional planning should be based on the revised patient placement criteria published by the American Society of Addiction Medicine. A history of alcohol withdrawal delirium, withdrawal seizures, complicated detoxifications, and unstable medical conditions should prompt inpatient hospitalization for close monitoring and detoxification. In general, benzodiazepines with short half-lives and no active metabolites are used for acute detoxification. Specific protocols used to treat alcohol withdrawal are described elsewhere.

Disulfiram should be used with extreme caution in the elderly given its side effect profile. There is evidence to support the efficacy of naltrexone in improving relapse to heavy drinking (42). Also, recent data point to the potential benefits of acamprosate in specific elderly subgroups with AUD (43). Despite this growing literature suggesting a role for AUD pharmacotherapy, there is no indication to start these medications in the ED or PES.

Older adults are most likely to receive a prescription for opioids and benzodiazepines in the primary care settings, making the potential misuse of these medications a public health concern. Over one-fourth of benzodiazepine prescriptions are written for persons older than 65 years, and long-term use of these medications results in development of physical dependence. Abrupt termination of benzodiazepines may result in rare but significant withdrawal symptoms, including delirium, psychosis, and seizures. Therefore, gradual tapering of these drugs is recommended, sometimes over months. Dependence on prescription opioid analgesics is also not uncommon in the elderly, especially in individuals with chronic pain disorders or significant psychopathology (44). Unexplained sedation, gait abnormalities, falls and fractures, or cognitive impairment should prompt the ED staff to inquire regarding benzodiazepine and opioid use. ED providers should also be aware of the age-related pharmacokinetic changes and the potential for drug-drug interactions involving benzodiazepines and opioids given the higher number of medications prescribed in the elderly.

ACUTE BEHAVIORAL EMERGENCIES IN LONG-TERM CARE FACILITIES

The prevalence of psychiatric disorders among new SNF admissions is reported to be over 80%, with the most common diagnoses being dementia and depression. Dementia, the most common psychiatric diagnosis among SNF residents, is found in approximately 50% of SNF residents in the United States; some studies have reported even higher rates. Depression is the second most common psychiatric diagnosis among SNF residents, with the prevalence rate ranging from 15% to 50%. Delirium is present in 6% to 7% of SNF residents, and approximately 10% of residents with dementia have superimposed delirium. In addition, psychotic symptoms are prevalent in 13% to 50% of SNF residents with dementia. Behavioral disturbances are present in approximately 75% of SNF residents; these include verbal abuse, socially inappropriate behaviors, wandering, and physical abuse. The presence of disruptive behaviors can make providing care extremely difficult in the SNF (45).

ED and PES staff frequently encounter SNF referrals during nights and weekends and often face tough dispositional situations. It is useful to be aware of the factors at play. SNF staffing levels tend to be lower during weekends and the covering nurses and aides are generally less familiar with the residents' baseline psychopathology and usually lack training in dealing with acute agitation or suicide threats. Moreover, psychiatric consultation is often lacking at the SNF, and the doctors who are called on to treat these patients—primary care physicians and geriatricians—may not be well versed in managing acute behavioral disturbances. Agitated elderly patients can be dangerous to themselves, other residents, or staff and require a higher level of staff monitoring than the facility may be able to provide (46).

ED personnel often perceive LTC referrals as potential "dumps" because these facilities sometimes refuse to accept residents back. It is also not unusual for these patients to be calm and pleasant in the emergency room, minimizing or denying any discomfort or presence of psychiatric symptoms, while attempts by the ED staff to obtain collateral information from LTC facilities often go in vain. Elderly referrals from LTC facilities to the ED or PES should undergo systematic evaluation as detailed in Table 35.1. The geriatric psychiatric assessment will not be complete until one obtains corroborative information from the family members, SNF staff, or primary care providers.

PSYCHIATRIC HOSPITALIZATION FOR THE OLDER ADULT

An older adult will need psychiatric hospitalization for many of the same reasons as a younger adult who is hospitalized. These include (1) physically assaultive behaviors toward caregivers and peers, (2) repetitive threats by a patient with a history of serious physical aggression, (3) psychosis with the potential for dangerous behaviors to self or others, (4) severe depression, and (5) acute suicidality. If inpatient psychiatric admission is warranted, brief hospitalization for stabilization is enough under most circumstances. Hyperactive or mixed delirium can result in acute agitation and may require medical hospitalization. Other reasons for hospitalization include self-neglect syndromes, pre-LTC placement, acute caregiver burnout, and diagnostic observation of significant behavior problems. These indications are similar for community-dwelling elderly and the older adults residing at LTC facilities.

Several issues need to be addressed by the ED or PES physician considering psychiatric hospitalization for an older adult. Are there specific geriatric psychiatry units available in the service area? These may provide expertise and treatment advantages over the general adult psychiatric units, yet they exist mainly in the larger metropolitan areas (47). If there are no geriatric psychiatry units, are there general psychiatry units available in the area that can safely accommodate the older adult? One certainly does not want to see an 85-year-old with agitation and dementia fall

and break a hip in an altercation with a manic 19-year-old patient. Many general adult units have attempted to physically separate the older adult population from others as much as design permits.

Lengths of stay for older adults in specialty psychiatric hospitals and general hospital behavioral health units are generally longer than those of younger adults (14.1 vs. 7.9 days) (48,49). This most likely reflects complex physical and social problems as well as conservative medication use.

Deciding whether to hospitalize the older adult in a medical or a psychiatric facility entails consideration of several issues. Generally, patients with delirium should be admitted to a medical facility. "Failure to thrive" admissions are best cared for in medical facilities. Patients who will need a more comprehensive workup including access to imaging, procedures, or medical specialist consultation are not well suited for a free-standing psychiatric hospital but may be appropriate for a psychiatric unit within a general hospital. Some patients object to admission to a psychiatric hospital, or a psychiatric facility may not be available in a rural area. Occasionally these patients with primary psychiatric issues can be admitted to a medical floor with orders for a sitter or 15-minute behavioral checks. Social services can later address a potential transfer.

Psychiatric facilities have the advantage of often being locked, which not only provides safety but also protects the wandering dementia patient. Patients are also not confined to a room and a bed. Psychiatric facilities always have specific programming throughout the day, which can be quite therapeutic for many older adults. Unfortunately, unless the facility has specific programming for dementia patients, this subpopulation is often not able to participate. Ideal outcomes of psychiatric hospitalization include medication review and adjustment, behavioral stabilization, family education, and more appropriate placement if indicated.

THE ISSUE OF MEDICAL CLEARANCE

Medical clearance becomes a concern when the on-call psychiatrist is contacted by the ED for an after-hours admission of an 82-year-old patient with new onset of agitation. The psychiatrist wants to ensure that an admission to a psychiatric facility is not based on an acute medical problem. At times a reluctant psychiatrist will keep questioning about possible medical etiologies of the behavioral disturbance. This can be irritating for the ED physician when no acute medical problem is found. Table 35.1 serves as an outline of a complete evaluation of a geriatric patient in the ED. If a good-faith attempt is made to cover items in this evaluation and no acute medical basis for the behavioral problem is found, admission to a psychiatric floor is appropriate.

One should remember that there is no such thing as "absolute medical clearance" in the evaluation of a patient in the ED. The tests and examinations suggested in Table 35.1 have their limitations. It is possible to miss the prodrome of a developing infection, a more exotic medical problem, or an unusual presentation of an existing medical issue. When the patient is admitted to the psychiatric hospital, he or she should be closely monitored both behaviorally and medically so that if a previously undetected medical problem declares itself, appropriate transfer can be arranged.

A urinary tract infection is one of the most common reasons for older women to experience a change in mental status. Yet even obtaining a urine collection in an uncooperative, agitated individual in the ED is problematic. This can, however, be medically dealt with in most psychiatric facilities. Another common scenario is that of a patient developing an infection with some confusion at an SNF and subsequently being treated with an antibiotic, only to have mental status continue to be abnormal even after the antibiotic treatment ends. The patient is sent to the ED or PES for evaluation. All medical tests are normal. Often forgotten is that delirium in the elderly can take weeks to months to fully resolve even if the contributing condition is eliminated (50). Additionally, pain is an often-overlooked factor as a cause of agitation in the older adult, especially in patients with aphasia or dementia with compromised communication ability. Although medical clearance is not absolute, it does provide a reasonable level of certainty that a geriatric patient is medically stable for admission to a psychiatric facility.

GERIATRIC EMERGENCY PSYCHOPHARMACOLOGY

Geriatric patients are more vulnerable to adverse drug reactions because of age-related pharmacokinetic and homeostatic changes. The reduced concentrations in plasma albumin seen with aging can lead to an increased concentration of "free" drug levels. The decline in glomerular filtration rate and decreased hepatic blood flow result in decreased renal and hepatic clearance of medications. These factors often lead to higher medication serum levels, with the same doses, than for younger adults. Decreased reactivity of homeostatic mechanisms such as blood pressure and postural control makes the addition of medications with sedating or orthostatic side effects more likely to contribute to falls and subsequent hip fractures. Additionally, a decline in dopamine and acetylcholine function in the elderly causes increased sensitivity to extrapyramidal symptoms with antipsychotics and impaired cognition with anticholinergic agents (51).

Despite the increased risk of adverse reactions, pharmacotherapy is often necessary to treat potentially dangerous and disruptive behaviors when behavioral interventions prove unsuccessful. It is important to note that appropriate and judicious use of psychotropics to treat underlying symptoms (ie, psychosis) or targeted behaviors (ie, physical violence) is not chemical restraint. Psychopharmacotherapy should be considered if the elderly agitated patient is exhibiting a potential to harm self or others or is impeding the medical evaluation and management, or both. Calming the patient without sedation is the goal of psychopharmacologic interventions for acute behavioral emergencies (52). Elderly persons are highly susceptible to adverse drug reactions. Therefore, each geriatric patient in the ED should only receive those medications that are clinically effective, in minimum doses and for the duration needed to treat the acute behavioral emergency. Once the emergency has passed, need for medications should be reassessed. The American Psychiatric Association recommends that "...nonemergency antipsychotic medication should only be used for the treatment of agitation or psychosis in patients with dementia when symptoms are severe, are dangerous, and/or cause significant distress to the patient" (53).

A 2012 systematic review of the available guidelines for behavioral and psychological symptoms of dementia (BPSD) noted that antipsychotic drugs have the strongest evidence, specifically supporting the use of haloperidol, risperidone, or olanzapine (54). The recommended starting dosage of haloperidol is 0.5 mg twice daily. There is some evidence for using between 1 and 3.5 mg of haloperidol per day to treat agitation and aggression in dementia, but adverse events are quite common. It is unclear if the benefits outweigh the risks. The use of conventional first-generation antipsychotics (FGAs) has been associated with sedation, orthostatic hypotension, increased risk for falls and hip fractures, extrapyramidal symptoms, and tardive dyskinesia (52). Currently, there is no evidence to support the use of low-potency FGAs in elderly patients.

A systematic review of published randomized controlled trials or meta-analyses between 1966 and 2004 that evaluated the efficacy of pharmacologic agents used in the treatment of the neuropsychiatric symptoms of dementia demonstrated modest, but statistically significant, evidence for the efficacy of olanzapine and risperidone. Olanzapine 5 mg and risperidone 1 mg were efficacious doses and well tolerated, except for somnolence. In the frail elderly, the starting dose is recommended at half these just-mentioned doses. Risperidone has a dose-dependent increase in adverse events, with 2 mg or above leading to significant extrapyramidal side effects. Olanzapine has shown efficacy at doses between 5 and 10 mg (but not at 15 mg); somnolence and gait abnormalities were commonly encountered side effects (55). Aripiprazole has also been noted to be efficacious in the treatment of psychosis and other neuropsychiatric symptoms associated with AD and is generally well tolerated. The initial dose used was as low as 2 mg/d, gradually titrated up to 15 mg/d (mean dose at endpoint = 10 mg) (56). Tariot et al. (57) reported on a double-blinded, placebo-controlled study using flexibly dosed quetiapine (median of the mean daily dose: 96.9 mg) and haloperidol (1.9 mg) in treating psychosis in patients with AD. Although both medications did not improve psychosis when compared with placebo, quetiapine was found to be efficacious in treating agitation and was better tolerated than haloperidol (57). Other quetiapine studies have

been negative, and the requirement for titration of this medication to therapeutic doses limits its use in the ED and PES settings. Currently, the evidence for the use of newer atypical antipsychotics in the ED and PES (paliperidone, iloperidone, lurasidone, brexpiprazole, cariprazine) is minimal. Brexpiprazole, a dopamine partial agonist developed from aripiprazole, is being studied for agitation in Alzheimer's disease in current clinical trials and may have a role in the future.

The Clinical Antipsychotic Trials of Intervention Effectiveness—Alzheimer's Disease (CATIE-AD) assessed the effectiveness of second-generation antipsychotics (SGAs) (risperidone, olanzapine, and quetiapine) versus placebo in outpatients with psychosis, aggression, or agitation and AD. Although the phase 1 trial did not demonstrate a large clinical benefit of treatment with SGAs as compared with placebo, the time to discontinuation due to a lack of efficacy favored olanzapine and risperidone. However, time to discontinuation due to adverse events favored placebo, and the authors concluded that the side effects offset the advantages in the efficacy of atypical antipsychotics in treating AD-associated neuropsychiatric symptoms (58). The results of the CATIE-AD trial suggest that the side effects of antipsychotics in the outpatient treatment of the neuropsychiatric symptoms of AD may outweigh the benefits.

Additionally, SGA use for BPSD has been associated with increased risk for cerebrovascular adverse events (59). In 2005, the FDA issued black box warnings stating that older adults treated with SGAs for dementias have an approximately 1.6- to 1.7-fold increased risk of mortality compared with placebo (60). In 2008 this warning was extended to include FGAs as well. The risk for ischemic stroke with FGAs is similar to that with SGAs, and older antipsychotics appear to carry the same or maybe even higher risk of mortality when compared with SGAs (61,62). The mortality risk of antipsychotics may in part depend on the medication used. A study through the Veterans Administration of 46,008 elderly patients with dementia who were receiving antipsychotics between 1998 and 2009 found that haloperidol had the highest mortality with a number needed to harm (NNH) of 26. This was followed by risperidone with an NNH of 27. Next was olanzapine with an NNH of 40, and quetiapine with an NNH of 50. Atypical antipsychotics also demonstrated a dose-response increase in mortality risk with a 3.5% increase in mortality in the high-dose subgroup compared to the low-dose group (63).

Despite the adverse effects of antipsychotics for BPSD, there are times when these medications may be necessary. In emergency situations when behavioral management has been ineffective it is important to utilize careful clinical judgment as well as communicating the risks and benefits of antipsychotics with families, patients, and caregivers. The expert consensus panel guidelines for the treatment of behavioral disturbances in dementia recommend the use of SGAs over FGAs (64). Overall, risperidone has the strongest evidence base for the treatment of BPSD and a treatment algorithm has been developed which uses risperidone as the first step (55,65). Although all antipsychotic use for treating BPSD in the United States is off label, in some non-US countries such as Canada, risperidone has regulatory approval (66). Quetiapine and aripiprazole have less robust evidence than risperidone, but meta-analysis has demonstrated superiority to placebo for both (55,67). However, most of the clinical trials using SGAs in the treatment of the neuro-psychiatric symptoms in dementia demonstrated clinical benefit over a course of days to weeks. Limited literature exists on the use of SGAs in the immediate control of acute agitation in this population.

In a systematic review, FGAs (mainly haloperidol) and SGAs were found to be equally efficacious and safe in the treatment of delirium in medically or surgically ill patients older than 60 years without cognitive disorders. Haloperidol at initial doses of 0.5 to 1 mg daily, olanzapine at 2.5 mg daily, risperidone at 0.5 to 1 mg daily, and quetiapine at 50 mg were used, and further titration was based on clinical judgment and patient tolerability (68). *See the chapter on delirium for additional information.*

Rapid orally disintegrating formulations of risperidone and olanzapine are currently available and may provide an advantage in the ED setting. There is some evidence to support the use of intramuscular injections of olanzapine to treat acute agitation secondary to dementia. In a double-blind study, acutely agitated elderly patients with

AD or vascular dementia or both were randomized to receive either intramuscular olanzapine (2.5 mg or 5.0 mg), intramuscular lorazepam (1 mg), or intramuscular placebo. Olanzapine (2.5 and 5 mg) and lorazepam demonstrated superiority to placebo at 2 hours in reducing agitation. At the end of 24 hours, the clinical superiority continued to exist for both olanzapine doses but not for lorazepam. Olanzapine was found to be both safe and efficacious in elderly patients with agitation (69). Some evidence also exists to support the use of intramuscular ziprasidone in the agitated geriatric patient and its use in EDs is becoming relatively routine (70).

Combining nonpharmacologic interventions with the use of psychotropic medication may decrease the total dose of medication needed to effectively treat agitation. Delirium should be assumed as the possible etiology for agitation, and the search for the cause of the delirium should be continued. Appropriate treatment interventions directed at both the underlying cause and agitation itself should be combined in effectively caring for the agitated elderly. The rationale for continued pharmacologic treatment should be regularly reassessed in the ED.

Benzodiazepines have a limited role in geriatric emergency psychopharmacology. Benzodiazepines that have long half-lives or ones with active metabolites have no role in the treatment of agitation in the elderly. Intramuscular lorazepam, a short-acting benzodiazepine without active metabolites, has been well studied in the agitated elderly. There is literature that argues against the use of lorazepam in elderly cognitively impaired individuals because of the increased risk of falls, respiratory depression, worsening cognition, and paradoxical disinhibition. However, cautious use of lorazepam at 0.5 mg doses (up to 2 mg total) for acute temporary management of agitation in the elderly may be advantageous in alcohol or benzodiazepine withdrawal (51). Also, if antipsychotic monotherapy fails, combining benzodiazepines and neuroleptics might curb acute agitation. There is virtually no indication for using long-acting antipsychotics, lithium, or antidepressants in the ED or PES.

Newer pharmacologic treatments for BPSD are being studied. Pimavanserin, a novel 5-HT2a receptor inverse agonist, is approved in the United States for psychosis in Parkinson's disease. It is being studied in other dementia-related psychoses and has one major advantage of not increasing fall risk (71). Prazosin, an alpha-1 adrenoreceptor antagonist, seems to have preliminary evidence of efficacy in agitation and aggression in Alzheimer's disease (72). Dextromethorphan/quinidine, currently approved for pseudobulbar affect, also is showing efficacy and safety in BPSD studies (73). The usefulness of these potential agents for BPSD in the acute settings of the ED or PES will need to be determined over time.

SELF-NEGLECT SYNDROMES IN THE OLDER ADULT

Self-neglect occurs in several psychiatric disorders. The most common is neglect seen as part of the negative symptoms in schizophrenia. Many of these patients, as they become older, live in CBRFs or other supportive supervised living situations. The other common diagnoses where self-neglect occurs are the dementias. These individuals are usually brought into the health care system before life-threatening neglect occurs. The cases of severe self-neglect in individuals living alone are often first contacted by the police doing "welfare checks" or social service agencies that are contacted by a neighbor, family, or landlord.

Another self-neglect syndrome seen in the elderly has been coined "Diogenes syndrome". Clark et al. in 1975 reported on 30 cases seen in his hospital of patients with extreme self-neglect who did not display any concern of their condition themselves (74,75).

The following describes a local case of "Diogenes syndrome":

A 78-year-old man was found dead in his home of 45 years. He was extremely emaciated, found wearing unwashed clothes, and surrounded by orderly stacks of pre-prepared meals that almost filled the room. When police explored his home, there was no running water; rooms were filled with old papers, letters, and other items to the point where only a walkway existed in some rooms. Neighbors reported that he always said hello and never voiced any complaints. Autopsy revealed death by starvation, with a neuropathology report diagnosing Binswanger dementia.

Diogenes syndrome is reported to occur in previously well-functioning individuals, most often without a history of a chronic psychiatric disorder. The syndrome is characterized by extreme self-neglect, social withdrawal, and hoarding behavior. Individuals often have some insight that something is wrong but are generally apathetic about the situation. There is speculation that this behavior can be due to a neurodegenerative process causing frontal lobe dysfunction (76). These individuals usually come to attention of the medical community when police or a social services agency find an older adult living in squalor and subsequently brings him or her to the ED or PES. When presenting at the ED or PES, these patients often show no distress or clear psychiatric symptoms. Often the lack of concern about their living situation along with an almost normal cognitive exam and reports of extreme self-neglect are diagnostic of this syndrome. On neuropsychological testing, impairment in recognition memory, executive functioning, and conceptualization were predictive of harm resulting from self-neglect (77). These individuals should be hospitalized and undergo both medical and psychiatric evaluations. Many will need protective placement and/or supportive care. They should not be discharged from the ED or PES with an outpatient evaluation arranged for the future which would certainly never be kept.

REFERENCES

1. Center for Medicare & Medicaid Services. (2015). *Nursing home data compendium 2015 edition*. Baltimore, MD: Centers for Medicare & Medicaid Services. Retrieved October 19, 2018, from https://www.cms.gov/Medicare/Provider-Enrollment-and-Certification/CertificationandComplianc/Downloads/nursinghomedatacompendium_508-2015.pdf.
2. Harris-Kojetin, L., Sengupta, M., Park-Lee, E., et al. (2016). Long-term care providers and services users in the United States: Data from the National Study of Long-Term Care Providers, 2013–2014. *Vital and Health Statistics, Series 3*, (38), x–xii, 1–105.
3. Moss, A. J., Harris-Kojetin, L. D., Sengupta, M., et al. (2011). Design and operation of the 2010 National Survey of Residential Care Facilities. *Vital and Health Statistics, Series 1*, (54), 1–131.

4. U.S. Census Bureau. (2017, April). *Facts for features: Older Americans month: May 2017*. Retrieved October 29, 2018, from https://www.census.gov/newsroom/facts-for-features/2017/cb17-ff08.html.

5. Rui, P., & Kang, K. *National Hospital Ambulatory Medical Care Survey: 2015 emergency department summary tables*. Retrieved October 20, 2018, from http://www.cdc.gov/nchs/data/ahcd/nhamcs_emergency/2015_ed_web_tables.pdf.

6. Conwell, Y. (1994). Suicide in elderly patients. In Schneider, L. S., Reynolds, C. F., Lebowitz, B. D., et al. (Eds.), *Diagnosis and treatment of depression in late life* (pp. 397–418). Washington, DC: American Psychiatric Association.

7. Kennedy, G. J., & Lowinger, R. (1993). Psychogeriatric emergencies. *Geriatric Emergency Care, 9*, 641–652.

8. Serper, M. R., & Allen, M. H. (2002). Rapid screening for cognitive impairment in the psychiatric emergency service. I: Cognitive screening batteries. *Psychiatric Services, 53*, 1527–1529.

9. Allen, M. H., Currier, G. W., Carpenter, D., et al. (2005). The expert consensus guideline series. Treatment of behavioral emergencies. *Journal of Psychiatric Practice, 11*(Suppl. 1), 1–108.

10. Loewenstein, D. A., & Mogosky, B. J. (1999). The functional assessment of the older adult patient. In Lichtenberg, P. A. (Ed.), *Handbook of assessment in clinical gerontology*. New York, NY: John Wiley and Sons.

11. Cohen, C., Meesters, P., & Zhao, J. (2015). New perspectives on schizophrenia in later life: For treatment, policy, and research. *Lancet Psychiatry, 2*, 340–350.

12. Maglione, J. E., Vahia, I. V., & Jeste, D. V. (2015). Schizophrenia spectrum and other psychotic disorders. In Steffens, D. C., Blazer, D. G., & Thakur, M. E. (Eds.), *The American Psychiatric Publishing text-book of geriatric psychiatry* (5th ed., pp. 309–332). Washington, DC: American Psychiatric Publishing.

13. Howard, R., Rabins, P. V., Seeman, M. V., et al. (2000). Late-onset schizophrenia and very-late-onset schizophrenia-like psychosis: An international consensus. *American Journal of Psychiatry, 157*, 172–178.

14. Soares, J. C., & Gershon, S. (1997). Therapeutic targets in late-life psychoses: Review of concepts and critical issues. *Schizophrenia Research, 27*, 227–239.

15. Piechniczek-Buczek, J. (2006). Psychiatric emergencies in the elderly population. *Emergency Medicine Clinics of North America, 24*, 467–490.

16. Zayas, E. M., & Grossberg, G. T. (1998). The treatment of psychosis in late life. *The Journal of Clinical Psychiatry, 59*(Suppl. 1), 5–10.

17. Tueth, M. J., & Zuberi, P. (1999). Life-threatening psychiatric emergencies in the elderly: Overview. *Journal of Geriatric Psychiatry and Neurology, 12*, 60–66.

18. Naughton, B. J., Moran, M. B., Kadah, H., et al. (1995). Delirium and other cognitive impairment in older adults in the emergency department. *Annals of Emergency Medicine, 25*, 751–755.

19. Thakur, M. E., & Gwyther, L. P. (2015). Agitation in older adults. In Steffens, D. C., Blazer, D. G., & Thakur, M. E. (Eds.), *The American Psychiatric Publishing text-book of geriatric psychiatry* (5th ed., pp. 507–526). Washington, DC: American Psychiatric Publishing.

20. Carlson, D. L., Fleming, K. C., Smith, G. E., et al. (1995). Management of dementia-related behavioral disturbances: A nonpharmacologic approach. *Mayo Clinic Proceedings, 70*, 1108–1115.

21. Cummings, J., Mintzer, J., Brodaty, H., et al. (2015). Agitation in cognitive disorders: International Psychogeriatric Association provisional consensus clinical and research definition. *International Psychogeriatrics, 27*(1), 7–17.

22. Jeste, D. V., Blazer, D., Casey, D., et al. (2008). ACNP White Paper: Update on use of antipsychotic drugs in elderly persons with dementia. *Neuropsychopharmacology, 33*, 957–970.

23. Sultzer, D. L., Davis, S. M., Tariot, P. N., et al., for the CATIE-AD Study Group. (2008). Clinical symptom responses to atypical antipsychotic medications in Alzheimer's disease: Phase 1 outcomes from the CATIE-AD effectiveness trial. *American Journal of Psychiatry, 165*, 844–854.

24. Sullivan-Marx, E. M. (2001). Achieving restraint-free care of acutely confused older adults. *Journal of Gerontological Nursing, 27*, 56–61.

25. Marks, W. (1992). Physical restraints in the practice of medicine. Current concepts. *Archives of Internal Medicine, 152*, 2203–2206.

26. Xu, J. Q., Murphy, S. L., Kochanek, K. D., et al. (2018). Deaths: Final data for 2016. *National Vital Statistics Reports, 67*(5), 1–75.

27. Conwell, Y., Duberstein, P. R., Caine, E. D., et al. (2002). Risk factors for suicide in later life. *Biological Psychiatry, 52*, 193–204.

28. Joiner, T. (2007). *Why people die by suicide*. London: Harvard University Press.

29. Conejero, I., Olie, E., Courtet, P., et al. (2018). Suicide in older adults: Current perspectives. *Clinical Interventions in Aging, 13*, 691–699.

30. Dombrovski, A. Y., Butters, M. A., Reynolds, C. F., et al. (2008). Cognitive performance in suicidal depressed elderly: Preliminary report. *The American Journal of Geriatric Psychiatry, 16*(2), 109–115.

31. Van Orden, K., & Conwell, Y. (2011). Suicides in late life. *Current Psychiatry Reports, 3*, 234–241.

32. Beck, A. T., Kovacs, M., & Weissman, A. (1979). Assessment of suicidal intention: The scale for suicide ideation. *Journal of Consulting and Clinical Psychology, 47*, 343–352.

33. Bommersbach, T. J., Lapid, M. I., Rummans, T. A., et al. (2015). Geriatric alcohol use disorder: A review for primary care physicians. *Mayo Clinic Proceedings, 90*(5), 659–666.

34. Oslin, D. W. (2004). Late-life alcoholism issues relevant to the geriatric psychiatrist. *The American Journal of Geriatric Psychiatry, 12*, 571–583.

35. Barry, K. L., Blow, F. C., Walton, M. A., et al. (1998). Elder-specific brief alcohol intervention: 3-month outcomes. *Alcoholism: Clinical and Experimental Research, 22*, 32A.

36. Callahan, C. M., & Tierney, W. M. (1995). Health services use and mortality among older primary care patients with alcoholism. *Journal of the American Geriatrics Society, 43*, 1378–1383.

37. Joseph, C. L., Ganzini, L., & Atkinson, R. (1995). Screening for alcohol use disorders in the nursing home. *Journal of the American Geriatrics Society, 43*, 368–373.

38. Oslin, D. W., Streim, J. E., Parmelee, P., et al. (1997). Alcohol abuse: A source of reversible functional disability among residents of a VA nursing home. *International Journal of Geriatric Psychiatry, 12*, 825–832.

39. Brower, K. J., Mudd, S., Blow, F. C., et al. (1994). Severity and treatment of alcohol withdrawal in elderly versus younger patients. *Alcoholism: Clinical and Experimental Research, 18*, 196–201.

40. Blow, F., Gillespie, B., Barry, K., et al. (1998). Brief screening for alcohol problems in elderly populations using the Short Michigan Alcoholism Screening Test–Geriatric version (SMAST-G). *Alcoholism: Clinical and Experimental Research, 22*, 31A.

41. Mayfield, D., McLeod, G., & Hall, P. (1974). The CAGE questionnaire: Validation of a new alcoholism instrument. *American Journal of Psychiatry, 131*, 1121–1123.

42. Oslin, D. W., Liberto, J. G., O'Brien, J., et al. (1997). Naltrexone as an adjunctive treatment for older patients with alcohol dependence. *The American Journal of Geriatric Psychiatry, 5*, 324–332.

43. Gueorguieva, R., Wu, R., Tsai, W. M., et al. (2015). An analysis of moderators in the COMBINE study: Identifying subgroups of patients who benefit from acamprosate. *European Neuropsychopharmacology, 25*(10), 1586–1599.

44. Finlayson, R. E., & Hofmann, V. (2002). Prescription drug misuse: Treatment strategies. In Gurnack, A. M., Atkinson, R. M., & Osgood, N. J. (Eds.), *Treating alcohol and drug abuse in the elderly* (pp. 155–174). New York, NY: Springer-Verlag.

45. Streim, J. E., & Katz, I. R. (2004). Psychiatric aspects of long-term care. In Sadavoy, J., Jarvik, L. F., Grossberg, G. T., et al. (Eds.), *Comprehensive textbook of geriatric psychiatry* (3rd ed., pp. 1071–1102). New York, NY: WW Norton.

46. Thienhaus, O. J., & Piasecki, M. P. (2004). Assessment of geriatric patients in the psychiatric emergency service. *Psychiatric Services, 55*, 639–640, 642.

47. Yazgan, I. C., Greenwald, B. S., Kremen, N. J., et al. (2004). Geriatric psychiatry versus general psychiatry inpatient treatment of the elderly. *American Journal of Psychiatry, 161*(2), 352–355.

48. National Association of Psychiatric Health Systems. (2006). *2005 annual survey: National trends in behavioral health care* (p. 35). Washington, DC: National Association of Psychiatric Health Systems.

49. Blank, K., Hixon, L., Gruman, C., et al. (2005). Determinants of geropsychiatric inpatient length of stay. *Psychiatric Quarterly, 72*(2), 195–212.

50. Siddiqi, N., House, A. O., & Holmes, J. D. (2006). Occurrence and outcome of delirium in medical inpatients: A systematic literature review. *Age and Ageing, 35*, 350–364.

51. Roose, S. P., Pollock, B. G., & Devanand, D. P. (2009). Treatment during late life. In Schatzberg, A. F., & Nemeroff, C. B. (Eds.), *The American Psychiatric Publishing textbook of psychopharmacology* (4th ed.). Arlington, VA: American Psychiatric Publishing.

52. Nassisi, D., Korc, B., Hahn, S., et al. (2006). The evaluation and management of the acutely agitated elderly patient. *Mount Sinai Journal of Medicine, 73*, 976–984.

53. American Psychiatric Association. (2016). *Practice guideline on the use of antipsychotics to treat agitation or psychosis in patients with dementia.* Retrieved September 1, 2018, from http://psychiatryonline.org/doi/pdf/10.1176/appi.books.9780890426807.

54. Azermai, M., Petrovic, M., Elseviers, M., et al. (2012). Systematic appraisal of dementia guidelines for the management of behavioural and psychological symptoms. *Ageing Research Reviews, 11*(1), 78–86.

55. Sink, K. M., Holden, K. F., & Yaffe, K. (2005). Pharmacological treatment of neuropsychiatric symptoms of dementia: A review of the evidence. *JAMA, 293,* 596–608.

56. Schneider, L. S., Dagerman, K., & Insel, P. S. (2006). Efficacy and adverse effects of atypical antipsychotics for dementia: Meta-analysis of randomized, placebo-controlled trials. *The American Journal of Geriatric Psychiatry, 14,* 191–210.

57. Tariot, P. N., Schneider, L., Katz, I. R., et al. (2006). Quetiapine treatment of psychosis associated with dementia. A double-blind, randomized, placebo-controlled clinical trial. *The American Journal of Geriatric Psychiatry, 14,* 767–776.

58. Schneider, L. S., Tariot, P. N., Dagerman, K. S., et al. (2006). Effectiveness of atypical antipsychotic drugs in patients with Alzheimer's disease. *The New England Journal of Medicine, 355,* 1525–1538.

59. Schneider, L. S., Dagerman, K. S., & Insel, P. (2005). Risk of death with atypical antipsychotic drug treatment for dementia: Meta-analysis of randomized placebo-controlled trials. *JAMA, 294,* 1934–1943.

60. FDA. *Atypical antipsychotic drugs information.* Retrieved September 5, 2018, from https://www.fda.gov/Drugs/DrugSafety/ucm094303.htm.

61. Gill, S. S., Rochon, P. A., Herrmann, N., et al. (2005). Atypical antipsychotic drugs and risk of ischemic stroke: Population based retrospective cohort study. *BMJ, 330,* 450.

62. Wang, P. S., Schneeweiss, S., Avorn, J., et al. (2005). Risk of death in elderly users of conventional vs. atypical antipsychotic medications. *The New England Journal of Medicine, 353,* 2335–2341.

63. Maust, D. T., Kim, H. M., Seyfried, L. S., et al. (2015). Antipsychotics, other psychotropics, and the risk of death in patients with dementia: Number needed to harm. *JAMA Psychiatry, 72,* 438–445.

64. Alexopoulos, G., Jeste, D., Chun, H., et al. (2005). The expert consensus guideline series. Treatment of dementia and its behavioral disturbances. *Postgraduate Medicine*, (Spec No), 6–22.

65. Davies, S. J., Burhan, A. M., Kim, D., et al. (2018). Sequential drug treatment algorithm for agitation and aggression in Alzheimer's and mixed dementia. *Journal of Psychopharmacology, 32*(5), 509–523.

66. Health Canada. *Risperidone–Restriction of the dementia indication.* Retrieved September 2, 2018, from http://healthycanadians.gc.ca/recall-alert-rappel-avis/hc-sc/2015/43797a-eng.php.

67. Cheung, G., & Stapelberg, J. (2011). Quetiapine for the treatment of behavioral and psychological symptoms of dementia (BPSD): A meta-analysis of randomized placebo-controlled trials. *The New Zealand Medical Journal, 124,* 39–50.

68. Lacasse, H., Perreault, M. M., & Williamson, D. R. (2006). Systematic review of antipsychotics for the treatment of hospital-associated delirium in medically or surgically ill patients. *Annals of Pharmacotherapy, 40,* 1966–1973.

69. Meehan, K. M., Wang, H., David, S. R., et al. (2002). Comparison of rapidly acting intramuscular olanzapine, lorazepam and placebo: A double-blind, randomized study in acutely agitated patients with dementia. *Neuropsychopharmacology, 26,* 494–504.

70. Rais, A. R., Williams, K., Rais, T., Singh, T., & Tamburrino, M. (2010). Use of intramuscular ziprasidone for the control of acute psychosis or agitation in an inpatient geriatric population: An open-label study. *Psychiatry, 7*(1), 17–24.

71. Cummings, J., Ballard, C., Tariot, P., et al. (2018). Pimavanserin: Potential treatment for dementia-related psychosis. *The Journal of Prevention of Alzheimer's Disease, 5,* 253–258.

72. Wang, L. Y., Shofer, J. B., Rohde, K., et al. (2009). Prazosin for the treatment of behavioral symptoms in patients with Alzheimer disease with agitation and aggression. *The American Journal of Geriatric Psychiatry, 17*(9), 744–751.

73. Cummings, J. L., Lyketsos, C. G., Peskind, E. R., et al. (2015). Effect of dextromethorphan-quinidine on agitation in patients with Alzheimer disease dementia. *JAMA, 314,* 1233–1254.

74. Clark, A. N., Mankikar, G. D., & Gray, I. (1975). Diogenes syndrome: A clinical study of gross neglect in old age. *Lancet, 1*(7903), 366–368.

75. Reyes-Ortiz, C. A. (2001). Diogenes syndrome: The self-neglect elderly. *Comprehensive Therapy, 27*(2), 117–121.

76. Cipriani, G., Lucetti, C., Vedovello, M., & Nuti, A. (2012). Diogenes syndrome in patients suffering from dementia. *Dialogues in Clinical Neuroscience, 14*(4), 455–460.

77. Tierney, M. C., Snow, W. G., Charles, J., et al. (2007). Neuropsychological predictors of self-neglect in cognitively impaired older people who live alone. *American Journal of Psychiatry, 15*(2), 140–148.

36

The Psychiatric Emergency Care of the Patient With Intellectual Disability

Mark J. Hauser, Robert Kohn

Clinicians who work in psychiatric emergency services (PES) are likely to encounter individuals with an intellectual disability (intellectual developmental disability, ID). The term intellectual disability encompasses many disorders that are defined in the *Diagnostic and Statistical Manual of Mental Disorders*, 5th Ed. (DSM-5) in the chapter "Neurodevelopmental Disorders." Intellectual disability or intellectual developmental disability is defined as a disorder with onset during the developmental period that includes both intellectual and adaptive functioning deficits in conceptual, social, and practical domains (1). DSM-5 no longer utilizes intelligence quotient (IQ) test scores exclusively in defining severity of intellectual disability; instead it focuses on deficits in intellectual function, such as reasoning, problem solving, planning, abstract thinking, judgment, academic learning, and learning from experience, confirmed by both clinical assessment and individualized, standardized intelligence testing; and on deficits in adaptive functioning that result in failure to meet developmental and sociocultural standards for personal independence and social responsibility. Individuals with autistic spectrum disorder (ASD) have deficits in social communication and social interaction and impairments in social emotional responsivity, nonverbal communicative behaviors used for social interaction, and deficits in developing, maintaining, and understanding relationships (1). One prevalence study of ASD in the United States found that approximately one-fourth have ID (2). The severity specifiers for intellectual disability are based on adaptive functioning: mild, moderate, severe, and profound.

The prevalence of intellectual disability in the United States is estimated to be between 1.1% and 3.2% (3,4). The National Comorbidity Survey Adolescent Supplement found that compared to those without ID, individuals with ID had a significantly higher prevalence of mental disorders in particular specific phobia, agoraphobia and bipolar disorder; 65% had a comorbid lifetime mental disorder (4). In addition, adolescents with ID have comorbid disorders with more severe impairment than those without ID. Similarly, adults with ID experience higher rates of mental disorders than the general population (5). In particular, individuals with Down syndrome are at high risk for developing neurocognitive disorder at an early age, an Alzheimer disease–like pattern. These comorbid mental disorders persist into adulthood and old age, as individuals with ID are living longer and healthier lives (6).

Individuals with ID might present for emergency psychiatric evaluation at any point in the life cycle and are twice as likely than the general population to present to the emergency department for a medical or mental disorder (7). Individuals with ID or other forms of neurodevelopmental disorders rarely present for emergency evaluation because of the neurodevelopmental disorder diagnosis. Rather, they present because of an acute problem that has occurred in addition to their ID.

Typically, evaluation, assessment, and treatment are complicated by the impairments inherent in an ID diagnosis. Many clinicians feel uncomfortable by the prospect of evaluating or treating patients with intellectual disabilities, as medical education often lacks specific training about patients with ID (8). During the initial encounter with such patients, many clinicians may feel unqualified to evaluate or treat the patient. Competent evaluation of the patient with ID requires clinicians to adapt their usual approach to account for the unique characteristics of the patient. This chapter focuses on intellectual disability as the primary form of neurodevelopmental disorder. The strategies and techniques presented are relevant and applicable with other neurodevelopmental disorders as well.

THE PATIENT WITH INTELLECTUAL DISABILITY

Intellectual disability refers to deficits in cognitive and adaptive functioning with onset during the developmental period (up to age 18). The diagnosis of ID has diverse etiologies, and in many cases the etiology is not known. ID is an enduring condition that persists over time. However, persons with ID continue to grow and develop over time, frequently displaying developmental progress, but at times punctuated by developmental setbacks. The cognitive impairment itself is unlikely to be the cause of presentation for emergency psychiatric evaluation or visits to the emergency department. The relevant issue is how ID complicates the presenting problem, evaluation, emergency management, and treatment planning. This discussion presumes, then, that an acute condition is present that becomes the focus of evaluation and treatment, conducted in the context of a longstanding intellectual or other neurodevelopmental disorder.

EPIDEMIOLOGY AND ETIOLOGY

Intellectual disability occurs in all socioeconomic groups around the world. The prevalence of intellectual disability is, however, inversely associated with parental socioeconomic status (4). Many studies have found a higher prevalence in males (2). Advances in biology and genetic analysis have resulted in the detection of more than 700 genes linked to ID, explaining only 15% of cases thus far (9). With testing, a biologic cause can be detected in a large proportion of affected individuals, yet the cause can remain unknown or be nonbiologic, as in the case of psychosocial factors. Known etiologic factors include the following:

clearly defined genetic causes (eg, Angelman syndrome, Down syndrome [Trisomy 21], fragile-X syndrome, phenylketonuria, Prader-Willi syndrome, Rubinstein-Taybi syndrome, Smith-Magenis syndrome, tuberous sclerosis complex, Williams syndrome, chromosome duplication and deletions), maternal prenatal factors (eg, poor nutrition, fetal alcohol syndrome and other toxicity from substance abuse, advanced age, tobacco use, diabetes, hypertension, epilepsy, asthma, infections), perinatal factors (eg, cerebral anoxia during difficult delivery, preterm birth), neonatal factors (eg, low birthweight), acquired childhood diseases (eg, encephalitis, meningitis), head injury, environmental factors (eg, nutritional factors, toxins such as lead), and psychosocial factors.

PRESENTATION FOR EMERGENCY EVALUATION

Some PES clinicians may mistakenly fail to apply the usual goals of psychiatric emergency care for those patients with ID. The primary goals—namely, assessment of risk of harm to self or others; completion of biologic, psychological, and social assessment; development of a patient-centered treatment plan; and treatment in a less restrictive setting—apply to patients with ID in the same way as other psychiatric emergency patients. An individual with ID may demonstrate poor frustration tolerance, may become irritable and exhibit a behavioral decompensation, or may develop psychiatric symptoms that become the focus of evaluation. ID often results in increased vulnerability to stress and sensitivity to changes in the environment. Therefore, the presence of ID may set the stage for a decompensation that leads to an emergency psychiatric evaluation. Four functions of problem behavior should be considered in any evaluation, as follows (10):

- Socioenvironmental control. Aggression and self-injurious behavior can be reinforced (eg, removing a person from an unpleasant situation in response to such behavior will increase the probability that the person will react similarly in the future).
- Communication. Problem behaviors can be a nonverbal means of communicating a variety of messages (eg, attention, discomfort, needs).

- Modulation of physical discomfort. Medical conditions, including adverse effects of medications, can cause physical discomfort, leading to aggression or self-injurious behavior.
- Modulation of emotional discomfort. Problem behaviors can occur as a state-dependent function of disorders such as major depression or bipolar disorder, manic phase.

The following are among the reasons an individual with ID may be brought to a PES:

- A change in mental status—for example, confusion, agitation, or psychotic symptoms.
- A change in mood, energy, or sleep patterns.
- A change in behavior, such as a new onset of irritability or aggressive behavior toward others or self-destructive thoughts or behavior (eg, head banging).
- New physical complaints, such as pain, or behaviors, such as agitation, that might signify physical illness. Sorting out such problems can be extremely challenging. An unimpaired person might say, "My stomach hurts," whereas an individual with ID might become irritable and lash out at their family or residential staff as a result of some physical pain.
- Loss of a favored relative or caregiver.

Correlated with visits to PES are prior history of visits to the emergency department, involvement with the criminal justice system, living with family rather than in a group home, greater family distress, not having a family doctor, not having a crisis plan, recent life events, and severity of disability (11,12).

Table 36.1 lists short- and long-term stressors that may trigger behavioral problems or exacerbate a psychiatric disorder in individuals with ID (13).

CONDUCTING THE EVALUATION

When conducting an evaluation for a patient with a neurodevelopmental disorder, the psychiatrist must consider both the underlying condition and the acute presentation. This does not require evaluators to completely alter their usual approach to patients; rather, psychiatrists should adapt their usual approach to fit the unique circumstances. Certain strategies can improve the likelihood of a successful emergency evaluation, thus leading to an effective treatment plan.

In approaching a patient with ID, the emergency psychiatrist relies upon his or her training in medicine as well as psychiatry. The search for an underlying medical cause of the presentation is perhaps the most important role of the emergency clinician. Individuals with ID who are brought to the emergency department because of a change in mental status or a behavioral disturbance may actually have an underlying medical or surgical problem that has not previously been identified. Awareness of this possibility is a first step; conducting a physical exam and obtaining appropriate laboratory tests may result in a diagnosis. At times there are signs and symptoms of illness. Behaviors might provide clues, such as head banging that indicates a headache, or tugging at an ear that indicates an ear infection. In such cases the psychiatrist should make the appropriate medical or surgical referrals. Often the psychiatrist can contribute further as an advocate for the patient by helping nonpsychiatric clinicians understand the patient's behavior and the underlying precipitant. In this way the psychiatrist can help ensure that the patient receives the appropriate evaluation and treatment. Another strategy of the successful evaluator is to resist the temptation to reach a premature conclusion—specifically, to resist an inappropriate diagnosis of "behavioral outburst due to ID." It could lead to a catastrophic outcome to overlook an underlying medical cause of a change in mental status or behavioral decompensation.

This is not to say that there is always an underlying medical condition. Sometimes there are behavioral issues that are best dealt with by skilled behavioral staff conducting a functional assessment of maladaptive behaviors and implementing a thoughtful behavior plan. The assessment of maladaptive behaviors in an individual with ID can be challenging and rewarding. PES clinicians should be given additional training in such behavioral interventions, especially in situations in which communication deficits or impaired social relatedness exist.

The first step of a successful evaluation is to identify an appropriate location for the evaluation. The ideal location is in a safe setting that is quiet and private, where possible. Being in the emergency department can be frightening, distracting, or overstimulating to the patient with ID and the psychiatrist. A confounding variable is that some

TABLE 36.1 Stressors That May Trigger Behavioral Problems

Type of Stressor	Examples
Transitional phases	Change of residence, new school or work place, altered route to work Developmental landmarks (eg, going into puberty, achieving majority)
Interpersonal loss or rejection	Loss of parent, caregiver, friend, or roommate Breakup of romantic attachment Being fired from a job or suspended from school
Environmental	Overcrowding, excessive noise, disorganization Lack of satisfactory stimulation Reduced privacy in congregate housing School or work stress
Parenting and social support problems	Lack of support from family, friends, or partner Destabilizing visits, phone calls, or letters Neglect Hostility Physical or sexual abuse
Illness or disability	Chronic medical or psychiatric illness Serious acute illness Sensory defects Difficulty with ambulation Seizures
Stigmatization because of physical or intellectual problems	Taunts, teasing, exclusion, being bullied or exploited
Frustration	Due to inability to communicate needs and wishes Due to lack of choices about residence, work situation, diet Because of realization of deficits

Republished with permission of American Association on Intellectual Developmental Disabilities, from Rush, A. J., & Frances, A. (2000). The expert consensus guidelines: Treatment of psychiatric and behavioral problems in mental retardation. *American Journal of Mental Retardation, 105*(3), 159–228; permission conveyed through Copyright Clearance Center, Inc. With permission.

ID individuals obtain positive reinforcement from the attention received for disruptive behaviors (eg, throwing a tantrum), especially when other patients, families, and staff constitute an audience. Although noise and distractions are inevitable in the emergency setting, finding a quieter and more private place can lessen their impact.

An appropriate location to conduct the evaluation should be found without delay, because patients with intellectual disability may have a diminished capacity to cope with waiting. Having to wait may cause additional behavioral deterioration, which may make the subsequent evaluation and any intervention more difficult. During the evaluation, family or familiar residential or day program staff should be invited whenever possible to keep the patient company. This precaution serves a dual purpose. First, the patient benefits from the predictability fostered by the presence of someone familiar; second, the patient's regular caregivers will be needed to provide history. The emergency psychiatrist should take the time to explain any tests and procedures as simply and clearly as is necessary for the patient to follow what is happening and to reduce the patient's anxiety.

The evaluation must involve speaking to and involving the patient regardless of the severity of the intellectual disability, and whether the individual with ID can participate in a clinical interview. For those who can undertake a clinical interview, the psychiatrist should consider how to structure the interview of the patient prior to initiating the interview and commence with questions that will place the patient at ease (14). An assessment of the patient's communication ability should be conducted at the outset. Leading questions should be avoided to minimize suggestibility. Phrases and questions should be short simple sentences stated one at a time avoiding metaphors, idioms, medical jargon, or other words that the patient might not understand. Obtain confirmation that questions were correctly understood before proceeding and if needed repeat the question. The use of visual aids may be appropriate in some cases.

Although the psychiatrist can begin an evaluation with limited information, obtaining information from collateral sources is vital. A comprehensive evaluation that encompasses many sources of information and includes both the recent and long-term history is valuable. In the assessment of a patient with ID, the concerns of the referring caregiver should be elicited. It is helpful to consider the context of the decision to seek emergency consultation. The caregiver's vantage point might or might not be comprehensive, and other vantage points might be relevant and supplement the assessment. Sometimes the caregiver of an individual with ID has been reluctant to involve medical personnel in the client's care. This reluctance may lead to delay until the problem is far advanced or at a point of crisis. Sometimes the decision to turn to the emergency department is reached when the caregivers are overly burdened and feel that they can no longer cope with the patient's behavior (15). Although they may come in grudgingly, caregivers expect the PES clinicians to solve the problem even though the behavioral issues are long-standing.

When the situation has deteriorated, one solution involves addressing the caregiver burden and arranging a much needed and appreciated respite. In other cases, respite represents wishful thinking and a desire to avoid tackling larger problems such as implementing appropriate behavioral management and sufficient residential staffing levels, or reconsideration of the residential placement. Another potential solution is a recommendation for medication that might help resolve the problem. One possible outcome of an emergency consultation is an acknowledgment of a problem that cannot be fixed in the PES. Another outcome is recognition that the solution

requires an array of interventions best implemented by outpatient crisis services, outpatient clinic providers, or hospitalization. When there is no immediate solution, caregivers may react with disappointment or frustration directed toward the emergency personnel. The clinician must be aware that such feelings may arise and must be prepared to manage these situations where there is no rapid resolution of the behavioral issues. Under pressure to resolve the situation, some clinicians will add or change a medication in order to do something, anything; even if it may not be appropriate. It often takes longer to have caregivers to accept a plan for nonpharmacological interventions when indicated rather than prescribing a medication that closes prematurely a discussion of nonpharmacological interventions and does not address the core issues.

Caregivers of patients with intellectual disability have characteristics that may influence their interactions with PES clinicians:

- Caregivers often have a long-standing involvement in the client's life and devotion toward that client. (Some caregivers are family members, whereas others are residential staff—paid or volunteer.)
- Caregivers may have an ideological perspective that medication is toxic and should be avoided. They may be skeptical about the role of medication and resist its use.
- Caregivers may yearn for a medication that could solve the entire problem.
- Caregivers may mistrust clinicians generally, as they may have had a bad experience in the past; while others may have great faith in clinicians and overvalue the potential for cure.
- Not all residential staff who present in the PES are caregivers, such as staff who may merely be transporting the client and hardly know the individual.

By understanding these characteristics and showing respect for the caregiver, it is possible to manage potential conflicts and promote proper care of the patient during the current episode and beyond.

Intellectual disability may obscure the standard diagnostic indicators of psychiatric disorders. For one thing, especially for the psychiatrist unaccustomed to the normal manifestations of intellectual disability, these manifestations may overshadow symptoms attributable to psychiatric illness (16). Moreover, impairments in cognitive and verbal skills make it difficult for many developmentally disabled individuals to articulate abstract or global concepts such as a depressed mood. Most DSM-5 diagnoses require the patient to describe his or her internal state. Asking an individual with a significant cognitive impairment or learning disability about hallucinations, delusions, or guilt is seldom productive. On the other hand, the person's disorganized behavior may have diagnostic significance (17). These are the challenges that individuals with ID often pose for psychiatric diagnosis.

Four aspects of intellectual disability may influence diagnosis (18):

- Intellectual distortion: Emotional symptoms are difficult to elicit because of deficits in abstract thinking and in receptive and expressive language skills.
- Psychosocial masking: Limited social experiences can influence the content of psychiatric symptoms (eg, mania presenting as a belief that one can drive a car).
- Cognitive disintegration: Decreased ability to tolerate stress can lead to anxiety-induced decompensation (sometimes misinterpreted as psychosis).
- Baseline exaggeration: Increase in severity or frequency of chronic maladaptive behavior after onset of psychiatric illness.

To allow for these possible distortions, diagnostic criteria for most DSM-5 disorders have been adapted for those with mild/moderate ID and severe/profound ID, which focus on biologic signs and symptoms and behavioral equivalents to subjective states (19).

The presence of an intellectual disability renders the person less well equipped to provide his or her history. In the face of communication difficulties, individuals frequently communicate through their behavior. Information should be obtained not only about the current problem and the events leading up to it but also about the patient's usual level of functioning. Behavioral changes may present as increased irritability or impulsivity, self-injury, or outbursts of aggression. A change from the usual level of functioning may be a clue to an underlying medical issue, such as constipation, a dental problem, a headache, or an infection (especially of the urinary tract). An underlying medical problem is perhaps the most important diagnostic possibility to rule in or rule out. Overlooking an underlying medical problem is a costly error, one likely to occur when the evaluator is distracted by the presence of a preexisting psychiatric problem or severe maladaptive behaviors.

On the other hand, when a careful evaluation yields no obvious underlying medical problem to account for the presentation, then the diagnosis of an onset or exacerbation of a psychiatric disorder should be considered. At times the diagnosis is simply behavioral, in that the patient is reacting to a psychosocial stressor, such as a change in the patient's environment. Examples of stressors include the loss of a favorite residential staff member; new staff who are not versed in the behavioral plan or how to interact with the individual; recent placement in a new residence; change in routine; disruption of the residential environment by the placement of a new resident; illness of a family member; change in frequency of family visits; or the developmental accomplishment of a sibling, such as graduation, marriage, or birth of a child. Effective intervention requires attention to these stressors, with appropriate use of adjunct medication when needed. Such a comprehensive approach may be outside the scope of a medical emergency department.

Medication side effects are another possible cause of behavioral deterioration. A high proportion of individuals with ID receive polypharmacy, three or more psychotropic medications concurrently (20). Benzodiazepines are commonly used as antianxiety medication. Benzodiazepines with long half-lives may accumulate and cause drowsiness and mental clouding. Short-acting benzodiazepines may cause interdose rebound with worsening of anxiety prior to the next scheduled dose. Individuals with ASD who take benzodiazepines may develop ataxia. In persons with communication deficits, such side effects may not be readily apparent or may persist undetected.

Antipsychotic medication can cause parkinsonism and akathisia, which patients with intellectual disability may have difficulty reporting because of communication deficits. Individuals with ID may be at greater risk of developing these side effects or having them exacerbated by inappropriate interventions. Akathisia can present as worsening agitation and can thus lead to increased dosage of an antipsychotic, causing further iatrogenic harm. Antipsychotic drugs can also interfere with alertness and overall performance.

It is important to maintain individuals with intellectual disability on the lowest effective dose of antipsychotic medication to control psychotic symptoms or target behaviors. Abrupt dose reductions can trigger problems such as agitation, behavioral deterioration, and worsening of abnormal involuntary movements, which may represent transient withdrawal dyskinesia. Therefore, dosage reductions are best accomplished when implemented slowly and carefully. Anticholinergic medications to counteract antipsychotic medication side effects should be used cautiously as they may further exacerbate cognitive impairment.

Other medications that may be missing from a list of current medications may cause acute psychiatric symptoms. These include antihypertensive drugs, eye drops for glaucoma (often beta-adrenergic blockers), and allergy medications.

It is important for the patient to undergo a thorough physical examination, performed systematically and patiently. This might be done by the medical emergency department or by the psychiatrist. The presence of familiar family or residential staff may help calm and reassure the patient during the physical exam. In some emergencies, when a patient cannot comply with examination, sedation may be necessary.

The PES clinician should take into account not only the presenting problem but also the patient's relationships with caregivers, family members, friends, and other clients. Individuals with ID are at risk of emotional, physical, or sexual abuse. At times, behavioral issues are a clue to an abusive situation. Therefore, the evaluator must be alert for signs of suspected or possible abuse and recognize their role as a mandated reporter.

A situation that arises repeatedly in the PES might be referred to as "the vanishing problem." That is, a person who presents for evaluation following a behavioral outburst has settled down by the time of the evaluation. A hospital emergency room is quite different from the patient's usual environment. A PES or free-standing crisis clinic may or may not be more homelike. In some cases, as discussed earlier, this change of environments exacerbates the immediate problem. In other cases, it allows the immediate problem to resolve. Even the ride to the emergency room can contribute to the resolution. If the residential staff person describes a behavioral outburst that has since resolved, it may be the case that stressors in the patient's environment, which are not present in the emergency department, triggered the behavior. This leaves the emergency department in the awkward position of having to conduct an evaluation after the problem has resolved.

For an individual with ID, a PES visit can be frightening, but it also can be perceived as enjoyable because of the increased attention without making demands. At worst, the PES is reinforced as the place to go when the individual is unhappy with their living situation and recognizes which behaviors will trigger a repeat visit in the future. A typical pattern then evolves, with recurrent PES visits and no resolution of the underlying issues. The residential staff may become reluctant to accept the person back, knowing that the circumstances there can be expected to trigger a recurrence of the problem. In a comprehensive psychiatric emergency system, the residential staff may be more accepting of discharge if they know that a mobile crisis team will be following up with the patient to ensure continuing treatment and linkage.

Emergency clinicians at times have excessive expectations of the capabilities of a residential program. At times there is a perception that the residential facility is a nursing home or approximates the round-the-clock staffing and services of a hospital. The typical residential program is more like a home with staff who assist with daily living skills and supports that overcome the challenges of the neurodevelopmental disorder. These supports do not substitute for a hospital level of care.

Psychopharmacologic treatment should be reserved for appropriate target disorders and syndromes. Medications should not be administered to the patient simply to diminish the caregivers anxiety. In such cases skillful management of family or residential staff expectations is beneficial. For example, the PES clinician can acknowledge that it would be ideal to have a medication that would effectively treat the symptoms without producing serious side effects, but such a medication may not exist. It is important to address possible environmental causes of problem behaviors. This will help the family or residential staff recognize the contexts in which such behaviors occur and make appropriate adjustments. One risk of prescribing antipsychotic medications for their nonspecific tranquilizing effect is that these medications will be continued indefinitely, resulting in the possibility of serious or long-term side effects.

In the presence of a psychiatric diagnosis, psychiatric medications are often necessary. Individuals with ID, as is the general population, are at risk for the full range of psychiatric disorders. They can suffer from major depressive disorder, bipolar disorder, obsessive-compulsive disorder, schizophrenia and other psychotic disorders, posttraumatic stress disorder, anxiety disorder, tic disorder/Tourette syndrome, eating disorders (pica, rumination), attention deficit disorder, and major neurocognitive disorders. In addition, pharmacologic treatment may be useful in treating certain symptoms that have not responded to reasonable behavioral and environmental interventions. Benzodiazepines, other sedating hypnotics, and some sedating antidepressants are helpful for the short-term treatment of sleep disturbances.

The treatment of impulsivity and aggression has two components: the acute psychiatric emergency and the management of chronic, persistent behaviors. The rate of aggression and impulsivity across studies ranges from 14% to 56% across studies of the ID population (21). In the acute treatment, medications must be chosen that will not oversedate the patient or cause disabling side effects. This may mask the more common reasons for aggression in this population, including hunger, pain, thirst, infection, fecal impaction, fear, recent abuse, and postictal confusion. Although oral antipsychotics are preferable, injectable antipsychotics may be used acutely. Benzodiazepines may cause disinhibition or oversedation but may be used as an adjunct to the antipsychotic if needed.

In the PES, the psychiatrist can initiate a psychotropic drug trial if he or she has ruled out nonpsychiatric etiologies or there is a need to temporarily address behavioral problems that have resulted from an underlying medical etiology. Few randomized controlled trials have been conducted for problematic behaviors, such

as aggression, psychotic symptoms, and self-injurious behaviors (22,23). Risperidone and olanzapine have randomized controlled trials showing them to be efficacious with patients with ID. Anticonvulsants such as valproic acid and carbamazepine, as well as lithium, buspirone, selective serotonin reuptake inhibitors (SSRIs), beta-blockers, and clonidine, have been reported in the literature to treat persistent impulsivity and aggression in patients with ID.

Self-injurious behavior occurs as a response to pain (infection of ear or sinus; dental disease; glaucoma; migraines; seizures; delirium; gastrointestinal problems, including impaction; menstruation or pregnancy) and medication side effects, among other medical etiologies. Such behavior in individuals with ID may occur in the context of psychosis, anxiety disorders, mood disorders, substance use, personality disorders, or an undefined cause. Behavior management and the treatment of underlying medical conditions should be accomplished first. Comorbid diagnoses such as psychotic disorders, bipolar disorder, depressive disorder, and compulsive disorders may also need to be treated with antipsychotics, anticonvulsants, and antidepressants if contributory (24).

In general, doses of medications for individuals with intellectual disability are guided by the same knowledge base as with other patients. In actual practice, one finds that it is usually better to begin with dosing strategies used in child psychiatry and geriatric psychiatry. Often it is better to start with a low introductory dose and increase the dose gradually, with subsequent dose decisions dependent on the patient's response.

DECISION REGARDING HOSPITALIZATION

The conclusion of an emergency evaluation requires consideration of the appropriate disposition of the patient with intellectual disability. It must be determined whether the patient requires a hospital level of care, and if so, whether he or she must be hospitalized involuntarily. Typically, inpatient psychiatry units are reluctant to accept patients with ID. They assert that the patient will not fit into the milieu or will not be able to participate in the usual therapeutic activities. Often this is true. Inpatient psychiatric care for individuals with ID requires some adaptation to individualized needs. Another frequent assertion is that inpatient staff lack specialized training in dealing with individuals with ID, and therefore are reluctant to undertake such treatment. It poses a challenge to the PES to determine whether these assertions represent valid considerations or convenient excuses. Inpatient units also reject admission for persons with ID because of a concern that there will be nowhere for them to go after the hospitalization. There are many examples of individuals who have remained nearly indefinitely on a psychiatric inpatient unit for want of an alternative destination, a circumstance that generates enduring reluctance to accept subsequent patients with ID. This issue can be resolved with advance planning in the form of interagency agreements that guarantee posthospital placement. Many individuals with ID have been receiving services from their state department of developmental disability or from an agency that provides residential care. Such a system should be available to resume ongoing care after the emergency treatment and often provides ID respite housing.

Some systems of care utilize their PES for an additional expanded role, as an overnight observation period and which may serve as a respite for both the patient and caregivers. Once demonstrating stability through the night, disposition back to the community may be more successful. The use of the PES in a respite and stabilizing role, can also obviate the need for inpatient hospitalization altogether, and greatly reduce the issues that arise in the referral process such as the reluctance of inpatient sites to accept this population.

In some cases, when the existing caregivers are not capable of caring for the person during the acute episode, PES clinicians must help develop an alternative plan. Such a plan may include temporary acute hospitalization. However, appropriate acute treatment coupled with long-term treatment strategies may make it possible for the individual to return to his or her prior environment.

COMPREHENSIVE TREATMENT PLANNING

In some cases, the emergency evaluation is a one-time interaction. In other cases, the clinician, or team of clinicians, is able to maintain involvement.

Some systems of care have established emergency teams to provide evaluation and consultation over time, with the goal of avoiding the use of emergency rooms and inappropriate hospitalizations. Some systems of care recognize the importance of establishing clinical services with the goal of avoiding overuse of the PES and avoiding inappropriate hospitalizations.

Comprehensive treatment planning includes consideration of a variety of categories of intervention. For example, a consultation regarding behavioral management strategies is likely to be helpful. PES clinicians may be able to call upon outpatient ID case management to come to the PES to provide such a consultation. Whereas behavioral management addresses the behaviors of the patient, effective strategies are designed to guide the actions of the family or residential or day program staff as they respond to recurrent behavioral issues. Family or staff responses should be purposeful, predictable, and consistent, with consistency applying to all staff interacting with the patient. Many residential programs are staffed 24 hours a day, and it is valuable for each staff person to present a consistent approach. With proper planning and training, residential staff are capable of collecting data over time using a data collection mechanism that focuses on target behaviors and target systems. These data can provide reliable information that is useful in the PES. One characteristic of the care of many persons with ID in the community who reside in supported programs is collection of data by staff that can be presented to the PES clinician. Such data may be useful instrumental in accessing and documenting the efficacy of behavioral and pharmacologic interventions.

LEGAL ISSUES

Various legal issues apply to all patients, but certain issues are of special concern in situations that involve an individual with intellectual disability (25). Informed consent presents a challenge in that the individual with ID has, by definition, substandard intellectual function and may have impediments to communication and learning. The diagnosis of ID, or other neurodevelopmental disorder, does not inevitably imply that the individual cannot consent to his or her own treatment.

Nonetheless, in many cases the capacity to consent may be compromised. In such cases, there may already be a legal guardian, who should be rapidly contacted by the PES. The PES clinician may assess capacity on a case-by-case basis, and a person may be deemed to have capacity to make some decisions and not others. In the emergency setting, life-threatening problems warrant emergency treatment even in the absence of informed consent. If someone clearly does not have capacity, a long-term caregiver or family member should be asked to consent to the evaluation and treatment. When there is a legal guardian, authorization for evaluation and treatment should be obtained from the guardian except in the case of life-threatening emergencies.

Many states have statutes that mandate the reporting of abuse, or suspicion of abuse, of persons with a disability. Clinicians should become familiar with their own state's laws, regulations, standards of practice, and procedural requirements.

CONCLUSION

Patients with intellectual disability and other neurodevelopmental disorders, such as ASD, pose special challenges when they present in psychiatric emergency settings. Patients with ID most often present because of an acute problem that has occurred in addition to their intellectual disability. The clinician must assess the patient's acute presentation in the context of the patient's intellectual disability and distinguish among an underlying medical illness, environmental stress, and the onset or exacerbation of a psychiatric disorder as potential causes of behavioral decompensation. Appropriate medical, surgical, or psychiatric referrals may follow the evaluation. The PES clinician may need to act as an interpreter and advocate to ensure that the patient receives adequate care. If medical or psychiatric hospitalization is indicated, the patient's posthospital placement (at the referring facility or elsewhere) should be planned in advance. Comprehensive treatment planning (which may include medications, behavior management strategies, and ongoing data collection) serves to promote effective care and minimize future emergencies.

Mental health professionals in the PES face many challenges in working with patients with intellectual disability. The PES is assessing and treating a population that in many ways is excluded from care in many other settings. Trained PES clinicians can work with this population to provide behavioral treatment planning so as to maximize patient function, allow for the least restrictive interventions, and develop plans to return patients safely to their family or community residential settings.

REFERENCES

1. American Psychiatric Association. (2013). *Diagnostic and statistical manual of mental disorders: DSM-5*. Arlington, VA: American Psychiatric Association.
2. Christensen, D. L., Braun, K. V. N., Baio, J., et al. (2018). Prevalence and characteristics of autism spectrum disorder among children aged 8 years – Autism and Developmental Disabilities Monitoring Network, 11 sites, United States, 2012. *Morbidity and Mortality Weekly Report, 65*(13), 1–23.
3. Zablotsky, B., Black, L. I., & Blumberg, S. J. (2017). *Estimated prevalence of children with diagnosed developmental disabilities in the United States, 2014–2016*. NCHS Data Brief, No. 291, 1–8.
4. Platt, J. M., Keyes, K. M., McLaughlin, K. A., & Kaufman, A. S. (2019). Intellectual disability and mental disorders in a US population representative sample of adolescents. *Psychological Medicine, 49*, 952–961.
5. Smiley, E., Cooper, S. A., Finlayson, J., et al. (2007). Incidence and predictors of mental ill-health in adults with intellectual disabilities: Prospective study. *British Journal of Psychiatry, 191*, 313–319.
6. Hauser, M. J., Kohn, R., Lerner, M. D., et al. (2018). Intellectual disabilities, autism, and aging: Medical-legal issues. In Holzer, J. C., Kohn, R., Ellison, J. M., & Recupero, P. R. (Eds.), *Geriatric forensic psychiatry: Principles and practice* (pp. 265–274). New York, NY: Oxford University Press.
7. McDermott, S., Hardin, J. W., Royer, J. A., et al. (2015). Emergency department and inpatient hospitalizations for young people with fragile X syndrome. *American Journal on Intellectual and Developmental Disabilities, 120*, 230–243.
8. Marrus, N., Veenstra-Vanderweele, J., Hellings, J. A., et al. (2014). Training of child and adolescent psychiatry fellows in autism and intellectual disability. *Autism, 18*, 471–475.

9. Vissers, L. E., Gilissen, C., & Veltman, J. A. (2016). Genetic studies in intellectual disability and related disorders. *Nature Reviews Genetics, 17*, 9–18.

10. Lowry, M., & Sovner, R. (1991). The functional existence of problem behavior: A key to effective treatment. *The Habilitative Mental Health Care Newsletter, 10*, 59–63.

11. Lunsky, Y., Balogh, R., & Cairney, J. (2012). Predictors of emergency department visits by persons with intellectual disability experiencing a psychiatric crisis. *Psychiatric Services, 63*, 287–290.

12. Lunsky, Y., Weiss, J. A., Paquette-Smith, M., et al. (2017). Predictors of emergency department use by adolescents and adults with autism spectrum disorder: A prospective cohort study. *BMJ Open, 7*(7), e017377.

13. Rush, A. J., & Frances, A. (2000). The expert consensus guidelines: Treatment of psychiatric and behavioral problems in mental retardation. *American Journal of Mental Retardation, 105*, 159–226.

14. Hastings, R. P. (2002). Do challenging behaviors affect staff psychological well-being? Issues of causality and mechanism. *American Journal of Mental Retardation, 107*, 455–467.

15. Deb, S., Matthews, T., Holt, G., & Bouras, N. (Eds.), (2001). *Practice guidelines for the assessment and diagnosis of mental health problems in adults with intellectual disability*. Brighton: The European Association for Mental Health in Mental Retardation.

16. Reiss, S., Levitan, G. W., & Szyszko, J. (1982). Emotional disturbance and mental retardation: Diagnostic overshadowing. *American Journal of Mental Deficiency, 86*, 567–574.

17. King, B. H., DeAntonio, C., McCracken, J. T., et al. (1994). Psychiatric consultation in severe and profound mental retardation. *American Journal of Psychiatry, 151*, 1802–1808.

18. Sovner, R. (1986). Limiting factors in using DSM-III criteria with mentally ill/mentally retarded persons. *Psychopharmacology Bulletin, 22*, 1055–1059.

19. Fletcher, R. J., Barnhill, J., & Cooper, S. A. (Eds.), (2016). *Diagnostic manual – intellectual disability: A textbook of diagnosis of mental disorders in persons with intellectual disability* (2nd ed.). Kingston, NY: National Association for the Dually Diagnosed.

20. Lunsky, Y., & Modi, M. (2018). Predictors of psychotropic polypharmacy among outpatients with psychiatric disorders and intellectual disability. *Psychiatric Services, 69*, 242–246.

21. Crotty, G., Doody, O., & Lyons, R. (2014). Aggressive behaviour and its prevalence within five typologies. *Journal of Intellectual Disabilities, 18*, 76–89.

22. Ji, N. Y., & Findling, R. L. (2016). Pharmacotherapy for mental health problems in people with intellectual disability. *Current Opinion in Psychiatry, 29*(2), 103–125.

23. McQuire, C., Hassiotis, A., Harrison, B., & Pilling, S. (2015). Pharmacological interventions for challenging behaviour in children with intellectual disabilities: A systematic review and meta-analysis. *BMC Psychiatry, 15*, 303.

24. Minshawi, N. F., Hurwitz, S., Morriss, D., & McDougle, C. J. (2015). Multidisciplinary assessment and treatment of self-injurious behavior in autism spectrum disorder and intellectual disability: Integration of psychological and biological theory and approach. *Journal of Autism and Developmental Disorders, 45*, 1541–1568.

25. Hauser, M. J., Olson, E., & Drogin, E. Y. (2014). Psychiatric disorders in people with intellectual disability (intellectual developmental disorder): Forensic aspects. *Current Opinion in Psychiatry, 27*, 117–121.

37

Psychiatric Emergencies During Pregnancy and Postpartum Patient

Lyle Barnes Montgomery, Erin J. Henshaw, Sheila M. Marcus

Pregnancy and the postpartum period are times of particular susceptibility to psychiatric illness. Sex differences for many psychiatric disorders have been attributed to genetics, gender role socialization, and hormonal influences (1). During the perinatal period, dramatic fluctuations in gonadal hormones influence the presentation of both mood and anxiety disorders. Accordingly, these are the psychiatric illnesses that are most likely to be seen in an emergency department setting during pregnancy and following childbirth. Undertreatment of anxiety and depressive disorders may adversely affect neonatal outcomes (2); thus, physicians are compelled to make rapid decisions about the use of appropriate pharmacotherapy in emergency settings. Women with psychotic illness struggle with the psychological challenges inherent in the birth process and transition to motherhood, and for these reasons may present to psychiatric emergency settings with worsening of delusional symptoms. Psychosis during the perinatal period presents a particular crisis when there are concerns about harm to the fetus or neonate. Likewise, excessive use of substances during pregnancy, which may be comorbid with psychiatric disorders, adversely affects fetal development.

Emergency physicians and psychiatrists must be aware that pregnant patients can present to the emergency department with psychiatric emergencies just as any other patient can, and that their risk of psychiatric problems may be higher than the general population. This chapter gives an overview of what emergency providers should keep in mind when treating pregnant or postpartum between patients.

PSYCHIATRIC DISORDERS DURING CHILDBEARING

Mood Disorders and Postpartum Psychosis

It is estimated that the period prevalence for any depressive disorder during pregnancy is 18.4%, and during 3 months postpartum it is 19.4% (3,4). For mood disorders, hormones drive increased symptomatology during the perinatal period (5). Estrogen and progesterone levels increase dramatically during pregnancy and then drop rapidly within hours of delivery rapidly, which affects the prevalence of both disorders during this time. The substantial increase in hospitalization postpartum has been attributed to mood disorders (6). Most postpartum psychosis is related to mood disorders, rather than primary psychotic disorders such as schizophrenia. For this reason postpartum psychosis is included in this section on mood disorders rather than with psychotic disorders.

Bipolar disorder in particular accounts for approximately half of the women hospitalized for postpartum psychosis in the 3 months following birth (7). Symptoms of depression may be confused with the normal pregnancy experience (eg, sleep and appetite disturbance, changes in energy and concentration), contributing to underdiagnosis and lack of treatment. Thus, careful screening for depression during pregnancy is essential. The 10-item Edinburgh Perinatal Depression Scale (EPDS) is the most commonly used screening questionnaire for depression in pregnancy (8,9). Patients who have a positive score on the EPDS should also be given the 17-item Mood Disorder Questionnaire (MDQ) to screen for preexisting bipolar disorder (10). In women with a positive EPDS, exclusion of the impairment criterion identifies 68% of postpartum women diagnosed with bipolar disorder by structured diagnostic interview (11).

There are suggested associations between depression in pregnancy and adverse birth outcomes. However, study findings have been inconsistent, and study design variability and limitations have made data comparisons difficult. Existing data suggest that depression in early to mid-pregnancy increases the risk of preterm birth, that there is a risk of low birthweight (LBW) babies in depressed mothers, and that early to mid-pregnancy depression increases the risk of small for gestational age (SGA) infants. There are no studies that link depression with congenital malformations. Newborns of mothers with depression have increased risk for irritability, fewer facial expressions, and decreased activity and attentiveness compared to babies of mothers with no depression (12). It is suggested that genetics or other prenatal factors cause this difference in behavior. Some studies demonstrate that babies of depressed women have similar physiologic profiles to their mothers' including elevated cortisol, decreased peripheral dopamine and serotonin, greater right frontal EEG activation, and lower vagal tone. Studies investigating maternal depression on child development have had design limitations and conflicting results (12).

Postpartum depression (PPD) is a common clinical disorder with symptoms identical to those of major depressive disorder in the general population, with the caveat that women with PPD are typically much more anxious, with frequent preoccupation about their ability to parent their new child and the health of the infant. Symptom onset is typically within 6 weeks of delivery (13), but the chronicity and duration may vary (14) with some women presenting up to 6 months postpartum. Prevalence rates are reported to be 13% to 19% within the first 3 months after delivery (15,16). Rates of relapse are particularly high in women with a prior history of depression. The risk of relapse for women with a history of major depression is 25%, and with a prior history of PPD the risk increases to 50% (17,18). As during other times, the risk of depression during postpartum is influenced by genetic vulnerability.

Factors such as single marital status, unplanned pregnancy, marital conflict, and preterm birth have been found to increase the risk of PPD (19,20). The onset of postpartum depressive symptoms can vary from several days after delivery to 6 to 12 weeks following delivery, and researchers have speculated that biological factors may have greater impact on early-onset PPD, and that psychosocial stressors may be of greater significance in later-onset PPD (21).

Bipolar illness is a severe recurrent illness, with a lifetime prevalence of between 1% and 2% (22). Although the course of this illness during pregnancy has not been as systematically studied as that of unipolar disorder (23), exacerbation of bipolar illness during the postpartum period is well documented. Women who stop mood stabilizing medication during pregnancy relapse soon after at a rate of 80% to 100%. This rate is two to three times higher than for pregnant women with bipolar disorder who continue their medication (24). Additionally, postpartum exacerbation of bipolar illness has been strongly associated with postpartum psychosis, and many women who have an index episode of postpartum psychosis will go on to develop bipolar illness (25-28).

Symptoms of postpartum psychosis may present within 48 to 72 hours following delivery and include rapid and dramatic deterioration with delusions, hallucinations, significant mood lability, profound insomnia, and obsessive, anxious preoccupation about infant well-being. Suicide risk for women with postpartum psychosis is 2 in 1,000, and the means used are often more lethal and violent compared with other women who complete suicide (29,30).

Whereas the initial risk of postpartum psychosis is estimated to be 0.1% to 0.2% (20), the risk of recurrence of postpartum psychosis after an index episode is estimated to be greater than 50% (31). Risk is similarly elevated for women with a history of bipolar disorder or a family history of postpartum psychosis. However approximately 50% of women who develop postpartum psychosis have no known risk factors (32-34).

For women with postpartum psychosis, aggressive treatment with mood stabilizers, antipsychotic medications, or electroconvulsive therapy (ECT) is indicated, and hospitalization is almost always necessary.

Given that sleep deprivation is a significant risk factor for bipolar mania relapse, women with a known history of bipolar disorder may want to consider enlisting help for nighttime feedings so that their sleep is less disrupted. This would not necessarily preclude breastfeeding that could continue during waking hours, supplemented by formula or pumped breast milk overnight.

Anxiety Disorders

Modest levels of anxiety are common during pregnancy as women adjust to this life transition. Recent reports have suggested rates of clinically significant anxiety of 22% (35); however, the course of specific anxiety disorders during pregnancy has not been systematically studied. Some reports (36,37) describe reduction in frequency of panic, whereas other reports (38) note worsening of panic symptoms during pregnancy. The study by Cohen et al. (38) suggests that women discontinuing medication were particularly susceptible to relapse of panic symptoms. Panic during pregnancy is a significant risk factor for postpartum exacerbation of anxiety, and relapse of panic symptoms postpartum is common (39,40), with 31% to 64% of women with antenatal symptoms experiencing a significant increase in panic symptoms following birth.

Obsessive-Compulsive Disorder

Obsessive-compulsive disorder (OCD), like panic, may present for the first time during pregnancy (41), and women with symptoms during pregnancy are at higher risk for postpartum exacerbation. In one studied group of patients with OCD, 43% relapsed during pregnancy in the context of medication discontinuation (42). Additionally, symptoms of OCD may be more problematic and distressing postpartum, and some women experience rapid and acute onset of OCD following birth (43). One of the most important tasks of the emergency department physician is differentiating postpartum OCD symptoms (ego-dystonic, obsessional, intrusive thoughts about harming the infant and attempts to avoid triggers for these thoughts) from the more psychotic, disorganized, or severely depressed symptoms of women who may be at much higher risk for infanticide.

Posttraumatic Stress Disorder

Posttraumatic stress disorder (PTSD) is approximately twice as common in women as in men. Moreover, because women are at significantly higher risk of sexual abuse during childhood and early adulthood, the intrusive procedures inherent in the management of pregnancy may trigger symptoms of PTSD. PTSD symptoms have also been described in women who have experienced prior losses during pregnancy as well as those who have had complicated prior deliveries (44).

Schizophrenia and Related Disorders

For nonaffective psychotic disorders, there does not appear to be a clear influence of hormones on illness presentation. Certainly the enormous psychological challenges inherent in pregnancy and postpartum may exacerbate psychotic symptoms in women with schizophrenia. Some case reports, and one study (45), suggested there is some improvement in women with chronic psychosis during pregnancy; however, many studies note that women who have psychotic symptoms requiring hospitalization during pregnancy are at risk approaching 40% for postpartum exacerbation (7). Despite these risks, brief psychotic disorder and exacerbation of schizophrenia occur much less frequently postpartum compared with postpartum psychosis related to bipolar disorder (46).

Studies have demonstrated that women with psychotic disorders during pregnancy are at higher risk for poor fetal outcomes, including prematurity, LBW infants, SGA, intrauterine fetal death, and neonatal infant demise (45). Several concurrent risk factors for poor perinatal outcomes are maternal tobacco, alcohol, and other substance use as well as low socioeconomic status. A population-based study from 2010 found that women with schizophrenia on no medication were at greater risk for LBW and SGA, compared with unaffected mothers, and adjusting for potential confounders. There was no significant difference in the risk of LBW, preterm births, large for gestational age (LGA), and SGA babies in mothers with schizophrenia receiving atypical antipsychotics during pregnancy and mothers with schizophrenia not receiving antipsychotics during pregnancy. However, mothers with schizophrenia receiving typical antipsychotics during pregnancy had slightly higher risk for preterm birth (47).

New-onset psychosis during pregnancy is both an obstetric and psychiatric emergency. The abrupt presentation of psychotic symptoms requires a full medical workup for possible organic causes. Thyroid anomalies may be particularly common during pregnancy and especially postpartum. Careful management of the illness (often requiring ECT), as well as assessment of a woman's ability to cooperate with prenatal care and her later capacity for caregiving to an infant, most often requires hospitalization.

PSYCHOTROPIC MEDICATION USE DURING PREGNANCY AND POSTPARTUM

Physicians attempting to balance maternal treatment with risk of exposure to the fetus are often reluctant to prescribe medication (48). This is a particular dilemma in the emergency department setting, where psychiatrically ill pregnant women may require emergent pharmacotherapy. As noted previously, untreated psychiatric illness is an important risk factor for unfavorable pregnancy outcomes, which suggests that optimal treatment during this time may affect a number of maternal and infant outcomes. Assessments of all medication during childbearing should include the potential for risk in three separate domains: teratogenic risk, direct neonatal toxicity, and longer-term neurobehavioral sequelae (49). They should be guided by the available literature, however sparse. It is critical to document that a careful discussion about risks, benefits, and available evidence or the lack thereof has taken place between the physician and the patient.

Risk Assessment and Drug Labeling

The US Food and Drug Administration introduced five pregnancy risk categories in 1979 (50) that are familiar to physicians treating women of childbearing age (Table 37.1). However these categories were found to be of limited usefulness, as they did not also address the issue of drug effects during lactation, and more importantly did not provide data of sufficient detail needed for informed decision-making. There was concern that use of the simplistic categories was not informative, in some cases causing increased risk to mother and baby by withholding medication. Most psychiatric medications are labeled Category C (and a few Category D), which may result in withholding of medication in cases in which the benefits clearly outweigh the risks, resulting in unnecessary morbidity and possibly mortality.

TABLE 37.1 US Food and Drug Administration Pregnancy Risk Categories

Category	Description
A	Adequate and well-controlled studies have failed to demonstrate a risk to the fetus in the first trimester of pregnancy (and there is no evidence of risk in later trimesters).
B	Animal reproduction studies have failed to demonstrate a risk to the fetus and there are no adequate and well-controlled studies in pregnant women.
C	Animal reproduction studies have shown an adverse effect on the fetus and there are no adequate and well-controlled studies in humans, but potential benefits may warrant use of the drug in pregnant women despite potential risks.
D	There is positive evidence of human fetal risk based on adverse reaction data from investigational or marketing experience or studies in humans, but potential benefits may warrant use of the drug in pregnant women despite potential risks.
X	Studies in animals or humans have demonstrated fetal abnormalities and/or there is positive evidence of human fetal risk based on adverse reaction data from investigational or marketing experience, and the risks involved in use of the drug in pregnant women clearly outweigh potential benefits.

These concerns led to the Pregnancy and Lactation Labeling Final Rule (PLLR) that went into effect in 2015. This new labeling requirement for package inserts is being phased in, with all medications approved after June 30, 2001 to be in compliance by 2020. Medications approved prior to June 30, 2001 are not subject to PLLR labeling, however were required to remove the previous pregnancy letter category by 2018. The new Pregnancy and Lactation Labeling Rule is narrative and is found in the Special Populations section of the package insert (Table 37.2).

Antidepressant Medication

Studies evaluating the risks of antidepressant medication in pregnancy are often limited by confounding factors that are not controlled for, such as severity of illness, substance use, smoking, and age. Although in a quantitative review miscarriage rates were 12.4% for women taking antidepressants, and 8.7% for women who were not, the confounding variables were significant enough to prevent an association between antidepressants and miscarriage. LBW and SGA effects are linked with SSRI use in pregnancy. Some studies statistically controlled for confounding factors, providing stronger evidence for a relationship between SSRI use and decreased infant birthweight. Although the difference was statistically significant, the absolute risk was small and of low clinical significance (51). A number of studies found that the risk of preterm birth is significantly higher in women using antidepressants; however, the difference in mean gestational age was small, generally 1 week or less compared with women not taking antidepressants. When confounding variables were controlled statistically, there was no difference in the rates of preterm births between those exposed or not exposed to antidepressants. Some studies have suggested that gestational age may be dependent on the duration of treatment with an antidepressant during pregnancy.

With the exception of paroxetine, there is no evidence that antidepressants (TCAs, SSRIs, bupropion, venlafaxine, duloxetine, mirtazapine) cause an increased rate of congenital

TABLE 37.2 Pregnancy and Lactation Labeling Final Rule (PLLR)

Category	Subcategories and Descriptions
Pregnancy (includes labor and delivery)	• **Pregnancy Exposure Registry:** if one exists, with contact information • **Risk Summary:** human, animal, and pharmacologic data in that order • **Clinical Considerations:** any known serious risks to the woman or fetus from the condition for which the drug is indicated, recommended dose adjustments during pregnancy and postpartum, maternal adverse reactions which are unique to pregnancy, fetal or neonatal adverse outcomes which are not developmental and are not discussed in the risk summary, and whether the drug is expected to affect labor and delivery • **Data**
Lactation	• **Risk Summary:** available data on the presence of the drug in breast milk, including drug, prodrug, and active metabolites, the effect of the drug on the breastfed child, the effect on breast milk production and excretion • **Clinical Considerations:** methods for minimizing exposure to the breastfed child, methods to monitor and mitigate effects on the breastfed child • **Data**
Females and males of reproductive potential	• **Pregnancy Testing:** recommendations, if any • **Contraception:** recommendations, if any • **Infertility:** drug effects on fertility and preimplantation loss

malformations. However, there is a greater amount of data for the SSRIs and TCAs (12). In regard to paroxetine, linked database reports found that infants exposed to paroxetine during the first trimester were at higher risk of cardiac malformations (52-54). However, other studies have disputed these findings (55-57).

Symptoms known as poor neonatal adaptation occurs during the days after birth in 15% to 30% of infants exposed to SSRIs in late pregnancy. The symptoms can include irritability, tachypnea, hypoglycemia, temperature instability, weak or absent cry, and seizures. The symptoms usually resolve in 2 weeks or less. Possible explanations for these symptoms include a discontinuation syndrome (58), toxicity related to increased SSRI levels (59), a gene–SSRI interaction (60), or sustained changes in brain function (61). Another neonatal complication of increased risk with late pregnancy exposure is persistent pulmonary hypertension. This condition results in right to left shunting of blood through the ductus arteriosis and foramen ovale and results in neonatal hypoxia. This condition occurs in about 0.5 to 2 per thousand births and is fatal in 10% of cases. Studies suggest that the rate is increased to 3 to 6 per thousand in infants exposed to SSRIs in pregnancy.

Benzodiazepines

Previous studies have suggested an association between benzodiazepines and cleft anomalies when used within the first trimester (62-64) with a risk of 0.6% which is approximately a 10-fold increased risk relative to the general population. Other studies have not demonstrated this association (65). A meta-analysis from 2011, with a cohort size of over 1 million, of which over 4,000 were exposed to benzodiazepines in pregnancy, yielded an odds ratio of 1.07 (95% CI 0.91-1.25), suggesting fetal safety in general. However, this same meta-analysis noted that synthesis of case-control studies suggested a twofold increase in oral clefts and therefore recommended counseling should include mention of an 80% increased risk of oral clefts associated with benzodiazepine exposure (66). A cohort study from the UK published in 2014 found no evidence for an increase in major congenital anomalies in children exposed to diazepam,

temazepam, and zopiclone. Based on current data, it appears that benzodiazepines may not be associated with an increased risk of oral cleft, but if they are, the risk is much lower than previously thought.

Frequent or high-dose use of benzodiazepines late in pregnancy may predispose the infant to neonatal withdrawal symptoms including hypotonia, neonatal apnea, and temperature instability (67-69). Whereas some authors concluded that third-trimester withdrawal was indicated to avoid these sequelae, most conclude that such withdrawal would unnecessarily predispose women to relapse of anxiety disorders. Clearly, the emergency department physician who may frequently be confronted with a highly anxious woman with poor sleep may need to consider the use of these agents.

Z Drugs (Hypnotic Benzodiazepine Receptor Agonists)

Sleep disturbances are reported in most patients who present with psychiatric emergencies, whether due to anxiety, psychosis, mania, or depression. There are little data on the safety of Z drugs (zolpidem, zopiclone, and zaleplon) used in pregnancy; however, the few studies to date have found no increased risk of teratogenicity (70).

Mood Stabilizers

Mood stabilizers are the primary treatment for bipolar disorder and include medications lithium, carbamazepine, oxcarbazepine, valproic acid, lamotrigine, and antipsychotic medications. Historically, lithium was thought to cause a 400-fold increased risk of Ebstein's anomaly, a tricuspid valve malformation (71). More recent studies have revised this risk to 20-fold (1 in 1,000 compared with a base rate of 1 in 20,000). Lithium use in the third trimester has been associated with cardiac dysfunction, diabetes insipidus, hypothyroidism, low muscle tone, poor sucking, lethargy, respiratory difficulties, and hepatic abnormalities in the newborn (72). These problems appear to be related to increased lithium levels at birth. As babies lose weight after birth, the risk of toxicity increases. Stopping lithium for 24 to 48 prior to delivery may reduce this risk. No long-term mental or physical effects have been demonstrated in children who were exposed to lithium during pregnancy. Dosages may need to be increased because of increases in extracellular fluid volume during pregnancy (73). Careful monitoring of serum levels and divided doses rather than once-daily dosing should be considered to increase safety. Following delivery, dosage may need to be decreased to prevent lithium toxicity in the postpartum woman. Caution is advised for women maintained on lithium who are breastfeeding as lithium does pass into breast milk. Monitoring of infant lithium levels and complete blood counts is recommended (74).

Valproic acid exposure during the first trimester has been found to increase the risk by 12- to 16-fold for spina bifida, and by 2- to 7-fold for atrial septal defect, hypospadias, cleft palate, polydactyly, and craniosynostosis. Long-term adverse effects in children exposed to valproic acid in pregnancy include: impaired cognitive function with dose dependent IQ reduction in 3 year olds (81), mild to significant developmental delay (114), and language impairment in school-aged children (76). No adverse effects from the use of valproic acid while breastfeeding have been reported (74).

Data indicate that the rate of major malformations related to carbamazepine exposure is 3.3% which is not much higher than the base rate of 2% to 3% in the general population. Babies exposed to carbamazepine were found to weigh 94 g (3.3 oz) less than controls (77). There is no evidence of impaired cognitive function in exposed children (75,112). No adverse effects from the use of carbamazepine while breastfeeding have been reported (74).

There is no evidence for teratogenesis related to lamotrigine use. Birthweights on average are 74 g (2.6 oz) less than controls. There is no evidence of impaired cognitive function or neurodevelopment in exposed children (78,79). No adverse effects from the use of lamotrigine while breastfeeding have been reported (74). However, one study found that infant serum levels were 30% of the maternal levels; therefore it is recommended that infants be monitored for rash (80).

For oxcarbazepine, one study found the risk of major malformations to be 2.8%, again within the base rate for the general population. However, it was noted that the study may have been underpowered (81).

Antipsychotic Medication

There is no evidence of teratogenesis in women taking typical (82) and atypical antipsychotic medications (83). There may be neonatal effects, including extrapyramidal symptoms, respiratory distress, difficulty feeding, floppy infant syndrome, and sluggish reflexes with typical antipsychotic exposure, but it typically resolves within a few days (84). Data have been conflicting regarding the effect of atypical antipsychotics on neonatal outcomes, demonstrating increased risk of LBW (83) as well as higher risk of being LGA (85). Metabolic effects, particularly gestational diabetes and weight gain, may indirectly increase the risk of associated neonatal outcomes, including macrosomia, hypoglycemia, shoulder dystocia, related birth injuries, and neural tube defects. There is evidence that gestational diabetes is almost twice as likely in women who used atypical antipsychotics (85). There is no evidence of long-term neurodevelopmental effects in children exposed to either typical or atypical antipsychotic medications in utero (79).

Psychotropic Medication Use during Lactation

All psychotropic medications pass into the breast milk and have the potential to affect the breastfeeding child. In 1994 the American Academy of Pediatrics issued a caution for all psychotropic drugs, given the unknown effects of these medications on the developing brain (86). With few exceptions, most psychotropic medications are excreted into breast milk in small concentrations, which are not likely to lead to adverse effects in the infant.

Most antidepressants are found in very small amounts in breast milk and may be undetectable. Rates of adverse events are low (113). The highest levels have been found for fluoxetine, citalopram, and venlafaxine. Nevertheless, it is recommended that they be continued if these have worked best in treating the mother's depression.

Typical and atypical antipsychotic medications are excreted at 3% to 5% of maternal levels. There have been a few reports of drowsiness and lethargy, but most reports indicate no adverse events. The exception is clozapine that is reported to be concentrated in breast milk and has been associated with sedation, decreased sucking reflex, restlessness, irritability, seizures, cardiac instability, and agranulocytosis in the infant. In cases in which the woman has achieved significant and lasting stability on clozapine after multiple failed medication trials (a frequent scenario for patients on clozapine), it may be safer to discontinue breastfeeding than to switch to a different antipsychotic medication.

The mood stabilizers valproic acid, carbamazepine, and lamotrigine appear safe for breastfeeding. Lithium, however, can pose risk to the infant. Serum lithium levels in the infant can be 10% to 50% of maternal serum levels and so are at risk of lithium toxicity if they should develop vomiting or diarrhea or if the mother develops lithium toxicity. Breastfeeding infants of women on lithium require more frequent pediatric assessment, including testing of lithium level, renal function, and thyroid function.

ACUTE AGITATION AND AGGRESSION: MANAGEMENT OF RESTRAINTS IN PREGNANT PATIENTS

For an acutely agitated pregnant woman who might require benzodiazepines or antipsychotic medication in an emergency department setting, often use of mechanical restraints is additionally considered. For women in the second and third trimester of pregnancy, the potential for the vena cava syndrome should be avoided; therefore, when mechanical restraints are used, careful positioning on the left side is essential. The inferior vena cava syndrome is caused by gradual compression and occlusion of venous return to the inferior vena cava. It may cause fall in blood pressure, tachycardia, and extreme anxiety in the woman and may predispose to fetal hypoxia. In pregnancy, this syndrome can be caused when a woman is placed on her back on a flat surface or on her right side and the gravid uterus reduces flow to the vena cava. This may occur if an acutely agitated woman is placed in four-point restraints on her back. Pregnant women who must be restrained should always have their bodies turned partway to the left, with a support under the right hip, to prevent this syndrome.

SUBSTANCE USE DURING CHILDBEARING

Substance use in a pregnant or breastfeeding woman can be the cause for significant morbidity, particularly for the fetus or infant. Many substances pass through the placenta causing fetal exposure. Some substances, like alcohol, are known to cause permanent damage to the developing fetal brain (fetal alcohol syndrome). For other substances, the long-term impact on the developing brain is still not clear. Depending on the substance the newborn may be at risk for substance withdrawal at the time of birth. Substance use while breastfeeding also poses risk to the infant due to the presence of substances in breast milk. Additionally, the use of substances can result in psychiatric emergencies in the mother including substance-induced psychosis, mania, depression, and increased risk of homicidal and suicidal behavior. Women who are actively using substances are at greater risk of poor nutrition, inadequate prenatal care, and other behaviors that put the fetus at greater risk. Ongoing substance use following birth may impair the woman's ability to care adequately for her infant. It is estimated that approximately 5% of pregnant women use at least one addictive substance during pregnancy. Problematic substances include alcohol, opioids, stimulants, cannabis, benzodiazepines, and tobacco. There is evidence that use of substances such as tobacco, cannabis, stimulants, and others can increase the risk of stillbirth by two to three times (87). For these reasons it is critical that pregnant and breastfeeding women are consistently screened for substance use, through interview and lab testing, so that appropriate and timely treatment can be offered.

LBW has been associated with maternal use of a number of substances including cannabis, cocaine, and tobacco. Stimulants such as cocaine and methamphetamine have been linked with placental abruption and hypertensive crisis, conditions which endanger the life of both mother and child.

The potential long-term effects for the child are particularly concerning. There is evidence that nicotine can make the brain more sensitive to other drugs such as cocaine, possibly increasing the child's vulnerability to future substance use. There is evidence that exposure to marijuana through breast milk in the first month of life can lead to decreased motor development at 12 months. THC (tetrahydrocannabinol) is passed into breast milk in moderate amounts and can become concentrated in breast milk with regular use. One study found that young pregnant women had a positive drug test for cannabis at a rate of 20%, which was twice the rate of self-reported cannabis use, demonstrating the importance of drug testing in addition to screening questions.

Neonatal abstinence syndrome is a neonatal condition that occurs following birth, when the infant is no longer exposed to the substances the mother was using during pregnancy. Substances of particular concern are opioids, alcohol, benzodiazepines, and barbiturates and require appropriate treatment. Some substances such as stimulants do not cause a withdrawal syndrome but may remain in the infant's system for up to a week causing symptoms such as irritability and hyperactivity due to the toxic effects of the substance rather than withdrawal from it.

Medical treatment is recommended for pregnant women who wish to stop using, to reduce risk to the fetus. Intensive Outpatient Programs have been particularly effective for pregnant women. Women are more likely to continue in programs, which also include prenatal care, childcare, parenting classes, and vocational training. For pregnant women addicted to opioids, treatment with methadone or buprenorphine as part of a comprehensive treatment plan, which includes drug treatment and prenatal care, can improve the outcome compared with untreated opioid use disorder. It is recommended that women who are already maintained on methadone or buprenorphine continue it during pregnancy (87). Buprenorphine appears to cause less dependence in the neonate compared with methadone, and so may be a preferred treatment in some patients. Infants born to mothers using methadone and buprenorphine are also at risk for withdrawal following birth.

THE ROLE OF PSYCHOTHERAPY AND REFERRAL FROM THE EMERGENCY SERVICE

For some women, the transition to motherhood presents a substantial personal challenge. The issues are myriad and might include alterations in professional aspirations; changes in the marital relationship; a disruptive, abusive, or absent partner; and social, housing, or economic instability. Although these issues are unlikely to be resolved in an emergency department setting, simply identifying the complexity of the issues that are contributing to the psychiatric illness may provide sufficient motivation to help a woman seek appropriate cognitive, supportive, or interpersonal psychotherapy to promote recovery. Several groups have investigated the effectiveness of interpersonal therapy and cognitive behavioral therapy in the treatment of depression during the puerperium, all suggesting positive outcomes when delivered by appropriately trained treatment providers (88,89). For those women who are reluctant to begin or continue pharmacotherapy, these treatments may be useful alternatives. Likewise, for women who choose to use pharmacotherapy but have significant psychosocial stressors, these treatments may be essential augmentation strategies.

EATING DISORDERS AND PREGNANCY

Eating disorders are common among women of childbearing age, and women with a history of either anorexia nervosa or bulimia nervosa are susceptible to symptom recurrence either during or after pregnancy (90-92). Clearly, women experience noticeable changes in their body shape during pregnancy and postpartum, and women with eating disorders in their history are particularly sensitive to experiencing depression or poor self-image triggered by these changes.

When compared with women without eating disorders, women with active eating disorders during pregnancy are at higher risk of miscarriages, congenital malformations, smaller infant head circumference, premature delivery, delivering by cesarean section, or delivering LBW or SGA infants (90,93-96). Among women with a history of eating disorders, those whose symptoms are in full remission before pregnancy may be less likely to experience negative infant outcomes or depression in pregnancy than women whose symptoms are not in full remission at the outset of pregnancy (97). Thus, health care professionals who have the opportunity to counsel women planning for pregnancy should recommend that women with histories of eating disorders take steps to engage in eating disorder treatment and wait to conceive until symptoms are in full remission.

Women with a history of both anorexia and bulimia are significantly more susceptible to PPD than nonsymptomatic women (90-92). Some women who suspend disordered eating behaviors during pregnancy for the protection of the fetus will return to previous restricting or bingeing behaviors soon after giving birth. Thus, care for women should include assessment of past and present disordered eating behavior and vigilant prenatal care with an emphasis on nutrition and healthy levels of exercise at various stages of pregnancy. Psychotherapy focusing on eating behaviors, body image, and coping with pregnancy-related stress is also recommended for reducing eating disorders in pregnancy and preventing PPD in susceptible women.

DOMESTIC VIOLENCE IN PREGNANCY

Domestic violence is a threat to the safety of an abused woman at any point in her life; however, the threat of domestic violence during pregnancy poses a significant risk to the pregnant woman as well as the fetus or infant. The reported prevalence of domestic violence during pregnancy ranges from 1% to 20.6% in studies, depending on the method of questioning and population characteristics (98-100). It is still unclear whether pregnancy is a time of increased risk for violence compared with other time points (101). A study of urban emergency department rates indicated that 79% of women reported at least one episode of being slapped, pushed, or kicked in their lifetime, and 15% reported at least one such episode while pregnant (102). In a sample of North Carolina emergency departments, domestic violence assaults accounted for 22% of the cases of pregnant patients seen for trauma (103), indicating that domestic violence may be a common reason for emergency visits during pregnancy.

Women reporting domestic violence in the year prior to becoming pregnant were found to be at higher risk for high blood pressure; vaginal bleeding; severe nausea, vomiting, or dehydration;

and kidney infection or urinary tract infection and were more likely to make hospital visits related to these symptoms during pregnancy (104). Women who experience abuse during pregnancy are more likely to miscarry (105), have lower gestational weight gain (106), or have preterm delivery of an LBW infant (104). Physical abuse is also related to the likelihood of delivering an infant who requires time in the intensive care unit after birth (104). Women in abusive relationships are more likely to delay prenatal care until the third trimester than nonabused women, increasing the risk to mother and fetus (100,107).

Reasons for the occurrence of domestic violence during pregnancy have not been thoroughly studied, although some risk factors have been identified for women. In a qualitative study of women abused during pregnancy, women identified several possible reasons for abuse during pregnancy, including jealousy or anger toward the unborn child, pregnancy-specific conflicts, or simply business as usual (108). Women reporting that the pregnancy was unwanted or unexpected for one partner may be more than four times as likely to experience domestic violence during the pregnancy (109), leading some to speculate that violence during pregnancy could be motivated by a perceived lack of control by the male partner or jealousy of the unborn child (101). Not surprisingly, women who report more severe and frequent abuse in their relationships prior to pregnancy are more likely to encounter domestic violence during pregnancy as well (108).

Domestic Violence Screening

Currently, the benefits and risks of routine screening for domestic violence in emergency care settings continue to be debated among researchers and clinicians (102,110). Certainly, emergency department care providers are in a unique position to identify and provide support to women experiencing domestic violence in pregnancy, especially concerning abuse-related injuries or pregnancy complications. Potential barriers to regular screening include care providers' fear of offending patients, limited time with patients to conduct screening during emergency visits, and, most important, inconclusive evidence that identification and intervention will result in positive outcomes for women being abused (110). In a review of the literature, Ramsay et al. (110) found that about one-half to three-fourths of women report that routine screening would be acceptable to them, and abused women were found more likely to approve of routine screening than nonabused women (110). It is widely suggested that an introductory statement may increase provider and patient comfort with screening, such as "Many women that we see happen to be in relationships with people who hurt them, and because it affects your health, I always ask about it. Are you in a relationship with a partner who physically hurts or threatens you?" Women are more likely to report incidents of violence when asked in a direct, brief, nonjudgmental manner by a health care professional than they are when self-report questionnaires are used (107).

The role of the provider in the emergency care setting is not to solve the problem of domestic violence for a patient or to convince the woman to leave her abuser. The process of leaving a domestic violence situation can be complicated and may pose a risk to the health of the woman or her children if sufficient planning, support, and resources are not involved. However, health care providers should consider their role an important one in identifying potential abuse and risk for serious injury (111), listening nonjudgmentally to women as they describe their concerns for their safety or that of their children (98), and providing support for women in a variety of ways as deemed appropriate by the woman. Providers should be familiar with specific local domestic violence resources and be willing to provide referral information if the patient finds this acceptable. Providers should be aware of potential risks in providing printed materials about domestic violence to abused women and may consider additional ways to facilitate connection with resources, such as allowing women to call domestic violence centers from the hospital phone rather than a home phone, or allowing the woman to arrange a meeting with social work providers during her emergency visit or a planned follow-up visit with another provider.

Furthermore, although women may not have immediate plans to press charges against the perpetrator, accurate medical documentation of abuse-related injuries can be very valuable if the abuse should ever be questioned in a legal setting (101). Espinosa and Osborne (98) suggest that notes should include specific descriptions of the abuse as reported by the woman when appropriate. Finally, providing access to resources targeting socioeconomic stressors may alleviate one of the potential triggers for increased violence or may facilitate a woman's ability to leave the relationship if desired. Counseling for abused women and their abusers may be available through state programming and can be useful if each individual is seen separately.

Women have a high risk of psychiatric symptoms peripartum and will present to the emergency department during this time. This chapter is meant to help guide emergency physicians and psychiatrists in providing appropriate care to this vulnerable population.

REFERENCES

1. Lewis-Hall, F., Williams, T. S., Panetta, J. A., et al. (Eds.), (2002). *Psychiatric illnesses in women: Emerging treatments and research.* Washington, DC: American Psychiatric Publishing.
2. Greden, J. F. (Ed.), (2001). *Treatment of recurrent depression.* Washington, DC: American Psychiatric Publishing.
3. Gaynes, B., Gavin, N., Meltzer-Brody, S., Lohr, K. N., Swinson, T., Gartlehner, G., et al. (2005). *Perinatal depression: Prevalence, screening accuracy and screening outcomes (Evidence Report/Technology Assessment No. 119. AHRQ Publication No 5-E006-2).* Rockville, MD: Agency for Healthcare Research and Quality.
4. Gavin, N. I., Gaynes, B. N., Lohr, K. N., Meltzer-Brody, S., Gartlehner, G., & Sinson, T. (2005). Perinatal depression: A systematic review of prevalence and incidence. *Obstetrics & Gynecology, 106,* 1071–1083.
5. Wisner, K. L., Perel, J. M., & Findling, R. L. (1996). Antidepressant treatment during breastfeeding. *American Journal of Psychiatry, 153,* 1132–1137.
6. Kendell, R., Chalmers, J. C., & Platz, C. (1987). Epidemiology of puerperal psychoses. *British Journal of Psychiatry, 150,* 662–673.
7. Harlow, B. L., Vitonis, A. F., Sparen, P., Cnattinglus, S., Joffe, H., & Huftman, C. M. (2007). Incidence of hospitalization for postpartum psychotic and bipolar episodes in women with and without prior prepregnancy or prenatal psychiatric hospitalizations. *Archives of General Psychiatry, 64,* 42–48.

8. Cox, J. L., Holden, J. M., & Sagovsky, R. (1987). Detection of postnatal depression: Development of the 10-item Edinburgh Postnatal Depression Scale. *British Journal of Psychiatry, 150*, 782–786.

9. Cox, J., & Holden, J. (1994). *Perinatal psychiatry. Use and misuse of the Edinburgh Postnatal Depression Scale.* London: The Royal College of Psychiatrists.

10. Hirschfeld, R. M., Williams, J. B., Spitzer, R. I., et al. (2000). Development and validation of a screening instrument for bipolar spectrum disorder: The Mood Disorder Questionnaire. *American Journal of Psychiatry, 157*, 1873–1875.

11. Clark, C. T., Sit, D. K., Driscoll, K., et al. (2015). Does screening with the MDQ and EPDS improve identification of bipolar disorder in an obstetrical sample? *Depression and Anxiety, 32*, 518–526.

12. Yonkers, K., Wisner, K., Stewart, D., Oberlander, T., Dell, D., Stotland, N., Ramin, S., Chaudron, L., & Lockwood, C. (2009). The management of depression during pregnancy: A report from the American Psychiatric Association and the American College of Obstetricians and Gynecologists. *Obstetrics and Gynecology, 114*(3), 703–713.

13. Stowe, Z. N., & Nemeroff, C. B. (1995). Women at risk for postpartum-onset major depression. *American Journal of Obstetrics and Gynecology, 172*, 639–645.

14. Wolkind, S., Zajicek-Colean, E., & Ghodsian, J. (1988). Continuities in maternal depression. *International Journal of Family Psychology, 1*, 167–181.

15. O'Hara, M. W., & Swain, A. (1996). Rates and risk of postpartum depression—A meta-analysis. *International Review of Psychiatry, 8*, 37–54.

16. Steiner, M. (1998). Perinatal mood disorders: Position paper. *Psychopharmacology Bulletin, 34*, 301–306.

17. O'Hara, M. W. (1995). *Postpartum depression: Causes and consequences.* New York, NY: Springer-Verlag.

18. Garvey, M. J., Tuason, V. B., Lumry, A. E., & Hoffmann, N. G. (1983). Occurrence of depression in the postpartum state. *Journal of Affective Disorders, 5*, 97–101.

19. Cox, J. L., Conner, Y. M., Henderson, I., McGuire, R. J., & Kendell, R. E. (1983). Prospective study of the psychiatric disorders of childbirth by self report questionnaire. *Journal of Affective Disorders, 5*, 1–7.

20. Kumar, R., & Robson, K. M. (1984). A prospective study of emotional disorders in childbearing women. *British Journal of Psychiatry, 144*, 35–47.

21. Suri, R., & Altshuler, L. (2012). Postpartum depression: Advances in recognition and treatment. *Focus, 1*, 15–21.

22. Kessler, R. C., McGonagle, K. A., Zhao, S., et al. (1994). Lifetime and 12-month prevalence of DSM-III-R psychiatric disorders in the United States. Results from the National Comorbidity Survey. *Archives of General Psychiatry, 51*, 8–19.

23. Viguera, A., Cohen, L., Baldessarini, R., et al. (2002). Managing bipolar disorder during pregnancy: Weighing the risks and benefits. *The Canadian Journal of Psychiatry, 47*, 11.

24. Viguera, A. C., Whitfield, T., Baldesserini, R. J., Newport, D. J., Stowe, Z., Reminick, A., et al. (2007). Risk of recurrence in women with bipolar disorder: Prospective study of mood stabilizer discontinuation. *American Journal of Psychiatry, 164*, 1817–1824.

25. Braftos, O. H. J. (1966). Puerperal mental disorders in manic depressive females. *Acta Psychiatrica Scandinavica, 42*, 285–294.

26. Reich, T., & Winokur, G. (1970). Postpartum psychosis in patients with manic-depressive disease. *The Journal of Nervous and Mental Disease, 51*, 60–68.

27. Brockington, I. F., Cernik, K. F., Schofield, E. M., et al. (1981). Puerperal psychosis. Phenomena and diagnosis. *Archives of General Psychiatry, 38*, 829–833.

28. Davidson, J., & Robertson, E. (1985). A follow-up study of post partum illness, 1946–1978. *Acta Psychiatrica Scandinavica, 71*, 451–457.

29. CEMD. (2001). *Confidential inquiries into maternal deaths: Why mothers die, 1997–99.* London: Royal College of Obstetricians and Gynaecologists.

30. Hawton, K. (2000). Sex and suicide. Gender differences in suicidal behaviour. *British Journal of Psychiatry, 177*, 484–485.

31. Robertson, E., Jones, I., Haque, S., Holder, R., & Craddock, N. (2005). Risk of puerperal and nonpuerperal recurrence of illness following bipolar affective puerperal (post-partum) psychosis. *British Journal of Psychiatry, 186*, 258–259.

32. Jones, I., & Craddock, N. (2001). Familiality of the puerperal trigger in bipolar disorder: Results of a family study. *American Journal of Psychiatry, 158*, 913–917.

33. Munk-Olsen, T., Laursen, T. M., Pedersen, C. B., Mors, O., & Mortensen, P. B. (2007). Family and partner psychopathology and the risk of postpartum mental disorders. *The Journal of Clinical Psychiatry, 68*, 1947–1953.

34. Blackmore, E. R., Rubinow, D. R., O'Connor, T. C., et al. (2013). Reproductive outcomes and risk of subsequent illness in women diagnosed with postpartum psychosis. *Bipolar Disorders, 15,* 394–404.

35. Heron, J., O'Connor, T. G., Evans, J., et al. (2004). The course of anxiety and depression through pregnancy and the postpartum in a community sample. *Journal of Affective Disorders, 80,* 65–73.

36. Villeponteaux, V. A., Lydiard, R. B., Laraia, M. T., et al. (1992). The effects of pregnancy on pre-existing panic disorder. *The Journal of Clinical Psychiatry, 53,* 201–203.

37. Klein, D. F., Skrobala, A. M., & Garfinkel, R. S. (1994–1995). Preliminary look at the effects of pregnancy on the course of panic disorder. *Anxiety, 1,* 227–232.

38. Cohen, L., Soares, C., Otto, M., et al. (2004). *Relapse of panic disorder during pregnancy among patients who discontinue or maintain anti-panic medication: A preliminary prospective study.* Presented at the 157th Annual Meeting of the American Psychiatric Association, New York, NY.

39. George, D. T., Ladenheim, J. A., & Nutt, D. J. (1987). Effect of pregnancy on panic attacks. *American Journal of Psychiatry, 144,* 1078–1079.

40. Cohen, L. S., Sichel, D. A., Dimmock, J. A., et al. (1994). Postpartum course in women with preexisting panic disorder. *The Journal of Clinical Psychiatry, 55,* 289–292.

41. Buttolph, M. L., & Holland, A. (1990). Obsessive compulsive disorders in pregnancy and childbirth. In Jenike, M. A., Baer, L., & Minichiello, W. E. (Eds.), *Obsessive-compulsive disorders: Theory and management.* Chicago, IL: Year Book Medical.

42. Sichel, D. A., Cohen, L. S., Dimmock, J. A., et al. (1993). Postpartum obsessive compulsive disorder: A case series. *The Journal of Clinical Psychiatry, 54,* 156–159.

43. Sichel, D. A., Cohen, L. S., Rosenbaum, J. F., et al. (1993). Postpartum onset of obsessive-compulsive disorder. *Psychosomatics, 34,* 277–279.

44. Ballard, C. G., Stanley, A. K., & Brockington, I. F. (1995). Post-traumatic stress disorder (PTSD) after childbirth. *British Journal of Psychiatry, 166,* 525–528.

45. Spielvogel, A., & Wile, J. (1992). Treatment and outcomes of psychotic patients during pregnancy and childbirth. *Birth, 19,* 131–137.

46. McGorry, P., & Connell, S. (1990). The nosology and prognosis of puerperal psychosis: A review. *Comprehensive Psychiatry, 31,* 519–534.

47. Lin, H. C., Chen, I. J., Chen, Y. H., Lee, H. C., & Wu, F. J. (2010). Maternal schizophrenia and pregnancy outcome: Does the use of antipsychotics make a difference? *Schizophrenia Research, 116,* 55–60.

48. Einarson, A., Portnoi, G., & Koren, G. (2002). Update on Motherisk Updates. Seven years of questions and answers. *Canadian Family Physician, 48,* 1301–1304.

49. Koren, G., Pastuszak, A., & Ito, S. (1998). Drugs in pregnancy. *The New England Journal of Medicine, 338,* 1128–1137.

50. Pernia, S., & DeMaagd, G. (2016). The new pregnancy and lactation labeling rule. *Pharmacy and Therapeutics, 41*(11), 713–715.

51. Oberlander, T., Warburton, W., Misri, S., Aghajanian, J., & Hertzman, C. (2006). Neonatal outcomes after prenatal exposure to selective serotonin reuptake inhibitor antidepressants and maternal depression using population-based linked health data. *Archives of General Psychiatry, 63,* 898–906.

52. Kallen, B. A., & Otterblad Olausson, P. (2007). Maternal use of selective serotonin re-uptake inhibitors in early pregnancy and infant congenital malformations. *Birth Defects Research, Part A: Clinical and Molecular Teratology, 79,* 301–308.

53. Kallen, B. A., & Otterblad Olausson, P. (2006). Antidepressant drugs during pregnancy and infant congenital heart defect. *Reproductive Toxicology, 21,* 221.

54. Cole, J., et al. (2007). Bupropion in pregnancy and the prevalence of congenital malformations. *Pharmacoepidemiology and Drug Safety, 16,* 474–484.

55. Louik, C., Lin, A., Werler, M., Hernandez-Diaz, S., & Mitchell, A. (2007). First-trimester use of selective serotonin-reuptake inhibitors and the risk of birth defects. *The New England Journal of Medicine, 356,* 2675–2683.

56. Alwan, S., et al. (2007). Use of selective serotonin re-uptake inhibitors in pregnancy and the risk of birth defects. *The New England Journal of Medicine, 356,* 2684–2692.

57. Einarson, A., et al. (2006). Evaluation of the risk of congenital cardiovascular defects associated with use of paroxetine during pregnancy. *American Journal of Psychiatry, 165,* 749–752.

58. Laine, K., Heikkinen, T., Ekblad, U., & Kero, P. (2003). Effects of exposure to selective serotonin reuptake inhibitors during pregnancy on serotonergic symptoms in newborns and cord blood monoamine and prolactin concentrations. *Archives of General Psychiatry, 60,* 720–726.

59. Oberlander, T., et al. (2004). Pharmacologic factors associated with transient neonatal symptoms following prenatal psychotropic medication exposure. *The Journal of Clinical Psychiatry, 65*, 230–237.

60. Oberlander, T., et al. (2008). Infant serotonin transporter (SLC6A4) promoter genotype is associated with adverse neonatal outcomes after prenatal exposure to serotonin reuptake inhibitor medications. *Molecular Psychiatry, 13*, 65–73.

61. Zeskind, P., & Stephens, L. (2004). Maternal selective serotonin reuptake inhibitor use during pregnancy and newborn neurobehavior. *Pediatrics, 113*, 368–375.

62. Aarskog, D. (1975). Association between maternal intake of diazepam and oral clefts [Letter]. *Lancet, 2*, 921.

63. Saxen, I. (1975). Associations between oral clefts and drugs taken during pregnancy. *International Journal of Epidemiology, 4*, 37–44.

64. Rosenberg, L., Mitchell, A. A., Parsells, J. L., et al. (1983). Lack of relation of oral clefts to diazepam use during pregnancy. *The New England Journal of Medicine, 309*, 1282–1285.

65. Altshuler, L. L. H. (1996). Pregnancy and psychotropic medication: Changes in blood levels. *Journal of Clinical Psychopharmacology, 16*, 78–80.

66. Enato, E., Moretti, M., & Koren, G. (2011). The fetal safety of benzodiazepines: An updated meta-analysis. *Journal of Obstetrics and Gynaecology Canada, 33*, 46–48.

67. Fisher, J. B., Edgren, B. E., Mammel, M. C., et al. (1985). Neonatal apnea associated with maternal clonazepam therapy: A case report. *Obstetrics & Gynecology, 66*, 34S–35S.

68. Gillberg, C. (1977). "Floppy infant syndrome" and maternal diazepam. *Lancet, 2*, 244.

69. Mazzi, E. (1977). Possible neonatal diazepam withdrawal: A case report. *American Journal of Obstetrics and Gynecology, 129*, 586–587.

70. Wikner, B. N., & Kallen, B. (2011). Are hypnotic benzodiazepine receptor agonists teratogenic in humans? *Journal of Clinical Psychopharmacology, 31*, 356–359.

71. Weinstein, M. R., & Goldfield, M. (1975). Cardiovascular malformations with lithium use during pregnancy. *American Journal of Psychiatry, 132*, 529–531.

72. Newport, D. J., Viguera, A. C., Beach, A. J., Ritchie, J. C., Cohen, L. S., & Stowe, Z. N. (2005). Lithium placental passage and obstetrical outcome: Implications for clinical management during late pregnancy. *American Journal of Psychiatry, 162*, 2162–2170.

73. Stotland, N. L., & Stewart, D. E. (Eds.), (2001). *Psychological aspects of women's health care. The interface between psychiatry and obstetrics and gynecology* (2nd ed., pp. 67–94). Washington, DC: American Psychiatric Press.

74. Eberhard-Gran, M., Eskild, A., & Opjordsmoen, S. (2006). Use of psychotropic medications in treating mood disorders during lactation: Practical recommendations. *CNS Drugs, 20*, 187–198.

75. Meador, K. J., Baker, G. A., Browning, N., Clayton-Smith, J., Combs-Cantrell, D. T., Cohen, M., Kalayjan, L. A., Kanner, A., Liporace, J. D., Pennell, P. B., Privitera, M., & Loring, D. W., for the NEAD Study Group. (2009). Cognitive function at 3 years of age after fetal exposure to antiepileptic drugs. *The New England Journal of Medicine, 360*, 1597–1605.

76. Nadebaum, C., Anderson, V. A., Vajda, F., Reutens, D. C., Barton, S., & Wood, A. G. (2011). Language skills of school-aged children prenatally exposed to antiepileptic drugs. *Neurology, 76*, 719–726.

77. The North American Antiepileptic Drug Pregnancy Registry. (2011). *Registry releases topiramate findings: Increased risk for malformations and low birth weight*. Somerville, MA: Massachusetts General Hospital.

78. Molgaard-Nielsen, D., & Hviid, A. (2011). Newer-generation antiepileptic drugs and the risk of major birth defects. *JAMA, 305*, 1996–2002.

79. Robinson, G. (2012). Psychopharmacology in pregnancy and postpartum. *Focus, 10*(1), 3–14.

80. Newport, D. J., Pennell, P. B., Calamaras, M. R., et al. (2008). Lamotrigine in breast milk and nursing infants: Determination of exposure. *Pediatrics, 122*, e223–e231.

81. McKenna, K., Koren, G., & Tetelbaum, G. (2005). Pregnancy outcome of women using atypical antipsychotic drugs. *The Journal of Clinical Psychiatry, 66*(4), 444–449.

82. Newham, J. J., Thomas, S. H., MacRitchie, K., McElhattan, P. R., & McAllister-Williams, R. H. (2008). Birth weight of infants after maternal exposure to typical and atypical antipsychotics: Prospective comparison study. *British Journal of Psychiatry, 192*, 333–337.

83. Yeager, D., Smith, H. G., & Altshuler, L. L. (2006). Atypical antipsychotics in the treatment of schizophrenia during pregnancy and the postpartum. *American Journal of Psychiatry, 163*, 2064–2070.

84. Altshuler, L. L., Cohen, L. S., Szuba, M. P., et al. (1996). Pharmacologic management of psychiatric illness during pregnancy: Dilemmas and guidelines. *American Journal of Psychiatry, 153,* 592–606.

85. Boden, R., Lundgren, M., Brandt, L., Reutfors, J., & Kieler, H. (2012). Antipsychotics during pregnancy: Relation to fetal and maternal metabolic effects. *Archives of General Psychiatry, 69,* 715–721.

86. American Academy of Pediatrics Committee on Drugs. (1994). The transfer of drugs and other chemicals into human milk. *Pediatrics, 93,* 137–150.

87. NIDA. (2019, June 19). *Substance use in women.* Retrieved from https://www.drugabuse.gov/publications/drugfacts/substance-use-in-women on 2019, August 3.

88. O'Hara, M. W., Stuart, S., Gorman, L. L., et al. (2000). Efficacy of interpersonal psychotherapy for postpartum depression. *Archives of General Psychiatry, 57*(11), 1039–1045.

89. Cooper, P. J., Murray, L., Wilson, A., et al. (2003). Controlled trial of the short- and long-term effect of psychological treatment of postpartum depression: I. Impact on maternal mood. *British Journal of Psychiatry, 182*(4), 412–419.

90. Franko, D. L., Blais, M. A., Becker, A. E., et al. (2001). Pregnancy complications and neonatal outcomes in women with eating disorders. *American Journal of Psychiatry, 158*(9), 1461–1466.

91. Abraham, S. (1998). Sexuality and reproduction in bulimia nervosa patients over 10 years. *Journal of Psychosomatic Research, 44*(3–4), 491–502.

92. Morgan, J. F., Lacey, J. H., & Chung, E. (2006). Risk of postnatal depression, miscarriage, and preterm birth in bulimia nervosa: Retrospective controlled study. *Psychosomatic Medicine, 68*(3), 487–492.

93. Micali, N., Simonoff, E., & Treasure, J. (2007). Risk of major adverse perinatal outcomes in women with eating disorders. *British Journal of Psychiatry, 190,* 255–259.

94. Bulik, C. M., Sullivan, P. F., Fear, J. L., et al. (1999). Fertility and reproduction in women with anorexia nervosa: A controlled study. *The Journal of Clinical Psychiatry, 60*(2), 130–135.

95. Brinch, M., Isager, T., & Tolstrup, K. (1988). Anorexia nervosa and motherhood: Reproduction pattern and mothering behavior of 50 women. *Acta Psychiatrica Scandinavica, 77*(5), 611–617.

96. Kouba, S., Hallstrom, T., Lindholm, C., et al. (2005). Pregnancy and neonatal outcomes in women with eating disorders. *Obstetrics & Gynecology, 105*(2), 255–260.

97. Stewart, D. E., Raskin, J., Garfinkel, P. E., et al. (1987). Anorexia nervosa, bulimia, and pregnancy. *American Journal of Obstetrics and Gynecology, 157*(5), 1194–1198.

98. Espinosa, L., & Osborne, K. (2002). Domestic violence during pregnancy: Implications for practice. *Journal of Midwifery & Women's Health, 47*(5), 305–317.

99. Norton, L. B., Peipert, J. F., Zierler, S., et al. (1995). Battering in pregnancy: An assessment of two screening methods. *Obstetrics & Gynecology, 85*(3), 321–325.

100. Parker, B., McFarlane, J., & Soeken, K. (1994). Abuse during pregnancy: Effects on maternal complications and birth weight in adult and teenage women. *Obstetrics & Gynecology, 84*(3), 323–328.

101. Jasinski, J. L. (2004). Pregnancy and domestic violence: A review of the literature. *Trauma, Violence, & Abuse, 5*(1), 47–64.

102. Datner, E. M., Wiebe, D. J., Brensinger, C. M., et al. (2007). Identifying pregnant women experiencing domestic violence in an urban emergency department. *Journal of Interpersonal Violence, 22*(1), 124–135.

103. Connolly, A. M., Katz, V. L., Bash, K. L., et al. (1997). Trauma and pregnancy. *American Journal of Perinatology, 14*(6), 331–336.

104. Silverman, J. G., Decker, M. R., Reed, E., et al. (2006). Intimate partner violence victimization prior to and during pregnancy among women residing in 26 U.S. states: Associations with maternal and neonatal health. *American Journal of Obstetrics and Gynecology, 195*(1), 140–148.

105. Jacoby, M., Gorenflo, D., Black, E., et al. (1999). Rapid repeat pregnancy and experiences of interpersonal violence among low-income adolescents. *American Journal of Preventive Medicine, 16*(4), 318–321.

106. Moraes, C. L., Amorim, A. R., & Reichenheim, M. E. (2006). Gestational weight gain differentials in the presence of intimate partner violence. *International Journal of Gynecology & Obstetrics, 95*(3), 254–260.

107. McFarlane, J., Parker, B., Soeken, K., et al. (1992). Assessing for abuse during pregnancy. Severity and frequency of injuries and associated entry into prenatal care. *JAMA, 267*(23), 3176–3178.

108. Campbell, J. C., Oliver, C., & Bullock, L. (1993). Why battering during pregnancy? *AWHONN's Clinical Issues in Perinatal and Women's Health Nursing, 4*(3), 343–349.

109. Gazmararian, J. A., Lazorick, S., Spitz, A. M., et al. (1996). Prevalence of violence against pregnant women. *JAMA, 275*(24), 1915–1920.

110. Ramsay, J., Richardson, J., Carter, Y. H., et al. (2002). Should health professionals screen women for domestic violence? Systematic review. *BMJ, 325*(7359), 314.

111. Bohn, D. K. (1990). Domestic violence and pregnancy. Implications for practice. *Journal of Nurse-Midwifery, 35*(2), 86–98.

112. Gaily, E., Kantola-Sorsa, E., Hiilesmaa, V., Isoaho, M., Matila, R., Kotila, M., Nylund, T., Bardy, A., Kaaja, E., & Granstrom, M. L. (2004). Normal intelligence in children with prenatal exposure to carbamazepine. *Neurology, 62,* 28–32.

113. Lanza di Scalea, T., & Wisner, K. L. (2009). Antidepressant medication use during breast-feeding. *Clinical Obstetrics and Gynecology, 52,* 483–497.

114. Cummings, C., Stewart, M., Stevenson, M., Morrow, J., & Nelson, J. (2011). Neurodevelopment of children exposed in utero to lamotrigine, sodium valproate and carbamazepine. *Archives of Disease in Childhood, 96,* 643–647.

38

The Psychiatric Emergency Care of the Transgender Patient

Laura Erickson-Schroth, Anderson E. Still

Psychiatric emergency departments (EDs) can be unpredictable and chaotic. At the same time, they require quick decisions about disposition and treatment. The combination of these forces with a general lack of knowledge about lesbian, gay, bisexual, transgender, and queer (LGBTQ) communities often leads to poor outcomes for these groups. Substandard care can range from missing important information to outright discrimination or violence. EDs are a last resort for many people and, in times of severe distress, should be safe havens. Instead, especially for marginalized groups, they can often be more traumatizing than the original mental health condition for which a patient sought care. Many psychiatrists, psychiatric registered nurses, and psychiatric nurse practitioners would like to learn more about LGBTQ communities. This interest in acquiring knowledge will likely lead to improved care in the future.

TERMINOLOGY

LGBTQ communities are often lumped together, but are extremely diverse. The words lesbian, gay, bisexual, and queer refer to a person's sexual orientation, the sex or gender of the people they are attracted to. Sexual orientation is distinct from gender identity, which is a person's internal sense of their own gender. Transgender, or trans, is an umbrella term used to describe those whose gender identities do not match their sexes assigned at birth. Trans people, like everyone else, may have any sexual orientation. Most people are familiar with the terms lesbian, gay, and bisexual, but not with the term queer. Those who describe themselves as queer may have a more open stance toward

who they could be attracted to, or may feel politically drawn to the term as opposition to heteronormativity, the expectation that everyone is heterosexual.

Terminology within LGBTQ communities is changing rapidly, and especially within trans communities (Table 38.1). The word transgender was not widely used until the 1990s, but has now largely replaced the older term, transexual. The term cisgender is now often used to describe those who are not transgender, in order to avoid making discriminatory comparisons, such as between transgender men or women and "real" or "biological" men or women.

Transgender women are those who were assigned male at birth and identify as female, while trans men are those assigned female at birth who identify as male. Trans women are sometimes referred to as MTF (male-to-female) and trans men as FTM (female-to-male). Although these abbreviations are not generally used within trans communities, they can be helpful in charting and communication between staff. For example, a history of present illness might begin: "The pt is a 37-year-old transgender man (FTM)...."

Not all people with gender identities different from those assigned at birth identify as male or female. Some view their genders as androgynous, both male and female, or neither. Common self-descriptors include genderqueer and nonbinary. Although most trans people use traditional pronouns (ie, "he" or "she"), some nonbinary people use "they" as their personal pronoun. This may, at first, seem difficult to adopt, but there are instances in English where "they" is already used in this way. For example, exiting a lecture hall, a person might find

TABLE 38.1 Transgender Terminology

Term	Description
Gender identity	A person's internal sense of their own gender.
Sexual orientation	The sex or gender of the people someone is attracted to.
Transgender	An umbrella term used to describe those whose gender identities do not match their sexes assigned at birth.
Cisgender	Describes those whose gender identities match their sexes assigned at birth.
LGBTQ	Lesbian, gay, bisexual, transgender, and queer.
Trans woman (MTF)	Someone who was assigned male at birth and identifies as female.
Trans man (FTM)	Someone who was assigned female at birth and identifies as male.
Genderqueer/nonbinary	A self-descriptor used by those who identify as androgynous, both male and female, or neither gender.
Pronouns	The words we use to describe someone's gender when we talk about them. These include he/him and she/her, but also they/them (used by many nonbinary people).
Gender-affirming surgery	Surgical procedures that change one's body to conform to one's gender identity.

a sweater left on a chair and ask, "Did anyone leave their sweater behind?"

Pronouns are important signifiers that a person's identity is being respected, and should be used correctly by staff even when the patient is not present. Although it may not seem like a top priority to some providers when dealing with a psychiatric emergency, referring to someone correctly can help decrease anxiety and provide a sense of comfort in an otherwise tense situation.

BACKGROUND

There are an estimated 1.4 million adults, or 0.6% of the total population, who identify as transgender in the United States (1). Studies have shown that transgender individuals face pervasive discrimination in every major area of life, including increased risks of homelessness, poverty, and discrimination in schools and workplaces. Moreover, these risks are often compounded for those transgender individuals who are also ethnic and racial minorities (2-5).

Despite recent victories, including marriage equality, for the LGBTQ community, transgender citizens remain particularly vulnerable. Notably, the Ninth Circuit Court wrote that "significant evidence suggests that transgender persons are often especially visible, and vulnerable, to harassment and persecution due to their often public nonconformance with normative gender roles" (6).

The National Transgender Discrimination Survey (NTDS), the largest completed survey of transgender individuals, found that survey respondents were nearly four times more likely to have a household income of less than $10,000/year compared to the general population. A staggering 90% reported experiencing harassment, mistreatment, or discrimination on the job, and one-fifth (19%) reported experiencing homelessness at some point because of their gender identity (2).

Transgender individuals also experience alarming levels of harassment and violence. For those in the survey who had expressed gender nonconformity during grades K-12, respondents reported extremely concerning rates of harassment (78%), physical assault (35%), and sexual violence (12%) (2). The National Anti-Violence Project, an organization dedicated to ending violence against LGBTQ and HIV-positive

individuals, recorded 52 reports of hate violence–related homicides in 2017, the highest
number ever recorded in their 21 years of collecting data. Risks were highest in transgender
individuals who were also people of color; 40%
of those 52 victims were transgender women of
color, which marked a 5-year rise in recorded
homicides within that population (4).

Given the prevalence and pervasiveness of
discrimination that transgender individuals face,
it is unfortunately not surprising that these experiences also carry into the health care setting.
Multiple studies have demonstrated that transgender patients often avoid the ED, even when they
require acute care, because of fears of discrimination and prior experiences (7). Importantly, these
fears may well be justified.

Transgender patients report negative interactions such as being misgendered, inadvertently
and purposefully outed, dealing with visibly
uncomfortable or poorly educated providers, and
witnessing health providers making jokes about
their gender expression. Even more unsettling,
one-fifth (19%) of NTDS respondents reported
being refused medical care because of their transgender or gender nonconforming status (2).

Transgender patients often struggle to access
health care because of cost and lack of insurance.
When they are able to access care, there are several
significant barriers to quality care. Lack of privacy in the ED frequently results in patients having to out themselves to other patients. Patients
need to present to the hospital at all stages of their
transition process, and, as such, discrepancies can
exist between patients' preferred names, identifying documentation, and the existing medical
record. This can lead to embarrassing or upsetting experiences for the patient, particularly when
providers appear uneducated or uncaring. Worse,
it can lead to situations in which the act of receiving health care exposes these patients to greater
risks of harassment and violence in their local
communities.

In one study, all participants reported experiences with providers who lacked knowledge
about gender identity or transgender care. Many
reported encounters in which hospital staff did
not even understand the meaning of the word
"transgender." They also reported enduring inappropriate and unnecessary questions regarding

their gender identity or genitalia and, at times,
inappropriate examinations (7).

Unfortunately, many health care providers
feel ill-equipped to provide quality care to transgender patients. Clinicians often receive only
minimal formal education regarding the needs
and care of LGBTQ individuals. According
to one survey of Emergency Medicine physicians, although 88% reported caring for gender
minority patients, only 17.5% of respondents had
received any formal training about this population. Moreover, most providers lacked medical
knowledge about common medications and surgeries in this population. Despite lack of training,
however, most providers (79.2%) did believe that
it was important to ask about gender identity and
include this information in the electronic health
record (8).

The lack of appropriate training for understanding and treating the health needs of transgender patients has been demonstrated at all
levels of training. In US and Canadian medical
schools, the median reported time dedicated to
teaching LGBT-related content in the entire
curriculum was only 5 hours. Thirty-three percent of schools reported no dedicated hours at all
during clinical years (9). In Emergency Medicine
residency programs, 26% of program directors
reported ever having presented a specific LGBT
lecture and 33% reported incorporating LGBT
health topics into the curriculum, with an average of 45 minutes of instruction in the last year.
Of note, program directors did express a desire
to include more hours dedicated to this topic (10).

Given the limited educational opportunities
for most hospital staff and clinicians, it is no wonder that many feel ill-prepared to understand and
treat transgender patients. But, given the vulnerability of this population, it is all the more important that providers receive the proper education to
ensure that such negative outcomes do not occur.

MENTAL HEALTH IN TRANS COMMUNITIES

Although there are not formal studies, anecdotal
evidence suggests that transgender clients present to psychiatric EDs in disproportionate numbers. Given the level of societal discrimination
and violence against transgender people, it is not

surprising that mental health issues are common in trans populations. Although data are scarce, researchers have repeatedly found increased rates of depression, suicidality, and substance abuse in trans populations (11).

In terms of mood disorders, depression is extremely common. Lifetime prevalence of depression among trans people in the United States is reported as being between 50% and 67%, much higher than the population average of 5.2% (11,12). Unsurprisingly, bipolar disorder, which is considered more biologically influenced, does not appear to be more prevalent in trans people compared to the general population, suggesting that environmental factors such as discrimination and abuse weigh heavily in depression.

Of note, many mental health providers erroneously believe that hormones taken for transition can lead to mood fluctuations that cause depression (estrogen) or mania (testosterone). They may even stop prescribed hormones in emergency or inpatient settings because of fear that these could be exacerbating a patient's mood disorder. There is no evidence that hormones taken at normal prescribed doses contribute to depression or mania. Alternatively, there is research suggesting that hormone treatment can decrease depression and anxiety, and improve quality of life (13). Discontinuing a patient's hormones can lead to worsening mood fluctuations as well as disrupt the therapeutic alliance. Hormones also have few interactions with psychiatric medications. Trans men typically take testosterone, which has little risk of interactions, and trans women often take estrogen in combination with an androgen-blocker such as spironolactone. Estrogen can interact with lamotrigine, decreasing its blood levels, requiring higher lamotrigine doses. Spironolactone can interact with lithium, and concomitant use should be avoided or monitored carefully so as to avoid lithium toxicity (Table 38.2).

Especially concerning to those working in emergency psychiatry are the incredibly high rates of suicidality in trans populations. In some studies, up to 76% of trans people report a history of suicidal ideation, similar to the percentage who report depression (11). In the NTDS, 41% of respondents reported a history of suicide attempts in their lifetimes (2). The general population rate in the United States is 4.6% (14). In most groups,

only a fraction of those with depression have suicidal thoughts or attempt suicide. This suggests that it is possible some trans people with suicidality do not have depression and, instead, consider suicide because of the enormous weight of living with marginalized identities in an unaccepting society.

It is extremely useful for emergency mental health practitioners to be able to separate suicide attempts from self-harming behaviors that are not carried out for the purpose of ending a person's life, as a history of suicide attempts is more likely to increase safety risk. Not enough is known about self-harm in trans populations, but the few studies that have been carried out suggest that rates may be high. Contrary to popular belief, most self-harm does not take place in genital or chest areas, but instead in the usual areas of the body where others self-harm, such as the arms, legs, or stomach (11).

In addition to depression and suicidality, research also shows increased rates of substance abuse in trans populations. Trans people may use substances for any of the reasons that others do and may also use them to cope with discrimination or facilitate sex work, which is more common in trans populations than the general public because of employment discrimination. Certain types of drugs, such as crystal meth, may be more popular among trans people, especially in cities, because of their cultural role as party drugs in LGBTQ communities. Unfortunately, studies show that trans people have a difficult time finding culturally competent substance abuse treatment services that allow for the circumstances needed for recovery. Less than 1% of substance abuse programs provide specialized care, and in many inpatient rehabs, trans patients are mistreated by staff and other patients, and forced to shower and sleep in facilities that do not match their gender identities (11).

Given the elevated rates of trauma in trans populations, it is likely that there are also increased rates of posttraumatic stress disorder, anxiety disorders, and personality disorders, although there is a lack of sufficient research to be certain. The majority of trans people with traumatic backgrounds likely faced repeated bullying and harassment rather than one isolated traumatic event. This type of chronic strain can lead

TABLE 38.2 Common Medications in Transgender Care

Medication	Desired Effects	Undesired Effects	Common Misconceptions	Psychiatric Drug Interactions
Estrogen (transgender women)	*Both estrogen and spironolactone:* breast growth/softening of skin/shift in fat storage to a more feminine appearance	*Estrogen only:* deep venous thrombosis or pulmonary embolism, especially in older women and those who smoke. *Spironolactone only:* hyperkalemia. *Both estrogen and spironolactone:* decrease in muscle mass (can be a desired effect)/decrease in sex drive and possible infertility (can be a desired effect)	While everyone reacts differently to hormones, and some trans people report fluctuations in mood on hormones, there is no evidence for increased risk of depression or mania. In fact, research suggests that hormone treatment can decrease depression and anxiety, and improve quality of life	*Lamotrigine:* estrogen can decrease lamotrigine levels. Trans women on estrogen may need higher than usual doses of lamotrigine. Consider blood levels if using typical lamotrigine dose without improvement in symptoms
Spironolactone (transgender women)				*Lithium:* Spironolactone can increase lithium levels, potentially leading to toxicity. Avoid combination or use with extreme caution
Testosterone (transgender men)	Increase in muscle mass/facial and body hair growth (can be an undesired effect if hair grows in unwanted areas)/masculinization of facial features/deepening of voice/clitoral growth/increase in sex drive (can be an undesired effect)	Male pattern balding/erythrocytosis/acne/possible infertility (can be a desired effect)		No significant drug interactions between testosterone and common psychiatric medications

to a complex array of symptoms, including anger, irritability, frequent mood swings, and poor coping with life stressors. These characteristics can make patients difficult to work with, and staff should remind themselves that abuse and trauma are at the heart of these behaviors.

Staff in psychiatric EDs do not always know trans people in their personal lives and may begin to believe that most or all trans people have the level of mental health difficulties as those who present to the ED. It is important to remember that there are many trans people who have faced discrimination and harassment and coped well because of resilience factors such as supportive families and connections to community. These people are rarely seen by psychiatric emergency services. Family and social support are especially important in building resilience. Studies of trans youth show that those with family support who are permitted to socially transition have similar rates of depression and anxiety to their cisgender peers (15).

There is no evidence of elevated rates of severe and persistent mental illness (SPMI) such as schizophrenia, schizoaffective disorder, or bipolar I disorder in trans populations (11). However, as in other groups, there is a small percentage of trans people with these major mental illnesses. Trans people with SPMI can face additional challenges when compared to cisgender people with SPMI because of a lack of culturally competent resources. Most LGBTQ resources are geared toward those without SPMI, and most SPMI resources are not LGBTQ-informed. There are a small number of organizations that work specifically with LGBTQ people with SPMI. In New York City, Rainbow Heights Club provides social activities, support groups, and meals specifically for LGBTQ people with major mental illness.

Many trans people with SPMI are prescribed hormones for transition. Hormone prescribers assess a patient's capacity for informed consent and, in general, do not start patients on hormones while they are experiencing an acute psychotic episode. However, patients who have periods without psychosis, or where psychosis is better controlled, can start hormones while they are able to make informed choices and should be continued on their prescribed hormones even while they are more psychiatrically ill.

CREATING A SAFE ENVIRONMENT IN THE EMERGENCY DEPARTMENT

Transgender patients often present to the ED not only with an acute medical or psychiatric concern but also with a history of harassment, discrimination, and prior negative experiences. Because of these fears, patients are often reticent to even present to the hospital, and when they do their experiences can have a significant and lasting impact on their future encounters with the health care system. This makes it imperative to provide a safe environment for these patients.

On an institutional level, hospital systems should make every effort to include preferred name and pronouns in the electronic medical record, intake forms, and on hospital bracelets, as well as including nonbinary gender options. Privacy is a significant concern for trans patients presenting to the ED, and these changes can decrease the number of encounters in which patients have to "out" themselves needlessly in front of staff or other patients. In turn, this makes patients feel more comfortable, respected, and safe.

In addition to clinical documentation, Lambda Legal recommends that hospitals amend their regulations to include gender identity and expression in nondiscrimination policies and patients' bill of rights, as well as utilizing all-gender restrooms (16). Allowing access to gender-affirming items, such as clothing and binders, should also be allowed unless there are specific safety concerns. Little things, such as putting up rainbow or LGBTQ-inclusive stickers, can also make patients feel more at ease.

Rooming is a common concern for trans patients, and should be a consideration when admitting them to the hospital. There are no requirements (legal or otherwise) that patients be roomed "by their genitalia." It is also important to consider that transgender patients do not always share the same preferences. Some may feel stigmatized in an individual room, while others may feel relief that they do not have to worry about disclosure issues or being placed in a room that is not congruent with their gender identity. Staff should respect patients' affirmed gender as well as their individual preferences whenever possible. It is also important that, once these changes have been made, hospital administration make staff members and the public aware of them.

Hospital systems, medical departments, and residency programs should also provide cultural competency training on the specific needs and considerations for this population. Transgender patients often report needing to provide education about these issues to providers, and this can put a strain on the patient-provider relationship. Increased education allows both providers and patients to feel more comfortable during the medical encounter and ensures a better quality of care.

In the ED, clinicians may want to consider screening everyone for gender identity (17). It is also important for staff to communicate (when clinically appropriate) any disclosures to ensure consistent use of the correct name and pronouns. Staff can use affirming language, asking such questions as "What name would you like me to call you?" and "What pronoun should we use when referring to you?" Although a patient's name and pronoun may not match all legal or insurance documentation, there is no reason that they cannot be respected. Mistakes do happen, and if providers do use incorrect names or pronouns, the best thing to do is acknowledge the error immediately and apologize before moving on.

Providers should also educate themselves on transition-related medications transgender patients routinely take, particularly when they are responsible for ordering these medications for patients admitted to the hospital. Whether purposefully or inadvertently, withholding a patient's hormone regimen will likely worsen gender dysphoria. Demonstrating this knowledge can also help patients feel more comfortable throughout the process, as well as ensuring appropriate medical and psychiatric care.

There can be situations in which other staff or patients are noted to be acting in an inappropriate manner toward trans patients. In addition to modeling appropriate behavior, it may be necessary to engage with other health care professionals or other patients directly if they engage in inappropriate or transphobic behavior. All efforts should be made to ensure that transgender patients feel safe within the ED.

Many staff members may feel uncomfortable pointing out where others are being disrespectful and may not know the best ways to broach this topic without alienating the person who made

the error. In our experience, it can be helpful to approach colleagues with an assumption that they are coming from a place of ignorance rather than purposeful ill will. For example, if another staff member calls a patient by the wrong pronoun, one might say, "Oh, it's not obvious in the chart but this patient goes by he/him. He's a trans man." Even if the colleague did purposefully use the wrong pronoun, that person is now in the position of responding to a clear but kind reproach.

If there is ongoing or systematic disrespect toward trans patients in a particular ED, there are a few options for working to improve the situation. If a particular staff member or members are displaying egregious behavior, this should be reported in the safest known way. However, if there is a culture of ignorance rather than hostility and the ED director is an ally, that person may be willing to organize a training. It is often helpful to bring in consultant from the outside to lead this kind of session, so that the employee with LGBTQ knowledge does not feel they are expected to educate others or disclose their own identity. In addition to hospital-based trainings, there are also in-person sessions on transgender mental health through the Philly Trans Wellness Conference (18), GLMA: Health Professionals Advancing LGBT Equality (19), and other organizations. An online curriculum on LGBT mental health is also available through a joint venture of the Association of LGBTQ Psychiatrists (AGLP) and Group for the Advancement of Psychiatry (GAP) (20).

TAKING A PSYCHIATRIC HISTORY WITH TRANS CLIENTS

The ED is a fast-moving and unpredictable environment. Providers have a limited amount of time with each patient, and typically there is no further relationship once the patient has been discharged or admitted. This can make rapport-building challenging.

Evidence has shown that the therapeutic relationship between patient and provider substantially impacts patients' follow-up on treatment recommendations. This is certainly no different with transgender patients. As basic as it might sound, demonstrating respect and compassion can go a long way in improving both the experience for trans patients as well as the likelihood that they will follow recommendations. Moreover, being aware of common life experiences and disparities these patients routinely face can help clinicians feel more comfortable when treating them.

The psychiatric interview is an essential step in fostering this patient-provider relationship. Providers should refer to transgender people by the name and pronouns that correspond with their gender identity. If unsure, asking politely for clarification is almost always appreciated. It is also imperative to remember that a trans patient's presentation to the ED may have nothing to do with their gender identity.

Transgender patients often report being asked inappropriate-seeming questions related to transgender status or surgical history. Keep in mind that there is no need to ask about surgical or genital status if it is unrelated to their care. When these questions are pertinent, providers should use inclusive and respectful language during the history taking process, and should ask these questions at the time they would ask any other patient their medical or surgical history. Explaining the rationale for these questions can also go a long way at putting transgender patients at ease.

CONCLUSIONS

Trans patients coming to psychiatric EDs often have a lot working against them. They may have histories of abuse or trauma that lead them to be wary of new people and environments, and the staff they meet when they arrive may have little knowledge about how to interact with them respectfully. Psychiatrists interested in ensuring a more supportive environment for trans patients in their emergency services can start by educating themselves and approaching patients with an open, warm stance. They may also want to help their facilities to incorporate gender-neutral bathrooms and sleeping arrangements, and encourage administrators to bring in outside consultants to run trainings for staff. Finally, as patients leave the ED, they may want to provide warm handoffs to inpatient units and gather LGBTQ-friendly resources for shelters and outpatient care. In times of crisis, a welcoming environment with knowledgeable staff can make all the difference.

REFERENCES

1. Flores, A. R., Herman, J. L., Gates, G. J., & Brown, T. N. T. (2017). *How many adults identify as transgender in the United States?* Los Angeles, CA: The Williams Institute.
2. Grant, J. M., Mottet, L. A., & Tanis, J. (2016). *Injustice at every turn: A report of the National Transgender Discrimination Survey.* National Center for Transgender Equality. National Gay and Lesbian Task Force. Retrieved from https://transequality.org/sites/default/files/docs/resources/NTDS_Report.pdf.
3. Lambda Legal. (2010). *When health care isn't caring: Survey on discrimination against LGBT people and people living with HIV* (pp. 5–6). New York, NY: Lambda Legal. https://www.lambdalegal.org/sites/default/files/publications/downloads/whcic-report_when-health-care-isnt-caring.pdf.
4. National Coalition of Anti-Violence Programs (NCAVP). (2018). *Lesbian, gay, bisexual, transgender, queer and HIV-affected hate and intimate partner violence in 2017.* http://avp.org/wp-content/uploads/2017/06/NCAVP_2016HateViolence_REPORT.pdf.
5. Grubb, H. M. (2016). Marginalization of transgender identities: Implications for health equity. *Psychiatric Annals, 46*(6), 334–339.
6. Avendano-Hernandez v. Lynch, 800 F.3d 1072, 1081 (9th Cir. 2015).
7. Chisolm-Straker, M., Jardine, L., Bennouna, C., Morency-Brassard, N., Coy, L., Egemba, M. O., & Shearer, P. L. (2017). Transgender and gender nonconforming in emergency departments: A qualitative report of patient experiences. *Transgender Health, 2*(1), 8–16.
8. Chisolm-Straker, M., Willging, C., Daul, A. D., McNamara, S., Sante, S. C., Shattuck, D. G., II, & Crandall, C. S. (2018). Transgender and gender-nonconforming patients in the emergency department: What physicians know, think, and do. *Annals of Emergency Medicine, 71*(2), 183–188.
9. Obedin-Maliver, J., Goldsmith, E. S., Stewart, L., White, W., Tran, E., Brenman, S., Wells, M., Fetterman, D. M., Garcia, G., & Lunn, M. R. (2011). Lesbian, gay, bisexual, and transgender-related content in undergraduate medical education. *JAMA, 306*(9), 971. doi:10.1001/jama.2011.1255.
10. Moll, J., Krieger, P., Moreno-Walton, L., Lee, B., Slaven, E., James, T., … Heron, S. L. (2014). The prevalence of lesbian, gay, bisexual, and transgender health education and training in emergency medicine residency programs: What do we know? *Academic Emergency Medicine, 21*(5), 608–611.

11. Carmel, T. C., & Erickson-Schroth, L. (2016). Mental health and the transgender population. *Psychiatric Annals, 46*(6), 346–349.

12. Weissman, M. M., Bland, R. C., Canino, G. J., Faravelli, C., Greenwald, S., Hwu, H. G., ... Lépine, J. P. (1996). Cross-national epidemiology of major depression and bipolar disorder. *JAMA, 276*(4), 293–299.

13. White Hughto, J. M., & Reisner, S. L. (2016). A systematic review of the effects of hormone therapy on psychological functioning and quality of life in transgender individuals. *Transgender Health, 1*(1), 21–31.

14. Kessler, R. C., Borges, G., & Walters, E. E. (1999). Prevalence of and risk factors for lifetime suicide attempts in the National Comorbidity Survey. *Archives of General Psychiatry, 56*(7), 617–626.

15. Olson, K. R., Durwood, L., DeMeules, M., & McLaughlin, K. A. (2016). Mental health of transgender children who are supported in their identities. *Pediatrics, 137*(3), e20153223.

16. Lambda Legal. *Transgender-affirming hospital policies*. Retrieved from https://www.lambdalegal.org/know-your-rights/article/trans-affirming-hospital-policies.

17. The Fenway Institute. *Do Ask, Do Tell: A toolkit for collecting data on sexual orientation and gender identity in clinical settings*. Retrieved from http://doaskdotell.org/ehr/toolkit/stafftraining/.

18. Philly Trans Wellness Conference. Retrieved from https://www.mazzonicenter.org/trans-wellness.

19. GLMA: Health Professionals Advancing LGBT Equality. Retrieved from http://glma.org/.

20. Association of LGBTQ Psychiatrists (AGLP) and Group for the Advancement of Psychiatry (GAP). *LGBT mental health syllabus*. Retrieved from http://aglp.org/gap.

39

Immigrants and Refugees

Cecilia M. Fitz-Gerald, Joe Kwon

Immigrants and refugees represent a uniquely challenging patient population to evaluate and manage in the emergency setting. The immigrant population within North America is steadily increasing, and the emergency department is frequently the first point of contact for medical services for these individuals (1-3). Immigrants and their children currently comprise approximately a quarter of the total population of the United States. (4). Of note, Latinos encompass the majority of the immigrant population within the United States, followed by Asian immigrants (5). International studies have repeatedly demonstrated that immigrants have lower utilization rates of mental health services compared to natural-born citizens (1,2,4,5). In the United States, immigrants from Latin America, Asia, and Africa have consistently demonstrated lower rates of use of mental health services (4). Comparatively, refugees and asylum seekers have demonstrated an increased usage of mental health services (2,4).

Understanding the various challenges that immigrants and refugees face in moving to a new country and seeking medical care is paramount in developing appropriate management strategies for this unique patient population. It is crucial to have a fundamental knowledge of cultural competency in order to minimize health care disparities in the setting of ethnic, racial, and religious diversity and to understand the various stressors that immigrants and refugees face in moving to a new country. The barriers that prevent refugees and immigrants from seeking mental health care will be discussed in this chapter, as will various management strategies to optimize patient care.

UNDERSTANDING CULTURE

Providing culturally appropriate care, also termed culturally competent care, is vital as medical care should be consistent with the values and beliefs of patients and their families (6). Culture is described as a shared dynamic and learned group of values, beliefs, and behaviors held by a set of people, and it influences how they view themselves and interact with others (7). Thus, in order to provide culturally competent care, health care providers should acknowledge any potential biases that may occur in the treatment of a patient because of cultural differences, educate themselves regarding cultural dynamics, expand their cultural knowledge, and explore the patient's cultural identity, understanding, and beliefs regarding his or her psychiatric symptoms and treatment options. (6,7). Cultural formulation (discussed later) is an important aspect of the psychiatric interview and should be incorporated into the evaluation and diagnosis by the emergency psychiatrist (7). Additionally, culturally competent care necessitates understanding barriers to care in order to minimize or remove these barriers if possible (6).

UNIQUE STRESSORS

In order to more fully understand this patient population and the challenges that they have faced in their lives, it is important to discuss the motivations that drive immigrants and refugees to leave their native countries. Individuals may choose to move to a new country to seek economic prosperity, educational opportunities, refuge from political and social turmoil, or to follow family members or other loved ones who have already immigrated to another country. However, in moving to a new country, immigrants and refugees often face a strenuous future complete with numerous obstacles and hardship, which impedes their ability to assimilate into a new country and culture. Immigrants and refugees frequently struggle with decreased social support, obtaining employment due to low levels of education and lack of job skills, the need to reside in high crime/violence areas, poverty, discrimination, and trauma secondary to experiences prior to immigration and/or from the immigration process (6,8,9).

These stressors impact the physical and emotional well-being of immigrants and refugees. Immigrants face disparities in socioeconomic status and educational opportunities along with decreased access to health care, which will be explored in a later section. Additionally, they have higher morbidity and mortality rates compared to the general population (6). These stressors facing immigrant populations contribute to increasing rates of suicide for African-American and Latino male youths and Latino female youths. Living in high crime areas is associated with increased aggressive behavior in minority youth due to numerous factors, including substance use, poverty, domestic violence, etc. In particular, minority children are at a higher risk for child abuse (6).

BARRIERS TO CARE

Many immigrants and refugees are hesitant to seek not only psychiatric care but also general medical care because of numerous barriers. Often cited barriers to care include language, lack of medical insurance, high cost of medical care, stigma, religious beliefs, lack of awareness of resources, transportation limitations, legal concerns, preference for alternative services, distrust of providers, and wait time to see a provider (4,5,8,9). Immigrants who lack medical insurance have even lower rates of mental health utilization compared to immigrants with medical insurance (4,5,8,9). Establishing eligibility for Medicare is one example of a barrier to care, as non-US citizens, including Green Card holders, must establish residency within the United States for a minimum of 5 years to become eligible for the Medicare program. Individuals who are non-US citizens are also less likely to have employee sponsored health plans than US citizens (5). Studies in Asian, Latino, and African immigrants demonstrate that patients prefer to seek help from religious leaders rather than mental health professionals and that faith is often cited as a coping

mechanism (4). Immigrants may also prefer to use folk healers or alternative service providers or may initially present to a primary care physician with somatic complaints, such as chest pain, fatigue, or difficulty breathing, instead of directly seeking care for mental health symptoms (4,8,9). Of the Latino immigrants, undocumented Latino immigrants had the lowest rates of mental health service utilization. Undocumented immigrants expressed fear of seeking mental health service because of concerns regarding being asked for documentation and the possibility of being denied medical care and deported (4,8).

In comparing the most commonly reported barriers to mental health service care by immigrant populations within the United States, Latino immigrants commonly reported lack of insurance, cost of care, language, and undocumented legal status (4,8). However, Asian (Chinese, Cambodian, Korean, Vietnamese), African, Iranian, Iraqi, and Eastern European immigrants frequently cited stigma and norms as more prominent barriers to mental health care. Additionally, Asian and African immigrants cited preference for alternative care, lack of knowledge/inaccessibility to care, language, and cost as common barriers to care. Iranian and Iraqi immigrants reported lack of knowledge, cost, and preference for alternative treatments. Older Iranian immigrants also cited distrust in medication as a barrier to care (4).

OPTIMIZING PATIENT CARE

Use of Interpreters

As language is frequently reported as a barrier to care, efforts to use interpreters to assist with interviews should be used as often as possible in order to increase patients' comfort with the evaluation and to minimize the language barrier. Many providers are hesitant to use interpreters when patients seem to be partially fluent in English. Although patients may be able to respond appropriately to questioning, this does not indicate that the patient is able to participate in a meaningful evaluation. In some situations, a patient may express his or her desire to have the interview conducted in English; however, it is still highly likely that there will be miscommunication during the evaluation due to the patient's difficulty in comprehending certain questions, explaining his or her psychiatric symptoms and/or history in detail, and the desire to switch to his or her native language in stressful situations (6). All health care institutions that receive federal funding are required to provide language-appropriate services (7,10). Language services available in medical settings include telephone/video interpreters and hospital-trained interpreters. Patient satisfaction is greater when using hospital-trained interpreters compared to telephone interpreters and should be utilized whenever possible (3).

Cultural Formulation

It is also important to use the cultural formulation technique and inquire about patients' cultural beliefs of their psychiatric symptoms in order to avoid misdiagnosis (9). When patients provide vague responses to direct questioning, providers should ask for further details of their symptoms and/or history in order to avoid unintentionally missing an important piece of information. It is important to start with open-ended questions, such as "What does that mean?" or "Can you tell me more about that?" Further questioning should include culturally sensitive questions, such as "What do you believe is causing your symptoms? What do your friends and family say?"

Providers should conduct patient interviews without the patient's family or friends present in order to allow the patient to express himself or herself more openly without the fear of judgment from his or her loved ones (7). Although family members and/or friends may offer to serve as interpreters during the evaluation, this may lead to inaccurate responses due to family dynamics, minimization of symptoms by loved ones, and misinterpretation (3,7). However, family and friends are an important source of support for patients and with the patient's permission, should be involved with treatment planning and provided psychoeducation. In addition, as many immigrants report the importance of their faith to their well-being, providers may choose to invite patient's religious leaders to become involved in their care and provide spiritual support for the patients and their loved ones (6).

CARE FOR UNDOCUMENTED IMMIGRANTS

As stated previously, many immigrants avoid seeking medical care because of fear of disclosing their unauthorized legal status and potential deportation to their native countries (11). However, health care providers are not legally required to disclose the immigration status of patients to federal officials, unless under certain circumstances, such as with a warrant, and have the right to remain silent if questioned by federal agents. In addition, U.S. Immigration and Customs Enforcement (ICE) has defined hospitals as "sensitive locations" where undocumented immigrants are generally protected from immigrant enforcement actions. Exceptions to this rule include matter of national security or terrorism, imminent risk of death or harm, and pursuit of a felon or suspected terrorist (12). Although not legal citizens, undocumented immigrants may seek emergent medical care under the Emergency Medical Treatment and Active Labor Act (EMTALA) and primary care through numerous nonprofit community health clinics. While caring for undocumented patients, health care providers should avoid discrimination, treat these patients with the dignity and respect given to any other patient under their care, and serve as an advocate for their patients through public policy changes (13). Increasing public awareness of patient privacy and legal rights through media campaigns (educational pamphlets, social media, radio, television) could be of additional benefit (11).

COMMUNITY RESOURCES

Studies have demonstrated that many immigrants are unaware of culturally appropriate community resources, including interpretation services available in health care systems. In order to increase accessibility to mental health services, it is important to increase awareness of the unique needs of immigrants/refugees and increase the number of cultural diversity training programs available to providers so that they may provide culturally competent care. Treatment planning should take into account the various stressors that the patient is facing and include social workers and referrals to appropriate community providers, ie, Spanish-speaking psychiatrists, or community clinics which provide culturally appropriate care. If financial constraints are an issue, efforts should be made to recommend uninsured and indigent patients lower cost medications, minimize lab work and other testing, and offer medication assistance waivers if possible. Patient education is paramount and should include psychoeducation, discussion of coping strategies, and addressing of stigma. On a larger scale, increasing community awareness of mental health and local community resources through media campaigns and public education would greatly reduce several barriers to care as would advocating policy changes regarding insurance coverage (6,8,9).

CONCLUSION

Immigrants and refugees are a particularly vulnerable and rapidly expanding population in our society that have unique needs that must be appropriately identified and addressed by emergency providers. First, it is necessary for providers to identify and minimize barriers to care in order to encourage these individuals to seek medical care. Providers should provide culturally competent care through expanding their cultural knowledge base, offering language interpreter services, assessing patients using cultural formulation principles, and educating and referring patients to appropriate community resources. Lastly, it is imperative that health care providers be cognizant of their own legal rights and those of their patients in order to create a safe environment for medical care and offer assurance to patients and their families.

REFERENCES

1. Abebe, D. S., Lien, L., & Elstad, J. I. (2017). Immigrants' utilization of specialist mental healthcare according to age, country of origin, and migration history: A nation-wide register study in Norway. *Social Psychiatry and Psychiatric Epidemiology, 52*(6), 679–687. doi:10.1007/s00127-017-1381-1. PMID: 28378064.

2. Sarría-Santamera, A., Hijas-Gómez, A. I., Carmona, R., & Gimeno-Feliú, L. A. (2016). A systematic review of the use of health services by immigrants and native populations [Review]. *Public Health Reviews, 37*, 28. doi:10.1186/s40985-016-0042-3. eCollection 2016. PMID: 29450069; PMCID: PMC5810113.

3. Ramirez, D., Engel, K. G., & Tang, T. S. (2008). Language interpreter utilization in the emergency department setting: A clinical review [Review]. *Journal of Health Care for the Poor and Underserved, 19*(2), 352–362. doi:10.1353/hpu.0.0019. PMID: 18469408.

4. Derr, A. S. (2016). Mental health service use among immigrants in the United States: A systematic review [Review]. *Psychiatric Services, 67*(3), 265–274. doi:10.1176/appi.ps.201500004. PMID: 26695493; PMCID: PMC5122453.

5. Chen, J., & Vargas-Bustamante, A. (2011). Estimating the effects of immigration status on mental health care utilizations in the United States. *Journal of Immigrant and Minority Health, 13*(4), 671–680. doi:10.1007/s10903-011-9445-x. PMID: 21286813; PMCID: PMC3132313.

6. Pumariega, A. J., & Rothe, E. (2003). Cultural considerations in child and adolescent psychiatric emergencies and crises. *Child and Adolescent Psychiatric Clinics of North America, 12*(4), 723–744.

7. Lim, R. F. (Ed.). (2015). *Clinical manual of cultural psychiatry* (2nd ed.). Washington, DC: American Psychiatric Publishing.

8. Bridges, A. J., Andrews, A. R., III, & Deen, T. L. (2012). Mental health needs and service utilization by Hispanic immigrants residing in mid-southern United States. *Journal of Transcultural Nursing, 23*(4), 359–368. PMID: 22802297; PMCID: PMC4060822.

9. Thomson, M. S., Chaze, F., George, U., & Guruge, S. (2015). Improving immigrant populations' access to mental health services in Canada: A review of barriers and recommendations [Review]. *Journal of Immigrant and Minority Health, 17*(6), 1895–1905. doi:10.1007/s10903-015-0175-3. PMID: 25742880.

10. Litzau, M., Turner, J., Pettit, K., Morgan, Z., & Cooper, D. (2018). Obtaining history with a language barrier in the emergency department: Perhaps not a barrier after all. *The Western Journal of Emergency Medicine, 19*(6), 934–937. doi:10.5811/westjem.2018.8.39146. PMID: 30429924; PMCID: PMC6225939.

11. Maldonado, C. Z., Rodriguez, R. M., Torres, J. R., Flores, Y. S., & Lovato, L. M. (2013). Fear of discovery among Latino immigrants presenting to the emergency department. *Academic Emergency Medicine, 20*(2), 155–161. doi:10.1111/acem.12079. PMID: 23406074.

12. Health Care Providers and Immigration Enforcement. *Know your and your patients' rights*. National Immigration Law Center. Retrieved February 11, 2019, from https://www.nilc.org/issues/immigration-enforcement/healthcare-provider-and-patients-rights-imm-enf/.

13. Berlinger, N., & Raghavan, R. (2013). The ethics of advocacy for undocumented patients. *Hastings Center Report, 43*(1), 14–17. doi:10.1002/hast.126. PMID: 23315847.

40

The Psychiatric Emergency Care of People who are Homeless: Intervention and Linkage

Van Yu, Ilana Nossel, Carlos Almeida, Hunter L. McQuistion

People who are homeless are among the highest utilizers of emergency services, and this high utilization has been linked to high rates of mental illness and medical illness (1-3). Homelessness is also associated with other social determinants of emergency service utilization including poverty, social isolation, safety concerns, and forensic involvement (4). Unfortunately, emergency department (ED) care and services are often ill-suited to help a person who is homeless address the myriad social determinants of their illnesses. This chapter describes the clinical features and social determinants that must be addressed in order for effective emergency care for people who are homeless and are living with mental illnesses to both reduce the likelihood of recurrent emergency service utilization and help people move on to higher functioning in their personal recovery.

HOMELESSNESS IN AMERICA

There are about 550,000 homeless people in the United States at any given time and it is estimated that there are about 3 million episodes of homelessness in the United States each year (HUD Annual Homelessness Assessment Report 2017). Reliable estimates indicate that 3% of Americans will experience homelessness at least once in their lives (5,6). People who are homeless suffer from more mental illness and substance use disorders than the general population (7), and mentally ill homeless people are often sicker than their housed counterparts (8) and use recreational drugs more than people with mental illnesses who are not homeless (9). Especially among single adults, comorbidity is the rule, rather than the exception. Between one-third and one-half of single homeless adults are believed to have a major psychiatric disorder: approximately 20% to 30% with major mood disorders and 10% to 15% with schizophrenia (10-12). Over the past 20 years, there is indication that affective disorders and especially substance use and dependence have risen among the single adult homeless population, the latter afflicting up to 84% of men and 58% of women (13).

Substance and alcohol misuse is not viewed as a primary cause of either first-time or recurrent homelessness (14,15) but is implicated in its chronicity (16). These individuals also benefit less from hospitalizations, are more frequently discharged against medical advice, and have less robust aftercare plans compared to nonhomeless mentally ill people (9). In addition to suffering a greater burden of behavioral health issues, there is higher morbidity and mortality due to medical illnesses compared to the general population (17).

People who are homeless do not constitute a homogeneous population in terms of gender, age, ethnicity, tenure of homelessness, or clinical characteristics. For example, single, homeless people tend to be psychiatrically more ill and engage in more substance use than members of homeless families (18). On the other hand, social factors, such as domestic violence, are more frequent causes of homelessness in families compared to single adults. People who are homeless are also heterogeneous in terms of pattern and longevity of homelessness.

For example, many people are homeless for short periods of time, but a cohort of "long-term shelter stayers," accounting for about 10% of the homeless, use over 50% of the resources in the shelter system (5). Although the characteristics of people living on the streets have not been studied as extensively as those who are sheltered, these characteristics appear to be similar with unsheltered people suffering from higher levels of mental illness, substance use disorder, medical illness, and trauma (19-21). Furthermore, unsheltered people tend to access acute care rather than routine preventive care for their health conditions (22).

THE NATURE OF PSYCHIATRIC CARE FOR PEOPLE WHO ARE HOMELESS

People who are homeless and living with serious mental illnesses face many barriers to care in fragmented traditional service settings that are not able to provide continuity of care (23-25). Also, people with homelessness and mental illnesses are often reluctant to engage in behavioral health care considering it as relatively unimportant compared to other, more immediate concerns, and severity of psychiatric illness seems to be negatively correlated to utilization of mental health services. For example, Koegel (26) showed that only one-fifth of severely mentally ill, homeless people in a sample in Los Angeles were engaged in psychiatric care and that only three-fifths of this sample had any such history. Recognizing this underutilization of psychiatric care, programs have developed to offer psychiatric care on-site at community-based sites where people who are homeless receive other services. This includes placing psychiatric and medical providers at shelters, drop-in centers, food programs, and on street outreach teams. Starting in the 1980s, community-based nonprofits such as the Project for Psychiatric Outreach to the Homeless and Project Renewal in New York City started placing psychiatrists in homeless shelters. Engagement with this on-site psychiatry has been associated with improved clinical and housing outcomes (27). Organizations such as Healthcare for the Homeless opened clinics in shelters, and more recently street medicine teams have been developed to bring medical care to people outdoors (28,29).

Active outreach is a bedrock clinical tool for people who are homeless. Such programs designed to locate and engage people have yielded increased access to services and housing. Psychiatrists integrating into these programs have been able to bring evaluation and treatment to homeless people who would otherwise not receive these services. Morris and Warnock (30) demonstrated improvements in psychiatric symptoms and psychosocial functioning in a group of homeless, mentally ill people who were not utilizing traditional outpatient treatment but were instead engaged with outreach services based on an Assertive Community Treatment model. Similarly, Stergiopoulos (27) demonstrated a positive correlation between clinical improvement and housing stability as related to number of visits with a shelter-based psychiatrist and treatment adherence.

THE STRUCTURE OF PSYCHIATRIC EMERGENCY MODALITIES FOR PEOPLE WHO ARE HOMELESS

Emergency services for people who are homeless and living with mental illness may be divided into two phases: prehospital and hospital-based emergency interventions. Prehospital modalities include specialized outreach programs and mobile crisis services which at times can obviate the need for hospital-based emergency services.

Prehospital: Outreach and Mobile Crisis Services

A homeless person who is experiencing a psychiatric emergency or who is seeking emergency psychiatric services will often have an opportunity to receive care from community-based services that may obviate the need for evaluation in a hospital-based ED. This care may come from mental health providers working with homeless service teams, mobile crisis programs, or law enforcement agencies.

In some communities, social service teams that serve people in shelters or on the street employ mental health providers. In addition to providing routine evaluation and care, these clinicians can evaluate an acute crisis to determine if hospital-based emergency care is needed versus providing or coordinating access to care and other services to adequately address the acute problem.

Mobile crisis teams, which may or may not be a mobile unit of a hospital-based ED, assess people in crisis to determine the most appropriate and least restrictive interventions. They are typically able to link people with an array of behavioral health, medical, and social services, including hospital-based emergency care if necessary. In some communities, the mental health providers working with homelessness service teams or mobile crisis teams are also empowered to have people who are homeless and acutely mentally ill transported, even involuntarily, to a hospital emergency room. Typically, the criteria for such involuntary transport are the same or similar to the involuntary commitment criteria of the jurisdiction.

Some police departments employ mental health providers, or partner with agencies that do, to create co-response or Crisis Intervention Teams to respond to people seemingly in psychiatric crisis in the community (31,32). This model of law enforcement response, also known as the "Memphis Model," includes specially trained police officers in mental illness and de-escalation techniques (33). The participation of a mental health provider on such a law enforcement team helps with professional support, including as a resource for clinical alternatives to arrest or other police action. In a similar model, the San Francisco Fire Department has created a Homeless Outreach Medical Emergency Team consisting of specially trained paramedics, which has reduced emergency service use among some previously high utilizers (34).

People who are homeless and in acute crises often decline services and care forcing clinicians to decide when to favor coercive versus noncoercive measures to address crises—when ought a homeless person be involuntarily treated or transported to a hospital? The first goal of outreach work is to create and nurture an effective working relationship through developing trust and familiarity, and this can be a painstaking process taking weeks, months, or even years. In the mean time, a homeless person can be living with untreated behavioral or physical health conditions that cause significant morbidity and suffering. It is not clear, however, that involuntary care improves clinical conditions or housing

outcomes as people often reject care that started as involuntary once it is no longer involuntary. Furthermore, chronic institutional care in state hospitals no longer exists as an alternative to homelessness because of a significant reduction in state hospital beds and lengths of stay (35). There is very little research comparing outcomes for either position with respect to successful long-term introduction to services that started as involuntary. A 1993 qualitative analysis of a project combining involuntary transport of people living on the street and commitment to acute, and then intermediate, hospitalization yielded mixed outcomes. In this New York City program, 27% of homeless acute inpatients were discharged to stable domiciliary environments, and 67% were transferred to a state hospital for intermediate care (36). In turn, of patients who were transferred, 29% were lost to follow-up via elopement or discharge against medical advice (37). Both individual engagement issues and systems limitations, especially a dearth of housing, may have resulted in relatively high dropout rates. More recently, Compton and colleagues (38) showed a decreased risk of homelessness after involuntary hospitalization for 4 months for people living with serious mental illness who were enrolled in involuntary outpatient commitment upon hospital discharge. Study participants, however, were not homeless prior to hospitalization.

Although involuntary care can be effective in certain situations, the painstaking work of outreach is the sensitive application of incentive and influence to engage people in care and services (39). Dyches and colleagues (40) retrospectively examined the effectiveness of Cleveland, Ohio's, community-based mobile crisis service by comparing users of this service with a matched sample of ED patients. People not already connected to mental health service providers were more likely to receive community mental health follow-up within 90 days. Compared with the ED group, mobile crisis service recipients were also more likely to be homeless and have serious mental illness. An extension of this study also indicated that mobile crisis contacts were less likely to be hospitalized (41), a finding consistent with other studies of mobile crisis services (42).

Hospital Psychiatric Emergency Services

People who are homeless use ED services disproportionately. In one large epidemiological study, Kushel (24) reported that almost one in every three homeless people visit a general ED in a given year, three times the rate of the general population (4). Another multisite study of chronically homeless adults found that in a 3-month period 30% of participants had moderate ED use (1-2 visits) and 12% had high ED use (3 or more visits) (1). In another study drawing on a sample in San Francisco, 55% of all reported ED encounters in a 1-year period were made by the 7.9% of homeless respondents who used the ED four or more times (4). A national study by Ku and colleagues estimated that homeless individuals made 550,000 ED visits annually, or 72 visits per 100 homeless people in the United States per year (43).

Because of this high utilization, homeless people often make up a significant percentage of ED patients. In one large urban public hospital located near a shelter, between 20% and 30% of visits were of homeless people (44). A study in 3 EDs in Northern Pennsylvania found that 7% of patients were homeless (45).

Among homeless people who utilize emergency care there is a high burden of mental illness. D'Amore (46) reported high rates of depression (81%), schizophrenia (27%), and alcohol use (70%), among a group of homeless ED utilizers who did not even present with a psychiatric chief complaint. Despite a high burden of mental illness, poor engagement in outpatient care contributes to ED utilization. McNeil and Binder (47) reported that at a public hospital in San Francisco patients who were homeless and mentally ill were more frequently hospitalized and often had a tenuous connection to outpatient services that resulted in a costly cycle of acute psychiatric admission and discharge. A study of 10,340 patients in the San Diego mental health system revealed that homeless patients used emergency, crisis residential, and inpatient services at steeply higher rates than their non-homeless counterparts, while participating in significantly fewer outpatient, day treatment, and case management services (48).

Substance use seems to be a predictive factor of ED utilization among homeless people. One study of homeless individuals with chronic public intoxication noted that the ED is their most frequent health care contact (49). In the sample of Kushel (4), surveyed from 1996 to 1997, substance misuse in the past year was strongly associated with ED use and multiple encounters. McNeil and Binder (47) echoed this by noting that the most frequent ED users in their study were homeless and with co-occurring substance misuse and mental illness. However, in a 1987 sample taken from the public shelter system in New York City, substance dependence and alcoholism were insignificant and negative predictors in ED appearance, respectively (50). The discrepancy may result from a number of causes, including a general increase in substance misuse among homeless populations, contemporaneously less aggressive health care outreach and transport by law enforcement and crisis services, and the possibility that a particular cluster of high-risk factors may augur repeat encounters with emergency services. A recent study of synthetic cannabis (K2) users in an urban psychiatric ED found that 84.5% were homeless (51). Additional factors among homeless people may include concurrent mental illness, chronicity of homelessness, medical comorbidities, victimization, arrest history, and history of violence (1,4,47,50,52).

Utilizing the ED as "primary provider" can be conceptualized as a sign of disaffiliation and poverty. Homelessness is disaffiliation in extremis and a perception of meager to nil social support is clearly linked to homelessness (53,54). Patients who are homeless have, in turn, been critical of ED staff behaviors (55). However, some authors have argued that comprehensive and sensitively managed ED contact is an ideal opportunity to nurture meaningful engagement (56) and to meld health and human services systems (57). Strong social work capacity is a central feature of well-designed psychiatric EDs. Lee and colleagues (58) describe a paradigm of a psychiatric ED as the center of a hub-and-spoke model, responsible for proactively engaging and connecting patients to care. As an outgrowth of this model applicable to homeless persons, there have been experiments with creating and expanding ED case management functions. Such interventions have been shown to improve emergency department recidivism in homeless people with chemical dependency (59,60). They have also been advocated for use with mentally ill populations (61). Some psychiatric emergency programs routinely employ postdischarge short-term case management as a function of their mobile crisis units (62). Newer models of care, such as medical homes specific to individuals who are homeless, have been developed which have demonstrated improvements in engaging individuals in primary care and decreasing use of the ED (63).

PREHOSPITAL ASSESSMENT AND INTERVENTION

Community-based emergency interventions with people with mental illness and homelessness typically occur in public spaces and in drop-in or shelter environments. In addition to the clinical features of the crisis, the setting of the crisis influences evaluation and emergency referral to a hospital. We present two illustrative clinical situations here that offer insight into the decision-making issues that prehospital crisis intervention clinicians frequently face (Case Examples 40.1 and 40.2).

Assessment and Management Skills and Techniques

The scope of crisis assessments of people with mental illness and homelessness is broad: issues of homicidality, clearly escalating agitation, and suicidality often yield relatively uncomplicated decision making with regard to personal or community safety. Threatening or agitated behavior presents a relatively low threshold for involuntary intervention, especially when the person is unable or unwilling to report a history. Furthermore, without knowledge of baseline behavior or thinking—often the case with homeless persons in the street—there is a tendency to select the safest clinical course of action. In such cases, third parties, such as the police or the public, may often contact crisis teams. They may themselves witness risky behavior, such as a person walking in traffic, or elicit information concerning suicidality through interviews with unknown bystanders.

Gil and Henry, however, present another commonly encountered challenge: personal danger through self-neglect. Conditions of self-neglect present special issues technically, ethically,

---

 CASE EXAMPLE 40.1: Gil

Gil had episodic contact with the street outreach team. Living in a city park during the summer, he would only occasionally use showers at a drop-in center, staying no more than an hour or so. When the weather turned cold, he would travel "out west." His style was pleasant, even chatty, but he shared nothing about himself except to say that he sometimes got food late at night when restaurants closed because they knew about his "important work." He reported owning numerous Internet businesses, stressing that he knew a famous software entrepreneur, from whom he was awaiting an imminent call for an offer to run a business empire. He declined housing, saying his pending business deal would not require him to receive help for "the needy." Gil drank wine and would become raucous when intoxicated, sometimes yelling obscenities to passersby, triggering calls to police, who would either move him along from his usual spot or take him to a hospital—never resulting in a psychiatric admission.

During one November, he did not travel, became more evasive and irritable, and did not visit the drop-in center. Then he disappeared for a week—until 1 day when the weather turned prematurely cold. The street outreach team found Gil lying curled on his side on a curb in the park, bedraggled, with alcohol on his breath and his parka very soiled. His face was gray with dirt, but ruddy, and his fingers cold and pink. He passively said "I'm okay" but would not get up. The team determined that he would likely succumb from hypothermia without involuntary transport to an emergency room.

The team psychiatrist contacted emergency medical services (EMS) and a special police unit. A team member contacted the local ED, alerting it to their arrival. Gil was brought by ambulance to the ED; his blood alcohol level was 22 and blood glucose was 420. He was admitted to the medical service for treatment of diabetes and alcohol withdrawal and was subsequently transferred under involuntary legal status to psychiatry.

CASE EXAMPLE 40.2: Henry

Henry, 32 years old, had lived quietly in the municipal shelter system for over a year, but was transferred to another shelter where there was a mental health team. He arrived with his belongings slung over his back in a large duffel, carrying it everywhere, declining to use a locked locker. He never changed his jean jacket and black pants. Although his rangy stature and stern demeanor seemed ominous, he was never threatening; instead, his manner was serious and courteous, albeit laconic with a monotone voice. Trained in graphic arts, Henry would spend hours writing and drawing well-crafted illustrations in a notebook, stating that he was working on a book, but unable to speak about its topic. Over months, staff tried to engage him, but he consistently declined all services. Psychiatric medication was emphatically, if politely, declined, saying he had no illness, was not interested in housing, and would be okay to leave the shelter for the street, if asked. Meanwhile, he had periods in which his hygiene became particularly poor and he wore the same clothing for weeks, bordering on being a health hazard for others. During one of these episodes, he was so withdrawn that he became mute and stopped eating. The team's psychiatrist believed Henry to be unable to care for himself, and contacted the police to involuntarily transport him to the local ED (he resisted passively). Henry was admitted and treated voluntarily with antipsychotic medication, agreeing to do so only as long as he was in the hospital. Over a period of 2 years this situation repeated twice. Although Henry never continued medication while in the shelter, for several weeks after each hospital discharge he was more voluble and flexible in applying for benefits, each time with incremental improvement in engagement with the team. After 3 years, he opted to enter a transitional housing program.

and legally and warrant special illustrative focus in this section. Although self-neglect presents a range of severity, in both situations presented in the case examples, team members assessed that without immediate intervention there would be an irreversible course toward significant self-harm.

To determine *when* to intervene in this regard, crisis teams rely on the patient's preexisting historical data, their observational skills, and manifest interview data (Table 40.1). One clear marker for intervention is a significant shift in behavioral adaptation to the environment, often marked by changes in personal routine. As a basic premise, homeless living is clearly difficult and some manage with remarkable survival skills. A person's relative ability to secure clothing, food, some form of safe shelter, and to attend to their health care and hygiene while homeless is a good indication of a person's capacities, especially in the face of serious mental illness or substance use disorders. Some people living with significant psychiatric symptoms take excellent care of themselves, making it difficult to justify involuntary evaluation or treatment, thus requiring careful and patient clinical, engagement (64). Yet, some

people who seemingly have few or mild symptoms are unable to attend to basic needs, requiring careful determination of capacity. Gil and Henry led unhealthful existences at baseline, but maintained a survival homeostasis that had changed dramatically by the point of crisis encounter. In Gil's case, an important variable was ambient temperature. For Henry, the immediate stressors were less clear, but he could no longer sustain the routines of the shelter.

Because these patients are often unable or unwilling to engage in a historical interview, clinicians may rely heavily on basic sensory observational skills of sight, sound, and smell to make these determinations. Clinicians note cognitive orientation, relatedness and interactive capacity, and self-appreciation of distress as they attempt to engage the person to elicit clinical data. But even prior to this, assessment typically begins with a period of observation at a distance. Is the person displaying threatening or odd behavior? Is he or she responsive to others? Then the focus zooms down to close observation, evaluating personal hygiene and appearance and noting odors. The existence of parasitic infestations and lower extremity cellulitis are important examples in this

TABLE 40.1 Prehospital Crisis Assessment

Before Encounter
Information from prior team contacts
Referral data
During Encounter
Sensory observations
   Visual and auditory: behavior
   Visual: personal appearance
   Visual: presence of infestations and/or infection
   Olfactory: breath and body odor
Orientation to place, time, person
Relatedness and interactive behavior
Self-appreciation of distress
Evaluate
Current behavior: disorganized, aggressive, impulsive, withdrawn
Homicidal and suicidal ideation
Change in personal routine or level of functioning within environment
Accessibility for in situ follow-up and voluntary interventions
Medical acuity

regard in that untreated medical conditions are common among people who are homeless. In fact, there is evidence that many involuntary interventions, especially among the street homeless, are significantly motivated by medical acuity (65). In such circumstances, psychiatric symptoms may cause people to neglect life-threatening medical illness, and identifying that such a person does not have capacity to refuse care may supply sufficient rationale to legally support involuntary transport. This becomes especially relevant in some communities during extreme weather. For example, the City of New York will declare weather emergencies in cold and hot weather to encourage first responders to involuntarily transport people with homelessness for hospital evaluation who are not adequately protecting themselves from the weather.

As noted, both Gil and Henry presented functional changes, but Henry lived in a setting where his exacerbation was more observable. The team knew him and had an even clearer view of his current baseline, permitting them to observe his illness and enabling intervention relatively early. In addition to executing the intervention in a more controlled environment, the team was able to follow up after Henry's hospitalizations, using each intervention to advance rehabilitative efforts. In contrast, crisis management in public spaces

often presents more ambiguities. Street-based clinicians must frequently render judgments with less baseline data. From a practical vantage point, for example, in cases of self-neglect, it is most useful to balance the team's estimation of clinical gravity with a sense of whether the person will be accessible to subsequent observations and resultant chances for voluntary engagement, including assistance in arriving at an ED. Regardless, it is important to ascertain as much demographic and clinical information as possible and to design evaluation and potential intervention options prior to actual face-to-face evaluation (39). This is particularly true when police or EMS is involved. Efficient and coordinated intervention is crucial in that the street may offer opportunity for a person to evade involuntary transport or, less frequently, for the distractive involvement of (a) passersby who wish either to help or to enable the person to elude transport. In this manner, different team members assume roles of working with the public or with the patient.

Whether on the street or in a more controlled environment, the team's function as a unit is critical. Especially in mobile crisis and street outreach environments, clinicians share long hours with each other and develop intimate knowledge of each others' clinical strengths and challenges. Successful teams use this knowledge in their clinical roles. For example, one team member may be particularly adept at engaging patients with personality disorders. In the end, the unit evolves a "team persona": a set of professional behaviors that characterizes the way it performs its work (39). To arrive at this, team leaders must be sensitive to encourage discussion of clinical disagreement, as well as exploring countertransference (66).

Legal and Ethical Issues

Even if there is a clinical determination that a person ought to have a hospital emergency evaluation, there can be significant structural obstacles to getting that person to the hospital. EMS first responders and law enforcement personnel are generally instructed to not involuntarily take a person to a hospital (unless, in the case of police, there is a determination to make an arrest), so they may be reluctant to involuntarily transport anyone who clearly communicates his or her wishes, even in the context of clear psychiatric symptoms. As a practical manner in such situations, a clinician can frequently access EMS or police supervisory personnel who may overrule a field-level decision when a clinician on the scene makes the case that a person does in fact not have decisional capacity. Also, in some communities, some mental health clinicians are legally empowered—effectively deputized—by local authorities to direct first responders to transport homeless persons for hospital evaluations.

In both Gil's and Henry's situation, could earlier interventions have changed their outcomes? Could Gil have been taken at an earlier encounter when he had alcohol on his breath? Could Henry's earlier episodes of poor personal hygiene been argued to be a community health problem for the shelter? Clinical teams pursue goals of long-term engagement and rehabilitation. In doing so, they struggle with issues such as these case by case, evaluating when coercive measures serve to advance engagement and recovery, as opposed to undermining it. Therefore, in addition to customary clinical decision making regarding community safety or violence potential, safety to self may extend beyond suicidal risk to a realm frequently encountered with people who are homeless and severely mentally ill. As previously noted, extreme self-neglect owing to lack of mental capacity can approach dangerousness to self and thus be justification for involuntary transport for a hospital evaluation, though there is wide variation among jurisdictions as to what degree this constitutes a legal standard for involuntary transport to a hospital.

HOSPITAL ASSESSMENT AND INTERVENTIONS

This section describes the processes of ED evaluation of the patient who is homeless. Conducting a psychiatric evaluation of homeless patients in the ED follows the format of any emergency psychiatric evaluation, but careful attention should be paid to the following critical areas.

Mode of Arrival

People who are mentally ill and homeless arrive to the ED alone or, not infrequently, accompanied by outreach, shelter, mobile crisis, EMS, or law enforcement personnel and may not be able to provide critical historical details. It is of utmost importance to ask whoever arrived with the patient for a detailed description of the circumstances leading to presentation, as well as whatever may be known about the individual's baseline level of functioning and illness.

First Step: Medical Evaluation

Patients who are homeless have less access to primary medical care and may have untreated, undertreated, or undiagnosed medical issues. Therefore, any patient presenting with evidence of an acute medical complaint, unstable vital signs, symptoms of chemical intoxication or withdrawal, delirium, or new-onset psychotic symptoms is first triaged for evaluation and stabilization by the medical ED. Homeless people have high rates of medical comorbidities, including HIV infection, tuberculosis, and medical complications related to substance abuse (67). Other medical problems to consider include injuries, hepatitis, anemia, malnutrition, skin and foot problems, chronic health issues such as hypertension and diabetes, respiratory disease, seizures, and head trauma (68,69). The clinician must aggressively assess for medical illness. A physical exam and basic laboratory tests should be performed, including complete blood count, comprehensive chemistry panel, liver function tests, blood alcohol level, and urine drug screen. Other tests should be performed as indicated, such as thyroid function, electrocardiogram, and chest radiograph. Gil's case, described in the previous section, is illustrative of the frequency with which homeless patients with diabetes have poor glucose control and are at high risk for complications. If an arriving patient is first triaged to the medical ED, a psychiatric concern may be identified either through self-report or because the ED physician identifies altered mood, thinking, or behavior.

Identifying Information

Starting an interview by asking for basic demographic information helps in obtaining a general context for the patient's symptoms and current presentation. For example, where has the patient been staying: a city shelter, private shelter, drop-in center, on the street, in the subways, on a couch or floor of a friend or family member, or in an abandoned building? How long has the patient been homeless? How does he or she spend his or her days? How does he or she meet basic needs?

Understanding the context of the patient's homelessness will provide an understanding of symptoms, level of adaptive functioning, and severity of psychosocial stressors. Has homelessness been a part of the patient's life for years, or is the patient newly homeless because of a recent housing crisis? For instance, has the person recently been ejected from his or her home as a result of family difficulties? Similarly, has he or she been unable to work because of depression or psychosis (and therefore been unable to pay rent)?

Chief Complaint and History of Present Illness

The clinician asks about the patient's symptom constellation, its chronology, and how he or she came to the ED. Whose idea was it and what help is being sought—and why today? If someone else called 911, it is also important to determine the patient's understanding of this occurrence. This helps engagement.

Past Psychiatric History

Homeless patients have decreased access to outpatient care. Key areas to cover in the interview are whether he or she has a current treatment provider

and, if so, the nature of the relationship and level of engagement. As with all patients presenting to an ED, asking about past hospitalizations, suicide attempts, and a history of suicide attempts and violence is critical. People who are homeless are at higher risk of social comorbidities, such as incarceration (70) and physical and sexual trauma (71). Acquiring a legal history, including treatment while incarcerated, can both inform assessment and perhaps indicate how the patient will react to an often highly structured ED setting. Symptoms of posttraumatic stress disorder may be less obvious on initial interview, but acquiring a history of exposure to trauma can be diagnostically informative and sensitizes the interviewer to a risk of experiential retraumatization during the ED visit itself, which would further distance the patient from collaborating with the assessment and consequent offers of assistance.

Alcohol and Substance Use History

It is critical to inquire about present and past alcohol and substance use and whether the patient has received treatment for a substance use disorder. If actively using alcohol or drugs, the patient's current motivation for treatment should be assessed, using the transtheoretical model (72).

The presentation of substance dependence is an important issue in the ED, and its significance may be either overappreciated or underappreciated. For example, it is important to not prematurely evaluate a patient's suicidal or aggressive impulses by assuming simple intoxication, as opposed to a frequently co-occurring mental illness. In our experience, many of these patients are alexithymic, or use severe forms of denial or affective isolation to defend against revealing the painful experiences they have when sober. Conversely, patients with prominent affective and psychotic symptoms with comorbid substance misuse may often be treated for these symptoms and not be assessed adequately for or given aggressive treatment of their substance or alcohol usage.

Psychosocial History

Asking patients about their upbringing, social network, educational history, employment history, sources of financial support, and linkage with community agencies is integral to the evaluation because some homeless patients may have family members or others who are able to provide history and support. Probing the patient's psychosocial history will help the clinician understand the link between the patient's mental illness and homelessness. Similarly, the clinician must sensitize himself or herself to the patient's cultural background and values. This enhances engagement and tunes interventions by enabling the clinician to better understand how homelessness is experienced and what social supports may be available. For example, a male immigrant Latino patient who is homeless may experience the burden of machismo, with a sense of shame concerning his impoverished state inhibiting an ability to reach out to family who may, in fact, be more available than he fears.

Mental Status Examination

Careful attention is focused on the patient's appearance, thus providing data on his or her ability for self-care. The patient's attitude toward the interviewing clinician indicates a willingness to engage with treatment providers, which may be useful in predicting whether he or she is likely to follow up with outpatient treatment. Because patients who are homeless have high rates of cognitive impairment (73), cognitive functioning should be assessed, including orientation, attention, memory, and calculating ability. In addition to informing the most helpful interventions, cognitive functioning provides additional data regarding a basic ability to care for self.

Collateral History

Especially in cases where transport to the ED is involuntary, it is absolutely critical to obtain collateral history from anyone who knows the patient—family members, case managers, shelter staff, outreach personnel, psychiatrists, or others. This clarifies the patient's history and current functioning and has crucial potential to facilitate clinical and social linkage, creating engagement with the patient's social system. This cannot be underestimated, because disposition is typically challenging with this patient population.

Assessment

After evaluating the patient, the clinician assesses the need for immediate intervention and determines an appropriate level of care. A key component of that decision is assessing safety—whether there is imminent risk of harm to self or others, or severe self-neglect as a result of impaired mental status. Understanding the nature of the immediate precipitants heralding presentation in both a psychosocial and diagnostic framework is imperative. It is especially important to deliberately evaluate adaptive personal strengths in that they inevitably modify the understanding of the patient's needs. The resourcefulness of many people who are homeless, for instance, is a factor in evaluating their ability to get their basic needs met.

Disposition

Depending on the assessment, patients may need to be observed and stabilized in the ED prior to disposition, sometimes avoiding premature decisions for inpatient admission. Although it is difficult to truly address a psychiatric illness or substance use disorder while a person is in the existential flux of homelessness, the availability of extended observation capacity, with the opportunity to observe patients for 72 hours or more, is particularly useful for at least acutely stabilizing these patients. This window of time can enable coalescence of complex amalgams of mental health, substance misuse, medical, and social resources. In determining the most appropriate disposition for the patient, the least restrictive environment should be selected and the concept of procedural justice should be employed. *Procedural justice* is defined as a process by which the patient feels that he or she has been involved in decision making regarding care and feels that the process has been collaborative and fair (74) (Case Example 40.3).

Finally, as with any person leaving the ED, taking into account a person's setting and situation in the community is crucial in formulating an effective disposition plan for a person who is homeless. The ED clinician must consider the following for a person who is homeless:

- How well does a person attend to his or her basic needs of safety, food, clothing, hygiene, and shelter?
- Where will the person be sleeping? Is he or she staying at a shelter or other transitional living program, or sleeping outdoors or in another location not otherwise intended for human habitation?

CASE EXAMPLE 40.3: Sheila

Sheila is homeless and suffers from schizoaffective disorder and alcohol and cocaine abuse. She frequently presents to the ED with complaints of auditory hallucinations in the context of medication nonadherence and substance use. Her symptoms typically resolve rapidly in the ED as she clears from toxic states and is restarted on antipsychotic medication. She has been encouraged to attend inpatient rehabilitation for treatment of her substance use disorder, but has declined such referrals. Sheila has also not followed up on past referrals for outpatient psychiatric and substance abuse treatment. At each ED visit, social workers contact the members of the Homeless Outreach Program requesting they meet with Sheila. They attempt to engage her, using a nonjudgmental approach, helping her to identify her goals and offering services to help her meet these goals. Over time, Sheila has built an alliance with the Homeless Outreach Program staff and is beginning to work with them to apply for housing and benefits.

Sheila's situation is an example of the ED stabilizing an acute event and then actively negotiating with the patient, and finally linking the patient to specialized follow-up. In this sense, the ED served as a hub, helping link a patient to community services (58). The ED social worker has a critical role in this, performing a needs assessment and implementing necessary social services interventions, including assistance in applying for benefits or referral to shelter, housing, case management, and outpatient treatment services.

- Whether in shelter or outdoors, how safe is the location, for both the person and his or her belongings and is there a safe place to store and take medication?
- How will the person access any prescriptions that are being provided? Will he or she go to the pharmacy or will the pharmacy deliver to the shelter or social service program that the person utilizes?
- Does the person have health insurance? How will the person follow up with any outpatient appointments that are offered? Does he or she have a means of travel to appointments?
- If the person is being served by a social service or government agency, what supports does that agency provide and how effectively is he or she actually engaged with those services and supports?

Countertransference Issues Relevant to Caring for Homeless Patients in the Psychiatric Emergency Service

As with all challenging relationships, working with patients who are homeless can elicit complex countertransference reactions—the overwhelming nature of their environmental, social, psychological, and psychiatric/medical needs understandably affects workers who come in contact with them. Inevitably, clinicians may struggle with the hopeless, helpless, and despairing conditions these persons experience every day. It is important to understand how one's feelings (eg, frustration, desire to help) can impact thoughtful, independent clinical assessment of an emergency situation.

It is important to appreciate that systemic factors external to the patient (such as ED overcrowding, or lack of bed availability) may be a confounding variable. Tensions may arise between ED staff and outreach clinicians who transport a recidivist person to the ED for evaluation and admission. Outreach staff can feel frustrated feeling that an ED staff is dismissive of their client while an ED staff can feel frustrated by recidivism that seems immune to their efforts.

Clinicians may also have feelings about secondary gain while evaluating people who are homeless and whose basic needs are so vast. Clinicians may feel angry about people reporting symptoms in an attempt to obtain food or shelter. Considering the challenges for homeless people of attending to basic needs, however, such "malingering" activity can instead be viewed as adaptive survival behavior. Furthermore, it is often the case that people who are "malingering" are also suffering from clinical problems that require urgent evaluation and care— a patient may be experiencing psychiatric symptoms but may not be able to articulate effectively about that and instead expresses other needs. Reacting only to a patient's manifest chief complaint will often result in missing significant clinical problems.

SYSTEMS ISSUES AND CLINICAL CARE

The challenges a person without a home faces are often overwhelming, intensely magnifying the struggle of financial problems, and exacerbating mental illness and substance use disorders. He or she must navigate multiple systems that are not coordinated: housing, entitlements, and medical and behavioral health. Clinicians on crisis teams or within the ED often find themselves caught between the overwhelming needs of patient, their sometimes manifest resistance to treatment, and the impediments imposed by these overarching systems. As a result, it is important for clinicians to avoid unintentionally aligning themselves with the patient's sense of hopelessness, helplessness, and despair, resulting in shuttling the person in and out of emergency services.

Because effective linkage is so important, services such as outreach teams, intensive case management, peer support, and ACT teams are particularly beneficial tools for treatment and rehabilitation. Outreach teams specifically working with people who are homeless and mentally ill are extremely useful as sources of history and have insight into shifts from baseline functioning that patients may be unable to provide. As discussed previously, these teams, as well as ACT programs and intensive case managers, become experienced in understanding the experiential life of the individual. Through their flexible roles in follow-up, linkage, and treatment, they are often the most useful contacts for the ED concerning this patient population. Coordination of care helps minimize unnecessarily frequent PES encounters and an important dimension of this is cultivating active networking relationships between the ED and these programs.

As an example, one urban hospital has had daily structured liaison with its Homeless Outreach Team and the clinical staff of a shelter across the street, itself operated by a community-based organization. Morning interdisciplinary rounds are conducted in the ED that include psychiatric attendings, residents, social workers, substance abuse counselors, and members of the outreach team. After rounds, communication is established with the clinical director of the shelter program to ascertain collateral history on patients. If needed, clinical interventions can be made while in the ED prior to disposition back to the shelter.

Communication within the general ED structure is equally important. In addition to comprehensive ED sign-out rounds, there must be regular and routine communication between the medical and psychiatric emergency departments and, at minimum, interdisciplinary rounding twice daily. One solution is to have a designated "medical/psychiatric district" staffed by a medical attending physician and a minimum of two registered nurses. Designated attending psychiatrists and psychiatric nurse practitioners serve as liaisons between the distinct medical and psychiatric emergency departments concerning patient care.

CONCLUSION

Emergency mental health services constitute one component of a constellation of services serving homeless populations. These services—entitlements, housing, employment, health, and mental health—receive a range of typically uncoordinated public funding that varies in breadth and depth, depending on the community. In addition to advocating for improved systems coordination, the key for clinicians is to create practical means to connect patients with what they need.

An important finding of the federal Access to Community Care and Effective Services and Supports (ACCESS) program, which evaluated homelessness services among multiple national sites, comparing specially integrated service macro-level systems with those that were not, was that client outcomes were actually indistinguishable, prompting an analysis that smaller groupings of service providers might be the most effective mechanisms for integrating and improving health and social outcomes (25,75). People with homelessness and mental illness often encounter emergency services at a point where other delivery structures have been unable to engage them. Through diligent clinical assessment of patients' personal crises, mental health professionals working in emergency services are often uniquely poised to identify systemic breakdown and act as effective agents in advancing client-level change, doing so by using small service networks of providers who are accustomed to working with each other and linking a common set of consumers to treatment and rehabilitation.

REFERENCES

1. Moore, D. T., & Rosenheck, R. A. (2016). Factors affecting emergency department use by a chronically homeless population. *Psychiatric Services, 67*, 1340–1347.

2. Moore, D. T., & Rosenheck, R. A. (2017). Comprehensive services delivery and emergency department use among chronically homeless adults. *Psychological Services, 14*(2), 184–192.

3. Thakarar, K., Morgan, J. R., Gaeta, J. M., Hohl, C., & Drainoni, M.-L. (2015). Predictors of frequent emergency room visits among a homeless population. *PLOS One, 10*(4), e0124552. doi:10.1371/journal.pone.0124552.

4. Kushel, M. B., Perry, S., Bangsberg, D., et al. (2002). Emergency department use among the homeless and marginally housed: Results from a community-based study. *American Journal of Public Health, 92*, 778–784.

5. Culhane, D. P., Dejowski, E. F., Ibanez, J., et al. (1994). Public shelter admission rates in Philadelphia and New York City: The implications of turnover for sheltered population counts. *Housing Policy Debate, 5*, 107–140.

6. Link, B. G., Susser, E. S., Stueve, A., et al. (1994). Lifetime and five-year prevalence of homelessness in the United States. *American Journal of Public Health, 84*, 1907–1912.

7. Fazel, S., Khosla, V., Doll, H., & Geddes, J. (2008). The prevalence of mental disorders among the homeless in western countries: Systematic review and meta-regression analysis. *PLOS Medicine, 5*(12), e225.

8. Lamb, H. R., & Bachrach, L. L. (2001). Some perspectives on deinstitutionalization. *Psychiatric Services, 52*, 1039–1045.

9. Lauber, C., Lay, B., & Rössler, W. (2006). Homeless people at disadvantage in homeless health services. *European Archives of Psychiatry and Clinical Neuroscience, 256*, 138–145.

10. Breakey, W. R., Fischer, P. J., Kramer, M., et al. (1989). Health and mental health problems of homeless men and women in Baltimore. *JAMA, 262*, 1352–1357.

11. Koegel, P., Burnam, M. A., & Farr, R. K. (1988). The prevalence of specific psychiatric disorders among homeless individuals in the inner city of Los Angeles. *Archives of General Psychiatry, 45*, 1085–1091.

12. Susser, E., Struening, E. L., & Conover, S. (1989). Psychiatric problems in homeless men. *Archives of General Psychiatry, 46*, 845–850.

13. North, C. S., Eyrich, K. M., Pollio, D. E., et al. (2004). Are rates of psychiatric disorders in the homeless population changing? *American Journal of Public Health, 94*, 103–108.

14. McQuistion, H. L., Gorroochurn, P., Hsu, E., & Caton, C. L. M. (2014). Risk factors associated with recurrent homelessness after a first homeless episode. *Community Mental Health Journal, 50*, 505–513.

15. VanGeest, J. B., & Johnson, T. P. (2002). Substance abuse and homelessness: Direct or indirect effects? *Annals of Epidemiology, 12*, 455–461.

16. Breakey, W. R., Susser, E. S., & Timms, P. (2001). Mental health services for homeless people. In Thornicroft, G., Brewin, C. R., & Wing, J. (Eds.), *Measuring mental health needs* (2nd ed.). London: Gaskell.

17. O'Connell, J. J. (2005). *Premature mortality in homeless populations: A review of the literature* (p. 19). Nashville, TN: National Health Care for the Homeless Council, Inc.

18. Shinn, M., Rog, D. R., & Culhane, D. P. (2005). *Family homelessness: Background research findings and policy options*. Retrieved from http://repository.upenn.edu/spp_papers/83.

19. Levitt, A. J., Culhane, D. P., DeGenova, J., O'Quinn, P., & Bainbridge, J. (2009). Health and social characteristics of homeless adults in Manhattan who were chronically or not chronically unsheltered. *Psychiatric Services, 60*, 978–981.

20. Montgomery, A. E., Szymkowiak, D., Marcus, J., Howard, P., & Culhane, D. P. (2016). Homelessness, unsheltered status, and risk factors for mortality: Findings from the 100,000 homes campaign. *Public Health Reports, 131*(6), 765–772.

21. Stergiopoulos, V., Dewa, C. S., Tanner, G., Chau, N., Pett, M., & Connelly, J. L. (2010). Addressing the needs of the street homeless. *International Journal of Mental Health, 39*(1), 3–15.

22. O'Toole, T. P., Gibbon, J. L., Hanusa, B. H., & Fine, M. J. (1999). Utilization of health care services among subgroups of urban homeless and housed poor. *Journal of Health Politics, Policy and Law, 24*(1), 91–114.

23. Kim, M. M., Swanson, J. W., Swartz, M. S., Bradford, D. W., Mustillo, S. A., & Elbogen, E. B. (2007). Healthcare barriers among severely mentally ill homeless adults: Evidence from the five-site health and risk study. *Administration and Policy in Mental Health and Mental Health Services Research, 34,* 363–375.

24. Kushel, M. B., Vittinghoff, E., & Haas, J. S. (2001). Factors associated with the health care utilization of homeless persons. *JAMA, 285,* 200–206.

25. Rosenheck, R. A. (2004). Back to the future: Funding, integrating, and improving mental health services. *Psychiatric Services, 55,* 1141–1142.

26. Koegel, P., Sullivan, G., Burnam, A., Morton, S. C., & Wenzel, S. (1999). Utilization of mental health and substance abuse services among homeless adults in Los Angeles. *Medical Care, 37*(3), 306–317.

27. Stergiopoulos, V., Dewa, C. S., Rouleau, K., Yoder, S., & Chau, N. (2008). Collaborative mental health care for the homeless: The role of psychiatry in positive housing and mental health outcomes. *Canadian Journal of Psychiatry, 53*(1), 61–67.

28. Withers, J. (2016). Street medicine: An example of reality-based health care. *Journal of Health Care for the Poor and Underserved, 22*(1), 1–4.

29. Howe, E. C., Buck, D. S., & Withers, J. (2009). Delivering health care on the streets: Challenges and opportunities for quality management. *Quality Management in Health Care, 18*(4), 239–246.

30. Morris, D. W., & Warnock, J. K. (2001). Effectiveness of a Mobile Outreach and Crisis Services unit in reducing psychiatric symptoms in a population of homeless persons with severe mental illness. *The Journal of the Oklahoma State Medical Association, 94*(8), 343–346.

31. Kirst, M., Francombe Pridham, K., Narrandes, R., Matheson, F., Young, L., Niedra, K., & Stergiopoulos, V. (2015). Examining implementation of mobile, police-mental health crisis intervention teams in a large urban center. *Journal of Mental Health, 24*(6), 369–374.

32. Compton, M. T., Broussard, B., Munetz, M., Oliva, J. R., & Watson, A. C. (2011). *The Crisis Intervention Team (CIT) model of collaboration between law enforcement and mental health.* Hauppauge, NY: Nova Science Publishers, Inc.

33. Dupont, R., Cochran, S., & Pillsbury, S. (2007). *Crisis intervention team core elements.* The University of Memphis, School of Urban Affairs and Public Policy, Dept. of Criminology and Criminal Justice, CIT Center. Retrieved from http://cit.memphis.edu/CoreElements.pdf.

34. Tangherlini, N., et al. (2016). The HOME team: Evaluating the effect of an EMS-based outreach team to decrease the frequency of 911 use among high utilizers of EMS. *Prehospital and Disaster Medicine, 31*(6), 603–607.

35. Fuller, D. A., Sinclair, E., Geller, J., Quanbeck, C., & Snook, J. (2016, June). *Going, going, gone: Trends and consequences of eliminating state psychiatric beds, 2016 (updated for Q2 data).* Arlington, VA: Treatment Advocacy Center. Retrieved from http://www.tacreports.org/storage/documents/going-going-gone.pdf.

36. Nardacci, D., Caro, Y., Milstein, V., et al. (1993). Bellevue population: Demographics. In Katz, S. E., Nardacci, D., & Sabatini, A. (Eds.), *Intensive treatment of the homeless mentally ill* (pp. 51–70). Washington, DC: American Psychiatric Publishing.

37. Schrage, H. E., Silver, M. A., & Oldham, J. M. (1993). Role of the state mental health system. In Katz, S. E., Nardacci, D., & Sabatini, A. (Eds.), *Intensive treatment of the homeless mentally ill* (pp. 167–182). Washington, DC: American Psychiatric Publishing.

38. Compton, S. N., Swanson, J. W., Wagner, H. R., et al. (2003). Involuntary outpatient commitment and homelessness in persons with severe mental illness. *Mental Health Services Research, 5,* 27–38.

39. Ng, A. T., & McQuistion, H. L. (2004). Outreach to the homeless: Craft, science, and future implications. *Journal of Psychiatric Practice, 10,* 95–105.

40. Dyches, H., Biegel, D., Johnsen, J. A., et al. (2002). The impact of mobile crisis services on the use of community-based mental health services. *Research on Social Work Practice, 12,* 731–751.

41. Guo, S., Biegel, D. E., Johnsen, J. A., et al. (2001). Assessing the impact of community based mobile crisis services on preventing hospitalization. *Psychiatric Services, 52,* 223–228.

42. Hugo, M., Smout, M., & Bannister, J. (2002). A comparison in hospitalization rates between a community-based mobile emergency service and a hospital-based emergency service. *Australian and New Zealand Journal of Psychiatry, 36,* 504–508.

43. Ku, B. S., Scott, K. C., Kertesz, S. G., & Pitts, S. R. (2010). Factors associated with use of urban emergency departments by the U.S. homeless population. *Public Health Reports, 125,* 398–405.

44. Goldfrank, L. (1991). Caring for homeless patients: Challenge for the 90's [Abstract]. *Hospital Physician, 4*, 13.

45. Feldman, B. J., Calogero, C. G., Elsayed, K. S., Abbasi, O. Z., Enyart, J., Friel, T. J., Abunamous, Y. H., Dusza, S. W., & Greenberg, M. R. (2017). Prevalence of homelessness in the emergency department setting. *The Western Journal of Emergency Medicine, 18*, 366–372.

46. D'Amore, J., Hung, O., Chiang, W., et al. (2001). The epidemiology of the homeless population and its impact on an urban emergency department. *Academic Emergency Medicine, 8*, 1051–1055.

47. McNiel, D. E., & Binder, R. L. (2005). Psychiatric emergency service use and homelessness, mental disorder, and violence. *Psychiatric Services, 56*, 699–704.

48. Folsom, D. P., Hawthorne, W., Lindamer, L., et al. (2005). Prevalence and risk factors for homelessness and utilization of mental health services among 10,340 patients with serious mental illness in a large public mental health system. *American Journal of Psychiatry, 162*, 370–376.

49. Dunford, J. V., Castillo, E. M., Chan, T. C., et al. (2006). Impact of the San Diego Serial Inebriate Program on use of emergency medical resources. *Annals of Emergency Medicine, 47*, 328–336.

50. Padgett, D. K., Struening, E. L., Andrews, H., et al. (1995). Predictors of emergency room use by homeless adults in New York City: The influence of predisposing, enabling, and need factors. *Social Science & Medicine, 41*, 547–556.

51. Manseau, M. W., Rajparia, A., Joseph, A., Azarchi, S., Goff, D., Satodiya, R., & Lewis, C. F. (2017). Clinical characteristics of synthetic cannabinoid use in a large urban psychiatric emergency setting. *Substance Use & Misuse, 12*, 822–825.

52. Albert, M., & McCaig, L. F. (2015). Emergency department visits related to schizophrenia among adults aged 18-64: United States, 2009-2011. *NCHS Data Brief, 215*, 1–8.

53. Breakey, W. (1987). Treating the homeless. *Alcohol Health and Research World, 11*, 42–47.

54. Wu, T., & Serper, M. R. (1999). Social support and psychopathology in homeless patients presenting for emergency psychiatric treatment. *Journal of Clinical Psychology, 55*, 1127–1133.

55. Ambrosio, E., Baker, D., Crowe, C., et al. (1992). *The Street Health Report: A study of the health status and barriers to health care of homeless women and men in the City of Toronto*. Toronto, ON: Street Health.

56. Redelmeier, D. A., Molin, J.-P., & Tibshirani, R. J. (1995). A randomized trial of compassionate care for the homeless in an emergency department. *Lancet, 345*, 1131–1134.

57. Morris, D. W., & Gordon, J. A. (2006). The role of the emergency department in the care of homeless and disadvantaged populations. *Emergency Medicine Clinics of North America, 24*, 839–848.

58. Lee, T.-S. W., Renaud, E. F., & Hills, O. F. (2003). An emergency treatment hub-and-spoke model for psychiatric emergency services. *Psychiatric Services, 54*, 1590–1594.

59. Okin, R. L., Boccellari, A., Azocxar, F., et al. (2000). The effects of clinical case management on hospital service use among ED frequent users. *American Journal of Emergency Medicine, 18*, 603–608.

60. Witbeck, G., Hornfeld, S., & Dalack, G. W. (2000). Emergency room outreach to chronically addicted individuals: A pilot study. *Journal of Substance Abuse Treatment, 19*, 39–43.

61. Forster, P., & King, J. (1994). Definitive treatment of patients with serious mental disorders in an emergency service, Part 1. *Hospital and Community Psychiatry, 45*, 867–869.

62. Sullivan, A. M., & Rivera, J. (2000). Profile of a comprehensive psychiatric emergency program in a New York City municipal hospital. *Psychiatric Quarterly, 71*, 123–138.

63. Jones, A. L., Thomas, R., Hedayati, D. O., Saba, S. K., Conley, J., & Gordon, A. J. (2018). Patient predictors and utilization of health services within a medical home for homeless persons. *Substance Abuse, 39*(3), 354–360. doi:10.1080/08897077.2018.1437500.

64. McQuistion, H. L. (2012). Homelessness and behavioral health in the new century. In McQuistion, H. L., Sowers, W. E., Ranz, J., & Feldman, J. M. (Eds.), *Handbook of community psychiatry* (pp. 407–422). New York, NY: Springer.

65. Tsemberis, S. J., Cohen, N. L., & Jones, R. M. (1993). Conducting emergency psychiatric evaluations on the street. In Katz, S. E., Nardacci, D., & Sabatini, A. (Eds.), *Intensive treatment of the homeless mentally ill* (pp. 71–89). Washington, DC: American Psychiatric Publishing.

66. McQuistion, H. L., & Gillig, P. M. (2006). Mental illness and homelessness: An introduction. In Gillig, P. M., & McQuistion, H. L. (Eds.), *Clinical guide to the treatment of the mentally ill homeless person* (pp. 1–8). Washington, DC: American Psychiatric Publishing.

67. Kerker, B., Bainbridge, J., Li, W., et al. (2005). *The health of homeless adults in New York City.* New York, NY: Departments of Health and Mental Hygiene and Homeless Services.

68. Hwang, S. W. (2001). Homelessness and health. *CMAJ, 164,* 229–233.

69. Kulik, D. M., Gaetz, S., Crowe, C., & Ford-Jones, E. L. (2011). Homeless youth's overwhelming health burden: A review of the literature. *Pediatrics and Child Health, 16,* e43–e47.

70. Burt, M., Aron, L., Douglas, T., et al. (1999). *Homelessness: Programs and the people they serve. Summary report: Findings of the National Survey of Homeless Assistance Providers and Clients.* Washington, DC: The Urban Institute.

71. Christensen, R. C., Hodgkins, C. C., Garces, L. K., et al. (2005). Homeless, mentally ill and addicted: The need for abuse and trauma services. *Journal of Health Care for the Poor and Underserved, 16,* 615–622.

72. Prochaska, J. O., & DiClemente, C. C. (1982). Transtheoretical therapy: Toward a more integrative model of change. *Psychotherapy: Theory, Research and Practice, 19,* 276–288.

73. Solliday-McRoy, C., Campbell, T., Melchert, T. P., et al. (2004). Neuropsychological functioning of homeless men. *The Journal of Nervous and Mental Disease, 192,* 471–478.

74. Fishkind, A., & Zeller, S. (2006). Psychiatric emergency services. In Gillig, P. M., & McQuistion, H. L. (Eds.), *Clinical guide to the treatment of the mentally ill homeless person.* Washington, DC: American Psychiatric Publishing.

75. Goldman, H. H., Morrissey, J. P., Rosenheck, R. A., et al. (2002). Lessons from the evaluation of the ACCESS program. *Psychiatric Services, 53,* 967–970.

41

The Psychiatric Emergency Care of Prisoners

Jonathan G. Dunlop, Debra A. Pinals

At times, psychiatrists working within psychiatric emergency services (PES) may be called upon to evaluate patients who have active involvement with the criminal justice or correctional systems. General psychiatry training may have provided limited exposure to correctional environments or limited opportunities to become familiar with the criminal justice system or how to collaborate with law enforcement. The correctional and criminal justice systems are themselves complex and multifaceted, as are the interactions of these systems with mental health care systems. However, the populations served by these systems overlap frequently and significantly. One retrospective cohort study of recently released former inmates showed, for example, significant utilization of emergency department visits for mental health and substance use complaints (1). The purpose of this chapter is to provide a foundation for psychiatrists within PES about patients who present as referrals from correctional institutions or with active criminal justice involvement. To that end, information regarding the prevalence and the treatment of mental illness within correctional settings will be provided. Case examples will be utilized to illustrate clinical and conceptual considerations relevant to patients in custody and referred while en route to correctional institutions or patients who are sent to emergency departments from correctional institutions. Although the terms have more specific meaning, for the purposes of this chapter "prisoners," "detainees," and "inmates" will be used to include anyone brought to the emergency department with some type of custody status. Of note, this chapter focuses on adult populations and the adult justice system.

A PRIMER ON CORRECTIONAL SYSTEM STRUCTURES AND SUPERVISION

We begin by providing definitions of terminology used within the correctional and criminal justice systems that can be subject to lay misperceptions, such as the conflation of "jails" and "prisons." Helping to clarify the meaning of these terms can elucidate the context of an individual patient's criminal justice involvement. This context may be highly relevant in determining the disposition of a given patient who presents to PES as differing resources may or may not be available to a patient depending on the nature of their criminal justice involvement. The following definitions provided are adapted from definitions utilized by the Bureau of Justice Statistics, a division of the United States Department of Justice (2).

Correctional institutions for adults are typically conceptualized as three distinct classes of institutions: lock-ups, jails, and prisons. **Lock-ups** are generally local municipal law enforcement facilities that temporarily detain individuals after arrest until business hours when courts are open or until the individual placed in police custody can be released. People are brought to lock-ups shortly after arrest, and individuals with acute emotional distress, or acute substance use or withdrawal, may be held in these environments. In some jurisdictions lock-ups are contiguous with jails, but in others they are stand-alone sites operated by the local municipality, such as those found in a police station. Lock-ups generally have no health services.

Jails are institutions run by local counties and house individuals who are either detained pretrial or who have been sentenced to a period of incarceration for generally less than 1 year. For some individuals, time spent awaiting trial can be prolonged, and multiple 1-year sentences can follow sequentially. Thus, given individuals can be in jails for longer than 1 year total. Jails are typically not part of a larger correctional system structure that would allow for referral to facilities within the system to provide specialized psychiatric care, although some jails have designated areas for individuals with psychiatric care needs. All jails are required to provide some constitutionally adequate mental health services as further discussed below in the select legal cases pertaining to psychiatric services in jails and prisons.

Prisons are state or federal run institutions that house individuals who have generally been sentenced to incarceration for 1 year or longer. As all of the inmates within a prison have been sentenced to longer defined periods of incarceration, prisons tend to have a more stable population of individuals compared to jails, which have a high rate of turnover of admissions and releases. Additionally, as part of a larger system such as a statewide department of corrections, prisons are able to refer inmates with acute mental illness to specialized facilities or units for acute psychiatric care within the corrections system and therefore inmates from prisons are less likely to be referred to PES.

One reason for the more transient population in jails compared to prisons is that jails house both pretrial detainees and sentenced inmates who are there for shorter periods of time. Pretrial detainees may be released upon posting bond or after a court hearing rendering a disposition of their legal case, such as being sentenced to time served within the jail. The date of release may therefore be unknown in advance for jail staff and even for the individual pretrial detainees. Upon release, these individuals may or may not be subject to ongoing supervision by the criminal justice system.

Beyond institutional corrections, there is correctional supervision in the community. **Probation** can be a predetermined part of a sentence issued by the judge at trial, and an individual can receive probation alone or probation following a period of incarceration. A person on probation receives ongoing supervision of compliance with terms and conditions by the criminal justice system

while remaining in the community, and violation of the conditions of probation may result in incarceration in a jail.

Upon release from prison, individuals may be subject to **parole** supervision (some may also be on probation related to other offenses). Parole includes specific conditions and violation of parole can result in a return to prison. Certain individuals may be ineligible for release on parole for reasons such as the original sentence might not be parole-eligible, or because of ongoing behavioral problems within the prison. Such individuals might "max out" or serve the maximum duration of their sentences such that upon release from prison they are not subject to ongoing criminal justice parole supervision.

PSYCHIATRIC SERVICES IN JAILS AND PRISONS

According to the Bureau of Justice Statistics, the point prevalence of individuals under criminal justice supervision in the United States in 2016 was 6.6 million individuals, or 1 in every 38 persons in the United States (3). The majority of these individuals (56%) were probationers, with parolees accounting for an additional 13% of this population (3). The total population of prisoners, or individuals held or incarcerated in jails or prisons as previously defined, was 2.1 million individuals, 1.5 million of whom were incarcerated within prisons with the remainder in jails (3). Although estimates regarding the degree of prevalence vary, there is consensus that individuals with serious mental illnesses are overrepresented within the 2.1 million incarcerated inmates and those on community supervision within the United States (4,5). Some have termed this phenomenon the "criminalization of mental illness" (6,7). A full discussion of the historical reasons for the development of the phenomenon of criminalization of serious mental illness is beyond the scope of this chapter. The policy developments often cited as relevant include the process of deinstitutionalization without subsequent funding for adequate community care resulting in the "transinstitutionalization" of individuals with serious mental illness into jails and prisons; however, this is increasingly recognized as only one factor among many (4). Other important but often overlooked factors leading to the overprevalence of individuals with mental illness and substance use disorders in the justice system include trends in sentencing of drug-related offenses that have increased overall rates of incarceration (4).

Data published in 2017 found a prevalence of as high as 50% of prisoners and 64% of jail inmates who either reported a mental health history or met a self-reported threshold of serious psychological distress within the past 30 days (8). Similar data were published in 2006, finding more than half of jail inmates and prisoners had some kind of mental health problem, based upon the self-report of inmates of either psychiatric symptomatology or a psychiatric diagnosis over the previous 12 months (9). Overall, the most frequently cited estimate of prevalence of mental illness is 16% of both jail inmates and state prisoners, with a higher prevalence in both female jail inmates (22.7%) and female state prisoners (23.6%); these data were similarly based on self-report of a mental condition or a psychiatric hospitalization (10). Overall, these data, while varied, tell us that the incarcerated population as well as the population of individuals under correctional supervision have high rates of mental illness compared to the general population.

In addition to the prevalence of mental illness in correctional settings, the incidence of suicide in correctional institutions merits specific mention in the discussion of challenges for psychiatric services within the United States correctional system. Suicide is the single leading cause of death in United States jails, accounting for 31% of the reported deaths in jails from 2000 through 2014 and occurring at a rate of 50 suicides per 100,000 inmates in 2014 (11). Within state and federal prisons, suicide accounted for 6% and 4%, respectively, of the reported deaths from 2001 through 2014 (12). Although recent data indicate death due to suicide within correctional institutions has increased year to year, one study noted a significant decrease in the incidence of jail suicide comparing data from 1986 to 2006 (11-13). That study, in comparing data about jail suicide from 20 years previous, found a decrease in the proportion of suicides that occurred during the first 24 hours of confinement as well as a decrease in the proportion of victims of suicide with evidence of intoxication as a contributing factor (13). The study noted that 8% of completed

suicides in 2005 and 2006 occurred while an inmate was monitored on suicide precautions and noted that many of the completed suicides occurred within 2 days of a court hearing (13).

Monitoring of inmates with suicidal ideation or other acute mental health problems poses a challenge for jails, and prisons as correctional institutions were primarily designed with a focus on institutional security rather than on preventing suicide or fostering a therapeutic milieu. Jails and prisons may, under the auspices of suicide precautions, utilize suicide prevention strategies that community providers would find surprising or potentially below the standard of care in a community setting, such as the use of safety smocks (made of heavy nylon which is difficult to tear) or the monitoring of acutely suicidal patients via closed circuit television or by fellow inmates employed to observe suicidal inmates in lieu of monitoring via 1:1 staff supervision (14). Decisions to place an inmate on suicide monitoring precautions or when to remove suicide precautions might be made by correctional staff or mental health professionals within the correctional setting, and these decisions may also be subject to competing considerations and dynamics within the jail or prison, such as staffing needs and institutional security considerations (14). Interestingly, one expert argues that jails have become overly reliant on admission screenings and the use of suicide precautions as the primary means of reducing jail suicides rather than developing a robust method of identifying suicidal inmates who are or may become at ongoing risk for suicide but do not self-report their suicidal ideation (14).

Given the high prevalence of individuals with mental illness and substance use disorders as well as the elevated suicide rates in correctional settings, mental health services for these populations are critical. Legal cases are described below that outline contours of minimum legally defined standards for these services. That said, psychiatric care in jails or prisons varies substantially from one correctional institution to another often depending on the allocation of resources within strained public budgets (15). For example, one study examining the delivery of evidence-based correctional psychiatric care in jails across a single state found that each jail within the state utilized its own suicide screening tool and none of them used a formal evidence-based screening tool (16). Another study examined the question of how well one state's prison mental health system was meeting the treatment needs of prisoners with mental illness and found that an estimated 65% of the prisoners experiencing mental health symptoms were not receiving treatment (17).

Within jail and prison settings, the issue of the treatment of inmates with antipsychotic medication over the patient's objection illustrates many of the potential complexities of psychiatric care within the correctional system. Although most inmates take their medications, including psychotropic medication willingly, both within and outside correctional institutions, when an inmate refuses medication, there are approaches to delivering needed medication that follow state protocols and laws. The protocols within a particular criminal justice setting, as well as the patient's legal status, may determine or contribute to which set of rules apply. Typically, individuals in jails will not be given psychotropic medication over objection for long-term treatment and may not even be given medications over objection in emergencies, whereas this is more commonly seen in prisons. In addition to the governing legal considerations, the variability of access to multidisciplinary providers and general care among correctional institutions can lead to variable approaches to the involuntary administration of antipsychotic medications. Many facilities may simply be unequipped or unable to administer antipsychotic medication without a patient's consent. This may have both upstream and downstream effects on psychiatric emergency services.

It should also be noted that in correctional settings, differing rules of restraint and seclusion apply compared to those in health care settings. Thus, when policies and practice allow for treatment over objection, the actual delivery of the medication may be done in the context of a hold applied by correctional staff outfitted in protective gear, concomitant videotaping to ensure proper procedure, and the like. Thus, given the numerous challenges in approaching medications in adult psychiatric patients who may not be able or willing to consent and a host of other challenges in correctional settings, emergency departments

outside of the correctional context may become a default location where an individual is evaluated and treatment is sought.

SELECT LEGAL CASES PERTAINING TO PSYCHIATRIC SERVICES IN JAILS AND PRISONS

Psychiatric care within jails or prisons occurs within a specific legal and regulatory framework, including state and local laws or administrative regulations that may vary from one jurisdiction to another. The legal context of psychiatric care within a correctional environment differs from some relevant legal considerations regarding care in PES discussed in Chapter 46: Common Legal Issues in Emergency Psychiatry. To provide a brief overview of the legal context of correctional psychiatric care, relevant landmark legal cases typically serve to establish minimum standards or "floors" required by the United States Constitution, though jurisdictions may adopt their own higher standards or "ceilings" for particular issues. In 1976, the US Supreme Court held in *Estelle v. Gamble* that "deliberate indifference" to an inmate's medical condition, a standard beyond typical negligence, is a violation of the Eighth Amendment prohibition against cruel and unusual punishment (18). In this holding, the Court affirmed that inmates have a constitutional right to treatment based on the US Constitution (18). The involuntary treatment with psychotropic medication of a prisoner within a prison setting was addressed by the US Supreme Court in 1990 as the Court held in *Washington v. Harper*, a case that established that administrative procedures were sufficient within the prison as long as specific criteria were met, such as medical appropriateness of the treatment for an inmate showing dangerousness to self or others that would otherwise compromise institutional security (19).

OVERVIEW OF RELEASE PLANNING AND DIVERSION FROM JAILS AND PRISONS

An additional challenge for the provision of psychiatric care in jails and prisons is adequately linking inmates to appropriate mental health services upon release from a correctional institution. The transition from incarceration to the community for sentenced inmates is commonly referred to as "reentry," and there are a host of services and supports, including medical care, that an individual might need in the community to maximize a successful transition. Data support that this period of transition is extremely high risk, with death rate magnitudes higher than the general population. One retrospective cohort study of former prison inmates found that in the first 2 weeks post release the risk of death was 12.7 times that of other state residents and the risk of death by overdose was 129 times that of other state residents (20). Additionally, the rate of suicide was 14 times greater than expected in another retrospective cohort study of former prison inmates 2 to 4 years post release (21). Although these are studies involving prisoner releases and not jail releases, both scenarios present challenges. Given the potential uncertain duration of time for pretrial detainees and the high degree of turnover in population, jails face challenges in coordinating programming and appointments upon release. For prisons, there are additional complexities as they may house inmates from across a given state who will return to geographically diverse areas with varying local community mental health resources. Even with the best planning efforts prior to release, the transition can lead to stress and distress, and inmates just released from incarceration can present in an emergency room for a variety of reasons.

As discussed above regarding probation and parole, inmates may also vary in the conditions of their release, which may or may not include mandatory participation in mental health and substance use treatment, as well as the degree of their ongoing supervision by the criminal justice system while in the community. Prisoners may or may not be released on parole supervision, and some serve the maximum duration of their sentence and would then be subsequently released without ongoing criminal justice supervision (5). For those on parole, coordination between treatment providers and the parole officers can be challenging.

Transition planning for individuals returning to their communities from jails and prisons generally also includes connecting inmates to health benefits, which often include access to benefits in the public system. One area of concern that many states and counties have tried to tackle includes the challenge that in some instances Medicaid benefits may be terminated rather than suspended upon incarceration (5). The significance of this is that if benefits are terminated, the individual needs to complete a reenrollment and eligibility determination, which can take time and coordination. When benefits are "suspended," they can be "turned on" more readily upon release (since benefits are not distributed during the incarceration period). Even with suspended Medicaid benefits, inmates returning to their communities may have to present at a benefit enrollment office with proper ID or take other steps to ensure their enrollment in a health plan is active.

Some community mental health systems have made efforts to enhance care through coordinated strategies such as forensic assertive community treatment (FACT) teams. These teams operate on a collaborative model wherein staff are knowledgeable and able to navigate supports between mental health and justice systems for the individual person served. (22). Some studies where FACT programs have been coordinated have shown decreased jail returns, but more research is needed and the applicability across jurisdictions is still quite variable (22,23).

One option available in some states for the linkage of released prisoners with mental illness to community resources is for civil commitment of eligible persons with mental illness who meet particular commitment criteria to be court ordered to outpatient services, sometimes referred to as "assisted outpatient treatment" or AOT (24). This is a mechanism that is used outside of criminal processes for an identified subset of individuals with mental illness and thus may or may not be widely applicable.

The difficulty in finding appropriate community resources after release from a correctional institution may be even more pronounced for those inmates with mental illness and a comorbid substance use disorder, a phenomenon sometimes attributed as the "triple stigma" of criminal justice involvement, mental illness, and substance use problems (25).

To provide a systems framework for how many communities are making efforts to divert individuals from courts, jails, and prisons, and developing better pathways for people being released from correctional supervision, psychiatrists in PES may benefit from a basic familiarity with the Sequential Intercept Model. This model aligns with a quasi-public health perspective with a stated goal of reducing the criminalization of mental illness. It posits that each point of interaction for an individual with mental illness with the criminal justice system is considered an opportunity to redirect these individuals out of the criminal justice system and into the mental health care system (7). Within the Sequential Intercept Model, the gatekeeping function of law enforcement in considering a referral to emergency services for an individual with mental illness who has come to the attention of law enforcement, and the subsequent disposition by emergency services, is termed Intercept 1, an initial point of filtration of individuals with mental illness from the criminal justice system to the mental health system (6,7). For a PES department with a large volume of referrals from law enforcement and corrections, use of the Sequential Intercept Model to map a given community's points of interaction between the criminal justice and mental health systems and corresponding resources can help facilitate communication and collaboration among these at times diffuse and disparate systems. For further discussion of jail diversion programs, readers should refer to the chapter on the crisis intervention model in the first edition of *Emergency Psychiatry: Principles and Practice* (30).

CORRECTIONAL AND EMERGENCY DEPARTMENT CASE EXAMPLES

We present now two case examples as applications of the material presented above regarding correctional psychiatry systems of care and as illustrations of additional clinical and conceptual considerations specific to the evaluation of a patient referred to PES from a correctional institution or with other active criminal justice involvement. The case examples are meant to illustrate the relevant principles regarding correctional psychiatry and PES rather than to present a full discussion of a workup of each case (Cases 41.1 and 41.2).

A consideration for a psychiatrist in PES evaluating an individual presenting in the custody of law enforcement or corrections with a complaint of suicidal ideation is performing an appropriate suicide risk assessment, particularly given that suicide is the leading cause of death in jails. A suicide risk determination for the correctional population should include consideration of risk factors contextual to the patient's legal status, such as court dates or potential adverse legal outcomes, as well as consideration for the capabilities of the correctional institution to maintain the patient's safety (26). As the availability and nature of psychiatric care can vary from one correctional institution to another, psychiatrists in PES should consider contacting the receiving correctional facility regarding their management of suicidal inmates and the access to ongoing psychiatric evaluation and treatment (26). Should inpatient psychiatric hospitalization be indicated for this patient,

 CASE 41.1

A 42-year-old man with an unknown psychiatric history presents to PES in the custody of law enforcement. The police report that the patient was arrested 1 hour ago for assault of a public official. The police utilize space at the local county jail to detain the individual until court opens and initial court hearings can begin the formal court processing of the charges. While being transported by police to the county jail, the prisoner/patient reported that he planned to kill himself if he were to be detained in jail. The police report they are seeking "clearance" to transport the patient to the county jail. On interview, the patient is irritable and minimally engaged with the assessment but reports a past history of suicide attempts and a current plan to hang himself if detained in the county jail.

disposition of the case may be complicated by his legal status, an issue which will be discussed in the next case example. Local emergency rooms may have protocols established with law enforcement and jails regarding management of cross-system cases. Because the individual may need to return to the correctional setting, acute clinical information sharing will be a critical component to ensure proper monitoring of an individual, regardless of what is discussed in the ED. Contracts for safety, as in all settings, should not be relied upon as dispositive of the absence of suicidal risk (27). Monitoring in the correctional institution should often remain the default next step if the person's symptoms are not felt to require or their legal status is precluding inpatient level of care.

Case 41.1 also raises concern for the potential that the patient may be malingering, or reporting suicidal ideation in order to avoid an undesired outcome of incarceration (26). Malingering has been shown to occur more frequently within correctional settings, when the perceived incentive to malinger may include obtaining desired medications or to avoid undesired placements within a facility, as compared to criminal forensic evaluations when the perceived incentive would be to be adjudicated incompetent to stand trial or not guilty by reason of insanity (28). A full discussion of the evaluation and management of malingering in PES is beyond the scope of this chapter, but the potential perceived incentive of the patient above to avoid incarceration is a relevant consideration in the evaluation and management of such a patient. With clinically suspected malingering, there are also risks that the patient's distress will not be taken seriously. It is critical to remember that clinical needs in an emergency department context are different from those in a correctional environment, so conveying "disbelief" of symptoms to correctional staff could result in a minimization of concern for what could be a patient's actual risk at the place of detention. Given the difficulties in assessing malingering versus adjustment and negative coping to incarceration, and that mental status presentations can vary across settings, the importance of monitoring of a potentially suicidal patient in a correctional environment cannot be underestimated.

The individual presenting to the emergency room in Case 41.1 might be eligible for diversion. Yet, at the point of assessment in PES, a diversion option might not be readily available, unless the community has developed specific pathways for such diversion, such as might have been done via a Sequential Intercept Model framework. For the PES psychiatrist, it is important therefore to know that a discharge from PES back to the custody of law enforcement would not necessarily leave the individual in an environment with ongoing care beyond suicide monitoring (although again, this may be different if the individual is sent to a jail where there is health care, versus a lock-up, where there likely is no health care). Furthermore, it is important to realize that a pretrial detainee may remain in jail for a variable period and may be released due to various potential legal dispositions (7). This could include a release the following day. Thus, the PES psychiatrist must evaluate the individual for their current presentation and may wish to give them instruction for resources to access if released from custody.

Finally, the Case 41.1 illustrates the potential issue of managing the presence of law enforcement personnel within psychiatric emergency services. Responses to the presence of law enforcement may vary from one institution to another based on institutional norms and historical practices. Ideally, the clinical and administrative leadership of PES will have promulgated policies for staff regarding the expectations for interactions with law enforcement with relevant input from law enforcement agencies. Notable considerations include determining whether or not officers will have weapons and clarifying the respective roles and responsibilities of law enforcement and hospital security for the management of a behavioral disturbance by a patient presenting in custody. Additionally, the presence of law enforcement in a potentially crowded and highly acute treatment setting could be alarming to other patients, therefore determining how to minimize such disruption of the milieu may benefit the PES.

Case 41.2 illustrates some of the potential limitations correctional institutions may face in the treatment of acute psychiatric illness.

CASE 41.2

A 27-year-old man with an unknown psychiatric history is brought to PES from a local jail where he has been sentenced to 90 days of incarceration owing to resisting arrest. Deputies report that while incarcerated, the patient has not been sleeping and he has been acting increasingly erratic and agitated. The deputies report that after the patient smeared feces on the wall of his cell he was moved to a locked cell in the medical wing of the jail to allow for closer observation, but his behaviors have continued to escalate. The deputies report the jail does not have a dedicated mental health unit and the patient has seen a psychiatrist within the jail once but has refused the recommended antipsychotics. The deputies report the jail has no means of administering involuntary antipsychotic medications. On interview, the patient is acutely disorganized and appears to be responding to internal stimuli and limited meaningful history can be obtained.

Although, as discussed above, the involuntary treatment of such a patient within a correctional setting may be permissible under the governing legal considerations for correctional psychiatry, some correctional facilities such as county jails may not have the ability to implement forms of involuntary treatment with antipsychotic medications. Given the potential mismatch between the patient's need for treatment and the level of care that can practically be provided within the correctional institution, the evaluating psychiatrist may benefit from a conceptual framework to determine an appropriate disposition. One model proposed to determine when a patient inmate may require inpatient psychiatric care outside of the correctional system is to examine both the patient's needs and the system's capacity to manage those needs. Although a "fitness for imprisonment" has been described (29), this concept raises other issues as the fitness of the system may collide with the individual's needs. If and when a determination has been made that the patient requires inpatient psychiatric hospitalization, psychiatrists in PES may encounter difficulty finding an appropriate disposition on an inpatient psychiatric unit. In some settings, working arrangements between local inpatient units and correctional institutions can help pave the way for hospitalization when needed. In other jurisdictions, correctional facilities have geared up specialized mental health staff and units to assist in the management of these types of situations. The disposition of such a patient may be complicated by their legal status and the question of whether the patient would require active supervision by custodial deputies while hospitalized, a question that may or may not be addressed by existing policies of the correctional institution. Additionally, the disposition of such a patient may be complicated by institutional countertransference toward patients with criminal justice involvement, who may be considered by receiving inpatient psychiatric units as more dangerous or less desirable to treat because of their legal status, regardless of the severity of the crime that resulted in their incarceration.

Psychiatrists working within PES should also be aware for their own potential countertransference or the potential countertransference of PES staff toward individuals referred from correctional institutions or with active criminal justice involvement. In the case described above, there may be no option other than to assess the patient with a proper screening for medical concerns and formulating a diagnostic assessment that can be conveyed back to the jail mental health staff, with guidance regarding strategies to enhance patient engagement and proper patient monitoring. In these types of scenarios, it would behoove the psychiatrist working in the ED to understand what pathways for accessing care exist for the patients in the particular jurisdiction, and to continue to advocate for appropriate levels of care and communications protocols across facilities and institutions.

SUMMARY AND CONCLUSIONS

The psychiatrist evaluating a patient in PES either referred from a correctional institution such as a jail or with other active criminal justice involvement may benefit from knowledge of the correctional and criminal justice systems and correctional psychiatry. Lock-ups, jails, prison, probation, and parole are terms whose specific meaning can be unfamiliar to health care professionals, but they delineate the context of a given patient's legal position within the criminal justice system. Mental illness is overrepresented in the populations of both jails and prisons, and suicide is the leading cause of death in jails. Correctional institutions such as jails and prisons may vary in their ability to refer inmates with acute psychiatric illness to specialized treatment facilities within the correctional psychiatry system or in their providing basic aspects of care. Approaches to acute episodes of psychiatric distress in correctional settings can be unfamiliar to clinicians working in health care settings. For inmates leaving jails or prisons, linkage with appropriate resources for mental health follow-up upon transition out of the correctional environment provides an additional challenge for both the correctional psychiatry and the community psychiatry systems. Individuals presenting to emergency services after incarceration reflect some of the most high risk individuals, and opportunities to help foster supports and aftercare are critical.

In the evaluation of a patient presenting with active criminal justice involvement, the psychiatrist in PES should account for the legal context of the patient in determining an appropriate disposition, including considering the actual psychiatric resources available within a given correctional institution or the potential complications in pursuit of inpatient psychiatric care outside of the correctional systems. Additionally, as PES is a potential point of interaction between the criminal justice and mental health systems, on a policy and advocacy level, the use of a conceptual framework such as the Sequential Intercept Model discussed above may facilitate intersystem communication and collaboration.

REFERENCES

1. Frank, J. W., Andrews, C. M., Green, T. C., et al. (2013). Emergency department utilization among recently released prisoners: A retrospective cohort study. *BMC Emergency Medicine, 13*, 16.
2. Bureau of Justice Statistics. *All terms & definitions.* Retrieved November 1, 2018, from https://www.bjs.gov/index.cfm?ty=tda. Last revised October 18, 2018.
3. Kaeble, D., & Cowhig, M. (2018, April). *Correctional populations in the United States, 2016.* U.S. Department of Justice, Office of Justice Programs, Bureau of Justice Statistics Bulletin, NCJ 251211.
4. Prins, S. J. (2011). Does transinstitutionalization explain the overrepresentation of people with serious mental illnesses in the criminal justice system? *Community Mental Health Journal, 47,* 716–722.
5. Baillargeron, J., Hoge, S. K., & Penn, J. V. (2010). Addressing the challenge of community reentry among released inmates with serious mental illness. *American Journal of Community Psychology, 46,* 361–375.
6. Lamb, H. R., Weinberger, L. E., & Decuir, W. J. (2002). The police and mental health. *Psychiatric Services, 53,* 1266–1271.
7. Munetz, M., & Griffin, P. (2006). Use of the sequential intercept model as an approach to decriminalization of people with serious mental illness. *Psychiatric Services, 57,* 544–549.
8. Bronson, J., & Berzonsky, M. (2017, June). *Indicators of mental health problems reported by prisoners and jail inmates, 2011-12.* U.S. Department of Justice, Office of Justice Programs, Bureau of Justice Statistics Special Report, NCJ 250612.
9. James, D. J., & Glaze, L. E. (2006, September). *Mental health problems of prison and jail inmates.* U.S. Department of Justice, Office of Justice Programs, Bureau of Justice Statistics Special Report, NCJ 213600.
10. Ditton, P. M. (1999, July). *Mental health and treatment of inmates and probationers.* U.S. Department of Justice, Office of Justice Programs, Bureau of Justice Statistics Special Report, NCJ 174463.
11. Noonan, M. (2016, December). *Mortality in local jails, 2000-2014 - Statistical tables.* U.S. Department of Justice, Office of Justice Programs, Bureau of Justice Statistics Statistical Tables, NCJ 250169.

12. Noonan, M. (2016, December). *Mortality in state prisons, 2001-2014 - Statistical tables*. U.S. Department of Justice, Office of Justice Programs, Bureau of Justice Statistics Statistical Tables, NCJ 250150.

13. Hayes, L. M. (2012). National study of jail suicide: 20 years later. *Journal of Correctional Health Care, 18*, 233–245.

14. Hayes, L. M. (2013). Suicide prevention in correctional facilities: Reflections and next steps. *International Journal of Law and Psychiatry, 36*, 188–194.

15. Felthous, A. R. (2013). Prisons and mental health: Introductory editorial: Hospitalizing mentally ill patients. *International Journal of Law and Psychiatry, 36*, 185–187.

16. Scheyett, A., Vaughn, J., & Taylor, M. F. (2009). Screening and access to services for individuals with serious mental illnesses in jails. *Community Mental Health Journal, 45*, 439–446.

17. Fries, B. E., Schmorrow, A., Lang, S. W., et al. (2013). Symptoms and treatment of mental illness among prisoners: A study of Michigan state prisons. *International Journal of Law and Psychiatry, 36*, 316–325.

18. Estelle v. Gamble. 429 U.S. 97 (1976).

19. Washington v. Harper. 494 U.S. 210 (1990).

20. Binswanger, I. A., Stern, M. F., Deyo, R. A., et al. (2007). Release from prison – A high risk of death for former inmates. *New England Journal of Medicine, 356*, 157–165.

21. Jones, M., Kearney, G. D., Xu, X., et al. (2017). Mortality rates and cause of death among former prison inmates in North Carolina. *North Carolina Medical Journal, 78*, 223–229.

22. Marquant, T., Sabbe, B., Van Nuffel, M., et al. (2016). Forensic assertive community treatment: A review of the literature. *Community Mental Health Journal, 52*, 873–881.

23. Smith, R. J., Jennings, J. L., & Cimino, A. (2010). Forensic continuum of care with assertive community treatment (ACT) for persons recovering from co-occurring disabilities: Long-term outcomes. *Psychiatric Rehabilitation Journal, 33*, 207–218.

24. Tamburello, A. C., & Selhi, Z. (2013). Commentary: Bridging the gaps for former inmates with serious mental illness. *Journal of the American Academy of Psychiatry & the Law, 41*, 510–513.

25. Hartwell, S. (2004). Triple stigma: Persons with mental illness and substance abuse problems in the criminal justice system. *Criminal Justice Policy Review, 15*, 84–99.

26. Foote, A., & Ostermayer, B. (2017). Legal and ethical challenges in emergency psychiatry. Part 2: Management of inmates. *Psychiatric Clinics of North America, 40*, 555–564.

27. Reid, W. H. (2005). Contracting for safety redux. *Journal of Psychiatric Practice, 11*, 54–57.

28. McDermott, B. E., Dualan, I. V., & Scott, C. L. (2013). Malingering in the correctional system: Does incentive affect prevalence? *International Journal of Law and Psychiatry, 36*, 287–292.

29. Vogel, T., Lanquillon, S., & Graf, M. (2013). When and why should mentally ill prisoners be transferred to secure hospitals: A proposed algorithm. *International Journal of Law and Psychiatry, 36*, 281–286.

30. Dupont, R. T. (2008). The crisis intervention team model: an intersection point for the criminal justice system and the psychiatric emergency service. In Glick, R. L., Berlin, J.S., Fishkind, A.B., Zeller, S.L. (Eds.), *Emergency psychiatry: Principles and practice* (1st ed.). Philadelphia: Wolters Kluwer Health/Lippincott Williams & Wilkins.

42

The Psychiatric Emergency Care of VIPs and Athletes in Crisis

Carla D. Edwards, Jon S. Berlin

PSYCHIATRIC EMERGENCY OF THE VERY INFLUENTIAL PERSON

Psychiatric emergencies of "very influential persons," or VIPs, are yet another illustration of the maxim that the psychiatric emergency service (PES) is the final safety net of the mental health system. When a fellow practitioner, celebrity, or otherwise prominent and influential person becomes too mentally ill, dangerous, and uncooperative for care in a private setting, a police transport to a psychiatric emergency setting is usually the next step. This is standard operating procedure, and the only time that deviations from it are likely to occur is when the target of the threatened violence is so prominent (eg, the President), or the VIP's connections and resources so exceptional, that back channels quickly materialize to whisk them away to a special treatment setting, sometimes before their arrival at a standard emergency site, sometimes after.

Although many might be used to the more common iteration of "very important person," we have chosen VIP to indicate "very influential person." All patients and persons are important, but some are more likely to exert a powerful influence than others.

An influential patient whose attributes, behavior, and/or status have the potential to influence a doctor's judgment or behavior is a "VIP patient" (1). Such high-profile referrals to a PES are fairly uncommon, but staff must be prepared for them. Certain adjustments are necessary to prevent disruption and ensure good care. Case examples run the gamut from persons who are only local celebrities all the way up to international stars: a CIT (Crisis Intervention Team) policeman who becomes suicidal (Case Example 42.1); a fellow psychiatrist experiencing a psychotic break; a visiting politician in a manic episode that appeared on social media earlier in the day; a famous writer that the PES psychiatrist admires; and a prominent attorney who calls his own attorney from a telephone on the waiting room wall and says to call the Governor and threatens to sue if not immediately released.

Davies (2) enunciates the key principle in managing all of these cases: "Doctors should treat a VIP patient just as they would any other." She elaborates the **top tips for treating a VIP patient**:

- Remember the person you are treating is—first and foremost—a patient
- Be aware that your objectivity may be clouded and that preferential treatment may not always be in the best interests of your patient
- Make sure that decisions about access to treatment are made based on clinical need
- A patient cannot insist you provide treatment you do not consider to be in their best interests
- Be prepared to justify your decisions and seek a second opinion if necessary
- The same rules of confidentiality apply whoever your patient is

Guzman, Sasidhar, and Stoller concur (3). They list nine well-thought-out principles in caring for VIPs: 1) "Don't bend the rules," 2) "Work as team, not in silos," 3) Communicate constantly with all stakeholders, 4) Have a careful plan for communication with the media, 5) "Resist 'Chairperson's Syndrome'" (where a case is given to the highest ranking physician administratively but not necessarily the one most qualified clinically), 6) Deliver care where it is most appropriate, 7) "Protect the patient's security," 8) "Be careful about accepting or declining gifts," and 9) Collaborate with the patient's personal physicians.

Nurok and Gewertz refer to a "VIP syndrome" when staff alter their usual operating

CASE EXAMPLE 42.1

The following is a composite case designed to illustrate some of the above points and to protect patient confidentiality.

A CIT police officer well-known for bringing patients to the PES is brought in on second shift by his police partner and two other officers after making a suicidal statement and refusing voluntary evaluation. He is now agreeable to talking, but humiliated about his appearance in PES. The adjacent walk-in clinic might be available. It is closed for the night but could easily be opened up for a more discreet interview. All three of his police coworkers are willing to stand by, and a nurse and clerk could come over for triage and registration. If the patient does not need admission or if a necessary admission can be arranged quickly, he would be spared the embarrassment of returning to PES where he might also encounter patients in the waiting room that he has worked with in a professional capacity. A psychiatrist therefore initially screens him at the front door. A determination is made that he is unarmed, nonviolent, sufficiently cooperative, and medically stable. A judgment call is made that special use of the walk-in clinic is warranted.

Comment: A minor bending of the rules can have more positives than negatives. In this case, an attempt to accommodate understandable self-esteem issues and to protect the officer's professional status with other patients may facilitate rapport, engagement, self-disclosure, assessment, and crisis reduction. This man is going to be seen in an unsecured area, but appropriate precautions have been taken. On the negative side, catering to a VIP patient can be disruptive to staff. It may hinder nursing's workflow, reduce the psychiatrist's availability to handle other patient care issues that need his attention, and cause staff resentment due to perceptions of favoritism or patient entitlement. But in this instance, PES was not overly busy, and staff appreciated that the exception being made was consistent with their mission of treating every patient as an individual. They may have also imagined receiving the same respect and professional courtesy for themselves if the roles were ever reversed.

The officer presented as calm and reasonable but superficial. He denied suicide ideas or risk. However, given the referring officers extreme worry about high risk, the psychiatrist assumed that the patient was minimizing his condition. He also noticed the patient made frequent use of psychiatric jargon; he attributed it to difficulty relinquishing control and transitioning from the caregiver role to the patient role (7). Emotionally, the evaluator noticed a conflicting urge within himself to avoid asking his customary follow-up questions and to collude with what he believed was the patient's denial. Fortunately, however, he persevered and obtained collateral history from the patient's police partner. The partner revealed that the patient had unholstered his weapon that evening during a verbal outburst of rage and despair about his wife's suspected infidelity. The patient had made specific suicidal and homicidal statements. Other relevant history included the fact that he had recently developed a problem with work absenteeism due to heavy drinking. When the psychiatrist presented this new information to the patient, he continued to minimize and expressed impatience with the evaluation process.

The psychiatrist decided to admit the patient involuntarily, but he was not looking forward to announcing his final decision. He (the psychiatrist) taught CIT classes at the police academy and had been making a special point to the class of promoting the concept of collaborative care. Internally, he felt himself trying to justify nonadmission, yet knew it was irrational. Ultimately, he decided to offer the patient the choice of admission to the PES observation area or to the acute inpatient service where fewer staff would know him. The patient opted for the former. Later, in reflecting on the episode of care, the psychiatrist concluded that, in this case, use of the walk-in clinic had not facilitated greater patient trust and openness in the evaluation but had perhaps mitigated an explosive reaction to involuntary hospitalization.

Comment: As stated, VIPs have the potential to influence a doctor's judgment, and the emergency psychiatrist's task was subtle and nuanced: he tried to be flexible but not pliable. Here, various things pressured him to initially underdiagnose clinical acuity and see

CASE EXAMPLE 42.1 *(continued)*

the patient in a more private but perhaps less safe space: overidentification with a fellow caregiver, a desire to build an innovative partnership with law enforcement, and a fear of physical violence. In a similar vein, when evaluating another physician, there can be the urge to let the physician diagnose himself.

Conversely, when evaluating a case that will come under intense public scrutiny, medicolegal and publicity fears may lead to the opposite tendency, to practice defensive medicine and overly conservative management. Psychiatry residents in particular often need help with this. They learn it is natural to visualize defending oneself in court, but in the end, they must decide if they would rather defend clinical care based on liability considerations or what was believed to be in the patient's best interest.

---

procedures to the point that patient care suffers (4). The appearance of a high-profile celebrity can be as disruptive to a hospital as a "disaster," and Smith and Sheffer recommend having a written VIP protocol with the same detail as a disaster plan (5). They advise taking pains to restrict access of nonessential personnel to avoid a "circus atmosphere," postponing any conversation with the patient about matters "extraneous" to the presenting complaint, and making an explicit statement to the patient that "I am going to treat you as I would any other patient," which in their experience high-profile individuals find reassuring. Such a statement may also help treating physicians to ground themselves and focus the doctor-patient dyad on the important task at hand. Other authors note that outside prurient interest can be so intense that it becomes necessary to use a pseudonym for the patient in the medical record (6). In the present era, Health Insurance Portability and Accountability Act of 1996 (HIPAA) training should make this unnecessary, yet even that may be insufficient to curb the voyeuristic impulses of some individuals.

This is a brief survey of caring for the VIP patient in the emergency psychiatry setting. It touches on well-described pressures arising from staff psychology, novelty within the institutional structure, and some of the characteristics of a high-profile individual. Obviously, much more could be said, for example, about the impact on staff of overweening pride that certain VIPs may exhibit. Narcissism cuts two ways, tempting some practitioners to give in to the flattery and mystique, and others to be dismissive of a patient's sense of entitlement. Emergency psychiatrists

who have made a commitment to people who are severely ill and marginalized may find it difficult to empathize with a famous person if they perceive in them a tendency to feel superior and devalue others. However, pathology of the self comes with its own set of troubles, and problems such as these notwithstanding, illustrious individuals can experience major mental illness and distress that are just as serious or painful as for the average person.

ATHLETES IN CRISIS

Not all athletes are VIPs as defined above; in this sense, we are dealing with overlapping Venn diagrams. However, many athletes, if not all, share some of the VIP's characteristics: natural gifts, a drive for excellence, and awareness of having a critical audience. It should also be noted that by no means do all of the athletes' psychiatric emergencies require care in a high-acuity PES: their crises may often be handled quite ably in an outpatient or inpatient clinical setting. But this discussion is a sobering reminder of the potential seriousness of the psychiatric issues that high-performing individuals can face.

There is a common misconception that elite athletes experience mental illnesses at lower rates than the general population. In fact, some studies have supported this assertion (8-10). Athletes are idolized, and their gold medals, endorsements, and multimillion-dollar salaries create an illusion that they do not face the same problems as the rest of the "average" general population. However, it can be argued that the unique stressors faced by elite athletes create significant challenges that are exclusive to that population; and as a result, they have a higher likelihood of experiencing mental illness and psychiatric emergencies.

The concept of "crisis" in sport has been defined in a variety of ways. The psychology literature has described athletic crises as transitions in an athlete's career— conceptualizing age, career, and situation-related transitions as crises. "Psychiatric emergency" was defined by the American Psychiatric Association's Task Force on psychiatric emergency service as "an acute disturbance of thought, mood, behavior or social relationship that requires an immediate intervention as a defined by the patient, family or the community. A psychiatric emergency might also be defined as a set of circumstances in which (1) the behavior or condition of an individual is perceived by someone, often not the identified individual, as having the potential to rapidly eventuate in a catastrophic outcome and (2) the resources available to understand and deal with the situation are not available at the time and place of the occurrence. Central to the concept of an emergency are the subjective quality, the unscheduled nature, lack of prior assessment or adequate planning and resultant uncertainty, severity, urgency and conflict or failure of natural or professional supports, all of which contribute to the need for immediate access to a higher level of care"(11).

A crisis is understood as a transient mental state in which the individual does not have the capacity to manage the stressors or circumstances they are in (11). It may be associated with suicidal thoughts, self-harm behavior, and early functional impairment. Crises can evolve into psychiatric emergencies; thus, it is important to have services available to provide assessment and management of crises. The significant role of stigma, as well as the relative lack of specialized sport psychiatry support, likely delays access to care for these athletes in crisis.

When these athletes present with psychiatric emergencies, it is important for the assessment and treatment team to have a competent sports-related line of questioning to better understand the contribution of sport to the athlete's presenting condition. It is also important to understand the influence of their sport (including training and competing) on their wellness and illness states, as well as any major events they are working toward or competing in. As sports are typically the central focus or profession for these athletes, it is important to incorporate their participation into the treatment and recovery plan. Collaborating with the athlete's interdisciplinary support team will also be important for ongoing support and management.

In the following sections, common types of psychiatric crises and emergencies in athletes will be described; special considerations for assessment and management plans will be discussed.

Suicide

Athletes are at risk for mental illness and suicide. In 2016, the World Health Organization (WHO) reported that suicide accounted for 1.4% of all deaths worldwide, and that it was the 18th leading cause of death (12). Suicide occurs throughout the lifespan and is the second leading cause of death among 15- to 29-year olds globally. This aligns with the athletic careers of most elite and professional athletes.

Studies designed to evaluate suicide risk in athletes have been inconclusive. When athletes are commodified, organizations try to predict which athletes fall into the "high-risk" category. For many decades, the National Football League has used a number of screening tools to generate psychological profiles of their athletes in order to better understand personality, leadership, aggressiveness, reaction styles, and off-field character. A literature review looking at athlete suicide spanning several decades indicated that risk factors that appear to have a significant influence on athlete suicide are injury, psychosocial stressors, pressure to win, substance abuse, retirement, Axis I psychopathology, and anabolic steroid use (13). An athlete presenting in crisis with any of these risk factors should be considered at an elevated risk for suicide.

Numerous professional athletes who died by suicide were given a diagnosis of chronic traumatic encephalopathy (CTE) on postmortem examination of their brains. CTE is a neurodegenerative disease that is postulated to develop years after repetitive head trauma (14). At this time there is no way to diagnose CTE in a living person; however, several neuropsychiatric symptoms have been described premorbidly in those individuals. These include memory loss, impaired judgment, cognitive impairment, impulse control problems, paranoia, confusion, disorientation, aggression, depression, tremors, changes in their speech, sensory impairment, and impaired concentration and attention. An association has been made between a history of head trauma and the subsequent diagnosis of CTE. Athletes who have a history of concussion and who exhibit significant neuropsychiatric symptoms should be considered at a higher risk for adverse outcomes and possibly suicide.

Mood Disorders

Empirical studies have demonstrated that athletes are as likely to experience depression as the general population (8,15-17). In 2015, the WHO estimated that nearly 6% of females and more than 4% of males in the age range 20 to 24 years experienced depression globally; and the prevalence rates continued to increase in every subsequent age interval until the sixth decade for women and the seventh decade for men. Depression has also been identified by the WHO as the major contributor to suicide (18). Studies have looked specifically at the prevalence rates of depression in college athletes as well as elite athletes. Reported findings suggest that depression prevalence rates in college athletes ranges from 15.6% to 25.6% (8,15,19,20), and rates in both groups are typically higher in female athletes (which is also consistent with the general population). Prevalence rates for depression in one population of elite athletes were consistent with WHO estimates as reported above (20).

Risk factors for depression in competitive athletes include female gender, freshman status in college, and pain (19). Additional risk factors include sports failure, concussion, significant injury, and the demand of intense training in combination with academic responsibilities (9,19,21-23).

There are no known studies examining prevalence data for bipolar disorder in athletes, although there are numerous cases of professional athletes with bipolar disorder who either attempted or completed suicide because of sports-related factors (13).

Failure-Based and Situational Depression; Postcompetition "Crash"

Sports crowns "champions" and brands "losers." Sport failures can be so catastrophic that they lead to depression and suicide (13). Failure in sport can take many forms, from losing a championship match to not being selected to a team. The athlete's response to sport failure will be subjective and individualized, based on their personal histories, coping styles, ability to manage losses, and how strongly their identities are tied to winning. Some athletes fear the loss of identity and purpose in the aftermath of a loss. After losing an Ultimate Fighting Championship (UFC) bout to Holly Holm in 2016, mixed martial artist and former champion Ronda Rousey stated, "what am I anymore if I am not this?" She described sitting in the corner of the postfight medical room pondering suicide after losing the fight (24). Depression rates in elite athletes have demonstrated significant increases in the aftermath of poor performance and a subsequent sport-failure experience (9).

Numerous stressors affect athletes, such as performance execution, maintaining health and healthy lifestyles, balancing academics, managing injuries, facing retirement, adjusting to success, management performance expectations, and anxiety. Although there is a long list of potential stressors that an athlete can face, failure in competition is one form of stressor that seems to increase negative affect and mood disorders such as depression (9).

In some sports, fan reactions to losses can impact the personal safety of athletes. During the 2018 Soccer World Cup in Moscow, Russia, Colombian footballers received death threats after missing penalty kicks in their loss to England (25). During the 2018 Winter Olympics in PyeongChang, South Korea, Canadian speed skater Kim Boutin also received death threats after winning a bronze medal in the short track event when the Korean skater was disqualified (26).

Elite athletes spend innumerable years throughout their adolescence and young adulthood training for world championships and Olympic Games. Throughout those years, they sacrifice many important life elements, including romantic relationships, school, employment, friendships, and starting families. Many of those relationships do not survive the intensity, frequency, and demand of the athlete's travel and competition commitments. Training, earning competition points for Olympic qualification, attending training camps and competitions around the world consume most of the athlete's life in the years leading up to major Games.

The Olympic Games are viewed as the "pinnacle" of what that athlete is trying to attain. Athlete experience at the Olympic Games is extremely variable. Incredible success can result in elation, big boosts in self-confidence, and relationships with sponsors and endorsements. However, there are many more athletes who *do not* win medals. Imagine training for many hours per day, every day of the week, and missing out on an Olympic medal by 0.01 second. Or crashing during a race and not being able to finish after many years of training.

The dedication leading to Olympic Games contributes to athlete identity and purpose. Elements such as lack of success at the Olympics, inability to complete competition because of disqualification, injury or crash, poor athletic performance, and trying to adjust to "regular life" after the Games are over can be quite difficult for athletes. Some develop significant "post Games crash" after the conclusion of their Games. Their trajectories can follow a number of different pathways at that time: retirement from the sport at the National Team level, a break from training and competition with the possibility of returning to training as the next Games approach, or continuing to train throughout the next Olympic cycle.

Anxiety

Elite athletes are at a comparable risk of experiencing anxiety disorders as the general population (17). Numerous studies have focused primarily on the performance aspect of anxiety symptoms as opposed to clinical elements of noncompetitive anxiety. Elevated levels of anxiety were found to be related to negative patterns of perfectionism (17), and a focus on performance (versus mastery) was predictive of athlete worry. Athletes who develop a more adaptive approach to the appraisal and interpretation of anxiety states are less likely to experience negative outcomes.

Athletes commonly experience anxiety as a result of internal and external demands to perform at optimal levels (10). Anxiety can be experienced under regular training conditions when pressure, expectations, and comparisons are leveled on a regular basis, in addition to preceding and during competition. Most elite athletes describe "normal nerves" before competition, which they interpret as typical, and feel that the energy generated is adaptive and conducive to optimal performance. Anxiety can sometimes surpass the optimal threshold, however, and interfere with performance.

Athletes who make significant errors in competition (particularly those that influence the outcome of a game) can develop anxiety that can interfere with their ability to effectively return to competition. Internalization of blame for losses can lead to panic attacks, fear of competition, and anxiety-related crises.

Traumatic Brain Injury

Concussion is the most common brain injury in young adults (27) as well as the most frequent type of head injury incurred in sports (10). The Centers for Disease Control and Prevention in the United States estimated that between 1.6 and 3.8 million concussions occur in sports and recreational activities annually (14). Concussion is associated with a heterogeneous symptom profile including physical (headache, dizziness), cognitive (memory impairment, poor concentration, and attention), affective (depression, anxiety), sensory (sensitivity), vestibular dysfunction, and oculomotor changes (28). It has been linked to major depression, generalized anxiety disorder, suicide, and other chronic neuropsychiatric sequelae (14,27,29-39). Although the vast majority of concussion sufferers recover without lasting effect, 10% to 20% of concussion sufferers have a prolonged, complicated, or incomplete recovery (29,33). Mental disorders experienced by concussion sufferers may occur at higher rates than the general population. Postconcussion depression has been reported at rates as high as 40% and anxiety at 24% (14,29-33,35-37). Studies have explored the rates of depression following multiple head injuries. A study of retired football players found that those with three or more concussions were 24.4% more likely to develop major depression

(36). Depression was also more likely to occur at an earlier age for athletes who have experienced a concussion.

Undiagnosed concussion is one of the strongest predictors for opioid misuse among athletes (29,40). Individuals with a history of concussion are also at an increased risk of developing cannabis abuse (29,41).

There is growing literature on the linkage between head trauma and the neuropsychiatric symptoms of CTE (described in the earlier section on Suicide). CTE has been associated with symptoms such as cognitive impairment, mood disturbance, "challenging behaviors," impaired executive function, impulsivity, depression, apathy, emotional lability, aggression, substance abuse, and suicidal ideation (14).

The relationship between concussion and suicide is well described (29,38,39). Individuals who have experienced head injuries have higher frequencies of suicide attempts and have a higher risk of death by suicide than those who have not experienced head injuries (39). If the mental health challenges that develop post concussion are not properly assessed and treated, they may lead to suicidal thoughts and intent (28). In addition to Axis I pathologies that can follow diagnoses of head trauma and concussion, the impact of the life changes that occur as a result of symptom load and impairment can be extremely difficult or even catastrophic. Athletes often depend on their sports as cathartic outlets for them, or that their athlete persona defines them. Missing entire (or multiple) seasons or being medically advised to not return to their sport can result in forced transitional crisis.

Owing to the high correlation of concussion with mental illness, every athlete presenting for mental health evaluation should be asked about their history of head injuries.

Response to Injury

Physical injury can be devastating to an athlete for a variety of reasons, depending on the timing and nature of the injury. Injuries occurring early in a sport season or Olympic cycle may give the athlete time to recover, rehabilitate, and compete in their desired events. Injuries that interfere with the athlete's ability to compete in a major event, create a significant interruption in training and

competition, or that are career-altering (or career-ending) may have a larger impact on their mental health. Characteristics of injuries that increase the risk of suicide include preinjury success, injury requiring surgical intervention, lengthy recovery and rehabilitation process with restriction from their sport, inability to attain preinjury success, and positional replacement by teammates (13,23). Stress has also been identified as an antecedent to injuries and can subsequently influence an athlete's response to injury as well as their approach to rehabilitation and subsequent recovery (22). Injuries can trigger or unmask mental health issues such as depression, anxiety disorders, disordered eating, substance use disorders, and suicidal ideation. In addition, athletes commonly utilize their sport as a means of expressing their talents, energy, and emotions. While injured, they lose access to this outlet, and their overall identity and purpose can become challenged (21).

Androgenic-Anabolic Steroids

Androgenic-anabolic steroids (AASs) are synthetic derivatives of the male hormone testosterone. These substances were introduced into the sporting arena in the middle of the 20th century, with the ultimate goals of improving physical performance and giving the user a competitive advantage. Targeted outcomes included increasing the time and intensity that an athlete could compete, as well as reducing the recovery time needed between workouts. AASs are believed to increase lean body mass, strength, and aggressiveness; however numerous adverse effects are also well-known. Aggression, hostility, rage, violence, mood disturbance (depression, hypo/mania), and psychosis have been described (42,43).

Some athletes engage in a practice referred to as "stacking," in which they use two or more AASs together, mix oral and/or injectable types, and sometimes add other drugs such as stimulants, painkillers, or growth hormones. Many commercially available workout supplements have high doses of caffeine, thyroid hormone, growth hormone, prohormones, and other similar substances as ingredients (which claim to produce explosive energy, increased mass and strength, aggression, and increased sex drive). Individuals who use these supplements and drugs believe that the use of multiple different drugs will produce greater strength or muscle size than they will get from a single drug; however, they do not appreciate the damage that these agents can cause to the body (44).

Studies have demonstrated that AASs have numerous central nervous system effects. The characteristics of these effects are influenced by several factors, including duration and dose of AAS use, concurrent organic diseases, use of other medications, consumption of alcohol or illegal substances, and the athlete's resilience (45-49). Athletes using supraphysiological doses of AASs demonstrated higher rates of clinical mood disorders (depression, mania, hypomania). Female AAS users endorsed more polysubstance use than nonusers, as well as more depressive symptoms during withdrawal and hypomanic symptoms while using AASs (50).

Suicidal ideation and completion are not uncommon in AAS users (45,51). Several case series have been published that illustrate the presence of significant mental illness in current or former AAS users who subsequently committed suicide. The authors postulated that chronic AAS use may induce severe psychopathology, which could influence suicidality in predisposed individuals. Numerous case reports of violent deaths (homicide, suicide, accidents, undetermined causes) in AAS users have also been published (45). One case series illustrated that deaths among AAS users usually concerned young male polysubstance users whose AAS- or polysubstance-related aggressive, disinhibited, and depressive behavior may increase the risk of premature death.

The concept of "roid rage" describes changes in behavior resulting from AAS use, such as sudden and exaggerated aggression, hostility, and unprovoked rage attacks. AAS users have heightened levels of alertness, lower frustration tolerance, and loss of impulse control (52,53). Increased incidence of violent crimes and physical partner abuse during AAS use has also been reported.

Athletes who use AASs can develop serious mental illnesses and experience significant behavioral disturbances that can end in tragedy. Athletes who present with mood or behavioral disturbances or suicidal/homicidal ideation should be asked about AAS and other supplement use.

Eating Disorders

Eating disorders have been well-studied in the athletic population. Numerous studies have identified higher rates of eating disorders in "leanness" and "aesthetic" sports (endurance running, gymnastics, and figure skating) (14,54-56). One study of Australian elite female athletes demonstrated the presence of anorexia or bulimia nervosa in 15% of those involved in leanness sports, 2% in nonleanness sports, and 1% of controls (16,57). Among Australian elite male athletes, anorexia and bulimia nervosa were found in 5% of those in leanness sports, whereas no athlete fulfilled criteria for eating disorders in the nonleanness sport and no-sport controls. In a large Norwegian study, the overall prevalence of eating disorders (including anorexia nervosa, bulimia nervosa, and eating disorder, not otherwise specified) was 13.5% in the elite athlete group versus 4.6% in the control group (55,58). Nearly one-third of the respondent cases who fulfilled criteria for an eating disorder were male.

Weight and leanness are significant issues for athletes in leanness, aesthetic, and aerial sports. Some sports require athletes to fit into a certain weight category for competition (for example, rowing, wrestling, taekwondo, judo, boxing, kickboxing, mixed martial arts). "Making weight" can be a very stressful time for athletes and they may have to cut their weight rapidly prior to "weigh-ins" for competition. Athletes in aesthetic sports and those whose "uniforms" are tight-fitting or revealing often experience internal and external pressure to lose weight. "Anorexia athletica" describes the concept of an athlete exhibiting many of the signs and symptoms of anorexia nervosa other than having a "significantly low body weight" (as intense training can result in increased muscle mass, which would mask this aspect). The psychological features of an eating disorder can be fixed and long lasting in these athletes. The pressure to lose or maintain low weight is often also reinforced by parents and coaches.

Eating disorders can become psychiatric emergencies if the disordered eating compromises the athlete's physical health, and the psychological components place the athlete at further risk for medical crisis because of ongoing insistence on restricting or purging. In addition, the thought of having to gain weight for an underweight athlete who believes he or she has to either maintain or lose weight can lead to severe anxiety and suicidal thoughts. The mortality rate associated with anorexia nervosa in 2005 was 9% to 12%, with one-third of those deaths attributable to suicide (3). Comorbidities commonly co-occur with eating disorders, with a significant portion of patients also endorsing mood disorders, anxiety, and/or substance abuse (56,59-61). One study reported that patients who endorsed bulimia nervosa comorbid with other psychiatric illnesses were more likely to report suicidal ideation and history of suicide attempts (62).

BRINGING IT ALL TOGETHER

Elite athletes can experience a variety of psychiatric illnesses at similar rates as the general population; however, certain situations can place them at higher risk for mental illness and suicide. Injury, sport failure, and concussions are experienced frequently in all levels of sports and have been associated with higher rates of suicide. AASs can severely affect mood, behavior, anxiety, judgment, and overall health. Sport-specific factors can create additional critical factors that should be considered during emergency psychiatry assessments. Elements related to the sport or competition may have a direct bearing on the reason for presentation, and inquiry about their sport should be incorporated into assessment and treatment planning. Most elite athletes have an interdisciplinary support team (IST) which can be involved to provide collateral information and assist with the treatment plan and follow-up.

REFERENCES

1. Alfandre, D., Clever, S., Farber, N. J., Hughes, M. T., Redstone, P., & Lehmann, L. S. (2016). Caring for "very important patients"—Ethical dilemmas and suggestions for practical management. *American Journal of Medicine, 129*(2), 143–147.
2. Davies, M. (2016). Do you know who I am? Treating a VIP patient. *BMJ, 353,* i2857.
3. Guzman, J. A., Sasidhar, M., & Stoller, J. K. (2011). Caring for VIPs: Nine principles. *Cleveland Clinic Journal of Medicine, 78*(2), 90–94.
4. Nurok, M., & Gewertz, B. (2019). The high-profile patient—Ensuring good care for the entire hospital. *JAMA Surgery, 154*(2), 105–106.
5. Smith, M. S., & Shesser, R. F. (1988). The emergency care of the VIP patient. *New England Journal of Medicine, 319*(21), 1421–1423.
6. Pourmand, A., LeSaux, M., Pines, J. M., & Shesser, R. (2018). Caring for VIPs in the emergency department: Are they VIPs or patients? *American Journal of Emergency Medicine, 36*(5), 895–896.
7. Stoudemire, A., & Rhoads, J. M. (1983). When the doctor needs a doctor: Special considerations for the physician-patient. *Annals of Internal Medicine, 98*(5 Pt. 1), 654–659.
8. Wolanin, A., Hong, E., et al. (2016). Prevalence of clinically elevated depressive symptoms in college athletes and difference by gender and sport. *British Journal of Sports Medicine, 50,* 167–171.
9. Hammond, T., Gialloreto, C., et al. (2013). The prevalence of failure-based depression among elite athletes. *Clinical Journal of Sport Medicine, 23*(4), 273–277.
10. Esfandiari, A., Broshek, D. K., et al. (2011). Psychiatric and neuropsychological issues in sports medicine. *Clinics in Sports Medicine, 30,* 611–627.
11. Allen, M. H., Forster, P., Zealberg, J., & Currier, G. (2002, August). *Report and recommendations regarding psychiatric emergency and crisis services* (p. 8). APA Task Force on Psychiatric Emergency Services. Retrieved February 18, 2019, from http://citeseerx.ist.psu.edu/viewdoc/download?doi=10.1.1.473.167&rep=rep1&type=pdf.
12. World Health Organization. Mental Health. Suicide Data. Retrieved February 18, 2019, from http://www.who.int/mental_health/prevention/suicide/suicideprevent/en/.
13. Baum, A. L. (2005). Suicide in athletes: A review and commentary. *Clinics in Sports Medicine, 24,* 853–869.
14. Finkbeiner, N. W., Max, J. E., et al. (2016). Knowing what we don't know: Long-term psychiatric outcomes following adult concussion in sports. *The Canadian Journal of Psychiatry, 61*(5), 270–276.
15. Wolanin, A., Gross, M., et al. (2015). Depression in athletes: Prevalence and risk factors. *Current Sports Medicine Reports, 14*(1), 56–60.
16. Reardon, C., & Factor, R. (2010). Sport psychiatry: A systematic review of diagnosis and medical treatment of mental illness in athletes. *Sports Medicine, 40*(11), 961–980.
17. Rice, S. M., Purcell, R., et al. (2016). The mental health of elite athletes: A narrative systematic review. *Sports Medicine, 46,* 1333–1353.
18. *Depression and other common mental disorders: Global health estimates.* Retrieved February 18, 2019, from http://apps.who.int/iris/bitstream/handle/10665/254610/WHO-MSD-MER-2017.2-eng.pdf.

19. Yang, J., Peek-Asa, C., et al. (2007). Prevalence of and risk factors associated with symptoms of depression in competitive collegiate student athletes. *Clinical Journal of Sport Medicine, 17*(6), 481–487.

20. Gulliver, A., Griffiths, K. M., et al. (2015). The mental health of Australian elite athletes. *Journal of Science and Medicine in Sport, 18*, 255–261.

21. Masten, R., Strazar, K., et al. (2014). Psychological response of the athletes to injury. *Kinesiology, 46*(1), 127–134.

22. Putukian, M. (2016). The psychological response to injury in student athletes: A narrative review with a focus on mental health. *British Journal of Sports Medicine, 50*, 145–148.

23. Smith, A. M., & Milliner, E. K. (1994). Injured athletes and the risk of suicide. *Journal of Athletic Training, 29*(4), 337–341.

24. Griggs, B. (2016, February 17). Ronda Rousey: I thought about killing myself. *CNN*. Retrieved February 18, 2019, from https://www.cnn.com/2016/02/17/entertainment/ronda-rousey-feat/index.html.

25. Roper, M. (2018, July 5). World Cup 2018: Colombia players who missed penalties against England receive death threats from angry fans. *Independent*. Retrieved February 18, 2019, from https://www.independent.co.uk/sport/football/world-cup/colombia-penalty-death-threat-world-cup-2018-mateus-uribe-carlos-bacca-andres-escobar-a8431001.html.

26. Canada's Kim Butin subjected to online threats after winning short-track bronze. (2018, February 14). *CBC Sports*. Retrieved February 18, 2019, from https://www.cbc.ca/sports/olympics/speedskating/kim-boutin-death-threats-olympics-pyeongchang-1.4533757.

27. Fralick, M., Thiruchelvam, D., et al. (2016). Risk of suicide after concussion. *CMAJ, 188*(7), 497–504.

28. Kontos, A. P., McAllister Deitrick, J., et al. (2016). Mental health implications following sport-related concussion. *British Journal of Sports Medicine, 50*(3), 139–140.

29. Todd, R., Bhalerao, S., et al. (2018). Understanding the psychiatric effects of concussion on constructed identity in hockey players: Implications for health professionals. *PLOS One, 13*(2), e0192125. Retrieved February 18, 2019, from https://doi.org/10.1371/journal.pone.0192125.

30. Max, J. E. (2016). Concussion and psychiatric outcome in adults and children. *The Canadian Journal of Psychiatry, 61*(5), 257–258.

31. Busch, R., & Alpern, H. P. (1998). Depression after mild traumatic brain injury: A review of current research. *Neuropsychology Review, 8*, 95–108.

32. Schoenhuber, R., & Gentilini, M. (1998). Anxiety and depression after mild head injury. *Journal of Neurology, Neurosurgery and Psychiatry, 51*, 722–724.

33. Mooney, G., & Speed, J. (2001). The association between mild traumatic brain injury and psychiatric conditions. *Brain Injury, 15*, 865–877.

34. Moore, E., Terryberry-Spohr, L., et al. (2006). Mild traumatic brain injury and anxiety sequelae: A review of the literature. *Brain Injury, 20*, 117–132.

35. Epstein, R. S., & Ursano, R. J. (1994). *Neuropsychiatry of traumatic brain injury*. Washington, DC: American Psychiatric Press.

36. Guskiewicz, K. M., Marshall, S. W., et al. (2007). Recurrent concussion and risk of depression in retired professional football players. *Medicine & Science in Sports & Exercise, 39*, 903–909.

37. Solomon, G. S., & Kuhn, A. W. (2015). Depression as a modifying factor in sport-related concussion: A critical review of the literature. *The Physician and Sports Medicine, 44*, 14–19.

38. Teasdale, T. W., & Engberg, A. W. (2001). Suicide after traumatic brain injury: A population study. *Journal of Neurology, Neurosurgery and Psychiatry, 71*, 436–440.

39. Wasserman, L., Shaw, T., et al. (2008). An overview of traumatic brain injury and suicide. *Brain Injury, 22*(11), 811–819.

40. Cottler, L. B., Ben Abdallah, A., et al. (2011). Injury, pain, and prescription opioid use among former National Football League (NFL) players. *Drug and Alcohol Dependence, 116*, 188–194.

41. Tait, R. J., Anstey, K. J., et al. (2010). Incidence of self-reported brain injury and the relationship with substance abuse: Findings from a longitudinal community survey. *BMC Public Health, 10*, 171.

42. Hartgens, F., & Kuipers, H. (2004). Effects of androgenic-anabolic steroids in athletes. *Sports Medicine, 34*(8), 513–554.

43. Geddes, J. (1991). Anabolic steroids and the athlete: Counseling patients about risks and side effects. *Canadian Family Physician, 37*, 979–983.

44. New York State Department of Health. *Anabolic steroids and sports: Winning at all costs*. Retrieved February 18, 2019, from https://www.health.ny.gov/publications/1210/.

45. Piacentino, D., Kotzalidis, G. D., et al. (2015). Anabolic-androgenic steroid use and psychopathology in athletes: A systematic review. *Current Neuropharmacology, 13*(1), 101–121.

46. Rubinow, D. R., & Schmidt, P. J. (1996). Androgens, brain and behavior. *The American Journal of Psychiatry, 153,* 974–984.

47. Schmidt, P. J., & Rubinow, D. R. (1997). Neuroregulatory role of gonadal steroids in humans. *Psychopharmacology Bulletin, 33,* 219–220.

48. Zarrouf, F. A., Artz, S., et al. (2009). Testosterone and depression: Systematic review and meta-analysis. *Journal of Psychiatric Practice, 15,* 289–305.

49. Ebinger, M., Sievers, C., et al. (2009). Is there a neuroendocrinological rationale for testosterone as a therapeutic option for depression? *Journal of Psychopharmacology, 23,* 841–853.

50. Gruber, A. J., & Pope, H. G., Jr. (2000). Psychiatric and medical effects of anabolic-androgenic steroid use in women. *Psychotherapy and Psychosomatics, 69,* 19–26.

51. Brower, K. J., Blow, F. C., et al. (1989). Anabolic androgenic steroids and suicide. *The American Journal of Psychiatry, 146,* 1075.

52. Pope, H. G., & Katz, D. L. (1994). Psychiatric and medical effects of anabolic-androgenic steroid use. *Archives of General Psychiatry, 51,* 375–382.

53. Conacher, G. M., & Workman, D. G. (1989). Violent crime possibly associated with anabolic steroid use. *American Journal of Psychiatry, 146,* 679.

54. Calhoun, J. W., Ogilvie, B. C., et al. (1998). The psychiatric consultant in professional team sports. *Child and Adolescent Psychiatric Clinics of North America, 7*(4), 791–802.

55. Currie, A., & Morse, E. (2005). Eating disorders in athletes: Managing the risks. *Clinics in Sports Medicine, 24,* 871–883.

56. Joy, E., Kussman, A., et al. (2016). 2016 update on eating disorders in athletes: A comprehensive narrative review with a focus on clinical assessment and management. *British Journal of Sports Medicine, 50,* 154–162.

57. Byrne, S., & McLean, N. (2002). Elite athletes: Effects of the pressure to be thin. *Journal of Science and Medicine in Sport, 5,* 80–94.

58. Sundgot-Borgen, J., & Klungland Torstvelt, M. (2004). Prevalence of eating disorders in elite athletes is higher than in the general population. *Clinical Journal of Sport Medicine, 14*(1), 25–32.

59. American Psychiatric Association. (2013). *Diagnostic and statistical manual of mental disorders* (5th ed.). Arlington, VA: American Psychiatric Association.

60. Meng, X., & D'Arcy, C. (2015). Comorbidity between lifetime eating problems and mood and anxiety disorders: Results from the Canadian Community Health Survey of Mental Health and Well-being. *European Eating Disorders Review, 23,* 156–162.

61. Rosling, A. M., Sparen, P., et al. (2011). Mortality of eating disorders: A follow-up study of treatment in a specialist unit 1974-2000. *International Journal of Eating Disorders, 44,* 304–310.

62. Crow, S. J., Swanson, S. A., et al. (2014). Suicidal behavior in adolescents and adults with bulimia nervosa. *Comprehensive Psychiatry, 55,* 1534–1539.

43

The Psychiatric Emergency Care of College and University Students

Victor Hong, Rahael Rohini Gupta, Rachel Lipson Glick

Emergency departments (EDs) located near colleges or universities will inevitably provide care to undergraduate and graduate students. Although much of the emergency medical management of young adults is similar whether they attend college or not, providing behavioral emergency care to this student population can be complex. Most college and university students are legally adults, but many maintain strong ties to their parents in regards to issues such as finances, health insurance, and emotional support. Additionally, schools have some level of responsibility for student well-being, which can make it difficult to balance the student's right to privacy and independent decision-making versus the need to keep the student and their peers safe. The number of students seeking care at college and university mental health clinics has increased dramatically in recent years, and many campus providers have long waitlists for services, even for students experiencing significant symptoms (1). This chapter will review best practices for the emergency psychiatric care of college and university students addressing special issues of confidentiality, coordination with campus services and school administration, and common presenting problems.

UNIQUE CHARACTERISTICS OF COLLEGE AND UNIVERSITY STUDENTS

Certain differences between youth who do not attend college and their age-matched college attending peers can be expected and should be considered when evaluating college and university students in an emergency setting. For many students, college means being away from home for the first time and navigating new social environments and relationships. Stressors such as academic pressures, relationship problems, and financial burdens are related to students' increases in mental health diagnoses and suicide attempts (2). For graduate students in particular, rates of depression and anxiety are significantly higher than in the general population, with challenging supervisory relationships, problems with work-life balance, and job market issues being contributing factors (3).

Much like their noncollege attending peers, college students do not seek mental health services due to lack of insight, stigma, and limitations of available resources. Additional barriers potentially unique to the college population include confusion about where to access care and logistical issues with working treatment into their academic schedules (4). When considering how students present to the ED in crisis, it is notable that many college students with elevated suicide risk do not utilize outpatient mental health services (5). Vacations, study abroad programs, internships, and travel for research may further exacerbate the problem of untreated or undertreated issues.

The issue of substance use on campus is relevant to ED presentations, particularly given the higher use of alcohol in college students versus their noncollege attending peers and the corresponding increased risk of suicidal thoughts and behaviors (6-8). Additionally, nonmedical use of prescription pills has increased significantly on college campuses, with resulting consequences including intentional and accidental overdoses (9).

Collecting collateral information when assessing college students in the emergency setting may involve complex issues with contacting parents and family (Table 43.1). Although technically adults, with all of the concomitant medicolegal benefits, it is best to think of students, particularly

TABLE 43.1 Family Involvement in Emergency Psychiatric Management of College Students

Reasons it is important to contact family
Financial (parent's insurance/financial support may be needed for the student's care)
Collateral data to inform safety assessment
For risk management purposes, families are best be involved early in the process
Evidence that TAY do better with family involvement
To involve family in safety planning and the provision of ongoing support post ED discharge

Barriers to contacting family
Confidentiality rules
Poor family relationship/history of abuse or neglect
Student's desire to handle matters independently
Student's fear of family response/stigma
Student's fear of financially burdening family

those who are undergraduates, as transitional age youth or TAY (10). There is significant evidence of improved outcomes when families are involved in the care of TAY, but as most students are 18 years of age or older, matters can become complicated when these legal adults withhold permission to contact their families (11,12). Fears that their parents will not be supportive, that their families will incur financial hardship with care or hospitalization, or of not wanting to burden their parents with their mental health problems are all commonly stated reasons for blocking parental involvement in their mental health crisis. Motivational interviewing techniques are helpful here, to help students recognize the potential benefits of such contacts and assuage their concerns about the risks of parent involvement.

TYPICAL EMERGENCY PRESENTATIONS

When examining the issue of college and university student psychiatric emergencies, one must consider the most common types of presentations. Certainly, one of the most common types of crisis in college and university students involves suicidal thoughts or behavior (13). Although the suicide rate is lower among college students than their age-matched peers, suicidal thoughts, behaviors, and self-injury are common (14). In one compelling study, 12.1% of students surveyed reporting seriously considering suicide anytime in

the 12 months prior to the survey, 1.9% reporting attempting suicide, and 7.8% reporting self-harm behaviors (15).

Although generally, the approach to suicide risk management in the ED for college students is similar to that taken with the general public, there are notable nuances to consider. As with any patient presenting with suicidal or self-harm behaviors that result in apparent or suspected injury, immediate medical triage is necessary. The issue of safety planning to help manage suicidal risk may be especially challenging with college and university student population. Given that students often attend school outside of their home state or even country, they may present to the ED with friends, resident advisors, coaches, or campus personnel, not with family members. The student may not trust these people with sensitive information and may be reluctant to involve them in safety planning. Although a willing, collaborative approach is always favored, regardless of consent, if safety is in question, the emergency clinician should gather information from those who have direct and intimate knowledge of the student's situation (16). As aforementioned, reaching out to families is recommended whenever possible, particularly if a student with elevated suicide risk is to be discharged. Ideally the student would also communicate with their family about the emergency visit, despite possible fears about repercussions. Disposition outcome notwithstanding, it is recommended to contact the Dean of Students office or other appropriate campus resources when a student with elevated suicide risk is evaluated in the ED, so that they can provide additional support and advocacy. There are confidentiality concerns about such contact, however, which will be detailed in a later section.

As with any suicide risk assessment, risk and protective factors are important to evaluate. For college and university students in particular, one must consider several factors that increase suicide risk, such as identification as lesbian, gay, bisexual, transgender, and queer (LGBTQ), an alcohol use disorder, a history of abuse, limited social supports, and academic or relationship stress (6,17-20). Although in most US states, firearms are prohibited on campus, there are outliers, as well as the risk of students accessing firearms off campus, including at the homes of family members and friends (21). Regardless of campus policies regarding firearms, no assumptions should be made on the part of the clinician and typical means reduction discussions including those around firearms are warranted.

Many common presentations to the ED for college and university students mirror those of their age group, including depression, anxiety, mania, psychosis, and substance intoxication. The high prevalence of eating disorder symptoms among college students needs to be considered, particularly when medical problems result from restrictive or purging behaviors (22). Certainly if symptoms of depression and anxiety are mild to moderate, referring to the campus counseling service or university health service is indicated. With any initial episode of manic or psychotic symptoms, vital signs, laboratory tests, a thorough history and physical examination, and, when indicated, neuroimaging and lumbar puncture are needed to rule out medical causes (23). When history reveals a more subacute ramping up of manic symptoms or evidence of gradually increasing prodromal symptoms, one can be more confident that a psychiatric etiology is present. As always, some of the most important information can be gathered from outside sources such as roommates, professors, and others.

Given college and university students' notable use of alcohol and other drugs, many students who present to the ED are intoxicated or have substance use as a complicating factor in their psychiatric crisis (24). Students often believe that substance use, especially binge drinking, is simply a part of the college experience. However, when the drug or alcohol use is severe, it should not be normalized but instead should be treated as a potentially harmful, dangerous behavior (25,26). ED providers must also remember that an intoxicated student who is not a regular drinker is at high risk for alcohol poisoning and needs close medical observation until clinically sober, as in Case 43.1. Frank education about the risks of substance use with concomitant motivational interviewing techniques is warranted in these cases.

Another presentation is the student who has either verbally made threats of violence or is considered a threat to others (27). As with suicide risk assessment, evaluation of acute warning signs is the foundation upon which disposition decisions should be made when concerns for violence are in play. Acute warning signs include the presence of agitation and substance use, and certainly explicit threats should be taken seriously. Accounting for chronic risk factors such as a history of violence toward others and being a victim of violence will help contextualize the evaluation and inform consideration of longer-term risk (28). Law enforcement involvement is crucial when a threat is credible, as is notifying the Dean of Students, which often activates threat assessment teams, which are now prevalent on college campuses. A Tarasoff notification is also indicated in these situations when specific individuals have been identified as potential victims (29).

INVOLVING UNIVERSITY SUPPORTS

Best practice emergency care often involves mobilizing support systems, and for students on a college or university campus, that may involve university employees and officials. Resident advisors and housing directors, counseling and health services personnel, student affairs staff, coaches, and sometimes professors or fellow students may all serve as supports. Privacy laws including the Family Educational Rights and Privacy Act (FERPA) and the Health Insurance Portability and Accountability Act (HIPAA) are often cited as barriers for communication with university officials. Emergency services are not

CASE 43.1

Alexis is a 19-year-old sophomore who was brought to the ED in an intoxicated state by her roommate. She came to the ED willingly but was slurring her words, stumbling, and somnolent. Her roommate told the triage nurse that after drinking "way too much" at a party earlier in the evening, Alexis had taken a razor blade to her wrist and threatened to "end it all." The roommate does not know the details of Alexis' medical or psychiatric history but says she thinks maybe Alexis is taking a medicine for depression.

After treatment with fluids and close observation for alcohol poisoning, Alexis is clinically sober and the psychiatric provider is asked to see her. Alexis explains she has struggled with anxiety and depression since her parents' divorce when she was in middle school. She takes Prozac and has found it helpful but has recently had an increase in depressive symptoms following a breakup. She sees a therapist at home (1-hour drive from school which is why she has a car on campus) every 2 weeks, and finds this helpful, but wonders if her medication should be adjusted. She worries that her grades are dropping because of trouble with concentration. On mental status examination, she appears sad but is able to smile appropriately. The rest of her mental status examination and her psychiatric review of systems are negative.

She says that she drinks very little and usually avoids parties because she does not like "the drinking scene," but after her boyfriend broke up with her, she had to do something to feel better, so she acknowledges she just kept drinking the punch at the fraternity party, even though she was not sure what was in it. This is the first time in her life she has ever gotten drunk.

Alexis admits to thoughts of suicide but says she does not think she would ever act on them. She has no history of suicide attempts but does have a distant history of some cutting behavior when she was in high school. She says that she has worked with her therapist to learn ways to distract herself when she has suicidal thoughts. She denies that she is thinking of suicide now that she is sober and even says, "I guess it is really bad for me to drink that much."

The psychiatrist asks about her support system at school, and Alexis admits she feels isolated and does not have a lot of friends. She says she speaks to and texts her mother every day but is not close to her father and only sees him occasionally.

The psychiatrist believes Alexis can return to her dorm, follow up with her therapist, and see a psychiatrist as an outpatient to adjust her medication but wants to develop a safety plan. He suggests to Alexis that they work together to help her find more support on campus. He also tells Alexis he would like her to call and let her mother know what happened.

Alexis becomes angry and says that her depression is her business and she does not want others to know. She also does not want to upset or worry her mother. The psychiatrist allows Alexis to calm down and then explains the importance of other people to help her stay safe and to be there when she needs someone.

Together Alexis and the psychiatrist decide that her lab partner is someone she trusts and can call when she feels worse. Alexis calls this person and he agrees to come to the ED to talk to the provider and Alexis together about her safety plan. The psychiatrist also convinces Alexis to let her mother know that she is struggling, as it is clear Alexis is close to her mother and her mother provides her with ongoing support. After making this call, Alexis admits she feels relieved since her mother was supportive and offered to come to campus and take her out to dinner that evening.

Finally, the psychiatrist explains that there are several resources on campus that he thinks Alexis would benefit from, including the Office for Students with Disabilities and the Dean of Students Office that helps students with psychiatric issues navigate services on campus. She is reluctant to consider referrals to these services because she worries about her privacy and does not want school officials to know she has depression. The psychiatrist reassures her that these services offer confidential help and can interface with professors and others in a manner which maintains her privacy but gets

CASE 43.1 *(continued)*

her help or accommodations if she needs them. She takes written information about both services and says she will think about contacting them.

As Alexis leaves the ED with her lab partner and safety plan (and an appointment to see her therapist in 2 days and her psychiatrist next week), she thanks the psychiatrist and apologizes for getting angry. She says she is glad her mother will be here in a few hours and thinks she will call the Dean of Students Office to see if their services will be helpful.

bound by FERPA as it is a federal statute that applies to a student's educational records and does not prohibit all communication between school administrators and others as some have interpreted it to do (30). HIPAA, and sometimes more stringent rules around confidentiality of mental health records based on state laws, does complicate matters of communication with university staff.

Managing a campus behavioral emergency may involve explaining to the student the importance of collaborating with campus personnel while still protecting the student's privacy, allowing them to participate in deciding which details of their care are communicated (31).

Because college and university students are transitional age adults who are known to do better when family is involved in their care, their university supports can be viewed as a surrogate or extended family and included in the treatment plan for a behavioral emergency. It behooves emergency services on or near campus to have an ongoing working relationship with campus counseling and health services as well as student affairs officials (31). It is also very helpful for ED clinicians to know the academic calendar and resources for whom to contact regarding class drop/add deadlines and important dates related to financial aid. Furthermore, if the emergency provider can talk to the student in crisis in an honest and knowledgeable way about campus resources, as the psychiatrist did in the case above, they are more likely to credibly convince the hesitant student that these resources are truly designed to be helpful and not punitive.

Providers also need to be aware of the college or university's responsibilities for the student body at large. School administration must balance the care of the individual student with the safety of all students on campus and any potential liability the school will face. In addition to having a working relationship with school officials and services, it is important for providers to understand that institutions have varying strategies when managing students in crisis, making suicidal or homicidal threats, or appearing unable to care for themselves because of severe symptomatology. Some schools may mandate leaves of absence or other interventions (32).

DISPOSITION MANAGEMENT

Certain factors, some of which are described in Table 43.2, should be considered when formulating the appropriate disposition for a college or university student in a behavioral health emergency. Certainly, inpatient psychiatric hospitalization is indicated when there is acute suicide or homicide risk, psychosis, or mania. That said, hospitalization may also be ideal in many other circumstances, due to students' distance

TABLE 43.2 Special Considerations When Evaluating/Discharging College Students

Academic calendar/financial aid issues
Availability of on and off campus mental health services
Local support system if family is far away
Involvement of university personnel in safety planning and/or follow-up
Student's relationship with parents/family and whether they should be part of safety plan
Screening for substance use and eating disorders

from primary social supports which compounds safety planning and makes difficult the provision of comprehensive support subsequent to the ED visit. Students who are new to campus (having not yet established a social support network), racial and ethnic minorities who may feel more isolated than their nonminority peers, and international students may feel especially unsupported. It can be very challenging when a student is hospitalized at a facility far away from campus, which can complicate transportation back to campus, communicating with school personnel, and arranging follow-up care. Ideally, if the campus has care managers, they would be involved to ensure adequate support post discharge from an inpatient unit. Partial hospital programs can be useful as a step-down level of care from the inpatient hospital or as a direct referral from the ED, but transportation and insurance issues are central here and often problematic.

Although many college counseling services treat the majority of students seeking mental health care, their structure and capacity may be poorly suited to manage urgent psychiatric issues. It is important for ED providers to have a good understanding of the scope of the campus counseling services, so as to refer the student to the most appropriate treatment setting. Many colleges and universities employ psychiatric providers to care for students, mostly within their broader student health services. When the disposition is to outpatient care at the student health service, knowledge of the referral system, typical wait times, ability to manage chronic and persistent mental illnesses, and whether they can see students for ongoing (versus short term) care is quite valuable. Ideally, counseling and health services leadership would collaborate with the ED on clarifying these issues and defining the scope of their care.

Although EDs can refer to community therapists and psychiatrists, helping college and university students navigate the labyrinth of insurance coverage is crucial, so as to minimize student frustration and their subsequent abandonment of efforts to seek care. Maintaining a current list of local providers experienced in managing this patient population, as well as what insurances they accept, can be very helpful. Follow-up contact with students post discharge to check in on the status of the outpatient care

and its establishment can bolster student follow through, in addition to potentially mitigating suicide risk.

Although substance use is widespread on college and university campuses, adequate substance use treatment options may not exist. There may be a recovery program on campus, with Alcoholics Anonymous (AA)/Narcotics Anonymous (NA) meetings and support services. These are important resources to share with students in need. On campuses where binge drinking or other sporadic substance use may be considered acceptable and normalized as part of student life, students may struggle to recognize their use as potentially serious. It behooves emergency clinicians to evaluate the frequency and intensity of the substance use, so as to not miss the opportunity to connect the student with indicated resources for treatment. Substance use can often exacerbate or unmask psychiatric issues such as mood problems, anxiety, mania, and psychosis.

SPECIAL POPULATIONS

There are numerous distinct populations of university students, with their own unique issues related to mental health crises. Several are highlighted here.

Medical Students

Although several graduate student groups including PhD candidates, law students, engineering students, and medical students are at increased risk of developing depression, as physician trainees who will at some time enter the ED as learners, medical students may have an inherently complicated relationship with hospital providers (33,34). Medical education is characterized by a unique set of stressors which may contribute to medical students' higher risk of suicide and suicidal ideation than age-matched populations (33). Medical students are more prone to harmful methods of coping such as excessive alcohol use (35). Many students experience rigorous and intellectually demanding academic and clinical obligations, often at the expense of their own health and personal relationships (36). After routinely witnessing severe illness and frequently supporting patients through painful and traumatic events, medical students may themselves incur trauma and distress. Indeed, acute and posttraumatic stress symptoms associated with clinical training are common in this population. Medical students' financial insecurities (with the majority of students graduating with profound debt) can prove stressful (37). In the context of professional and financial insecurity, and routinely demanding work, academic and personal shortcomings may feel devastating, contributing to psychiatric emergencies in the medical student population.

The emergency provider will be well served to be aware of and sensitive to mental health stigma in the physician and physician trainee populations (38). Students may worry that revealing a personal struggle with mental illness or being recognized as depressed by others will impair their candidacy for residency training positions or compromise how they are regarded by professional superiors and peers. Stigma is at least partly responsible for the fact that medical students are less likely than the general population to receive appropriate treatment for mental illness despite seemingly good access to health care (36).

Because a medical student may be highly concerned about disclosure due to stigma, the emergency clinician can provide strong reassurance about confidentiality. The clinical interview should never include medical student colleagues. Additionally, when possible, attending faculty or residents who have worked with—or are likely to work with—a medical student in a professional context (eg, core clerkship director, clerkship supervisors) should not be involved in their ED care. Because medical students are prone to maladaptive methods of coping such as excessive alcohol use, providers should maintain a high level of suspicion for underlying mental health issues when a medical student presents to the ED with alcohol intoxication. Providers should keep in mind medical students' financial insecurities when connecting students with postdischarge resources and recommendations for academic breaks.

Student Athletes

Student athletes are tasked with balancing their athletic, academic, and extracurricular obligations. Added pressure from coaches, peers, and parents to meet performance expectations can be sizable. Their athletic performance may be central to the student athlete's concept of identity and failure to perform can engender considerable stress and anxiety. When illness or injury precludes their athletic participation, the student athlete's self-worth and social structure may be disrupted (39). In addition, student athletes are more likely than their nonathlete peers to participate in binge drinking, an activity associated with impulsive behavior and suicidality (40). Eating disorders, as well as attention-deficit hyperactivity disorders (ADHDs), have also been found to occur more frequently among athletes than among the general population (41).

Given the increased prevalence of eating disorders in the student athlete population, the emergency clinician should maintain a high index of suspicion for this issue. Early identification, which is opportune in the ED, and early intervention are associated with better outcomes in patients with eating disorders. By connecting a student suspected of having an eating disorder with appropriate care, the emergency clinician can play an important role in supporting a student's recovery (42).

The emergency physician should be aware that prescribing or administering psychiatric medications to student athletes may be complicated for several reasons. First, student athletes may be hesitant to take medications due to reasonable concerns about psychiatric medications affecting their safety and performance. Secondly, oversight and governance bodies such as the National College Athletic Association (NCAA) and the World Anti-Doping Agency (WADA) have complicated and sometimes conflicting rules about athletes' use of controlled substances such as stimulants (43). As with all students, collaborating with campus supports (including athletic department staff) can be invaluable as they can be useful partners in the treatment plan.

International Students

The international student experience can present its unique host of challenges. Arriving and adjusting to life in the United States with little to no support, adapting to a new culture, pressure to perform academically, and potential financial strain associated with the costs of study abroad are all potential factors which could contribute to stress. Struggles with English proficiency can make it difficult to establish a supportive social network and succeed in their field of study. In the ED visit, language and cultural barriers may make it difficult for the student to accurately express their symptoms to providers. International students are less likely than domestic students to perceive a need for mental health help and to seek it out. Shame and stigma remain significant barriers to care for many international students, and the difficulties of involving families at a great distance and across cultures can be complex. Due to all of these issues and typically limited supports with whom to safety plan, hospitalization may need to be utilized more frequently (44).

Maintaining awareness of cultural differences in symptom presentation and considering the possibility that somatic symptoms may actually belie mental illness will be helpful for the ED provider. Interpreters should be used whenever possible to enhance communication and accurate understanding.

Racial/Ethnic Minorities

Students who are in the minority and marginalized are at higher risk of depression, anxiety, and other mental health disorders. A recent study indicated that students identifying as a racial/ethnic minority receive less treatment (both medications and therapy) than their White peers, with Asians having the lowest prevalence of treatment (45). Racial/ethnic minority students also have the lower perceived need for mental health treatment and lower rates of diagnosis than White students. It is therefore likely that when these students present to the ED, they may do so without any structured outpatient treatment in place, which will influence the ED disposition. More extensive psychoeducation regarding the need for psychotropic medications and other treatments may be needed for racial/ethnic minority students. Mental health stigma is reported as potent for racial and ethnic minorities, which could impact these students' disclosure of suicidal thoughts and behaviors in the emergency setting. These issues are exacerbated when these minority students are engaging with clinicians and staff of different racial/ethnic backgrounds than themselves. Being culturally humble and aware of one's own biases is crucial for rapid rapport development, accurate diagnosis, and informed disposition decisions.

LGBTQ Populations

Students who identify as LGBTQ are more likely to report significant distress and a greater prevalence of stressful life events than their heterosexual and cisgender counterparts (46). They are more likely to report social stressors such as isolation and frank harassment (47). Factors including stigma, discrimination, and the stress associated with being part of a minority group combine to increase the risk of poor mental health in this population (48). LGBTQ students have a greater risk of symptoms of anxiety and depression and are more likely to engage in self-harm and suicidal behaviors (49). While more likely to use mental health services than their heterosexual counterparts, there remains a high level of unmet treatment needs for LGBTQ students requiring additional attention and research. Given that issues and stresses related to gender identity, intimacy, and sex can contribute to symptomatology, it is wise for the ED provider to inquire specifically about the sexual orientation, gender preference, and unique sexual life experiences of all students who present to the psychiatric ED with depression, suicidal ideation, or attempted suicide (50). Specific training for emergency staff regarding appropriate terminology and LGBTQ issues, current understanding of sexual and gender identity (including gender fluidity), the importance of utilizing correct pronouns when addressing students, and approaching them in a nonjudgmental manner is indicated (51). Demonstrating awareness of and sensitivity to the unique struggles of LGBTQ students, as well as validating any struggles, may help foster better provider-patient rapport and enhance the quality of care. Failure to convey awareness and compassion can have a profoundly negative effect on the patient experience and will undermine a provider's ability to appropriately and safely assess the LGBTQ student in crisis.

CONCLUSION

College and university students represent a unique group of transitional age youth who have high rates of psychiatric symptomatology and live on the cusp of adulthood yet frequently still depend on a high level of support from family and others. Their crisis care needs may be complicated by barriers to communication with their families and school officials.

Graduate students, who are frequently older yet still reside in educational communities, also have high rates of psychiatric symptoms and struggle with their own unique issues. Minority student populations and special groups require even more nuanced consideration to provide optimal care. Although the psychiatric problems and care for college and university students are similar to that of other young adults, psychiatric emergency providers must be aware of the additional stressors these young people may face because of their student status. The complex process of safety planning without family involvement or when campus personnel must be included may further complicate treatment planning.

REFERENCES

1. Lipson, S. K., Lattie, E. G., & Eisenberg, D. (2018). Increased rates of mental health service utilization by U.S. college students: 10-year population-level trends (2007–2017). *Psychiatric Services, 70*(1), 60–63. doi:10.1176/appi.ps.201800332.

2. Liu, C. H., Stevens, C., Wong, S. H. M., Yasui, M., & Chen, J. A. (2019). The prevalence and predictors of mental health diagnoses and suicide among U.S. college students: Implications for addressing disparities in service use. *Depression and Anxiety, 36*(1), 8–17. doi:10.1002/da.22830.

3. Evans, T. M., Bira, L., Gastelum, J. B., et al. (2018). Evidence for a mental health crisis in graduate education. *Nature Biotechnology, 36*(3), 282–284. doi:10.1038/nbt.4089.

4. Czyz, E. K., Horwitz, A. G., Eisenberg, D., et al. (2013). Self-reported barriers to professional help seeking among college students at elevated risk for suicide. *Journal of American College Health, 61*(7), 398–406. doi:10.1080/07448481.2013.820731.

5. Eisenberg, D., Hunt, J., Speer, N., & Zivin, K. (2011). Mental health service utilization among college students in the United States. *The Journal of Nervous and Mental Disease, 199*(5), 301–308. doi:10.1097/NMD.0b013e3182175123.

6. Arria, A. M., O'Grady, K. E., Caldeira, K. M., Vincent, K. B., Wilcox, H. C., & Wish, E. D. (2009). Suicide ideation among college students: A multivariate analysis. *Archives of Suicide Research, 13*(3), 230–246. doi:10.1080/13811110903044351.

7. Lamis, D. A., Malone, P. S., Langhinrichsen-Rohling, J., et al. (2010). Body investment, depression, and alcohol use as risk factors for suicide proneness in college students. *Crisis, 31*(3), 118–127. doi:10.1027/0227-5910/a000012.

8. Blanco, C., Okuda, M., Wright, C., et al. (2008). Mental health of college students and their non-college-attending peers: Results from the National Epidemiologic Study on Alcohol and Related Conditions. *Archives of General Psychiatry, 65*(12), 1429–1437. doi:10.1001/archpsyc.65.12.1429.

9. Califano, J. A., National Center on Addiction and Substance Abuse at Columbia University. (2007). *Wasting the best and the brightest: Substance abuse at America's colleges and universities.* New York, NY: CASA.

10. Davis, M., & Vander Stoep, A. (1997). The transition to adulthood for youth who have serious emotional disturbance: Developmental transition and young adult outcomes. *Journal of Mental Health Administration, 24*(4), 400–427.

11. Livesey, C. M., & Rostain, A. L. (2017). Involving parents/family in treatment during the transition from late adolescence to young adulthood: Rationale, strategies, ethics, and legal issues. *Child and Adolescent Psychiatric Clinics of North America, 26*(2), 199–216. doi:10.1016/j.chc.2016.12.006.

12. Solky, H. J., McKeever, J. E., Perlmutter, R. A., et al. (1988). Involving parents in the management of psychiatric emergencies in college students far from home. *Journal of American College Health, 36*(6), 335–339.

13. Mortier, P., Cuijpers, P., Kiekens, G., et al. (2018). The prevalence of suicidal thoughts and behaviours among college students: A meta-analysis. *Psychological Medicine, 48*(4), 554–565. doi:10.1017/S0033291717002215.

14. Han, B., Compton, W. M., Eisenberg, D., et al. (2016). Prevalence and mental health treatment of suicidal ideation and behavior among college students aged 18-25 years and their non-college-attending peers in the United States. *Journal of Clinical Psychiatry, 77*(6), 815–824. doi:10.4088/JCP.15m09929.

15. *American College Health Association-National College Health Assessment II: Reference Group Executive Summary Fall 2017.* (2018). Hanover, MD: American College Health Association.

16. American Psychiatric Association. (2003). *Practice guideline for the assessment and treatment of patients with suicidal behaviors.* Retrieved January 14, 2019, from https://psychiatryonline.org/pb/assets/raw/sitewide/practice_guidelines/guidelines/suicide.pdf.

17. Mortier, P., Auerbach, R. P., Alonso, J., et al. (2018). Suicidal thoughts and behaviors among first-year college students: Results from the WMH-ICS project. *Journal of the American Academy of Child & Adolescent Psychiatry, 57*(4), 263–273.e1. doi:10.1016/j.jaac.2018.01.018.

18. Dvorak, R. D., Lamis, D. A., & Malone, P. S. (2013). Alcohol use, depressive symptoms, and impulsivity as risk factors for suicide proneness among college students. *Journal of Affective Disorders, 149*(1–3), 326–334. doi:10.1016/j.jad.2013.01.046.

19. Whitlock, J., Eckrode, J., & Silverman, D. (2006). Self-injurious behaviors in a college population. *Pediatrics, 117*(6), 1939–1948.

20. Joiner, T. (2005). *Why people die by suicide.* Cambridge, MA: Harvard University Press.

21. National Conference of State Legislatures. (2018). *Guns on campus: Overview.* Retrieved January 15, 2019, from http://www.ncsl.org/research/education/guns-on-campus-overview.aspx.

22. Eisenberg, D., Nicklett, E. J., Roeder, K., et al. (2011). Eating disorder symptoms among college students: Prevalence, persistence, correlates, and treatment-seeking. *Journal of American College Health, 59*(8), 700–707. doi:10.1080/07448481.2010.546461.

23. Keshavan, M. S., & Kaneko, Y. (2013). Secondary psychoses: An update. *World Psychiatry, 12*(1), 4–15. doi:10.1002/wps.20001.

24. Schulenberg, J. E., Johnston, L. D., O'Malley, P. M., et al. (2018). *Monitoring the Future national survey results on drug use, 1975–2017: Vol. II, College students and adults ages 19–55.* Ann Arbor, MI: Institute for Social Research, The University of Michigan. Retrieved January 15, 2019, from http://www.monitoringthefuture.org//pubs/monographs/mtf-vol2_2017.pdf.

25. Thompson, K. M., & Huynh, C. (2017). Alone and at risk: A statistical profile of alcohol-related college student deaths. *Journal of Substance Use, 22*(5), 549–554. doi:10.1080/14659891.2016.1271032.

26. Centers for Disease Control and Prevention. (2018). *Drug overdose deaths.* Retrieved January 15, 2019, from https://www.cdc.gov/drugoverdose/data/statedeaths.html.

27. Pollard, J. W., Nolan, J. J., & Deisinger, E. R. (2012). The practice of campus-based threat assessment: An overview. *Journal of College Student Psychotherapy, 26*(4), 263–276. doi:10.1080/87568225.2012.711142.

28. Resnick, M. D., Ireland, M. & Borowsky, I. (2004). Youth violence perpetration: What protects? What predicts? Findings from the National Longitudinal Study of Adolescent Health. *Journal of Adolescent Health, 35*(5), 424.e1–424.e10.

29. Felthous, A. R. (2006). Warning a potential victim of a person's dangerousness: Clinician's duty or victim's right? *Journal of the American Academy of Psychiatry & the Law, 34*(3), 338–348.

30. Schuchman, M. (2007). Falling through the cracks—Virginia Tech and the restructuring of college mental health services. *New England Journal of Medicine, 357*(2), 105–110. doi:10.1056/NEJMp078096.

31. Glick, R. L., & Schwartz, V. (2007). Assessment and management: Special considerations for college students in psychiatric crisis. *Psychiatric Issues in Emergency Care Settings, 6*(4), 7–13.

32. Appelbaum, P. (2006). Law and psychiatry: "Depressed? Get out!": Dealing with suicidal students on college campuses. *Psychiatric Services, 57*, 914–915.

33. Dyrbye, L. N., Thomas, M. R., & Shanafelt, T. D. (2006). Systematic review of depression, anxiety, and other indicators of psychological distress among U.S. and Canadian medical students. *Academic Medicine, 81*(4), 354–373.

34. Rotenstein, L. S., Ramos, M. A., Torre, M., et al. (2016). Prevalence of depression, depressive symptoms, and suicidal ideation among medical students: A systematic review and meta-analysis. *JAMA, 316*(21), 2214–2236. doi:10.1001/jama.2016.17324.

35. Montgomery, A. J., Bradley, C., Rochfort, A., et al. (2011). A review of self-medication in physicians and medical students. *Occupational Medicine, 61*(7), 490–497.

36. Roberts, L. W. (2010). Understanding depression and distress among medical students. *JAMA, 304*(11), 1231–1233. doi:10.1001/jama.2010.1347.

37. Steinbrook, R. (2008). Medical student debt – Is there a limit? *New England Journal of Medicine, 359*, 2629–2632.

38. Schwenk, T. L., Davis, L., & Wimsatt, L. A. (2010). Depression, stigma, and suicidal ideation in medical students. *JAMA, 304*(11), 1181–1190. doi:10.1001/jama.2010.1300.

39. Rao, A. L., & Hong, E. S. (2016). Understanding depression and suicide in college athletes: Emerging concepts and future directions. *British Journal of Sports Medicine, 50*(3), 136–137.

40. Reardon, C. L., & Creado, S. (2014). Drug abuse in athletes. *Substance Abuse and Rehabilitation, 5*, 95–105. doi:10.2147/SAR.S53784.

41. Joy, E., Kussman, A., & Nattiv, A. (2016). 2016 update on eating disorders in athletes: A comprehensive narrative review with a focus on clinical assessment and management. *British Journal of Sports Medicine, 50*(3), 154–162. doi:10.1136/bjsports-2015-095735.

42. Gulliver, A., Griffiths, K. M., & Christensen, H. (2012). Barriers and facilitators to mental health help-seeking for young elite athletes: A qualitative study. *BMC Psychiatry, 12,* 157. doi:10.1186/1471-244X-12-157.

43. Reardon, C. L., & Factor, R. M. (2016). Considerations in the use of stimulants in sport. *Sports Medicine, 46*(5), 611–617. doi:10.1007/s40279-015-0456-y.

44. Eisenberg, D., Golberstein, E., & Gollust, S. E. (2007). Help-seeking and access to mental health care in a university student population. *Medical Care, 45*(7), 594–601.

45. Lipson, S. K., Kern, A., Eisenberg, D., et al. (2018). Mental health disparities among college students of color. *Journal of Adolescent Health, 63*(3), 348–356. doi:10.1016/j.jadohealth.2018.04.014.

46. Przedworski, J. M., VanKim, N. A., Eisenberg, M. E., et al. (2015). Self-reported mental disorders and distress by sexual orientation: Results of the Minnesota College Student Health Survey. *American Journal of Preventive Medicine, 49*(1), 29–40. doi:10.1016/j.amepre.2015.01.024.

47. Przedworski, J. M., Dovidio, J. F., Hardeman, R. R., et al. (2015). A comparison of the mental health and well-being of sexual minority and heterosexual first-year medical students: A report from the medical student CHANGE study. *Academic Medicine, 90*(5), 652–659. doi:10.1097/ACM.0000000000000658.

48. Dunbar, M. S., Sontag-Padilla, L., Ramchand, R., et al. (2017). Mental health service utilization among lesbian, gay, bisexual, and questioning or queer college students. *Journal of Adolescent Health, 61*(3), 294–301. doi:10.1016/j.jadohealth.2017.03.008.

49. Taliaferro, L. A., & Muehlenkamp, J. J. (2015). Risk factors associated with self-injurious behavior among a national sample of undergraduate college students. *Journal of American College Health, 63*(1), 40–48. doi:10.1080/07448481.2014.953166.

50. Kitts, R. L. (2010). Barriers to optimal care between physicians and lesbian, gay, bisexual, transgender, and questioning adolescent patients. *Journal of Homosexuality, 57*(6), 730–747. doi:10.1080/00918369.2010.485872.

51. Landry, J. (2017). Delivering culturally sensitive care to LGBTQI patients. *The Journal for Nurse Practitioners, 13*(5), 342–347.

PART VI

Policy and Special Topics

Section Editor: Rachel Lipson Glick

44

Policy Issues Relating to the Treatment of People With Psychiatric Disabilities in Emergency Department Settings

Susan Stefan

If any group of stakeholders were to design a system [of emergency services for people in psychiatric crisis] a priori, the most common service currently available could not emerge from the deliberative process.

American Psychiatric Association Task Force on Psychiatric Emergency Services (2002).

The quotation that opens this chapter is a striking statement, and it is true. Hospital emergency departments (EDs) currently provide the bulk of emergency psychiatric care, serve as gatekeepers for inpatient mental health beds, and have had thrust upon them a virtual monopoly in determining whether an individual will be detained involuntarily and subject to commitment proceedings. Sometimes these tasks are performed by specialized or dedicated psychiatric emergency services (PESs), but for the most part, only larger urban areas with sufficient volume to make such a focus feasible have PESs. Thus, although there are about 4,600 emergency departments in the United States, only about 1,607 provide psychiatric care, described as "services and facilities available on a 24-hour basis to provide immediate unscheduled outpatient care, diagnosis, evaluation, crisis intervention and assistance to persons suffering acute emotional or mental distress" (1). However, many of those services are provided by doctors and nurses with little specialized training in mental health assessment and treatment. Only 150 PESs in the country are staffed 24 hours a day with psychiatrists, psychiatric nurses, and other mental health professionals (2).

Thus, it is fair to say that the vast majority of decisions to involuntarily detain an individual

with a psychiatric disability in an emergency department are not made by mental health professionals. Emergency department staff who make decisions about triage, assessment, treatment, and disposition of people with psychiatric disabilities often have relatively little formal mental health training or treatment experience. In addition, there is little time to spare from the pressures and demands of a busy ED to sit with patients and have the conversations necessary to evaluate more complex cases, let alone secure confirming information from available collateral sources. Yet the decisions made by ED staff about the assessment, treatment, and disposition of people in psychiatric crisis have a profound impact on the lives of those individuals, on the use of scarce emergency department resources and beds, and on the use of ever-diminishing mental health resources, including inpatient beds.

The resulting situation is an unpardonable waste of limited healthcare dollars. Emergency departments are by far the most expensive venue for the delivery of care for psychiatric crises, with Blue Cross/Blue Shield reporting that the average cost of an emergency department visit is $1,049 (3). Far less expensive alternatives are available, and many more would be available if current reimbursement policies were altered to encompass them. Beyond the misuse of scarce healthcare dollars and resources, the ED setting is rarely optimal for individuals in psychiatric crisis: Their needs for time, support, and a calm environment are difficult to meet in most urban EDs, and the specialized care and experience to respond to some of the more complex psychiatric issues may be lacking in rural areas. Finally, people in psychiatric crisis often need an array of social services and supports that hospital ED staff are ill-equipped to access, and formal, organized coordination with agencies that provide those services is rare.

It is common for hospital emergency staff to struggle under unsustainable workloads, while vulnerable, fragile psychiatric patients wait, sometimes for days, in claustrophobically small emergency department rooms or on gurneys in the hall, often in thin hospital johnnies. Psychiatric patients, unlike medical patients, are frequently forbidden to leave the hospital prior to assessment if it has been concluded at triage that they may pose a risk, even if they feel better or get tired of waiting. Those who try to leave prior to assessment may be escorted back and sometimes restrained, by hospital security guards. The use of restraints on psychiatric patients in emergency departments, and requirements of clothing removal that are sometimes enforced by forcible stripping, can make the ED experience extremely aversive and traumatizing to people already in psychiatric crisis.

The insights in this chapter are the results of 4 years of interviews, site visits, and meetings with emergency department physicians, nurse managers, nurses, social workers, psychologists, and psychiatrists that I performed as director of the Center for Public Representation's National Emergency Department Project.[*] The center assembled a national advisory panel that included representatives of urban, rural, and small city emergency departments; managed care; state mental health program directors; the research community; and people who identified themselves as consumers

of mental health services (two of whom had gone on to create innovative crisis alternatives to traditional emergency departments). In addition, I read more than 1000 accounts by people with psychiatric disabilities of their experiences with emergency departments across the country and scoured the medical, social science, and even anthropological research literature on emergency departments.

One of the major findings of this national project is that hospital emergency departments and people with psychiatric disabilities are joint victims of a system that is both shaped and driven by legal requirements and the incentive structures they create. The current dysfunctional situation is produced by the intersection of social control, embodied by state civil commitment laws; mandatory access, required by federal Emergency Medical Treatment and Active Labor Act (EMTALA) regulations; lack of alternatives, the result of federal and state reimbursement requirements and limitations; and the exaggerated perceptions of looming liability under state tort laws.

Thus, the power of the emergency department to detain, its powerlessness to impose restrictions on access to its services, pervasive staff concerns about tort liability for discharging an individual with a psychiatric disability, and the absence of viable crisis step-downs or alternatives interact to produce inevitable and unsustainable growth in presentations to EDs of individuals in psychiatric crisis, as well as an overstated need for inpatient beds to provide disposition for patients whom ED staff are reluctant to discharge. This mix is made even more complex by other regulatory and legal requirements, including Medicaid and Social Security eligibility restrictions on immigrants and people whose disability is due to substance abuse, that also drive use of emergency departments by people with psychiatric disabilities.

However, hospitals and emergency department staff share the responsibility for emergency department delays and boarding of psychiatric patients because they persistently and unnecessarily overadmit psychiatric patients. The scarcity of inpatient beds, although real, is not the sole source of the problem. Disproportionate admissions can stem from the following:

- Lack of staff with experience in mental health issues
- Exaggerated and misplaced liability fears

[*]The Center for Public Representation is a national litigation and advocacy organization for people with mental disabilities, including psychiatric disabilities, developmental disabilities, and brain injuries. The National Emergency Department Project was funded with grants from the Ittelson and van Ameringen Foundations.

- "Iatrogenic" admissions, in which a patient who arrived at the ED in relatively stable condition becomes agitated and out of control as a result of delays or other ED experiences
- Inpatient admissions that are essentially acts of compassion for poor, homeless, and substance-abusing people seeking respite or detoxification services. These acts, although well-meaning, are expensive and ineffective solutions to far broader systemic issues

It is clear that action at the national, state, and hospital levels is needed to alleviate the misuse of social resources and provide people in psychiatric crisis the care that EDs are not equipped to supply. Two crucial and complementary avenues to solving the current situation exist. The first is the addition and funding of alternative forms of psychiatric crisis care, from crisis houses and respite beds to peer drop-in centers, family foster care, and mobile crisis units (4). Accomplishing this is more difficult than may be apparent because these alternatives can rarely access traditional reimbursement dollars and often do not provide the social control function that makes EDs magnets for secondary users (see the section "State Commitment Laws and Secondary Users" later in this chapter for discussion of this term). Finally, the familiarity and accessibility of EDs are attractive features to people under great stress.

The second solution is for EDs to do all they can to reduce inappropriate and unnecessary psychiatric inpatient admissions. This will require a significant change in culture and support by hospital leadership. Reducing the current focus on liability issues and speed of disposition, resisting the pressures of secondary users such as police or family members to admit patients, working proactively with other social agencies that serve patients who appear frequently in the ED, and adopting a recovery and rehabilitation orientation—all of these proposals run fundamentally contrary to the culture in many EDs. Often, sheer exhaustion prevents staff from doing outreach and creating alliances, both with mental health systems and political representatives, that might result in better coordination, higher funding, the creation of crisis alternatives, and other measures to alleviate some of their burdens.

THE LAWS THAT DRIVE EMERGENCY DEPARTMENT USAGE AND POLICIES

Emergency departments are gatekeepers for two crucially important systems: the legal system of involuntary commitment and involuntary treatment, and the inpatient psychiatric treatment system. Yet staff in emergency departments have little training in assessing people with psychiatric disabilities, and generally even less knowledge of the laws that create the system in which they operate.

State Commitment Laws and Secondary Users

All states have statutes providing that people with mental illness who are dangerous to themselves or others as a result of their mental illness may be involuntarily detained. State commitment laws generally provide that there are three classes of individuals with the power and authority to detain a person involuntarily: judges, police, and medical professionals. Judges are generally not available after hours, and neither are most medical or mental health professionals. Therefore, when others—family members, group home providers, landlords, or school authorities—perceive that a person with a psychiatric disability needs to be involuntarily detained, there are two potential solutions to the problem: calling the police or going to the emergency department. Police, in turn, often use their powers of detention to bring a person displaying mental health symptoms to the emergency department and are in fact encouraged to do so when the perceived alternative is jail (5). Emergency departments are the gatekeepers for two crucially important systems—the legal system of involuntary commitment and the mental health treatment system of inpatient care—and they are always open.

The power of emergency departments to detain people with psychiatric disabilities, conferred by state civil commitment laws, is key to understanding a major component of ED use. The emergency department is open 24 hours a day, 7 days a week, and because of federal EMTALA requirements, it has no eligibility criteria, nor can it reject any initial presentations for assessment. Family members, case managers, police officers, group home operators, nursing homes, and others solve their own problems with individuals with psychiatric disabilities by bringing those individuals to the emergency department for evaluation and (more important) detention. This is an effective and efficient solution for these "secondary users" of emergency departments and is usually cost free for them.

It should be clear that not all family members, police officers, and others who accompany people with psychiatric disabilities to EDs are secondary users. Some come with the individual to provide comfort and advocacy; some police officers are genuinely trying to get treatment for someone who might otherwise be in a jail cell. The definition of *secondary user* requires that the ED visit be initiated by the secondary user to solve his or her problems created by an individual with a psychiatric disability.

Secondary users are not confined to those who bring an individual to the emergency department. When mental health professionals leave messages on their answering machines advising any patient calling after hours to go to the emergency department, they are not only acting unethically (6,7), they are also secondary users, solving their problem of after-hours emergencies by thrusting it on the local emergency department. When state mental health agencies cut the budgets of crisis services, they are transferring part of their professional responsibilities—to provide on-call coverage or to fund the full spectrum of mental health services for their clients—to emergency department staff without compensating the ED for taking on those responsibilities.

Secondary use may account for a substantial number of mental health–related visits to the emergency department, and policy solutions to emergency department problems must begin with data collection that identifies secondary users as such and begins to search for strategies regarding accountability. For example, community mental health providers could be required to report their use of emergency departments for mental health–related events, and use could be audited to see whether it reflected inadequate de-escalation skills on the part of provider staff. State mental health agencies might be legislatively required to assign case managers to any of their clients who used the emergency department more than six times a year.

But simply having the obligation to assess people for potential risk associated with psychiatric disabilities, and the opportunity to involuntarily detain those people, does not by itself lead to increased admissions. Emergency department staff do not *have* to involuntarily detain people with psychiatric disabilities just because they *can* involuntarily detain them. Rather, in many involuntary detentions, liability fears overshadow clinical judgment. In addition, it generally takes less time to do an assessment resulting in admission than to take the time to arrange discharge and outpatient follow-up. Thus, the pattern continues, in which the patient perceived as a problem is passed along to an inpatient unit, much as the person's presence in the ED may be the result of someone passing his or her problem along to the ED.

State Tort and Malpractice Laws and the Problem of Unnecessary Admissions

Decisions made by ED professionals to admit psychiatric patients to inpatient beds are driven by a complex mixture of factors. In addition to clinical concerns, pressure from secondary users such as family or police may increase the chances of inpatient admission regardless of clinical presentation. Finally, many emergency department staff acknowledge that liability concerns play a part in decisions to admit a psychiatric patient. Upon closer examination, a substantial number of these concerns appear to be both exaggerated and misplaced.

First, ED decision makers tend to focus almost completely on liability arising from failure to admit an individual. Inpatient admission is seen as the "safe" route, to avoid the risk that the individual might later commit suicide or harm someone else. This focus on psychiatric disposition may obscure or minimize other important clinical and liability issues, including inadequate assessment, failure to attach sufficient importance to an individual's medical symptoms or concerns, or the use of force in emergency departments to prevent an individual from leaving.

Furthermore, liability for patient suicide almost always results not from the simple failure to predict the suicide but from errors that are far easier to avoid, such as failure to read a psychiatric consult or failing to access readily available collateral information. In most cases where juries find liability, there is an apparent and egregious circumstance—for example, a patient requesting admission being told in virtually the same breath that she was not being admitted because she did not meet inpatient criteria and did not have health insurance, or a patient with suicidal ideation being discharged from the emergency department with a 30-day supply of drugs and an appointment 1 month later.

Ironically, ED staff may be unaware of state-of-the-art research that counsels that people who are chronically, consistently suicidal as a reflection of an underlying personality disorder rather than major depression should *not* necessarily be hospitalized (8,9). In addition, ED staff increase the likelihood of their own legal liability by accepting a model of complete responsibility for predicting dangerousness that does not reflect reality and that inappropriately assigns to mental health professionals all risk of adverse outcome. For example, a well-known risk factor for an adverse outcome is the presence of guns in the patient's household (10). ED staff should always inquire about whether there are guns in a patient's residence and document the response, advise family members or others who share the household to dispose of the guns (locking them in a cabinet is not sufficient to reduce risk), and document that advice. The ED cannot be held responsible for involuntarily detaining anyone who has guns in his or her household. This risk is the family's responsibility and to hospitalize someone because of it postpones a situation over which ED staff have no control because the person will go home sooner or later. ED staff can identify and fortify protective factors and identify and work to reduce risk, but unless an individual is truly incompetent, risk and responsibility should be shared with the patient and his or her family, who best know the circumstances of their environment and lives.

Often, ED staff err by documenting only the evidence supporting their conclusions. Good documentation shows that the professional appreciated and assessed for risk and, where appropriate, sought consultation. Good documentation cites both protective factors and risk factors and underscores the steps taken to enhance the former and reduce the latter. Good documentation reflects any available input from collateral sources regarding both risks and strengths, as well as an assessment of the reliability of the collateral source (some secondary users provide inaccurate information in an effort to obtain admission for a patient). All of these steps help insulate thoughtful dispositional decisions—whether the decision is to admit or to discharge a patient—from liability.

Contingent Suicidality and Unnecessary Admissions

A classic example of frequently unnecessary inpatient admission driven by fear of liability is the case of contingent suicidality. *Contingent suicidality* was first described by Michael Lambert and refers to patients who use threats of suicide as a means to gain hospital admission, by explicitly threatening to commit suicide if they are not admitted (11). Lambert followed a group of patients who made these threats, as well as a group of "noncontingently" suicidal patients, for 7 years. At the end of the 7-year period, 20 people had died, 18 of them in the noncontingently suicidal group. Of the 10 clear suicides, none of them were in the contingently suicidal group (12). The actual risk of suicide for contingently suicidal presentation is far lower than for noncontingently suicidal people.

There is a specific mode of presentation associated with people who are contingently suicidal, as well as specific correlates. People who are contingently suicidal tend to be "dramatic, complaint prone" and show "shelter-/refuge-seeking" behavior (13). They often include a request for hospitalization when describing their chief complaint, and they manifest "frequent help seeking exclusively for the most restrictive types of care" (14). They have "provocative or waxing reports of SI/HI/psychoses" as the interview progresses, while simultaneously demonstrating "overt evidence of future orientation or secondary gain" (14). They often have co-occurring substance abuse problems and may have legal involvement (11).

One way for EDs to reduce admissions to psychiatric inpatient beds is to educate staff to be aware of the phenomenon of contingent suicidality and to accept the recommendation of mental health consultants who are aware of the phenomenon to refuse admission to people who are contingently suicidal. At the same time, ED staff can try to assist the individual to solve whatever problem he or she is trying to solve by seeking inpatient admission, whether it is a legal problem or a need for respite.

JCAHO Suicidality Assessment Requirements and Overadmission

A recent development that may unintentionally and unnecessarily fuel psychiatric admissions is the requirement by the Joint Commission on Accreditation of Healthcare Organizations (JCAHO) to assess suicidality in all behavioral health patients (15). This requirement aims to make professionals pay attention to the possibility of suicidality because research has shown that thousands of people present to emergency departments with self-inflicted injuries and are never evaluated for mental health problems, let alone suicidality. It also aims at increasing the assistance that emergency departments offer to people with suicidality, including hotline phone numbers and referrals. These are worthy goals and do not require or necessarily lead to increased inpatient admissions.

EMTALA Regulations and Their Interaction With Psychiatric Patient Admissions

As most emergency department staff are aware, federal EMTALA regulations require that all patients who present to the ED be provided with screening for emergency conditions. Although someone who is unconscious or incompetent has "presented" at the emergency department if he or she is brought in by someone else, there are mixed regulations and court holdings about whether EMTALA applies to people who are brought involuntarily to the emergency department by police (16-18). It is not clear whether a person who does not seek evaluation but is brought by someone else for an evaluation is "presenting" at the ED.

The statutory definition of an "emergency medical condition" is one that, in the absence of medical attention, could reasonably be expected to result in "imminent danger of death or serious disability" (42 U.S.C. 1395dd[e][1]). The regulations make explicit that emergency medical conditions include psychiatric conditions (42 C.F.R. 489.24[b]). The Seventh Circuit held that a person can have an "emergency medical condition"

related to psychiatric disability, even if he or she is neither homicidal or suicidal, if the individual is still, in the opinion of the ED staff, in a condition to be harmful to self or others (19). The fact that someone is claiming to be suicidal does not create an obligation to treat if after screening the staff concludes that the person is not actually suicidal, any more than a person convinced he or she is having a cardiac problem is entitled to treatment if ED staff conclude that he or she does not have a cardiac problem.

A person may leave the emergency department after presenting for treatment at any time under EMTALA, even if screening determines that the individual needs treatment and stabilization (although the same may not be true under the state's civil commitment statutes). EMTALA does not require that involuntary treatment or tests be forced on a competent individual who refuses tests or treatment. Under 42 C.F.R 489.24, the hospital must ensure that the medical record contains "a description of the examination, treatment, or both if applicable, that was refused by or on behalf of the individual." In addition, the hospital must "take all reasonable steps to secure the individual's written informed refusal" (or that of the person acting on his or her behalf). Finally, the written record should indicate that "the person has been informed of the risks and benefits of the examination or treatment, or both." The same requirements apply to a refusal on the part of the individual to accept a transfer to another facility.

The EMTALA issue that ED staff sometimes ignore with psychiatric patients is the obligation to screen for emergency *medical* conditions, especially if that is the basis of the individual's complaint. Stories (and cases) of emergency department staff minimizing important medical complaints because of overattention to psychiatric concerns are numerous. At least one study shows that mentally ill people constitute a disproportionate number of people who die from medical conditions shortly after leaving an emergency department (20). This does not mean that the medical workup some inpatient facilities demand prior to accepting a patient who came in with a psychiatric complaint is necessarily justified. It does mean that if a patient presents with a medical complaint, the patient's psychiatric condition should not diminish or distract from the importance of screening for that complaint.

SOLUTIONS AND STANDARDS

The problems presented in this chapter have two kinds of solutions: systemic and regulatory solutions, which require alliances with other actors in the mental health field, and solutions that hospitals themselves can undertake. Emergency departments are difficult cultures to change because they operate both with insulated autonomy and under such stress that any kind of change is experienced as an overwhelming and untenable burden imposed from the outside by uncomprehending outsiders. It requires leadership, leadership support of staff taking risks, and involving staff in the process of change to make change possible. With that in mind, the following are suggested solutions to help reduce unnecessary inpatient psychiatric admissions.

Hospital- and Emergency Department–Based Solutions

Reduce Inappropriate and Unnecessary Inpatient Admissions by Reducing Iatrogenic and Liability-Based Inpatient Admissions

Many problems that emergency departments face in assisting people with psychiatric disabilities—boarding, searching for inpatient beds, agitated and unruly patients—could be reduced substantially simply by identifying and reducing unnecessary inpatient admissions. As discussed previously, many of these admissions are driven by fear of liability or are iatrogenic admissions—inpatient admissions of patients who were calm when they arrived at the ED but become agitated as a result of events in the ED.

The Center for Public Representation's National Advisory Council, which included ED psychiatrists, managed care, advocacy groups, researchers, consumers of mental health services, and representatives of the state mental health system, agreed on a number of findings and recommendations related to the treatment of people with psychiatric disabilities in emergency departments that would assist in reducing iatrogenic admissions. A selection of these standards is referenced below.

The following suggestions are aimed at increasing quality of care while reducing admissions. To increase the quality of care, it first has to be properly defined; therefore, the first suggestion for change is directed at how the hospital measures quality of care delivered to people with psychiatric disabilities.

Reconfigure Quality Assessment Standards in Assessing Care of People With Psychiatric Disabilities

Standard quality assessment measures do not readily apply to assess the quality of treatment of people with psychiatric disabilities in emergency departments. Because people with psychiatric disabilities make up such a small proportion of the overall patients seen in the ED, they are sometimes excluded entirely from quality assessment and sometimes included in ways that can create a perverse disincentive to provide quality care to people with psychiatric disabilities and increase inpatient psychiatric admissions.

For example, standard measures of ED quality include time from triage to disposition, recidivism, patients who leave without being seen, follow-up with care, patient satisfaction with care, and mortality. The emphasis on reducing total time in the ED might lead to more admissions because it may take more assessment time and planning to arrange for an outpatient discharge; sometimes taking additional time to observe a patient in the ED, or contacting family members and waiting for their arrival, can obviate the need for inpatient admission.

Recidivism with psychiatric patients is not necessarily voluntary, and using recidivism as a measure without carefully factoring in secondary use may be problematic. It may also indicate a positive result: A person with suicidal ideation might have been discharged on the basis of a promise to return if symptoms worsened.

Patient satisfaction with care, unless measured carefully, may be confounded by patient dissatisfaction with clinically appropriate admissions and refusals to admit. Mortality should definitely be a measure for psychiatric patients who die of *medical* conditions shortly after being seen in an ED. To use nonnatural deaths, such as being killed by police or suicide, may be problematic for a variety of reasons: Events in the patient's life or failures to alter the environment that are entirely beyond the ED's control may be implicated in the patient's death, and to automatically equate suicide with failure by the ED staff is to support the myth that suicide is so predictable and preventable by mental health professionals that the failure to do so is automatically a marker of low-quality care. This assumption in turn may encourage unnecessary or inappropriate admissions to inpatient units.

The center's National Advisory Council suggested both principles and benchmarks of quality care to people with psychiatric disabilities in EDs. Principles that should guide policy and practice are that care should be patient centered, minimize coercion, increase choice, and reduce or eliminate the need for force (4). Of particular importance, care should be individualized and enhance a patient's sense of safety, with a clear understanding that EDs should not assume that interventions intended to ensure safety enhance either a patient's sense of safety or actual safety. Finally, patients' dignity should be respected, including their needs for food, hydration, and hygiene.

More appropriate benchmarks include the following:

- Time between presentation and assessment, particularly for people brought in involuntarily under petitions for emergency detention; in those cases, an outside assessment has already been made that the person has an emergency psychiatric condition. No person under an involuntary detention order should wait more than 3 hours for complete assessment and evaluation and development of a disposition decision or treatment plan
- Specific measurement of and reduction in security guard use of force on persons with psychiatric disabilities in the emergency department
- Measurement of and ongoing, consistent reduction in use of restraint and seclusion in the ED
- Chart audits to ensure that individuals presenting with medical complaints were appropriately assessed for those complaints
- Reduction in inappropriate and unnecessary inpatient admissions

Emergency department staff and mental health consumer advocacy groups should be interviewed to suggest other ways of measuring excellent care of psychiatric patients in emergency departments.

Adopt Standards for the Treatment of People With Psychiatric Disabilities in Emergency Departments

The quality assurance measures described previously should result in changes in ED standards and practice. A selection of the most important changes includes issues regarding the use of security guards and the forcible removal of clothing.

Use of security guards: We have learned in working with EDs around the country that one reliable measure of whether people with psychiatric disabilities are receiving appropriate treatment in emergency departments is the frequency with which security guards or police are called to forcibly intervene, and the degree of force that they use. Entire panoplies of patient behavior that could be characterized as understandable frustration and anxiety or a result of psychiatric symptomatology are reframed as security problems when an ED staff does not have the time or mental health skills to intervene appropriately. These range from the patient who keeps emerging from his or her room to find out the status of his or her examination to the patient who attempts to leave; the patient who is pacing or standing on the gurney; the patient who resists giving up a watch, piece of jewelry, or other treasured item; and the patient who is yelling abuse. In all of these cases, we have seen nurses call security guards to institute restraints; more rarely, psychiatric patients have been pepper sprayed by security guards. In one famous case, King/Drew Hospital in Los Angeles came close to losing federal funding because it tasered psychiatric patients. On December 24, 2004, the hospital announced that in order to retain federal funding, it had "begun replacing police with mental health workers to calm patients" (21).

The center's National Advisory Council recommends that hospital security guards should not carry guns, pepper spray, or Tasers. (Only about 15% to 20% of hospital security guards carry guns, and less than a third carry pepper spray.) Although security guards should dress in distinctive clothing, full police uniforms may be frightening to people in psychiatric crisis, particularly those who have just been brought in by police and should be avoided if possible.

Security guards should receive training in interacting with people with psychiatric disabilities, including training in de-escalation and on the effects of stereotypes and stigma on perceptions of likely violence and unpredictability of persons with psychiatric disabilities. But most importantly, the use of force by security guards on people with psychiatric disabilities in the ED should be tracked, with identification of the staff person who called for security, to look for possible patterns and the need for additional training for staff to be able to handle these issues themselves.

Clothing removal: A common instance of security guard intervention is the blanket requirement that psychiatric patients remove all their clothing and change into johnnies. Some patients with sexual abuse histories resist this requirement. Ironically, the patients most disturbed by the requirement to remove their clothing are often the ones who are forcibly stripped by male security guards, resulting in retraumatization (and possible legal liability) (22,23). The National Advisory Council found that flight risk is not sufficient justification for removal of clothing and that a blanket policy of automatic disrobement based solely on psychiatric diagnosis was clinically unjustified, discriminatory, and illegal; it recommended that "care and treatment in emergency departments should not be conditioned on disrobing, except in extremely limited circumstances where professionally documented assessments weigh the emotional and physical risk to the individual of enforced clothing removal against the immediate medical necessity for such removal to provide treatment, and conclude that the requirement of disrobing is essential" (4).

Reduce Inpatient Admissions Based on Exaggerated and Misdirected Fear of Liability

Emergency departments can educate staff about contingent suicidality and accept the recommendations of psychiatric consultants not to admit individuals with contingent suicidality. In addition, staff can be trained to recognize secondary use of the ED and reframe what is needed from admission to conflict resolution or problem solving. Staff should also learn that the risk of legal liability is not as high as they fear for mistakes in prediction about suicidality or homicidality provided that the clinical evaluation is well documented. Rather, liability often turns on additional, and usually fairly egregious, omissions or negligence in care.

Reduction in admissions is difficult to accomplish unless leadership emphasizes that inpatient admission is a last-resort alternative, carrying possibilities of regression, stigma, or stereotype, as well as a message about the incapability of the individual to solve his or her own problems. Hospital and ED leaders should also readily acknowledge that good patient care sometimes requires taking risks, and that staff will be supported in taking those risks. Finally, hospital leadership can explicitly reject the paradigm that the ED professional is completely responsible for all risk associated with psychiatric patients and is able to predict and gauge all risk. Rather, exploring the nature of the risk with the patient and readily available collateral sources; sharing the risk with the patient and family members as appropriate; and documenting the assessment of risk factors as well as protective factors, the reason for selecting whatever dispositional option is selected and for rejecting the alternatives, and the specific steps taken to reduce risk are good steps to quality patient care as well as reduction of liability.

Reduce Inpatient Admissions Related to Secondary Users and High Users

Research shows that when people in psychiatric crisis are accompanied to the emergency department by family members or others who are determined to secure an inpatient admission, the rate of inpatient admissions increases (24,25). Several studies found that this was true regardless of other clinical factors (24,25). Sometimes, secondary users will bring someone to the emergency department who truly needs to be involuntarily detained for his or her own safety or the safety of others: The fact that detention solves the secondary user's problems does not automatically mean it is not the clinically appropriate alternative. But ED staff should be aware of and not unduly swayed by pressures to hospitalize an individual and be alert to ways in which methods of conflict resolution might be used to better handle the situation between the patient and the secondary user.

In particular, the ED should keep data on secondary users who are paid to provide mental health care to psychiatric patients. The distinction between group homes that unnecessarily resort to emergency departments to handle problem clients and group homes whose staff is able to de-escalate and handle issues is a quality indicator that is currently invisible and should be transparent. The identities of group homes that make frequent use of emergency departments are not protected and should be a matter of discussion between the hospital and the state mental health authority that contracts with the group homes. Of course, this requires actual communication between hospital ED staff, hospital authorities, and the state mental health system, which itself is rare. Simply establishing contact and coordination with other parts of the service system responsible for patients who frequently use the emergency department may itself lead to reduced admissions.

Collaboration and Communication With Other Systems of Care

Improve Coordination With State Agencies

In the last 10 years, state mental health agencies have retreated from involvement in acute psychiatric care, often without taking steps to ensure that the resulting vacuum is filled (26). These steps include increasing funding for community crisis alternatives as envisioned by the Community Mental Health Centers Construction Act of 1963 (27) and ensuring coordination with private facilities providing acute care beds. Perhaps most important, contractual or even regulatory or legislative enactments must prohibit or severely restrict private facilities that contract with state agencies to provide beds from refusing or rejecting individual patients (with exceptions for truly extraordinary circumstances).

In an environment of shrinking crisis services and private facilities cherry-picking patients for inpatient beds, emergency departments fill the vacuum, often keeping patients in tiny rooms or on gurneys for days at great expense while the patient's psychiatric condition deteriorates. In this situation, both patients and staff are frustrated, resentful, and angry. Although the source of much of the patient's agitation and escalation and anger is being cooped up in the ED, and might well diffuse if discharged, staff are reluctant to discharge an angry, frustrated, and escalating patient. The situation can be explosive.

ED staff are unhappy about these conditions, but the insular and overworked ED culture tends to result in insufficient collaboration with the state mental health system or alliance with consumer and family groups to solve problems at a systemic level. At the very least, the mental health and substance abuse system's most frequent users of emergency department services should be identified, and, with the patient's consent (and participation, if possible), representatives of the systems of care could meet to ensure that the individual has services in place, including case managers and primary care physicians, that the individual has been enrolled in the programs for which he or she is eligible, and that plans are made for predictable crises (eg, anniversaries of traumatic events). Collaboration with other parties leads to reduction of risk—both actual risk for the patient and liability risk for the ED, which is no longer making important disposition decisions blind to other factors in the individual's life and services.

Create Standard Medical Clearance Protocols for Psychiatric Patients

One of the most common complaints about delays in disposition involves medical clearance from the admitting hospital. (Of course, no clearance issues arise if the person is not admitted—yet another reason to reduce admissions.) When patients refuse tests that are required for disposition, EDs sometimes force blood draws and catheters, raising ethical, legal, and liability issues (16). A standard medical clearance protocol should be negotiated statewide among all stakeholders, including the insurers who have to pay for the tests, police who require medical clearance, and others. The Center for Public Representation's National Advisory Commission finds that "uniform medical clearance standards applicable to all patients presenting with psychiatric conditions are inappropriate" beyond "vital signs, medical history, and visual examination" (4). The commission has called for a national expert consensus panel to create a set of tests or algorithms depending on the nature of the patient's presentation. In the absence of a national panel, hospitals might press for a state panel to accomplish the same objectives, as has happened to some degree in a number of states, including Arizona (28), Illinois (29), and Massachusetts (30).

Creating Alliances to Bring About Change at the State and Federal Levels

Hospitals and emergency department staff rarely have dialogues with patient advocates and advocacy groups, although they are natural allies in many respects and the combination could wield effective results at the legislative and regulatory level.

Both hospitals and patient advocates strongly desire to develop alternatives to emergency departments for psychiatric crisis care; to prevent nursing homes, group homes, and other service providers from using emergency departments to dump unwanted patients; and to free up bureaucratic roadblocks that delay accessibility of inpatient beds when those are necessary. If a state hospital association and patient advocacy groups were to band together to achieve just these three results, it could make an enormous difference in the quality of care that patients received and EDs could provide. Although state legislatures cannot undo the requirements of EMTALA, they can begin by requiring transparency on the part of nursing homes and community providers regarding their emergency department use, investigate unnecessary use through licensing authority, and impose consequences through contracting.

CONCLUSION

The problems with emergency department care of people in psychiatric crisis are in many ways deeply embedded in the way that our country has chosen to fund (or not to fund) health care, especially mental health care. Many solutions are beyond the reach of individual hospitals. But some solutions *can* be implemented by hospitals themselves. Policy solutions require hospitals to focus on the specific needs of people with psychiatric disabilities in their emergency departments, work to reduce inpatient admissions, and reach out to and work with state agencies and advocacy groups on systemic solutions to specific problems of inappropriate reliance on emergency departments to perform crisis intervention and social services. Hospitals and advocacy groups must begin a dialogue and create the alliances necessary to work for legislative and regulatory changes for the benefit of both the psychiatric patients and the ED staff who suffer under the current structure of care.

REFERENCES

1. American Hospital Association. (2006). *Hospital statistics 2006*. Chicago, IL: American Hospital Association.
2. American Association for Emergency Psychiatry. (2005). *Psychiatric emergency services (PES) in the U.S.* Bloomfield, CT: American Association for Emergency Psychiatry.
3. Wellmark BlueCross/BlueShield. *Decisions count: What you can do*. Retrieved from http://www.wellmark.com/decisions_count/dc_emergencyroom.htm.
4. Stefan, S. (2006). *Emergency department treatment of psychiatric patients: Policy issues and legal requirements*. New York, NY: Oxford University Press.
5. Teplin, L. A. (2000). *Keeping the peace: Police discretion and mentally ill persons*. Washington, DC: National Institute of Justice.
6. American Psychiatric Association. (2001). Section 1-AA. In *Opinions of the Ethics Committee on the principles of medical ethics, with annotations especially applicable to psychiatry*. Washington, DC: American Psychiatric Association.
7. Colorado Board of Medical Examiners. *Guidelines regarding practice coverage outside of normal office hours* (No. 40-17). Retrieved from: http://www.dora.state.co.us/medical/policies.htm.
8. Paris, J. (2007). *Half in love with death: Managing the chronically suicidal patient*. Mahwah, NJ: Erlbaum Associates.
9. Jacobs, D. (2007). *A resource guide for implementing the Joint Commission on Accreditation of Health Care Organizations (JCAHO) 2007 patient safety goals on suicide*. Wellesley, MA: Screening for Mental Health.
10. Lambert, M. T., & Silva, S. (1998). An update on the impact of gun control legislation on suicide. *Psychiatric Quarterly, 69*, 127–134.
11. Lambert, M. T., & Bonner, J. (1996). Characteristics and six month outcome of patients who use suicide threats to seek hospital admission. *Psychiatric Services, 47*, 871–873.
12. Lambert, M. T. (2002). Seven year outcomes of patients evaluated for suicidality. *Psychiatric Services, 53*, 92–94.
13. Lambert, M. T. (2003). Suicide risk assessment and management: Focus on personality disorders. *Current Opinion in Psychiatry, 16*, 71–76.
14. Fitzgerald, A. (2004, November 5). *Assessing risk: Getting beyond "suicidal ideation, will not contract for safety."* Presented at Psychiatric emergencies: The case for diversionary care, Boston University School of Medicine, Cambridge, MA.

15. Joint Commission on Accreditation of Healthcare Organizations, (2007). Goal 15A. In *2007 National Patient Safety Goals*. Chicago, IL: Joint Commission on Accreditation of Healthcare Organizations.

16. Tinius v. Carroll County Sheriff's Department, 321 F.Supp.2d 1064, 1088 (N.D. Iowa 2004). (Questioning whether EMTALA applied when Sheriff's deputies brought an individual to an emergency department for care he did not want.)

17. Kraft v. Laney, No. CIV S-04-0129 GGH (E.D. Cal. Aug. 24, 2005). (EMTALA did not apply when neither the patient nor the police requested examination and it was not apparent that patient was suffering from an emergency medical condition.)

18. Evans v. Montgomery Hospital Medical Center, 1996 U.S.Dist.LEXIS 5785 (E.D.Pa. May 1, 1996). (Finding EMTALA applicable to an individual brought by police, but this decision predates revision of EMTALA regulations intended to clarify that individuals brought to the ED for blood tests by police are not necessarily covered by EMTALA unless they have a medical condition that would be obvious to a prudent layperson [42 C.F.R. 489.24(c)].)

19. Thomas v. Christ Hospital and Medical Center, 328 F.3d 890 (7th Cir. 2003).

20. Sklar, D. P., Loeliger, E., & Edmunds, K. (2006). Unanticipated death following discharge to home from the emergency department. *Academic Emergency Medicine, 13*(Suppl. 1), 132.

21. Police to stop using Taser guns at troubled hospital. (2004, December 24). *San Diego Union Tribune*.

22. Scherer v. Waterbury Hospital, 2000 Conn.Super. LEXIS 481 (Conn.Super.Ct. 2000).

23. Sampson v. Beth Israel Deaconess Medical Center, Dr. Kelly Corrigan and Heather Richter, CA No.06-10973 (D.Mass. filed June 5, 2006).

24. Segal, S. P., Laurie, T. A., & Segal, M. J. (2001). Factors in the use of coercive retention in civil commitment evaluations in psychiatric emergency services. *Psychiatric Services, 52*, 514–520.

25. Micheels, P., Cuoco, L. F., Lipton, L., et al. (1998). Criteria-based voluntary and involuntary psychiatric admissions modeling. *International Journal of Psychosocial Rehabilitation, 2*, 176–188.

26. New Freedom Commission on Mental Health. (2004). *Subcommittee on acute care: Background paper* (DHHS Publication SMA-04-3876). Rockville, MD: U.S. Department of Health and Human Services. Retrieved from http://www.mentalhealthcommission.gov/papers/Acute_Care.pdf.

27. P.L. 88-164 (1963).

28. Lippman, G., & Ali, S. (2003, March 18). *Medical clearance and screening of psychiatric patients in the emergency department* [Memorandum]. Available from the author.

29. Illinois Hospital Association, Behavioral Health Steering Committee, Best Practices Task Force. (2007). Appendix A. In *Final report: Best practices for the treatment of patients with mental and substance use illnesses in the emergency department*. Chicago, IL: Illinois Hospital Association.

30. Massachusetts College of Emergency Medicine and Massachusetts Psychiatric Society. (2003). *Consensus statement on medical clearance*. Waltham, MA: Massachusetts College of Emergency Medicine. Retrieved from http://www.macep.org/practice_ information/medical_clearance.htm.

45

Violence Prevention and Control: A Public Health Approach

Stephen W. Hargarten, Ann L. Christiansen, Sara A. Kohlbeck

Violence (which includes homicide, suicide and suicide attempt, assault, and unintentional firearm injury) poses a significant public health problem in the United States. Other sections and chapters of this book describe more thoroughly the complex challenge of violence and the clinical role that emergency psychiatrists have in working with people who are at risk for becoming violent either toward themselves or others. This chapter provides an overview of the unique role that emergency psychiatrists, as members of the healthcare community, have in preventing and controlling violence both at an individual and population level.

The World Report on Violence and Health, published by the World Health Organization (WHO), describes violence as a complex problem with multiple factors that influence whether an individual is prone to act in a violent manner (1). These factors can be biologic, behavioral, social, cultural, economic, environmental, and political. This understanding of violence is similar to the biopsychosocial model put forward by Engel to describe the role of biologic, psychological, and social factors and their influence on human behavior and disease (2). With regard to violence, WHO and agencies such as the Centers for Disease Control and Prevention use an ecologic model for understanding these factors and how they overlap to influence an individual's behavior (Figure 45.1). At one level, the model describes how biology and personal history influence individual behavior, including demographics, impulsivity, educational attainment, and substance abuse, as well as prior history of aggression and abuse. On another level, the ecologic model describes how close relationships with family, friends, intimate partners, and peers might increase or decrease the risk of being a victim or perpetrator of violence. This risk depends on one's exposure to violence, especially in the case of partner violence and child maltreatment, and for young people the acceptance or approval of violence by friends. A third level is the community in which those relationships occur. Potential risk factors at the community level include high incidence of unemployment, transient neighborhoods, and population density, to name a few. The fourth level of this model describes the broad societal factors whereby violence is either encouraged or inhibited. Examples of the risk factors at a societal level include the availability of weapons and the social norms surrounding

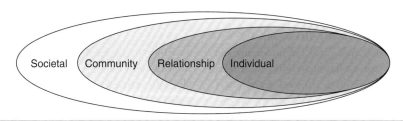

FIGURE 45.1 • Ecologic model for understanding violence.

their use. Other social factors include the social, economic, and institutional forces and policies that result in inequities between different population groups (1).

Traditionally, the responsibility for preventing and controlling violence has fallen on the judicial, law enforcement, and correctional systems. The healthcare field has been largely responsible for the medical and behavioral health treatment and care of individuals after an event or, ideally, the behavioral health treatment of individuals at risk of violence in order to prevent a violent event. With expanding knowledge regarding the multifaceted risk factors and prevention strategies for violence, the WHO states that those in the healthcare community have a special role in preventing and controlling violence and that this role would ideally be in collaboration with public health practitioners, researchers, law enforcement, those involved in the judicial system, and representatives from other sectors of civil society. Those in the healthcare field have a unique perspective regarding violence because of their proximity to the treatment and care of those who are potential and actual perpetrators and victims of violence. Healthcare personnel have access to data and information to assist with research and prevention strategies, as well as communicating to other stakeholders and policy makers about the burden of violence. Additionally, healthcare personnel can share their own stories and experiences in treating victims of violence. These stories can be a powerful advocacy tool for resources and for policy, system, and environmental changes.

The purpose of this chapter is to describe more thoroughly the public health approach to reducing violence and the opportunities that emergency psychiatrists have in using its tools to prevent and control violence for both individuals and populations.

PUBLIC HEALTH APPROACH FOR REDUCING VIOLENCE

The public health approach is an important framework to apply to violence prevention and control because it provides a systematic method for identifying and addressing a specific health issue and for evaluating efforts to address health issues. The public health approach leverages tools such as surveillance, epidemiologic analysis, intervention design, and evaluation to focus on recognizing the underlying risk and protective factors for health issues, identifying strategies to address these factors, and evaluating the impact that those strategies have made to reduce the biopsychosocial disease burden—in this case, violence (3).

The science of injury control and prevention builds on the public health model and is based on the understanding that injury is a disease rather than the result of fate or random occurrences (4,5). By employing this framework, injury is no longer seen as an "accident," but rather as a preventable disease. The fundamentals of injury control and prevention are constructed from the epidemiologic triad of host (injured individual), agent or vector (eg, kinetic energy from a car or gun), and environment (physical, socioeconomic, or policy). Injury control and prevention is the scientific discipline of understanding what prevents or attenuates the transfer of energy to the host, which can happen by separating the host from the agent through modification of the environment (eg, through policy changes), equipping the host with protections against the agent (eg, by providing safe storage for firearms), or eliminating or modifying the vector that transmits the energy (eg, by providing access to smart guns) (6-9). William Haddon developed a two-dimensional approach to injury analysis by combining the epidemiologic triad of agent, host, and environment with the three levels of prevention: primary (pre event), secondary (event), and tertiary (post event) (10). This phase-factor matrix, which was first utilized to analyze motor vehicle crash injury, has become the scientific underpinning of injury control and prevention. Any injury event can be broken down into the component factors of Haddon's matrix, allowing specific interventions to target specific factors and levels of prevention (11).

Traditionally, interpersonal violence has been considered the responsibility of the criminal justice system, and prevention has focused mainly on deterrence and means restriction. Suicide, on the other hand, has been viewed as a problem to be dealt with by the behavioral health sector, and the conventional strategy has been to facilitate access to treatment for behavioral health issues to prevent suicides. As the burden of both of these areas of violence continues to grow, the public health community, along with others, has realized that such a complex issue requires multifaceted approaches to reduce the impact of violence on our society (3,6).

BURDEN OF HOMICIDE AND SUICIDE

Suicides and homicides are a significant public health burden across the lifespan. Over the past 12 years, the number of suicides and intentional injuries from self-harm has increased substantially. In 2016, suicide was the 10th leading cause of death in the United States. In 2004, approximately 32,000 people died as a result of suicide, and in 2016, that number increased to 44,000. In 2004, approximately 400,000 had a nonfatal self-inflicted injury, and in 2016, this number grew to over 500,000. For American Indian, Alaska Native, and White individuals, aged 10 to 34 years, suicide was the second leading cause of death, behind all unintentional injuries. For Black individuals, suicide is the fifth cause of death for youth of age 10 to 14 years, the third for youth of age 15 to 24 years, and the fourth for young adults of age 25 to 34 years. The majority of suicide deaths, approximately 52%, were firearm related, whereas the majority of nonfatal, self-inflicted injuries were the result of poisoning (12). Studies of suicide and firearm ownership demonstrated that US residents are more likely to die by suicide if they live in areas with high rates of firearm ownership (13,14). Additionally, other studies have shown that firearm suicide rates are higher in rural communities than in urban communities (15,16).

The number of homicide deaths has risen slightly in the past 12 years. In 2004, homicide was the 15th leading cause of death, and in 2016, it was the 16th. In 2016, over 19,000 people died by homicide. An additional 1.6 million people were treated either in the emergency department or hospital as a result of some type of assault. Although homicide is ranked as the 16th leading cause of death for all race groups combined, it was the seventh leading cause of deaths for Blacks. Among Black youth and young adults aged 15 to 34 years, homicide was the leading cause of death. Seventy-nine percent of all homicides were firearm-related, and 81% of assaults were the result of being struck by or against an object (12). Studies of firearm-related homicides show that they primarily occur in large metropolitan areas and are largely the result of the kinetic energy (bullets) from handguns (3,15,16).

STRATEGIES FOR REDUCING FIREARM-RELATED DEATHS AND INJURIES

Preventing firearm-related morbidity and mortality is an important strategy for reducing the overall burden of violence because of the lethality of firearms. Several studies assessing case fatality rates indicate that events such as assault and self-harm are much more likely to result in a fatality when a firearm is used compared with other events involving injury mechanisms such as poisoning or suffocation (17,18). One study examining case fatality rates in the Northeast found that 91% of all suicide acts in which a firearm was used resulted in death, compared with 2% of suicide acts involving poisonings by drugs (17).

To reach the Healthy People 2020 objective of no more than 9.3 firearm-related deaths per 100,000 individuals, much more effort needs to be undertaken among all stakeholder groups (19). Evidence-based strategies to reduce firearm-related injuries and deaths exist. These strategies are described here and are framed by the public health model, highlighting the intervention opportunities regarding the host (individual), agent (kinetic energy) or vector (firearm), and environment.

Individual-level interventions that aim to reduce firearm-related injuries and deaths have largely focused on educational programs, including media campaigns and other forums to raise awareness of the burden of firearm-related homicides and suicides. Other educational programs focus on safe storage practices and disposal for firearms. In the case of suicide, there are a number of school-based programs designed to educate people on the signs of suicide, as well as to screen youth who may be at risk for suicide (20). Youth-oriented violence prevention programs focus on behavior management and teaching conflict resolution skills, as well as on increasing positive interactions with role models or other older peers through mentoring, tutoring, and work study (21).

A number of prevention opportunities can accomplish change by focusing on the disease vector, which in this case is the firearm. Some examples include mandating standardized safety devices, installing grip safeties, loaded chamber indicators, and magazine disconnect devices, and redesigning firearms to prevent unauthorized use by a child or another individual. Strategies that focus on safe storage of firearms, including gun locks, lock boxes, and gun safes, are another way to reduce the impact of firearm-related injuries and deaths in that they interrupt the "transmission" of the disease from the agent to the host by limiting or inhibiting access to the firearm. Often individuals who are not willing to remove firearms from the home are more willing to store a weapon so it is out of reach of unauthorized users (22,23).

Finally, a number of environmental changes can be implemented to reduce firearm-related injuries and deaths. These changes involve enforcement of laws to reduce illegal carrying or use of firearms, which can include legal sanctions such as an increased likelihood of arrest and punishment for unlawful carrying or use of a firearm. Another example is regulating the sales of firearms through mandatory background checks on all individuals, limiting the number of firearms an individual can purchase at a single time, and regulating firearm dealers (22,23). Policy and social environment changes that address upstream causes of violence, including interventions that address societal norms around violent behavior, may also reduce firearm-related injury and mortality.

ROLE OF EMERGENCY PSYCHIATRY PHYSICIANS

The WHO asserts that health care professionals have a unique role to play in preventing violence, specifically violence caused by firearms. Russell Gruen et al. (24) outline a model of physician responsibility that describes the domains of professional physician obligations to promote the health of the community members they serve. These obligations stem from the social status physicians maintain, as well as their perceived expertise on not only the biologic aspects of disease but also the social, behavioral, environmental, and economic conditions that affect health.

The primary and central domain is the physician's responsibility to provide individual patient care. Beyond this, Gruen et al. argue that physicians are also obligated to promote access to care, including increased insurance coverage and availability of care for the uninsured, because these system characteristics have a direct impact on the health of the community. The third domain of professional obligation is advocacy for socioeconomic influences that link directly to public policies and improved health outcomes, and where physician advocacy of such policies is likely to be feasible and impactful. One example would be a physician making a public statement advocating for policies that provide funding to educate the public on safe storage of firearms or promote evidence-based policies such as gun violence restraining orders. Other examples of advocacy and community participation opportunities presented by Gruen et al. include working to improve systems of care within an institution, raising awareness of a health or social issue by discussing with friends and family or participating in a public forum, participating in some form of public advocacy or lobbying, encouraging a medical society to act on a public health issue, and serving in a local organization or political group (24).

The following examples provide some additional opportunities to expand the role of emergency psychiatrists beyond providing individual patient care that has a broader impact on the public's health and on the prevention and control of firearm violence.

1. Collaborate with community partners such as crisis agencies, law enforcement, criminal justice, schools, businesses, public health, and other sectors of civil society through community coalitions to ensure a coordinated system for managing individuals at risk for suicide or homicide
2. Work with community stakeholders to adopt comprehensive strategies to increase access to inpatient and outpatient behavioral health treatment opportunities
3. Work with public health professionals and coroners/medical examiners to ensure that surveillance systems are collecting accurate information on the circumstances surrounding firearm-related injuries and deaths

4. Conduct research studies to develop potential primary and secondary violence prevention strategies

5. Work with court systems that order behavioral health treatment to ensure that these treatments are provided and that those treatment outcomes are measured and documented

6. Advocate for the reduction of access to lethal means, including firearms, by supporting modifications to the agent and the environment to reduce the misuse of firearms

7. Work with policy makers to ensure that mental health detentions and court decisions requiring treatment are reported, with appropriate confidentiality safeguards, so that background checks for firearm purchases include salient behavioral health-related information

8. Affiliate with organizations such as the Centers for Disease Control and Prevention's National Center for Injury Prevention and Control, the Society for the Advancement of Violence and Injury Research, and the State and Territorial Injury Prevention Directors Association to network with others dedicated to reducing the burden of violence

9. Partner with research scientists from the Centers for Disease Control and Prevention's academic-based Injury Control Research Centers and National Academic Centers of Excellence on Youth Violence Prevention

10. Help to push the firearm violence prevention upstream by openly discussing violence disparities and sharing personal experiences in treating patients who are victims of firearm violence

11. Advocate on a hospital-level for programming, including hospital-based interventions, that addresses the biopsychosocial needs of patients who are affected by firearm violence. This may include engaging with traumatically injured patients and social work to ensure the patient has adequate community-based support at the time of discharge from the hospital setting

Violence continues to be an issue that affects the health and well-being of communities.

By understanding the complexities of violence and the interrelations between individuals, their proximal social relationships, their communities, policy, and society, it is possible to consider opportunities to reduce violence by targeting each of these domains. Emergency psychiatrists are a critical part of the multifaceted array of stakeholders addressing these issues because of their role as physicians and their direct experience in the treatment and care of those who are potential and actual perpetrators and victims of violence.

ACKNOWLEDGMENTS

The authors wish to thank Rachel Glick and Jon Berlin for their helpful comments and review of this chapter.

REFERENCES

1. Krug, E. G., Dahlberg, L. L., Mercy, J. A., et al. (2002). *World report on violence and health*. Geneva: World Health Organization.

2. Engel, G. L. (1980). The clinical application of the biopsychosocial model. *American Journal of Psychiatry, 137*(5), 535–544.

3. Hargarten, S. W., Lerner, E. B., Gorelick, M., Brasel, K., deRoon-Cassini, T., & Kohlbeck, S. (2018). Gun violence: A biopsychosocial disease. *Western Journal of Emergency Medicine, 19*(6), 1024–1027.

4. Committee on Trauma, American College of Surgeons. (1999). *Resources for optimal care of the injured patient: 1999*. Chicago, IL: American College of Surgeons.

5. Committee on Injury Prevention and Control, Division of Health Promotion and Disease Prevention. (1999). *Reducing the burden of injury*. Washington, DC: National Academies Press.

6. Rosenberg, M., & Fenley, M. A. (Eds.). (1991). *Violence in America: A public health approach*. New York, NY: Oxford University Press.

7. National Committee for Injury Prevention and Control. (1989). *Injury prevention: Meeting the challenge*. Oxford, UK: Oxford University Press.

8. Mohan, D. (2000). *Injury control and safety promotion: Ethics, science and practice*. New York, NY: Taylor and Francis.

9. Robertson, L. (1992). The problem, history and concepts. In *Injury epidemiology*. New York, NY: Oxford University Press.

10. Haddon, W. (1972). A logical framework for categorizing highway safety phenomenon and activity. *The Journal of Trauma, 12*, 193.

11. Runge, J., & Hargarten, S. W. (2006). Injury prevention and control. In Marx, J., Hockberger, S., & Walls, R. (Eds.), *Emergency medicine: Concepts and clinical practice* (6th ed., pp. 940–951). St. Louis, MO: Mosby.

12. Centers for Disease Control and Prevention, National Center for Injury Prevention and Control. *Web-based injury statistics query and reporting system (WISQARS). Leading causes of death reports* (2004–2016). Retrieved September 21, 2018, from http://www.cdc.gov/ncipc/wisqars.

13. Siegel, M., & Rothman, E. F. (2016). Firearm ownership and suicide rates among US men and women, 1981–2013. *American Journal of Public Health, 106*(7), 1316–1322.

14. Miller, M., Lippmann, S. J., Azrael, D., et al. (2007). Household firearm ownership and rates of suicide across the 50 United States. *The Journal of Trauma, 62*(4), 1029–1035.

15. Branas, C. C., Nance, M. L., Elliott, M. R., et al. (2004). Urban-rural shifts in intentional firearm death: Different causes, same results. *American Journal of Public Health, 94*(10), 1750–1755.

16. Shiffler, T., Hargarten, S. W., & Withers, R. L. (2005). The burden of suicide and homicide of Wisconsin's children and youth. *WMJ, 104*(1), 62–67.

17. Spicer, R., Miller, T., Langley, J., et al. (2005). Comparison of injury case fatality rates in the United States and New Zealand. *Injury Prevention, 11*, 71–76.

18. Miller, M., Azrael, D., & Hemenway, D. (2004). The epidemiology of case fatality rates for suicide in the northeast. *Annals of Emergency Medicine, 43*(6), 723–730.

19. U.S. Department of Health and Human Services. (2006). *Healthy people 2010 midcourse review*. Washington, DC: U.S. Government Printing Office.

20. Knox, K. L. (2007). Interventions to prevent suicidal behavior. In Doll, L. S., Bonzo, S. E., Mercy, J. A., et al. (Eds.), *Handbook of injury and violence prevention* (pp. 183–201). New York, NY: Springer.

21. Gottfredson, D. C., & Bauer, E. L. (2007). Interventions to prevent youth violence. In Doll, L. S., Bonzo, S. E., Mercy, J. A., et al. (Eds.), *Handbook of injury and violence prevention* (pp. 157–181). New York, NY: Springer.

22. Karlson, T. A., & Hargarten, S. W. (1997). *Reducing firearm injury and death: A public health sourcebook on guns* (pp. 116–123). New Brunswick, NJ: Rutgers University Press.

23. Rivara, F. P., & Kellerman, A. L. (2007). Reducing the misuse of firearms. In Doll, L. S., Bonzo, S. E., Mercy, J. A., et al. (Eds.), *Handbook of injury and violence prevention* (pp. 311–331). New York, NY: Springer.

24. Gruen, R. L., Pearson, S. D., & Brennan, T. A. (2004). Physician citizens—Public roles and professional obligations. *JAMA, 291*(1), 94–98.

46

Common Legal Issues in Emergency Psychiatry

Debra A. Pinals, Kimberly Kulp-Osterland, Thomas Chaffee

Working with patients at times of crisis in a psychiatric emergency service (PES) or an emergency department (ED) can be a positive and rewarding clinical experience, yet a number of legal, regulatory, and ethical issues can be challenging to navigate for emergency psychiatric providers. Issues related to confidentiality, informed consent, involuntary treatment, and transfer of individuals from one level of care to another, as well as liability concerns, can add to the stress of working in this high-risk setting. In this chapter, we review common legal and regulatory issues psychiatric ED providers need to be aware of when caring for emergency psychiatric patients and we discuss how to best manage these challenging situations appropriately.

PRESENTATION TO THE EMERGENCY DEPARTMENT: LEGAL STATUS AND CLINICAL CONDITIONS

Individuals with mental health concerns arrive in the emergency setting in a variety of ways, both voluntarily and involuntarily. They can walk in on their own or be brought by family willingly or less than willingly. They can be referred by the medical ED team to be seen by psychiatry because of concerns about their mental state, psychiatric symptoms, or safety. They can be brought by police or ambulance, again on either a voluntary or involuntary status. Their concerns may range from a request for medication refills to seeking treatment referrals for a newly recognized psychiatric symptom. They may present asking for crisis support in a time of psychosocial upheaval. Or they may be exhibiting suicidal ideation or behaviors or other dangerous behavior in the community. Regardless of how they arrive or what help

is being sought, a key initial question that must be resolved when they present is whether they can be held, even against their will, until an assessment can be completed.

Individuals who arrive at the PES are generally able to leave at will unless certain parameters are met that allow them to be held involuntarily. For example, if someone has checked into triage and identified as a patient and there are concerns about their safety related to a psychiatric issue, there may be sufficient justification to hold them through the legal mechanisms authorized by state mental health laws related to temporary holds. A common example is when an individual expresses suicidal ideation to the medical staff during a medical examination and the medical staff refer the individual for psychiatric evaluation. If the patient then wants to leave before a psychiatric examination is completed, there is generally the authorization to hold the individual to allow time for further psychiatric assessment and determination of next steps.

Laws in the United States vary in terms of what criteria allow for the involuntary detention or hold of individual patients, often called "temporary holds" (1). These holds are generally based on mental health criteria and not just on dangerousness. In most states, some initial petitioning paperwork begins the process of involuntary hold and treatment. Initial petitions can be authorized generally by law enforcement and other individuals, depending on the state. In some states (eg, Michigan), initial petitions can be authorized by any individual over the age of 18 years, followed by an attestation or a certification by an authorized clinician that the person requiring treatment has a mental illness (defined in the law) and that the mental illness creates particular risks. The duration of a temporary hold can vary (1).

Eventually, to continue to hold a person involuntarily in psychiatric care, there must be a hearing and a court order to ensure that the individual's due process rights for deprivation of liberty are attended to properly. These court hearings usually occur after the period of emergency department hold and stabilization has ended and the patient has been admitted to the hospital. But with longer ED waits for hospital beds (see below), there can be issues as to how long a person can be held involuntarily in a PES or ED. Clinicians should seek legal guidance on their own jurisdiction's laws about how often there need to be renewals for temporary involuntary holds or whether such renewals are even allowed. In some jurisdictions, patients must be released in a certain time frame if they do not want to stay. Even when an involuntary hold is legally authorized, providers should always maximize patient engagement and foster voluntary participation in treatment to provide the best care.

Individuals brought to the ED for medical reasons who wish to leave against medical advice might require a consultation from a psychiatrist to determine their capacity to decline medical treatment and disposition. Such capacity assessments are often requested of psychiatric consultants by medical providers. Involuntary psychiatric hospitalization is one tool that might be used in these circumstances but only where there is evidence of a valid psychiatric issue, even in the face of significant medical problems (2).

USE OF SECLUSION AND RESTRAINT

Individuals experiencing a psychiatric emergency may also have behavioral dysregulation that cannot be managed with less restrictive means resulting in use of restraint or seclusion. Every state has regulations regarding the use of restraints, and Centers for Medicare and Medicaid Services (CMS) and other bodies have established criteria for the use of restraints and seclusion and the limits of their use in clinical settings (3). Efforts around the country to prevent and reduce the frequency and duration of seclusion and restraint are widespread (4). Providers should familiarize themselves with all federal, state, and institutional policies related to seclusion and restraint, including

the use of emergency involuntary medications in their jurisdiction when working in psychiatric emergency contexts. Although overall utilization levels vary, the use of seclusion or restraint can be a source of potential high risk for the patient both because of the accidental physical injury and the traumatizing nature of the intervention (4,5). In addition, staff injuries can occur during process of restraining patients, and there can be liability attached if the parameters of the situation did not warrant that level of intervention.

POLICE INTERACTIONS IN THE PSYCHIATRIC EMERGENCY SETTING

When police bring a patient into the ED, they may be doing so because a petition was filed with a local court and the police were sent to transport the patient to the ED for an evaluation. Alternatively, the police might initiate their own petition and bring the patient to the ED when they think the individual needs an assessment. Police are increasingly being trained in mental health issues and are working in partnership with mental health services (6). For example, Crisis Intervention Team Training teaches a specialized group of officers to manage mental health crises and helps create policies between local police and community mental health. In addition, arrangements for police "drop-offs" at the emergency department or at diversion centers are increasingly common to allow for a warm handoff of the patient to the proper clinicians and care (7). As there are jurisdictional variations of these system protocols, clinicians in emergency department settings should become familiar with what is happening in their region (8).

Regardless of the organizational framework, it is always a good idea for psychiatric staff to speak directly to police who are dropping a patient off in the ED. Police can often share useful information about what occurred in the community that brought the patient to attention. Police paperwork might not convey the rich details of the community encounter. For example, a patient might have engaged in a 12-hour barricade situation when police arrived to respond to a family call of concern that an individual was paranoid and had expressed suicidal threats. When the patient arrives in the ED looking calmer and the police paperwork states that the patient had "suicidal thoughts," the texture of the police interaction could be unknown to the evaluating psychiatrist. There are often silos between law enforcement and ED personnel, and information can be lost if these silos are not bridged.

CONFIDENTIALITY LAWS AND EXCEPTIONS

Confidentiality is a key tenet of all patient-physician relationships. This is uniquely import-ant in the field of mental health, as the information disclosed is often particularly sensitive. Patients may elect to share details with practitioners that they intentionally conceal from their friends and family. Creating an environment where informa-tion can be freely shared requires mutual trust. Thus it remains vital to respect patient confiden-tiality. This importance of confidentiality was rec-ognized in the landmark US Supreme Court case, Jaffe v. Redmond (1996) (9). The case revolved around a patient's psychotherapy notes, which were ultimately withheld from the court, citing psychotherapist-patient privilege. The major regulations governing privacy come from three primary sources: (1) Health Insurance Portability and Accountability Act of 1996 (HIPAA) (10), (2) state confidentiality statutes, and (3) codes of pro-fessional practice.

HIPAA is a law enacted by the federal gov-ernment to systematically respond to threats to medical privacy. It aims to protect the privacy of individual health information, and specifically for patients with mental illness, it helps protect confidential mental health treatment records. HIPAA requires patient authorization prior to the release of medical information and mandates that patients be informed as to how their medical information will be used. It is always best practice to get explicit, signed consent from patients before releasing information. Confidentiality is also reg-ulated by state confidentiality statutes, which may further prohibit disclosures that would otherwise be allowed under HIPAA.

For substance use–specific treatment, a sep-arate law for confidentiality, 42 C.F.R. Part 2 (11), is operationalized across the United States. Its provisions are generally more strict in terms

of privacy protections than HIPAA. Although perhaps not commonly encountered in the ED setting, it is important to realize that if patient information about substance use treatment ser-vices is requested from outside providers, specific authorization is required unless exceptions to 42 C.F.R. Part 2 are in place, but these exceptions tend to be limited.

Even with the rules about confidentiality, there can be situations where confidentiality is in conflict with patient safety or the safety of others, putting psychiatrists in a challenging situation. This is especially relevant in the ED or PES where such circumstances are typically more acute and the consequences are poten-tially severe when determining whether con-fidentiality or safety are the primary driver of a decision to communicate a concern to some-one other than the patient. For example, it is not uncommon for a suicidal patient, brought in by police, with no collateral information, to refuse to participate in the interview. How can one effectively triage, corroborate information, or safety plan without additional information? A psychiatrist may need to contact the patient's family, caregiver, friends, or treatment provid-ers in order to develop an accurate formulation and provide appropriate care. Exceptions to pri-vacy to assure safety might outweigh the privacy provisions.

Guidance from the US Department of Health and Human Services acknowledges that HIPAA provides some flexibility to privacy, including sit-uations when covered entities may disclose pro-tected health information because they believe such disclosure is necessary to prevent or lessen a serious and imminent threat to a person or the public (12). This necessitates the clinician use their best judgment. It is prudent also to docu-ment reasoning behind breaching confidentiality. Clinicians should document what was disclosed, to whom it was disclosed, and why it was dis-closed. Any disclosures made must be limited to information directly relevant to the person's involvement in the patient's care. For example, for care coordination, HIPAA allows in some circumstances disclosure without authorization as long as the disclosure is the "minimum neces-sary" (12). Notably, it is always permissible for a clinician to gather information about the patient from others (for example family and friends). However, clinicians must be careful about unintentionally revealing unnecessary information during these conversations.

In addition to HIPAA considerations, disclosures and breaches of confidentiality might be mandated or at least permitted by state law in certain circumstances when a patient may present a risk of harm to third parties or the public (see, for example, http://www.ncsl.org/research/health/mental-health-professionals-duty-to-warn.aspx). The issue originates from the California Supreme Court's decisions in the landmark case of Tarasoff *v. Regents of the University of California* cases (13,14). The Court in this case first determined that when a patient reveals ideas about harming a third party, the clinician might have a duty to breach confidentiality and warn the potential third party under certain circumstances (13). In a 1976 subsequent review of the first ruling, the California Supreme Court refined its decision, emphasizing the role of the mental health professional required protecting an identified victim, and warning might only be one action related to this duty to protect (14). The *Tarasoff* case is commonly referred to as the "duty to warn," but in actuality, it should be considered a "duty to protect" as elucidated in the second court ruling (14). The *Tarasoff* case was only relevant in California, but other states have since commonly adopted variations on its provisions. State laws typically provide guidance for what might be "reasonable precautions" to take to help protect a third party who might be at risk of harm due to the actions of a patient. Specifically, depending on the jurisdiction and clinical situation, a clinician may need to take actions that can reasonably lead to the protection of the third party, such as hospitalization and/or notification of police, warning the identified person(s) at risk, and/or other actions. With a proper release of information permitting contact to a third party (if the party is named by the patient), these warnings are not a privacy breach, but in situations involving particular potential victims, even approaching the patient for a release might be complicated. As one author notes, clinicians should examine both the laws in their state and the nuances of the clinical situation to determine the best course of action vis-à-vis the patient and the third party who is at risk (15).

As noted above, hospitalization can be one vehicle to discharge the duty to protect individuals who might be at risk due to actions of a patient (16). Hospitalization, however, still needs to be clinically indicated. As such, in the ED, if someone presents without a mental health issue, but expresses threats of harming others, there can at times be causes for notifying police as another form of "protecting" a third party who might be at risk. It can be difficult to sort out the issues from an ethical perspective of preserving the patient's trust and wanting to protect the public. These risks can be heightened when a patient's threat involves the use of a firearm that the patient has access to, and the clinical and ethical dimensions of how to approach these situations can be complex. Clinicians should consider seeking second opinions from other clinicians or legal advice in these challenging scenarios, as balancing the laws of confidentiality with the exception of when there might be a duty to protect someone else from harm is a complicated and high-risk situation (17).

CONSENT AND PATIENT ENGAGEMENT IN THE PES SETTING

Informed consent can be broadly defined as a process of obtaining permission prior to a medical intervention. It is an important aspect of medical ethics and has evolved as an essential component of treatment. Although it is well established in nonemergent settings, it is often more nuanced and challenging to apply during emergencies. Valid informed consent has three general components (18,19): 1) disclosure, 2) competence, and 3) voluntariness. Disclosure is the cornerstone of informed consent and requires a physician to provide a patient with certain information about a proposed intervention. Clinicians often have trouble deciding how much information they should disclose. A general principle is to ask what would a "reasonable" patient want to know. This typically includes information about the risks and benefits of the treatment, alternatives to the recommended treatment, and the risks of no treatment (20). A common example involves voluntary hospitalization, which is often initiated in the ED. Patients may assume they would be able to leave the hospital whenever they choose, but all states have provisions that allow a psychiatric patient to be held involuntarily for a defined and limited period of time if certain conditions apply (such as risk of harm to self or others due to mental illness). It is important to clearly disclose the basic information about this prior to the voluntary admission, otherwise the informed consent process can be considered invalid. The patient's ability to understand the information also can be questioned, thus highlighting the importance of good documentation of these issues.

A provider can and should determine if the patient is competent to make decisions or seek consultation to do so. In order to seek a patient's informed consent, the patient must be competent. If a physician determines that a patient lacks decision-making capacity, it may be necessary to find a surrogate decision maker, who then becomes the recipient of the information disclosed and decides on behalf of the patient. States vary in how they determine which surrogate decision makers can authorize psychiatric hospitalization or whether the law requires a different process such as a judicial hearing (21). Examples of surrogate decision makers for general medical and psychiatric decisions might include healthcare proxies, persons with durable power of attorney, guardians, and even courts, depending on the decisions at hand. In a guardianship proceeding, the court makes a formal adjudication regarding the patient's competency and approves a formal surrogate decision maker. Although guardianship determinations can be lengthy, they can also be obtained more expediently in emergency situations. Emergency guardianship is not usually sought in an ED, but it can be initiated there. Often an emergency will allow for the introduction of the medical intervention if it involves saving life or limb of the incapacitated person. Family input might be helpful in the steps related to seeking consent and if they are engaged with the patient, it is a good idea to bring them into the medical care as long as there are appropriate releases of information. However, there may be ethical and legal limitations to the role of family input that requires balancing as family members technically may not have the legal authority to make decisions for another individual unless they are officially designated as a surrogate decision maker by an advanced directive or by the court. Also, if the patient has refused communication with family, there would need to be a justification that would allow this. When there is a surrogate decision maker, the duty of informed consent shifts as providers must still disclose relevant information to that individual on behalf of the patient (19). Although the patient who is declared incapacitated can still "assent" or "dissent," they cannot "consent," but it can still be important to explain to the patient what is happening with the treatment.

Voluntariness implies that patients are given a voluntary choice among alternatives and are free from coercion. Although this seems obvious, there are many situations in the PES where this is relevant. For example, patients are often given the option to be admitted to the hospital "voluntarily," but providers use coercive language about moving toward involuntary commitment if they decline. In the emergency setting and elsewhere, it is important to explain choices without coercive language. This can be done by reviewing the voluntary hospitalization and its pros and cons, as well as explaining factually that a patient's risk would cause the clinician to pursue involuntary hospitalization, leaving the patient at least aware of the risks and benefits of declining to sign into the hospital voluntarily. In *Zinermon v. Burch* (22), the US Supreme Court examined the voluntary admission of an incompetent patient and determined that there should have been a mechanism to hospitalize this individual without having him sign a consent form that he did not understand. The provider in the ED should be familiar with the laws in their jurisdiction around psychiatric admission of the person who is not competent to sign into the hospital on a voluntary basis.

Emergencies can trigger a valid exception to getting full and informed consent from the patient (18,19). For example, the emergency administration of psychiatric medication where imminent risk must be averted could be one such situation. However, before administering medication involuntarily without consent, clinicians should assess the situation to determine if less restrictive and intrusive options would be sufficient and reasonable to address the emergency.

Any exception to informed consent should be carefully documented, clearly explaining the rationale for not providing consent. In the case of the psychopharmacologic intervention without consent, clinicians should document how less restrictive means were considered, and why they were not appropriate for the situation.

TRANSFER OF CARE

The Emergency Medical Treatment and Active Labor Act of 1986 (EMTALA) (23) is an important federal statute that attempts to ensure that all people presenting to the ED, regardless of ability to pay, will be stabilized and treated appropriately before discharge or transfer to another institution. EMTALA requires all hospitals receiving Medicare funds to adequately screen, examine, stabilize, and transfer patients, regardless of the patients' ability to pay. EMTALA mandates that before a patient transfer can take place, the patient must be evaluated and stabilized, and the receiving hospital must agree to the transfer and have facilities to provide the needed treatment. Psychiatric emergencies are covered under EMTALA, and care provided must adhere to EMTALA standards. This includes assuring medical stability before transfer to a psychiatric facility for inpatient care, as well as being sure transport of the at-risk patient is done in the safest way possible, that is, ambulance rather than family car. Although litigation around EMTALA in psychiatric matters is not as common as medical cases, psychiatrists should consider careful assessment and documentation that the condition under review is stabilized prior to transfer and assure transport is safe as the best method of adhering to the terms of EMTALA (24).

PSYCHIATRIC BOARDING AND THE POTENTIAL ROLE OF TECHNOLOGY AND EMTALA

Unfortunately, it has become the norm nationwide for patients awaiting psychiatric hospitalization to experience long wait times in the ED. These individuals may receive little to no mental health treatment while situated in a noisy, uncomfortable, and sometimes chaotic environment. The cause of the boarding problem is multifactorial; the mental health system is a complex and dynamic system which relies on the balance of many different parties and systems to operate successfully. Emergency departments and psychiatric hospitals are only two pieces in the puzzle. Although psychiatric inpatient bed access challenges may be one component in long emergency department wait times, other factors include lack of other options in the community such as crisis centers, crisis residential housing, or structured and supportive housing served by assertive community treatment services or crisis response teams (25). Additionally, access to open beds on acute psychiatric units has been identified as an issue especially for particular patients (26). Complicating matters further, the ability to estimate bed needs that are time and area (or region) specific is not an easy task.

Psychiatric patients requiring intensive treatment and services are often diagnostically complex and may have comorbid medical issues that delay placement. Studies have examined who is at risk for delayed access to inpatient care both for pediatric and adult psychiatric patients in PES settings (26,27). Delays related to insurance status, particular risk issues, and complexity of disposition are major drivers. In the authors' experience, placement may also be impeded by additional complexities as well as stigmatization of certain comorbidities such as substance use issue and personality disorders, intellectual or developmental disabilities, and other factors. Other circumstances that may hinder timely placement include criminal justice involvement, lack of insurance or ability to pay for hospitalization, lack of housing or family to provide for smooth discharge after hospitalization, and recent or ongoing agitation or aggression. Further exacerbating the problems, delays in transfer for one patient often result in longer waits for other waiting patients (28). In psychiatric care, facilities may not accept patients onto inpatient units from the ED due to factors such as a patient's insurance not covering care at a particular hospital or other barriers to the patient's ability to pay. This could be construed as an EMTALA violation, and as such, if the psychiatric unit has space, the patient may need to be accepted from the PES (29,30). EMTALA violations can lead to loss of Medicare dollars and may be a useful tool to force hospital units to accept patients if they have beds. Psychiatric bed registries are increasingly being developed to help use technology as one approach to identify where there might be psychiatric inpatient beds available and to also look systematically at any patterns of patient refusal that warrant further exploration (31). With these advances, psychiatric staff in the emergency department may have some further leverage and knowledge to access psychiatric beds in a timely manner, and inpatient units might be able to identify needs for additional staff or other resources to manage more complex patients.

DISCHARGING PATIENTS FROM PES SETTINGS

A decision to discharge a patient from a PES setting implies that there has been a careful assessment of the patient's psychiatric issues and reason for presenting for ED care, a risk assessment based on the information available or information that should be obtained during the course of the evaluation, and a determination of the proper level of care needed, if any, for the patient after the PES visit. Careful documentation of the decision, its reason, and recommended follow-up is important. Access to other means of care, such as more urgent outpatient appointment slots, partial hospitalization programs, or crisis stabilization units may be needed and available. Psychiatrists working in a PES should have knowledge of local resources to meet these patient needs. Patients may or may not be willing to take advantage of recommended services. If they are unwilling, a determination should be made as to whether an involuntary treatment option is needed and if criteria are met through legal standards. In this way, the psychiatric professional is required to analyze a given clinical situation and use their training and experience to make decisions that balance safety and patient autonomy. Careful documentation of these recommendations will help protect the psychiatrist from litigation should there be an unfortunate event such as a patient suicide following a decision to discharge the patient (18).

MITIGATING LEGAL LIABILITY

A thorough psychiatric evaluation with careful documentation is the best protection against malpractice. Also, there has been a growing literature on screening and examination of risk factors for

both suicide and violence risk, with some standardized tools being implemented (32,33). This is an important area of attention, with one study showing that residents in training could benefit from education about how to incorporate asking about known risk factors for violence into their risk assessments (34).

The potential for legal liability in psychiatric emergency settings can be anxiety-provoking for practitioners. Common reasons for liability include claims of negligent discharge after an unfortunate event, such as a patient suicide or an act of violence following an assessment in the ED. Although a physician can be sued at any time, successful litigation against a practitioner requires there to be proof that there was a dereliction of duty that directly leads to damages (18). Practitioners would do well to ensure that they have documented risk assessment and mental status assessment and made efforts to contact family or others to provide information about a patient in those situations where this information can be helpful to make a clinical decision about discharge or admission. Medical charting need not be long, but it should contain the relevant information (35) for patient care. It should also explain what occurred in the clinical encounter, should care be questioned later. Warm handoffs to outpatient clinics or crisis stabilization units and documentation of these are key. An explicit statement of the level of care needed for the patient and data supporting this recommendation should be included in the documentation. If a patient is being held involuntarily, it is important that proper paperwork is completed to authorize this. Although there are no absolute protections from legal liability, consultation from supervisors and colleagues knowledgeable in particular areas can be helpful. For example, when children are seen in a PES, having a child psychiatrist available to consult can be helpful in making emergency medication decisions or discharge decisions. Consultation with legal staff can also be helpful when issues arise related to legal regulation of psychiatric practice.

CONCLUSION

Psychiatrists practicing in emergency settings should possess an understanding of common legal and regulatory issues encountered in emergency psychiatry. Common issues such as ensuring that a patient's legal status is clear at all times, consideration of risk assessment for good risk management in triage decisions, as well as thinking about issues of confidentiality and its exceptions are broad areas with which the practitioner must feel comfortable. Good clinical judgment and common sense in the context of an understanding of the law should be the primary determinants of decision-making in the ED. Given the fast-paced nature of the emergency setting, some basic knowledge of common legal issues that arise is important. When necessary, consultation with hospital legal staff or colleagues is generally available at all hours and is encouraged when there are questions. Our hope is that the basic knowledge of legal issues, such as those outlined in this chapter, will help those who provide emergency psychiatric care feel more comfortable.

REFERENCES

1. Hedman, L. C., Petrila, J., Fisher, W. H., et al. (2016). State laws on emergency holds for mental health stabilization. *Psychiatric Services, 67*, 529–535.

2. Byatt, N., Pinals, D. A., & Arikan, R. (2006). Involuntary hospitalization of medical patients who lack decisional capacity: An unresolved issue. *Psychosomatics, 47*, 443–448.

3. Centers for Medicare & Medicaid Services (CMS), DHHS. (2006). Medicare and Medicaid programs; Hospital conditions of participation: Patients' rights; Final rule. *Federal Register, 71*, 71377–71428.

4. Hernandez, A., Riahi, S., Stuckey, M. I., et al. (2017). Multidimensional approach to restraint minimization: The journey of a specialized mental health organization. *International Journal of Mental Health Nursing, 26*, 482–490.

5. Terrell, C., Brar, K., Nuss, S., et al. (2018). Resource utilization with the use of seclusion and restraint in a dedicated emergency psychiatric service. *Southern Medical Journal, 111*, 703–705.

6. Pinals, D. A. (2015). Crime, violence and behavioral health: Collaborative community strategies for risk mitigation. *CNS Spectrums, 20*, 241–249.

7. Kubiak, S., Comartin, E., Milanovic, E., et al. (2017). Countrywide implementation of crisis intervention teams: Multiple methods, measures and sustained outcomes. *Behavioral Sciences & the Law, 35*, 456–469.

8. Pinals, D. A., & Price, M. (2018). Law enforcement and psychiatry. In Gold, L. H., & Frierson, R. L. (Eds.), *The American Psychiatric Association Publishing textbook of forensic psychiatry* (3rd ed., pp. 451–462). Arlington, VA: American Psychiatric Association Publishing.

9. Jaffee v. Redmond, 518 U.S. 1 (1996).

10. U.S. Department of Health and Human Services. *The Health Insurance Portability and Accountability Act of 1996 (HIPAA) privacy rule*. Retrieved April 1, 2019, from http://www.hhs.gov/ocr/privacy.

11. U.S. Department of Health and Human Services. *Code of Federal Regulations Title 42, Part 2*. Retrieved April 1, 2019, from https://www.govinfo.gov/content/pkg/CFR-2018-title42-vol1/xml/CFR-2018-title42-vol1-part2.xml.

12. U.S. Department of Health and Human Services. *HIPAA privacy rule and sharing information related to mental health*. Retrieved April 1, 2019, from https://www.hhs.gov/sites/default/files/hipaa-privacy-rule-and-sharing-info-related-to-mental-health.pdf.

13. Tarasoff v. Regents of the University of California, 118 Cal Rptr 129, 529 P2d 553 (1974).

14. Tarasoff v. Regents of the University of California, 17 Cal 3d 425, 131 Cal Rptr 14,551 P2d 334 (1976).

15. Weinstock, R., Bonnici, D., Seroussi, A., et al. (2014). No duty to warn in California: Now unambiguously solely a duty to protect. *Journal of the American Academy of Psychiatry & the Law, 42*, 101–108.

16. Herbert, P. B. (2002). The duty to warn: A reconsideration and critique. *Journal of the American Academy of Psychiatry & the Law, 30*(3), 417–424.

17. Barnhorst, A., Wintemute, G., & Betz, M. E. (2018). How should physicians make decisions about mandatory reporting when a patient might become violent? *AMA Journal of Ethics, 20*, 29–35.

18. Appelbaum, P. S., & Gutheil, T. G. (2007). *Clinical handbook of psychiatry and the law* (4th ed.). Philadelphia, PA: Wolters Kluwer/Lippincott Williams & Wilkins.

19. Pinals, D. A. (2009). Informed consent: Is your patient competent to consent to treatment? *Current Psychiatry, 8*, 33–43.

20. Murray, B. (2012). Informed consent: What must a physician disclose to a patient? *AMA Journal of Ethics (formerly Virtual Mentor), 14*, 563–566.

21. Boldt, R. C. (2015). The "voluntary" inpatient treatment of adults under guardianship. *Villanova Law Review, 60*, 1–58. Retrieved April 1, 2019, from SSRN: https://ssrn.com/abstract=2589715.

22. Zinermon v. Burch, 494 U.S. 418 (1979).

23. Center for Medicare and Medicaid Services. *Emergency Medical Treatment & Labor Act (EMTALA)*. Retrieved April 1, 2019, from https://www.cms.gov/regulations-and-guidance/legislation/emtala/.

24. Lindor, R. A., Campbell, R. L., Pines, J. M., et al. (2014). EMTALA and patients with psychiatric emergencies: A review of relevant case law. *Annals of Emergency Medicine, 64*, 439–444.

25. Pinals, D. A., & Fuller, D. A. *Beyond beds*. National Association of State Mental Health Program Directors 2017 Technical Assistance Papers. Retrieved April 1, 2019, from https://www.nasmhpd.org/sites/default/files/TAC.Paper_.1Beyond_Beds.pdf.

26. Stephens, R. J., White, S. E., Cudnik, M., et al. (2014). Factors associated with longer length of stay for mental health emergency department patients. *Journal of Emergency Medicine, 47*, 412–419.

27. Hoffmann, J. A., Stack, A. M., Monuteaux, M. C., et al. (2018). Factors associated with boarding and length of stay for pediatric mental health emergency visits. *American Journal of Emergency Medicine*. doi:10.1016/j.ajem.2018.12.041.

28. Heslop, L., Elsom, S., & Parker, N. (2000). Improving continuity of care across psychiatric and emergency services: Combining patient data within a participatory action research framework. *Journal of Advanced Nursing, 31*(1), 135–143.

29. Quinn, D. K., Geppert, C. M., & Maggiore, W. A. (2002). The Emergency Medical Treatment and Active Labor Act of 1985 and the practice of psychiatry. *Psychiatric Services, 53*, 1301–1307.

30. Saks, S. J. (2004). Call 911: Psychiatry and the new Emergency Medical Treatment and Active Labor Act (EMTALA) regulations. *Journal of Psychiatry & Law, 32*, 483–512.

31. Triplett, P., Harrison, S. D., Daviss, S. R., et al. (2015). Creating a statewide bed tracker and patient registry to communicate bed need and supply in emergency psychiatry: The Maryland experience. *Joint Commission Journal on Quality and Patient Safety, 41*(12), 569–574.

32. Brown, G. K., Currier, G. W., Hyman-Jager, S., & Stanley, B. (2015). Detection and classification of suicidal behavior and nonsuicidal self-injury behavior in emergency departments. *Journal of Clinical Psychiatry, 76*, 1397–1403.

33. Roaten, K., Khan, F., Brown, K., & North, C. S. (2016). Development and testing of procedures for violence screening and suicide risk stratification on a psychiatric emergency service. *American Journal of Emergency Medicine, 34*, 499–504.

34. Wong, L., Morgan, A., Wilkie, T., & Barbaree, H. (2012). Quality of resident violence risk assessments in psychiatric emergency settings. *Canadian Journal of Psychiatry, 57*, 375–380.

35. Gutheil, T. G. (1980). Paranoia and progress notes: A guide to forensically informed psychiatric recordkeeping. *Hospital and Community Psychiatry, 31*, 479–482.

47

The Crisis Call: Psychological Emergencies and Suicide Hotline Practices

John Draper, Gillian Murphy

It was not long ago nearly all voice mail greetings for mental health services—as well as messages on mental health and suicide prevention websites—offered an instruction like this: "If you are thinking about suicide, call 911 or go to your nearest emergency room." While this instruction has not vanished, it may now add "or call the National Suicide Prevention Lifeline (800-273-8255)." The circumstances under which a crisis hotline call or an emergency department visit is needed are not always clear. What are the similarities and differences in assessing and caring for a person in a suicidal crisis in an emergency setting as opposed to a service such as the National Suicide Prevention Lifeline? Given the overcrowding and expense commonly associated with emergency department care, these are essential questions for modern healthcare professionals and systems to consider.

In the vast majority of cases, thoughts of suicide do not warrant emergency service involvement, but provider anxiety associated with suicide risk can often lead to interventions that extend beyond immediate need. Contributing to this can be a lack of understanding of the role that community-based crisis hotlines can play in keeping individuals safe and supported within the community.

Suicide and crisis hotlines share a number of commonalities with emergency department practices. Generally, they both serve everyone in the community 24/7/365 (regardless of insurance status), they both assess for risk and severity of symptoms, and based on this assessment, they may provide brief intervention and resource referrals. Both services abide by the same rules of confidentiality, though crisis hotlines are typically anonymous, and do not require that callers provide any identifying information to receive care. A vital function of emergency department professionals is to perform triage (especially important in high utilization periods) and determine the need for admission to inpatient units or, alternatively, address discharge plans. Most suicide prevention and crisis hotlines do not perform triage per se, though a number of hotlines have strategies for efficiently serving and diverting callers with nonurgent needs.

After a brief historical review of suicide/crisis centers, this chapter will describe the research and best practices related to suicide/crisis hotlines, utilizing Substance Abuse and Mental Health Services Administration (SAMHSA)-funded evaluation findings and resulting industry standards established by the National Suicide Prevention Lifeline. Given the overlapping functions of crisis call centers and psychiatric emergency department work, a number of these best practices have implications for emergency physicians and staff.

THE HISTORY OF CRISIS CALL CENTERS IN COMMUNITY CRISIS CARE

In 1958, the first suicide hotline in the United States was established at the Los Angeles Suicide Prevention Center (LASPC). Over the decades that followed, suicide and crisis hotlines experienced significant growth, fueled largely by the 1963 Community Mental Health Act, which focused on shifting treatment and support services from institutions to community (1). Most of the early community crisis hotline efforts through the 1960s and 1970s were volunteer-driven and involved extensive training in "nondirective" care through the use of "active listening" techniques. An important distinction for these centers within their communities lay in the anonymity and ease of access they could provide. Individuals could engage care without the stigma and perceived barriers of the mental healthcare system.

As the number of suicide and crisis centers continued to grow, a parallel movement to bring professional crisis care into communities began to develop (2). Mobile crisis teams (or "psychiatric mobile outreach services") operated on a similar principle to hotlines, to the extent that a person in a psychiatric crisis, unwilling or unable to access care in clinical settings, could receive help without leaving his/her homes. With the increase of these clinically oriented mobile outreach services, data demonstrating their positive impact on diverting psychiatric patients from hospitals also began to appear (3,4). Groundbreaking professionally staffed crisis, information and referral hotlines with mobile crisis, and dispatch capabilities were soon established in major metropolitan areas (1). These programs served comprehensive public mental health needs by providing central access points to all crisis and behavioral health services in these urban communities.

By 2005, crisis hotlines had become so important within regional systems that they were recommended in a national public health technical assistance report as an essential component of a model community–based comprehensive psychiatric response service (1). It was not until 2007, however, that the US Joint Commission on Hospital Accreditation issued its first statement on this issue, when in their published National Patient Safety Goals on Suicide, they required that hospitals "provide information such as a crisis hotline to individuals and their family members for crisis situations" (NPSG.15.01.01).

THE NATIONAL SUICIDE PREVENTION LIFELINE

In 2001, Congressional funding was appropriated to the SAMHSA for a grant program to establish a national network of local crisis hotlines, linked to a single toll-free number, that could effectively reach and serve all those at risk of suicide. Now known as the National Suicide Prevention Lifeline, 1-800-273-TALK (8255), this network has been administered by Vibrant Emotional Health (formerly known as the Mental Health Association of New York City) since 2004. The Lifeline offers a free and confidential service that is available to anyone in emotional distress or suicidal crisis. By calling the Lifeline, individuals across the United States in need of immediate assistance are connected to the nearest available crisis center, within a national network of more than 160 such centers.

Crisis centers that participate in the Lifeline network are each independently owned and operated. Although these centers vary in size and structure, from small local volunteer-based centers to large state-funded entities, each center must submit a formal application to become a member center, be accredited by an approved accrediting body, and demonstrate competence in suicide assessment and intervention. All participating centers are required to adhere to Lifeline clinical standards of care, including a willingness to take all actions necessary, including emergency interventions with or without a caller's consent, in order to keep callers safe.

LIFELINE ESTABLISHES BEST PRACTICES FOR CRISIS HOTLINES

One of the most influential requirements of the Lifeline grant, and a key contributor to the subsequent growth and establishment of the Lifeline network as a core community resource, involves network center participation in ongoing SAMHSA-funded evaluation studies. This requirement provides Lifeline an opportunity to promote standards of practice that are developed from the combined expertise of crisis center staff and experts in the field of suicide prevention and directly informed by evaluation findings. To date, 68 network centers have participated in 11 separate evaluation studies. The iterative process through which crisis line practices are implemented, evaluated, refined, and evaluated once more is evident through a review of the SAMHSA-funded evaluation studies that have been undertaken since 2003. The findings from these evaluations of crisis hotlines have proven to be groundbreaking for the field of suicide prevention and crisis hotlines, both nationally and internationally.

Prior to the investment of SAMHSA in the Lifeline, very little was known about the effectiveness of crisis hotlines in supporting those at risk and reducing suicide. Earlier investigations lacked sufficient sample size, controls, rigorous methodologies, and follow-up contact with callers to clearly determine if hotlines were sufficiently reaching at-risk populations, effectively reducing risk, or linking callers to care (5). The SAMHSA-funded evaluations of crisis hotline processes and outcomes changed that, providing overall evidence in support of the role crisis hotlines played in responding to crisis and suicidal callers.

Initial SAMHSA-funded outcomes-oriented investigations were conducted by research teams led in 2003 and 2004 by Dr Madelyn Gould from Columbia University and Dr John Kalafat from Rutgers University. Dr Gould's team focused on 1,085 suicidal callers and Dr Kalafat's team explored the outcomes of 1,617 nonsuicidal crisis callers from eight crisis centers across the country (6,7). Callers' crisis and suicide states were assessed at the beginning and end of their calls and, for those who consented, at a follow-up call approximately 3 weeks after the original call to the center. Findings demonstrated that these hotlines were effective in reaching seriously suicidal callers; more than half of all callers had a suicide plan, nearly 60% had made past attempts, and over 8% called the line with an attempt in progress. Findings also indicated that significant reductions in crisis and suicide status occurred during the calls and continued to the follow-up. Notably, in response to an open-ended question as to what was helpful about the call, 11.6% (n = 44) of suicidal callers said that the call prevented them from killing or harming themselves.

Another research team from the University of Quebec, led by Dr Brian Mishara, focused on the process interaction between the counselor and caller to determine what practices affected call outcomes, positively or negatively. Mishara's team silently monitored 1,431 crisis and suicide-related calls at 14 crisis centers. Overall, when changes occurred from the beginning to the end of the calls, they were positive with nearly half of callers reporting less confusion, helplessness, and hopelessness by the end of the call (8).

Although these initial evaluation findings answered many longstanding questions about hotline efficacy and related practices, each discerned a number of marked shortcomings in counselor practices that required systematic attention. Mishara, Chagnon (8) noted that, of the 1,431 callers, 723 were not asked about suicidal thoughts. Of the 474 who were asked or spontaneously reported suicidal thoughts, no questions about the means were asked on 46% of the calls. Of the 159 calls in which the helper was aware that the caller was considering suicide and had determined what means to use, only 30 were asked if an attempt was in progress. Questions about prior attempts were asked of only 104 callers. Kalafat, Gould (7) noted similar concerns. Follow-up assessments conducted with 801 of the 1,617 callers who had been categorized by centers as nonsuicidal crisis callers indicated that 52 (6.5%) reported having suicidal thoughts when they had originally called the centers, and 17 of these callers said they had told the crisis worker of these thoughts yet no risk assessment had been conducted. Gould, Kalafat (6) noted that counselors did not initiate rescue services for 40% of suicidal callers who had engaged in either preparatory behavior or an actual action to hurt or kill themselves immediately prior to calling the center. In addition, although most suicidal callers reported improvement upon follow-up, about 43% remained suicidal and only 35% had been linked to care.

In all, findings from these studies identified three major areas as targets for practice improvement: the need for uniform standards and practices for *suicide risk assessment* among callers; a clear policy for necessary actions to take to maintain the safety of callers assessed to be at *imminent risk* of suicide; and a need for *follow-up* with callers at risk, to both de-escalate risk and promote linkages to community care.

BEST PRACTICES IN SUICIDE ASSESSMENT

In 2006, in response to these evaluation findings, the Lifeline, with guidance from the Standards, Trainings and Practices Committee (STPC), developed evidence-informed Suicide Risk Assessment Standards (SRAS), which served to group the wide range of available risk factors and warning signs into a more useful and useable framework through which to view the assessment process (9). These standards propose that the combination of suicidal desire with intent and acquired capability is associated with risk for suicide. The SRAS require that crisis center staff ask callers a minimum of three "prompt questions" which address current suicidal desire, recent (past 2 months) suicidal desire, and past suicide attempts. An affirmative answer to any of these would then require a full suicide risk assessment with the caller, consistent with the following four core principles:

- **Suicidal desire**—addresses the preoccupation with self-harm and suicide, often driven by a hopeless sense that no feasible alternatives could ameliorate the distress
- **Suicidal capability**—relates to the fearlessness of taking action that could be self-harming, a sense of competence, availability of means, specificity of plan, and preparation of attempt
- **Suicidal intent**—indicates the probability of enactment and encompasses certain factors, including an attempt in progress (the clearest indicator), an imminent plan to hurt self/others, preparatory behaviors, and intent to die
- **Buffers/connectedness**—focuses on immediate supports, planning for the future, engagement with the crisis counselor and core values can tip the scale of ambivalence more toward the wish to live

Although many of the factors present in the desire and intent principles of the Lifeline framework were common in risk assessments, the inclusion of factors related to capability and buffers were relatively new. The emphasis on capability factors emerged from research underpinning Joiner's Interpersonal Theory of Suicide (2005), which stipulated that suicidal capability, alongside thwarted belongingness and burdensomeness to others, were all necessary for a person to take serious suicidal actions. Specifically, Joiner observed that suicidal capability is "acquired"; past practices of risk-related behaviors and/or impaired cognitive states are necessary to "prepare" despairing individuals to act contrary to their natural instinct for self-preservation. The inclusion

of the buffers principle was essential for assessing the degree of a caller's ambivalence toward suicide (eg, "I could never do that to my mother") and for providing the counselor with life-preserving values stated by the caller that could be leveraged for further discussion, intervention, and safety planning.

Adopted throughout the network by 2007, the SRAS allowed for center-specific development of individual assessment processes, so long as each of the four core areas, and identified subcomponents (see Table 47.1), was addressed.

In 2006, Lifeline selected a suicide prevention training program that reflected many of the assessment principles and best practices suggested by evaluation findings, the Applied Suicide Intervention Skills Trainings (ASIST) by Living Works, Inc. ASIST trainings were made available to the Lifeline network and an evaluation implemented to determine the way in which these trainings and the national standards affected Lifeline counselor behaviors with callers. Between 2008 and 2009, Gould et al. evaluated 17 Lifeline crisis centers before and after they received the ASIST trainings. Callers with ASIST-trained counselors were found to be less depressed, less suicidal, and more hopeful by the end of the call (10). This finding was attributed to the ASIST model's success in helping the counselor build rapport with suicidal callers, as well as strengthening the counselor's ability to explore the caller's suicidal ambivalence, his/her reasons for living, and connecting the callers to informal supports in his/her life (10). Although Gould's evaluations since 2008 have consistently shown that Lifeline centers have improved markedly in asking callers about suicide, neither the standards alone nor the subsequent ASIST trainings have had a marked effect toward enhancing comprehensive risk assessment practices of counselors, such as exploring suicidal plans in greater detail or past suicidal behaviors (10). Nevertheless, research reported by the RAND Corporation on California-based crisis centers demonstrated that callers to Lifeline member centers were much more likely to be assessed for suicide risk and feel less distressed by the end of the call than callers contacting non-Lifeline crisis centers (11).

TABLE 47.1 Lifeline Four Core Principles of Suicide Assessment

	Desire	Intent	Capability	Buffers
Level 1	Suicidal ideation	Attempt in progress	History of attempts	Immediate supports
	Hopelessness	Plan—method known	History of self-harm (NSSI)	Reasons for living
		Preparatory behaviors	Available means	Ambivalence
		Expressed intent to die	Dysregulated	
			Currently intoxicated	
Level 2	Perceived burden		Substance abuse	Sense of purpose
	Feeling trapped		Exposure to another's attempt	Planning for future
	Self-hate		Acute symptoms mental illness	Engagement with helper
	Psychological pain		Sleep disturbance	Social supports
	Feeling intolerably alone (low belonging)		Increased anxiety	Core beliefs
			History of violence to others	

Safety Focus

In 2018, Lifeline began to reassess the content and guidelines provided to network centers around assessment of risk. Importantly, the focus for crisis center staff can be very different from that of the clinician in a face-to-face encounter and how information is presented in counselor training must reflect that. Crisis center staff must establish a connection, engage a caller, and gain trust all within in a very short period of time, all while addressing immediate safety. Is this caller safe enough to even continue this conversation? Has this caller already taken action to harm himself/herself? This is a very different scenario to that presented to the emergency department clinician who can witness the distress and engage physical formal or informal supports. The Lifeline STPC initiated a review of developments within the area of suicide assessment and recommended

that Lifeline: rename the SRAS to more clearly reflect the context in which the crisis counselor undertakes their assessment; maintain the four core principles of the SRAS and combine relevant elements of the IR guidelines; and develop a standard that emphasizes safety at its core with a focus on prevention over prediction.

This developing Safety Assessment model will address the particular needs of crisis center staff with a focus on the unique flow of crisis call flow. It will reinforce the importance of caller engagement and rapport building, collaborative problem solving, assessment of "safety now" (immediate), safety planning (longer term), and maintaining safety over time through linkage and follow-up. Training and guidance for center staff will also aim to reinforce the fact that even within the core principles outlined, some elements must always be addressed in the assessment process (see Table 47.1, Level 1).

BEST PRACTICE IN IMMINENT RISK INTERVENTION

Again in response to evaluation findings, the Lifeline Policy for Helping Callers at Imminent Risk of Suicide was developed (12) and focused on three core areas: *active engagement*, which requires that hotline staff make reasonable efforts to collaborate with callers at imminent risk and use the least invasive approach in maintaining safety; *active rescue*, which requires that staff take all action necessary to secure the safety of a caller, and initiate emergency response with or without the caller's consent, if they are unwilling or unable to take action on their own behalf; and *collaboration* with other community crisis and emergency services toward better assuring the continuous care and safety of Lifeline callers determined to be at imminent risk of suicide. In later determining the impact of this policy, Gould, Lake (13) reviewed 491 imminent risk calls at eight crisis centers in the Lifeline network. Crisis counselors actively engaged the callers in collaborating to keep themselves safe on 76.4% of calls, providing an array of successful interventions ranging from safety planning, offering follow-up, engaging third-party support, or making mobile crisis referrals. Emergency rescue services, without the callers' collaboration, were needed on 24.6% of calls. These "active rescues" were largely limited to calls where callers expressed many or strong reasons for dying and had little sense of purpose in their lives. Having an attempt in progress, being intoxicated at the time of the call, and a low level of engagement with the crisis counselor also increased the odds of active rescue. Overall, findings indicated that the IR policy had a marked impact on improving counselor interventions with imminent risk callers.

BEST PRACTICE IN FOLLOW-UP PRACTICE AND CARE COORDINATION

Low follow-through on referrals, as well as recurring suicidal ideation at follow-up (6), highlighted the need for crisis centers to support callers even after their call had ended. In 2008, SAMHSA began to provide Lifeline centers with funding specifically aimed at establishing follow-up services for high-risk Lifeline callers (later to include local emergency department discharges). To date, 44 follow-up grants to 41 crisis centers have been issued. In general, follow-up care can involve home visits, letters, phone calls, emails, or texts that are designed to check in with an individual who has recently experienced a suicide crisis in order to assess his/her well-being and level of risk. For crisis centers, follow-up is usually by telephone and typically occurs between 24 and 48 hours after the initial contact. Phone calls are brief, and while they can be tailored to the individual's need, they are structured and focus on continued assessment of risk and safety, review and revision of the established safety plan, status of any upcoming appointments, and problem-solving obstacles to linkage. Follow-up typically continues until a caller is connected to care, is determined to be stable and no longer in need of support, or refuses services.

Follow-up care has become central to Lifeline crisis center service provision. As with other Lifeline initiatives, follow-up practice within the network has been thoroughly reviewed by Lifeline and evaluated by researchers. Initial findings indicate significant benefits, with 79.6% of callers indicating that the crisis center follow-up intervention stopped them from killing themselves, whereas 90.6% reported that it kept them safe (14). Individuals who presented with higher levels of risk at the time of their initial call to the Lifeline perceived the follow-up intervention to be more valuable than those at lower suicide risk. In addition, those with demographic vulnerabilities, such as lower levels of education and time spent homeless, also perceived the intervention to be more valuable. Counselor activities, such as discussing distractors identified in the caller's safety plan, social contacts to call for help, and continued exploration of a caller's reasons for dying, were also found to be particularly helpful.

THE ROLE OF CRISIS HOTLINES AND FOLLOW-UP IN EMERGENCY PSYCHIATRIC CARE AND DISCHARGE

Despite the fact that many who attempt suicide or experience a suicidal crisis may be engaged (albeit briefly) within emergency and hospital care, there are few supports in place to ensure they pursue treatment or, once engaged in treatment, that they will receive the services they need. The risk of suicide attempts and death has been shown to be highest within the first 30 days following discharge from an ED or inpatient psychiatric unit (15,16), yet many never attend their first mental health appointment or maintain treatment for more than a few sessions (17). However, a variety of postdischarge follow-up contact approaches have been shown to reduce suicides and suicide attempts, and enhance linkages to care (18).

Beyond the benefits of follow-up contact with higher-risk hotline callers, following up with patients with a crisis team or by telephone within 1 month after an emergency department discharge for a suicide attempt has been shown to significantly reduce the likelihood that the person reattempts suicide (19,20). One recent study of over 1,300 participants from eight emergency departments across the United States found that follow-up by call-center staff, with assessment and safety planning review, significantly reduced suicide attempts by 30% over 1 year (21). These authors compared the impact of this intervention to other major public health issues, noting that the level of risk reduction was more than five times greater than the number of those needing statins to prevent heart attacks. In another study, also providing follow-up and safety planning for discharged suicidal patients from nine emergency departments, a 45% reduction in suicidal behaviors over a 6 month period was noted (22). Further, telephonic follow-up before a service appointment can result in improved motivation, a reduction in barriers to accessing services, and higher attendance rates (23).

Follow-up contacts not only saves lives, they save resources. The need for emergency departments to deploy special strategies for assisting patients has become more and more apparent. Between 2006 and 2013, emergency departments across the country saw a 12% increase in adult patients presenting with suicidal ideation (24) and an almost threefold increase in children and adolescents presenting with suicidal ideation or attempts (25). Given significant overcrowding in ED settings, repeat users negatively impact an already overburdened system. In fact, 45% of incurred costs for suicide attempt admissions have been attributed to readmissions to the ED (26). One study of the return on investment (ROI) of postdischarge follow-up calls for suicidal ideation or deliberate self-harm demonstrated that insurance providers could save money by investing in crisis centers to provide follow-up calls as both a measure to prevent suicidal behavior as well as the subsequent need for additional inpatient or emergency department intervention (27). Another study examining cost-effective intervention for suicide risk in emergency departments estimated that telephone follow-up with suicidal patients discharged from emergency departments significantly reduced suicide risk at a cost of $5,900 per life-year saved (28).

These findings, alongside the demonstrated follow-up expertise of crisis hotlines, have led to a key SAMHSA initiative focused on the establishment of working partnerships between Lifeline centers and their local hospital inpatient and emergency services. The Joint Commission's 2016 Sentinel Alert #56 indicating that the Lifeline number should be provided to all patients being discharged with recent suicide ideation underscores the potential role of crisis hotlines in promoting continuity of care in the community, following emergency department visits and inpatient stays. Because crisis centers provide 24/7 access to mental health professionals who are specifically trained in suicide assessment and crisis intervention, their support of high-risk individuals not only helps to keep individuals safe but can prevent the inappropriate use of 911, emergency departments, and crisis intervention services that results in an inefficient use of expensive and often limited resources. In a 2017 survey of Lifeline crisis center practices, of 141 centers sampled, 84% reported providing some form of follow-up service, with over 30% having a formal relationship with their local ED (29).

Since 2013, SAMHSA has provided grants to 18 Lifeline centers to partner with hospital emergency departments and inpatient units. The Gould team has been evaluating their impact on reducing suicidality, suicide attempts, ED visits, and inpatient readmissions, as well as linkages to community services. All research, partnership models, follow-up tools, and approaches can be found on the Lifeline website developed specifically to promote collaborative relationships across crisis and emergency services (http://followup-matters.suicidepreventionlifeline.org/). This website provides detailed information on follow-up services as well as sample protocols and procedures from crisis centers.

CRISIS HOTLINE PARTNERSHIPS IN COMMUNITY CRISIS AND EMERGENCY CARE

The provision of effective follow-up may entail not only engagement with local hospital and emergency systems but also with a wide range of community-based organizations. Included as a final component in the policy for helping callers at imminent risk of suicide, the element of collaboration with community service providers underscores the importance of working with services that are most likely to be involved with a center's suicidal callers. Although there are a wide variety of police/crisis center partnership models in the Lifeline network, the most common appears to be crisis center participation in training local officers in the Crisis Intervention Training (CIT) model. It is estimated that more than 400 CIT programs are operational across the country (30). The CIT model, pioneered by the Memphis, Tennessee Police Department, consists of a special training to a designated group of officers to respond to mental health-related crisis calls. The model invites partnerships with local mental health providers and consumers and promotes voluntary transports of persons at imminent risk and reduces the incidence of punitive, coercive tactics in police encounters with persons with a mental illness (30). In other approaches to relationship building, Lifeline centers provide training to hostage negotiators for police departments, training in crisis intervention for the police academy, and training for local 911 call takers in how to use crisis centers to assist those callers with nonemergent mental health needs. In 2013, the Lifeline, in collaboration with the National Emergency Number Association (NENA), developed a Suicide Prevention Standard Operating Procedure (SOP) for 911 call centers nationwide. This SOP was the first of its kind and serves to not only identify recommended practice for all Public Safety Answering Points (PSAPs or 911 centers) when assisting suicidal callers but also to facilitate crisis center implementation of the Lifeline Imminent Risk Policy which emphasizes crisis center collaboration with community service providers and, in particular, emergency responders.

FUTURE DIRECTIONS

The use of community-based crisis hotlines embodies an essential component of an affordable, accessible healthcare system which seeks to be patient-centered. Effective care transitions and collaboration between community-based behavioral health services are central components of the Zero Suicide initiative of the National Action Alliance as well as the 2012 National Strategy for Suicide Prevention (NSSP), and both emergency service providers and crisis call centers are ideally positioned to push this agenda forward. In addition to discharge follow-up models, there are growing federal, national, and state interests in positioning crisis hotlines as central access points in model programs for comprehensive community crisis care. Published recommendations from the SAMHSA (31), the National Action Alliance for Suicide Prevention (32), and the National Association of State Mental Health Program Directors (NASMHPD) (33) concur that a full continuum of community crisis care resources will be essential components to American behavioral healthcare systems in the years ahead, with crisis call centers providing a single point of access. On November 13, 2018, the Secretary of Health and Human Services released a statement to State Medicaid Directors that indicated the road ahead:

> Another strategy [for ensuring individuals with serious mental illness are provided with appropriate levels of care] is to increase availability of intensive outpatient and crisis stabilization programs designed to divert Medicaid beneficiaries from unnecessary stays in emergency departments and inpatient facilities as well as criminal justice involvement. Core elements of crisis stabilization programs include regional or statewide crisis call centers coordinating access to care in real time, centrally deployed mobile crisis units available 24 hours a day seven days a week, and short-term, sub-acute crisis stabilization programs.

There are further indications that the presence of a nationwide system of crisis hotlines will become increasingly ubiquitous for those with mental health and suicidal crises. In 2018, Congress passed the National Suicide Hotline Improvement Act, which seeks to explore the feasibility of designating a 3-digit number (n11) for a national mental health crisis and suicide prevention hotline (34). In the event such a 3-digit number were established, a cultural understanding would likely evolve that would help answer the question that began this chapter: "When should a person who is suicidal call 911 and when should he/she call a suicide hotline?"

What is clear is that a suicidal caller should expect a different response when calling the suicide hotline number than when calling 911. That response would not typically involve the dispatch of law enforcement or emergency medical authorities. Instead, the response would come from a crisis counselor who, if consistent with Lifeline's best practices, would provide good contact with the caller; assessment of the caller to ensure his/her safety; active efforts to collaborate with the caller to optimize his/her safety; offers to link the caller with additional care and supports, as needed; and offers to follow-up with the caller, especially if he/she is at any degree of risk. And, in many cases, this response might reduce the number of persons visiting emergency departments with suicidal thoughts and behaviors for years to come.

REFERENCES

1. Technical Assistance Collaborative. (2005). *A community-based comprehensive psychiatric crisis response service.* Retrieved from http://www.tacinc.org/media/13106/Crisis%20Manual.pdf.

2. Ruiz, P., Vazquez, W., & Vazquez, K. (1973). The mobile unit: A new approach in mental health. *Community Mental Health Journal, 9,* 18–24.

3. Bengelsdorf, H., et al. (1993). The cost effectiveness of crisis intervention. Admission diversion savings can offset the high cost of service. *Journal of Nervous and Mental Disease, 181,* 757–762.

4. Guo, S., et al. (2001). Assessing the impact of community-based mobile crisis services on preventing hospitalization. *Psychiatric Services, 52,* 223–228.

5. Lester, D. (2012). The effectiveness of suicide prevention and crisis intervention services. In Lester, D., & Rogers, J. (Eds.), *Crisis intervention and counselling by telephone and the Internet* (pp. 411–421). Springfield, IL: Charles C. Thomas.

6. Gould, M. S., et al. (2007). An evaluation of crisis hotline outcomes. Part 2: Suicidal callers. *Suicide and Life-Threatening Behavior, 37,* 338–352.

7. Kalafat, J., et al. (2007). An evaluation of crisis hotline outcomes. Part 1: Nonsuicidal crisis callers. *Suicide and Life-Threatening Behavior, 37,* 322–337.

8. Mishara, B. L., et al. (2007). Comparing models of helper behavior to actual practice in telephone crisis intervention: A silent monitoring study of calls to the U.S. 1-800-SUICIDE network. *Suicide and Life-Threatening Behavior, 37,* 291–307.

9. Joiner, T. E., et al. (2007). Establishing standards for the assessment of suicide risk among callers to the National Suicide Prevention Lifeline. *Suicide and Life-Threatening Behavior, 37,* 353–365.

10. Gould, M. S., et al. (2013). Impact of Applied Suicide Intervention Skills Training on the National Suicide Prevention Lifeline. *Suicide and Life-Threatening Behavior, 43,* 676–691.

11. Ramchand, R., et al. (2017). Characteristics and proximal outcomes of calls made to suicide crisis hotlines in California. *Crisis, 38*(1), 26–35.

12. Draper, J., et al. (2014). Helping callers to the National Suicide Prevention Lifeline who are at imminent risk of suicide: The importance of active engagement, active rescue, and collaboration between crisis and emergency services. *Suicide and Life-Threatening Behavior, 45,* 261–270.

13. Gould, M. S., et al. (2016). Helping callers to the National Suicide Prevention Lifeline who are at imminent risk of suicide: Evaluation of caller risk profiles and interventions implemented. *Suicide and Life-Threatening Behavior, 46*(2), 172–190.

14. Gould, M. S., et al. (2018). Follow-up with callers to the National Suicide Prevention Lifeline: Evaluation of callers' perceptions of care. *Suicide and Life-Threatening Behavior, 48*(1), 75–86.

15. Appleby, L., et al. (1999). Suicide within 12 months of contact with mental - services: National clinical survey. *BMJ, 318,* 1235–1239.

16. Qin, P., & Nordentoft, M. (2005). Suicide risk in relation to psychiatric hospitalization. *Archives of General Psychiatry, 62,* 427–432.

17. Mitchell, A. J., & Selmes, T. (2018). Why don't patients attend their appointments? Maintaining engagement with psychiatric services. *Advances in Psychiatric Treatment, 13*(6), 423–434.

18. Knesper, D. J. (2010). *Continuity of care for suicide prevention and research: Suicide attempts and suicide deaths subsequent to discharge from the emergency department or psychiatry inpatient unit.* Newton, MA: Education Development Center, Inc.

19. Motto, J. A., & Bostrom, A. G. (2001). A randomized controlled trial of postcrisis suicide prevention. *Psychiatric Services, 52,* 828–833.

20. Vaiva, G., et al. (2006). Effect of telephone contact on further suicide attempts in patients discharged from an emergency department: Randomised controlled study. *BMJ, 332,* 1241–1245.

21. Miller, I. W., et al. (2017). Suicide prevention in an emergency department population: The ED-SAFE study. *JAMA Psychiatry, 74*(6), 563–570.

22. Stanley, B., et al. (2018). Comparison of the safety planning intervention with follow-up vs usual care of suicidal patients treated in the emergency department. *JAMA Psychiatry, 75*(9), 894–900.

23. Zanjani, F., et al. (2008). Effectiveness of telephone-based referral care management: A brief intervention to improve psychiatric treatment engagement. *Psychiatric Services, 59,* 776–781.

24. Owens, P. L., et al. (2017). Emergency Department Visits Related to Suicidal Ideation, 2006–2013. HCUP Statistical Brief #220. Agency for Healthcare Research and Quality, Rockville, MD.

25. Plemmons, G., et al. (2018). Hospitalization for suicide ideation or attempt: 2008–2015. *Pediatrics, 141*(6), e20172426.

26. Gibb, S. J., Beautrais, A. L., & Fergusson, D. M. (2005). Mortality and further suicidal behaviour after an index suicide attempt: A 10 year study. *Australian and New Zealand Journal of Psychiatry, 39,* 95–100.

27. Richardson, J. S., Mark, T. L., & McKeon, R. (2014). The return on investment of postdischarge follow-up calls for suicidal ideation or deliberate self-harm. *Psychiatric Services, 65,* 1012–1019.

28. Denchev, P., et al. (2018). Modeling the cost-effectiveness of interventions to reduce suicide risk among hospital emergency department patients. *Psychiatric Services, 69*(1), 23–31.

29. National Suicide Prevention Lifeline. (2017). *Crisis center follow-up survey report.*

30. Compton, M. T., et al. (2008). A comprehensive review of extant research on Crisis Intervention Team (CIT) programs. *Journal of the American Academy of Psychiatry and the Law, 36,* 47–55.

31. Substance Abuse and Mental Health Services Administration (SAMHSA), Interdepartmental Serious Mental Illness Coordinating Committee. (2017). *The way forward: Federal action for a system that works for all people living with SMI and SED and their families and caregivers.* Rockville, MD: Substance Abuse and Mental Health Services Administration.

32. National Action Alliance for Suicide Prevention. (2016). *Crisis now: Transforming services is within our reach.* Washington, DC: Education Development Center, Inc.

33. National Association of State Mental Health Program Directors (NASMHPD). (2017). *Beyond beds: The vital role of a full continuum of psychiatric care.* Retrieved from http://bhltest2.com/wp-content/uploads/2018/05/TACPaper1-BeyondBeds.pdf.

34. National Suicide Hotline Improvement Act of 2017, H.R.2345.

48

Emergency Telepsychiatry

Avrim B. Fishkind, Flávio Casoy, Gonzalo Perez-Garcia, Robert N. Cuyler

Psychiatric conditions are estimated to account for 12.5% of emergency department (ED) admissions in the United States, with increasing frequency compared to prior decades. In addition to sheer ED volume, over 40% of mental health ED visits result in psychiatric hospitalization, significantly more than hospitalizations for other medical conditions (1).

Reasons for psychiatric admission to the ED are varied: psychiatric crises (eg, acute psychosis and suicidality, intoxication, and overdose), requests for psychotropic medication refills, lack of community treatment resources, and conditions such as altered mental status or panic attack that present with mixed medical and psychiatric symptoms. Psychiatric emergencies both add to overcrowding, diversion, and boarding as well as providing unique challenges to the medically oriented emergency department. Agitation, delusions, hallucinations, self-injury, and aggression are conditions that clash with the bright, crowded ED environment that is more geared toward managing cardiac events and auto accidents, as well as requiring significant time from staff that may detract from the care of other patients.

According to a poll of more than 1,700 emergency physicians at the 2016 meeting of the American College of Emergency Physicians, three-quarters of respondents report seeing at least one patient per shift requiring inpatient psychiatric hospitalization. One-quarter of respondents stated they have patients boarding in the ED for at least 2 days waiting for psychiatric beds (2).

Concern over psychiatric boarding has prompted efforts at regulatory remedy. The State of Washington in 2014 ruled that ED boarding of patients under civil commitment violates state law and directed increases in psychiatric bed capacity (3). The Joint Commission in 2012 introduced standards requiring protocols for reducing risk of self-harm and for initiation of a formal psychiatric treatment plan within the fourth hour of an ED admission (4).

With significant declines in psychiatric inpatient beds in private and public facilities over the past quarter century (5), transfer from the ED to an available psychiatric bed is often a long and arduous process in many communities. Placement is further impeded by homelessness, uninsured status, and specialty needs such as pediatric, geriatric, substance use, or developmental disability (6). Added to this complex mix is the absence or shortage of psychiatric specialists in most US hospitals, having mental health professionals neither on premises nor available on call.

The psychiatric manpower shortage is not unique to the emergency department. Numbers of US psychiatrists have declined in the past decade, both in total and per capita. Approximately half of US counties lack a practicing psychiatrist, with distribution of practicing psychiatrists significantly concentrated in large urban areas. Psychiatry is also an aging profession, with some 55% of doctors older than 55 years. Fueled by the scarcity of practitioners and unfavorable reimbursement rates in commercial, Medicare, and Medicaid plans, over 50% of office-based psychiatrists maintain "cash only" practices (7).

For the office practicing psychiatrist, maintaining hospital privileges creates obligations for rotating call. As fewer psychiatrists maintain privileges, frequency of call rotation increases, further inhibiting willingness to maintain consulting status which obligates ED response. In addition, the payer mix for psychiatric admissions in the ED skews toward Medicare, Medicaid (8), and uninsured populations, consequently at risk of being viewed unfavorably by physicians. The obligations to respond to psychiatric consult requests may interfere with practice schedule, evening or weekend activities, and sleep. Arguably, this mix of factors may be particularly unappealing to established practitioners in an aging, scarce profession.

The converging factors of psychiatric emergencies in the ED and shortage of available consulting psychiatrists have multiple consequences at the individual patient level as well as for the health system. Emergency department diversion rates, boarding of psychiatric patients, challenges in initiating stabilizing treatment, and shortage of available psychiatric beds have driven search for innovative delivery models in telemedicine.

TELEPSYCHIATRY IN THE EMERGENCY DEPARTMENT

Telepsychiatry has emerged along with other forms of telemedicine, jointly facilitated by search for solutions to medical access problems and the availability of increasingly affordable communication technologies (broadband, videoconference systems, and medical peripheral devices) (9). Telepsychiatry, or telemedicine via interactive live video teleconferencing with a psychiatrist, helps meet patients' need for convenient, affordable, and readily accessible mental health services. Its use was first pioneered in 1959 at the Nebraska State Hospital in Norfolk and in 1969 at Massachusetts General Hospital providing evaluations at the Logan Airport Health Clinic (10). Telepsychiatry expanded through the 1990s and 2000s. Its application allowed the implementation of numerous innovative health programs aimed at expanding access to care, facilitated by gradual recognition by payers as a covered service. Telepsychiatry has emerged as a well-accepted model for distributing psychiatric care, with numerous published case studies and clinical trials reporting equivalence of therapeutic engagement, quality/reliability of assessment, quality of care, outcomes, and patient/practitioner satisfaction as compared with in-person models of care (11). From 2004 to 2014, the number of telepsychiatry health visits of rural Medicare patients rose from 2,365 to 87,120 visits, with expectations for continued growth (12). The nature of the psychiatric encounter, which rarely requires a "hands-on" physical examination, is seen as a particularly favorable factor for videoconference-based patient interaction (13).

Telepsychiatry can serve a variety of functions in the emergency department: (1) consultation with the attending emergency physician to stabilize acute conditions and determine who most needs inpatient psychiatric hospitalization, (2) assessment of early discontinuation options for emergency psychiatric detentions placed by physicians or local law enforcement, (3) initiation of prompt, individualized treatment, and (4) consultation for patients with medical and psychiatric comorbidity.

LITERATURE, RESEARCH, AND OUTCOMES IN EMERGENCY TELEPSYCHIATRY

The earliest publication concerning emergency telepsychiatry appeared in 1997 (14). Meltzer discussed the future of the discipline, citing the need to establish interrater reliability with on-site doctors, diagnostic reliability, validity of risk assessment, and the ability to triage to the appropriate level of care. With demonstration of robust evidence base, he reasoned that emergency telepsychiatry would provide the best practice model for rapid access to expertise in emergency care. A 1998 report detailed results of a telemedicine link established between mainland Ireland and an offshore island (15). The island's primary care doctor had access to emergency psychiatry consultations and follow-up appointments. While only nine patients were seen, successful resolution of the acute presentation was reported, with satisfactory audio and video experience by patients and staff. Sorvaniemi *et al* (2005) summarized a series of 60 consecutive patients presenting to a psychiatric hospital in Finland assessed via teleconferencing (16). Mean consultation time was 37 minutes (range 15-120). Fifty-five patients preferred video consultation to in-person consultation because they did not have to wait for assessment. Staff and patients rated the experience with audio and video as satisfactory.

The first emergency management guidelines for telepsychiatry were published in 2007(17). The authors correctly noted the limited literature in the field. Four areas of interest were delineated. The first, administrative issues, indicated the need to know local regulations, resources and collaborators to ensure aftercare wraparound services post-crisis evaluation, and procedures for maintaining evening and weekend coverage. The second area, legal and ethical issues, pointed to the need to understand local commitment and duty-to-warn regulations. Third, analysis of general clinical issues emphasized working with local multidisciplinary teams as partners, effective engagement with law enforcement personnel, and recommendations for postencounter staff and patient safety. Finally, examination of rural issues included the need for more detailed assessment of firearm access, the inclusion of families in assessment and treatment, and the widespread prevalence of substance abuse without adequate local treatment options. The authors noted that that it was not yet known which diagnoses are most appropriate for treatment through videoconferencing and whether e-mail, texting, or other electronic technologies should augment telepsychiatry in emergencies.

Several studies have looked at boarding of psychiatric emergency patients in emergency departments (18,19). In 2012, Nicks and Manthey sought to define the financial impact of psychiatric boarding in the emergency department (20), reviewing all psychiatric (n = 1,438) and nonpsychiatric ED admissions over a period of 1 year in an academic medical center. Emergency department length of stay was 3.2 times longer for psychiatric admissions (1,089 minutes) than nonpsychiatric admissions (340 minutes). Boarding of psychiatric patients waiting for inpatient beds resulted in additional costs of $2,264 per patient based on calculations related to loss of bed turnover. The authors correctly noted that mechanisms were needed to decrease psychiatric patients coming to the emergency department (input), decrease the length of stay in the emergency department (throughput), and enable quicker discharge from the emergency departments to available inpatient and outpatient care (output). Notably, the metrics of this academic health system, with an inpatient psychiatric unit and availability of psychiatric consultants, may represent a particularly well-resourced health system compared with modal US hospitals.

Prompted by concerns about boarding, emergency telepsychiatry research in the last decade has looked at improving throughput in the emergency department. Seidel and Kilgus (21)

looked at 73 emergency psychiatry patients who were interviewed in-person or via teleconferencing. A second psychiatrist, acting as an observer, was in the room with the patient and completed a parallel assessment. Regarding disposition decisions, agreement between the observing psychiatrist and the assessing psychiatrist was 86% via telemedicine and 84% via in-person. There were no statistical differences in strength of disposition recommendation, diagnosis, or the HCR-20 dangerousness scale. Shortly thereafter, Southard and Neufeld studied whether emergency department telepsychiatry enhanced access and efficiency (22). They studied psychiatric patients presenting to the emergency department for 212 days prior to telemedicine and 184 days after. Using telemedicine, median time from consult order to start of consult decreased by 82%, from 14.2 to 2.6 hours. Door-to-consult time decreased by 69%, from 19.6 to 5.9 hours, and length of stay decreased 69%, from 26.3 to 8.2 hours.

In 2009, the state of South Carolina implemented an emergency department telepsychiatry initiative (23). As of October 2018, the program has been implemented in 24 hospitals, provides an average of 570 telepsychiatry evaluations per month, has 17 full or part-time telepsychiatrists, and operates 18 hours per day. In 2015, Narasimhan and colleagues (24) analyzed data from 9,066 telepsychiatry encounters, contrasted with a matched control group (n = 7,261). Compared with controls, inpatient admission rates were reduced by 34%, inpatient length of stay was reduced by 53%, and overall 30-day medical costs for treating mental health patients was reduced by $3,320 per episode of care. 30-day inpatient costs were $2,336 less in the telepsychiatry group. Regarding continuity of care, telepsychiatry consult patients were more likely to keep 30-day outpatient appointments (46% versus 16%) and 90-day outpatient appointments (54% versus 20%). Total 30-day healthcare costs after psychiatric evaluation were comparable between groups.

Emergency telepsychiatry is now moving outside of the hospital-based emergency department. In 2008, the Burke Center, a community mental health authority in Lufkin, Texas, opened the nation's first Mental Health Emergency Center (MHEC) with 24/7 coverage entirely staffed by telepsychiatrists (25). MHEC is a free-standing facility with a Psychiatric Emergency Service (PES), an involuntary Extended Observation Unit (EOU), a voluntary Crisis Residential Unit (CRU), and Mobile Crisis Outreach Teams (MCOT). Telepsychiatrists serve all four units, providing new evaluations, follow-ups, and rounds. On-site mental health staffing includes nurses, social workers, and psychiatric technicians. The MHEC model creates the opportunity to divert patients away from medical emergency departments when need for medical clearance is deemed unnecessary. Police officers may bring patients directly to MHEC following a phone triage protocol with an MHEC nurse. Ninety-five percent of patients who were previously sent to medical emergency departments now first come to MHEC, where the psychiatrists can treat many nonacute medical illnesses in addition to providing psychiatric assessment and management. Fewer than 20% of patients are transferred to inpatient psychiatric hospitals. Approximately 88% of patients report improvement at MHEC, and approximately 85% are satisfied with telepsychiatry (25). A recent study of cost avoidance to hospitals in the Burke MHEC service area showed $17.7 million in cost savings over 10 years for deferred visits to area hospital emergency departments (26).

Finally, more recent emergency telepsychiatry efforts focus on using telepsychiatry with first responders to prevent unnecessary transports of patients in crisis to emergency departments and instead to divert to available and appropriate community-based mental health resources. A recent project with the Houston, Texas, Sheriff's Department equipped six Crisis Intervention Team officers with iPads and modified teleconferencing software enabling access to psychiatric consultants. Thirty patients were evaluated via emergency telepsychiatry crisis calls. Forty-five percent of patients were diverted from an emergency room, a jail, or a psychiatric facility, translating into savings of $26,244 in transport and emergency responder costs for just 31 patients (27). A similar program in Charleston, South Carolina, called the Telehealth Mobile Crisis Program supports a masters-level clinician from the South Carolina Department of Mental Health who connects remotely with emergency medical service (EMS) supervisors. Data collected over a 7-month period shows that 56% of patients

assessed via telemental health are diverted from the emergency room (n = 722 calls). The estimated cost savings for the first year in decreased transport and emergency room visits is $1.1 million (28). Of note, in both systems, reduced cost is not the sole outcome: linkage to community crisis services, outpatient clinics, and residential units were defined as critical elements of program success.

TECHNOLOGY REQUIREMENTS

Telemedicine practitioners in early and many current applications use healthcare-grade video teleconferencing (VTC) systems to connect with patients. The units are placed in the physician's office and connected via available broadband to a companion system at the distant patient care location, typically a hospital or clinic. VTC units have desirable features including near-life image size allowing the physician and patient to see one another on large monitors. These units are also equipped with pan/tilt/zoom features, enabling the physician to take a close-up view (eg, for examination of tremor or pupillary size) or wide-angle view (eg, to include family members or staff in the visit). While initially cost-prohibitive in certain applications, the price-point for VTC's has declined dramatically, accompanied by widespread availability and affordability of high-speed internet service. Technology barriers have continued to fall as wireless connectivity has become ubiquitous: patients and physicians have become used to personal communication via video on tablets and smartphones, laptops have become more powerful, and people have become accustomed to work on multiple screens. As a result, the VTCs are ceding ground to the use of smaller units connected to wireless networks. It is common, for example, for medical emergency departments to employ wireless-enabled tablets mounted on carts. Physicians can sit in an office with a powerful system comprised of a laptop and several connected monitors that allow them to simultaneously videoconference with the patient, review the patient's medical record, and access reference materials as needed. Data security and privacy protection are embedded in available healthcare-grade solutions. Hospitals can place a laptop or a tablet on a rolling cart to enable services at the bedside or in multiple examination rooms. Available technology includes robotic systems giving physicians joystick control of motorized carts. As cellular data capacity improves, portable wireless systems can be used at the initial point of contact by police officers and other first responders, allowing for remote evaluation and triage by a telepsychiatrist, potentially improving civilian and first responder safety as well as decreasing emergency department or jail utilization for mental health crises.

Hospitals implementing a telepsychiatry program should provide guaranteed download connection speeds of 15 megabytes per second (Mbps) and upload speeds of 5 Mbps. Telemedicine programs must also establish compliance with HIPAA/HITECH regulations for data security, business associate agreements and confidentiality, as well as internal medical staff policies (29). Designated and accountable information technology (IT) staff who are actively involved in all stages of the program are essential for program success.

CLINICAL APPROACH

By definition, almost all emergency psychiatric patients arrive at some level of crisis. The initial step on arrival is evaluation by a triage nurse or physician to ensure that the patient is sufficiently medically stable for a psychiatric assessment. Suicidal individuals who have taken an overdose, for example, may need immediate acute medical stabilization. Intoxication, delirium, atypical cardiac problems, neurovascular accidents, epilepsy, and others can all present with initial behavioral manifestations. Also, individuals with serious mental illness often have comorbid serious medical illnesses that may be in need of acute stabilization, even if not the primary driver of the presentation. This triage includes obtaining vital signs, initial physical examination, and a brief mental status examination. At this point, it is also important to assess for imminent suicidal or homicidal risk in order to determine if close supervision is required pending completion of the full assessment.

There are many situations where it is appropriate to request a telepsychiatric assessment. These include (1) assessments for patients who present to the ED with primary psychiatric complaints, such as suicidality, depression, anxiety, agitation, or psychotic symptoms, (2) determining appropriate level of care for patients with psychiatric complaints, (3) evaluation and management of substance use disorders, (4) management of people with chronic serious medical illness whose depression or anxiety leads to poor treatment adherence and frequent readmissions, (5) management of delirium on medical or surgical floors, (6) guidance on issues of mental capacity, (7) addressing conflict within or between treating teams for patients with complex medical and biopsychosocial issues, (8) guidance on management of psychiatric medications when patients present for nonpsychiatric reasons, and (9) evaluation of involuntary status.

Some in the psychiatric community worry that telepsychiatry loses the intangible connection a doctor and patient develop during an interview. However, with on-site orientation to the visit and presence of high-quality audio/visual connection, the experience of interviewing a patient on video is quite similar to completing an in-person interview. Some situations may not be appropriate for telepsychiatry. For example, an on-site psychiatrist would be able to walk up to an immobilized patient and make eye contact at the bedside, which can be problematic with a laptop or tablet attached vertically to a cart. Similarly, a hoarse, recently intubated patient may not be able to speak loudly enough for the psychiatrist to hear on video unless an external microphone can be provided for the patient. However, creative solutions can often be found such as using an iPad held by a nurse and angled so eye contact can be established or with the bedside nurse repeating the hoarse client's verbalizations. There may be situations where the patient is opposed to seeing a psychiatrist via videoconferencing. Some patients are shy or sensitive to the speaker volume and may want greater privacy. These situations are similar to complaints by patients who present to the emergency department with a psychiatric complaint and the expectation for treatment in a private, contained office, not a busy, noisy ED. These concerns must be handled with care and compassion by local staff.

Once triage is complete, a request for a telepsychiatric assessment needs to be submitted to the telepsychiatrist on call. A request should include the results of the triage, any accompanying legal paperwork such as legal holds, EMS or police documentation, notes written by emergency department doctors or nurses since patient arrival, a face sheet to confirm identity, any available laboratory or imaging results, and a signed consent from the patient agreeing to a telemedicine assessment. In the case of a consultation to a hospitalist for a patient admitted to a medical floor, a clear consult question is necessary. Facilities have different arrangements for consultation requests. In some facilities, the ED clerk faxes the necessary information to the telepsychiatry services and follows up with a phone call requesting a consultation. Other facilities have integrated electronic health records, and the ED physician places an electronic order for a consultation. Other systems have secure online portals where the consult request and clinical information are exchanged electronically.

If the telepsychiatrist has any questions regarding the case, she may request a phone conversation with the requesting physician prior to seeing the patient. It is common practice for the telepsychiatrist to speak with the patient's nurse to obtain a close perspective on the patient's interactions and behaviors since arriving in hospital. The nurse or other staff member should obtain consent from the patient for an assessment and set up the equipment at the patient's bedside or in a consult room in a way that allows the telepsychiatrist and patient to see and hear each other clearly.

The psychiatric interview then proceeds much as any emergency psychiatric interview detailed in other chapters of this book. If the patient feels uncomfortable with the videoconference method, the psychiatrist can address these anxieties and normalize the situation. The psychiatrist needs to complete a mental status examination, address major areas of the psychiatric review of systems, take a careful history of the current crisis, prior episodes, and psychiatric treatments, and complete a safety assessment. If family and friends are present, they should be asked to step out for a portion of the interview to determine if the patient is currently experiencing abuse and to inquire about other sensitive areas, such as risky sexual behaviors or drug use. Presence of an in-person staff member can be helpful as well, particularly when it comes to the limitations of telemedicine, such as providing olfactory cues (detecting a malodorous patient with self-care neglect, detecting the smell of alcohol, etc) and tactile cues (eg, testing for rigidity). It is important to obtain urine drug screens to help differentiate psychiatric illnesses from substance use disorders. Urinalysis, complete blood counts, metabolic panels, and thyroid panels may be necessary to complete the assessment and make differential diagnoses. The hospital may send these results prior to requesting the assessment to expedite the final disposition process, or the psychiatrist can request these be sent for review once the results are obtained for final disposition and medication recommendations.

Several methods are used for medication management. In many situations, the telepsychiatrists serves as consultant and provides medication recommendations for the ED physician or hospitalist to incorporate in their treatment plan. In other cases, the telepsychiatrist directly orders medications. In the latter situation, formal follow-up mechanisms are vital for managing dosage adjustments and assessment of side effects and adverse reactions. In complex patients, a follow-up telephone conversation between the psychiatrist and attending physician is important to avoid medical errors.

It is helpful for the telepsychiatrist to be knowledgeable of community resources around the hospital. Level of care decisions need to be appropriate to the resources available to the patient. It is unhelpful for a psychiatrist to recommend a partial hospitalization program in lieu of an inpatient admission if there is no nearby program available. If a recommendation is given for inpatient admission, and if medication is indicated, telepsychiatrists should recommend starting a regimen to initiate treatment while placement is arranged, which may take several days. While the patient is boarding in the ED, it is helpful for there to be regular reassessments to determine continued need for admission. Patient improvement may make it possible to rescind an involuntary status, allowing for discharge and community follow-up.

ETHICS AND EMERGENCY TELEPSYCHIATRY

When using any new technology to assist with the delivery of health care, one must always ensure that the four basic principles of medical ethics—autonomy, beneficence, nonmaleficence, and justice (30)—are respected. The key benefit of telemedicine is allowing doctors to reach patients in remote areas, but some have expressed concern that the use of technology rather than in-person evaluations can cause patients to feel dehumanized, particularly those who do not fully understand the technology (31).

Recent joint recommendations by the American Psychiatric Association and American Telemedicine Association address a variety of best practice recommendations, many of which had ethical implications (32). In telemedicine as well as in any medical intervention offered to patients, informed consent becomes vitally important. In addition to the usual expectations for in-person encounters, informed consent for a telepsychiatry evaluation should cover the risks of technical difficulties, interruptions, and a very rare risk of breach of security affecting confidentiality. The informed consent should also assure the patient the right to omit sensitive information from their history, the right to request nonmedical personnel to leave the telemedicine examination room, and the right to terminate the consultation at any time. Respect for autonomy also requires an assurance of medical confidentiality. Telepsychiatrists, especially those who work from a home office, should offer patients the same respect and confidentiality that they expect to receive in any in-person clinical setting. This means the telepsychiatrist ensuring that nonclinical staff in their home (spouses, children, housekeepers, etc.) do not overhear, interrupt, or otherwise witness the encounter. It is vital that the psychiatrist working from home work behind a closed door and have the ability to use headphones or to mute microphones and speakers. People residing or working in the psychiatrist's home should be aware of the importance of respecting the privacy of the home office and telepsychiatry evaluations that take place there.

Telepsychiatry lends itself well to the principles of beneficence and nonmaleficence, as it increases access to providers, may reduce or optimize healthcare spending, improves quality of care, and offers reduced wait times for needed treatments. In emergency settings without on-site psychiatric staffing, telepsychiatry consultations provide improved emergency mental health care in rural hospitals as well in the numerous urban hospitals without comprehensive psychiatric coverage. By reducing ED length of stay and carefully evaluating continued need for involuntary hold, telepsychiatry may increase beneficence and nonmaleficence by allowing greater access to psychiatrists and reduce unnecessary inpatient psychiatric transfers for patients who have been sufficiently stabilized in the ED (33). A psychiatrist is more likely to be able to safely clear a psychiatric patient for discharge, as emergency department doctors have been shown to be more cautious when assessing the risks in a psychiatric patient who presents with a complaint of self-harm (34).

The use of teleconference technology expands the psychiatrist's choice of setting beyond the office or clinic. However, it is the responsibility of the psychiatrist to ensure compliance with state licensure laws and regulations (35). Default practice dictates that the psychiatrist must be licensed in the state where the patient is located. Exceptions include certain federal healthcare systems (Veterans Administration and Indian Health Service) that allow for single state licensure across multiple jurisdictions. Furthermore, the Interstate Medical Licensure Compact allows a rapid licensure process for physicians establishing practice in multiple states, allowing for licensure in 24 states and one territory (36). However, it is vitally important that a psychiatrist engaged in multistate practice be aware of applicable commitment laws to ensure that they are complying with the law and providing appropriate recommendations. For example, the amount of time that an emergency psychiatric hold lasts can vary from as little as 23 hours to as much as 140 days, depending on the state. Medical necessity for initiation of a psychiatric hold can vary greatly from state to state: almost every state allows for a hold for "danger to self" or "danger to others due to mental illness," but only a handful allow emergency detention for recent suicide attempt or inability to meet basic needs (37). Psychiatrists also need to be aware of any state laws surrounding privacy and security of medical information, the provision of telemedicine services, and availability of reimbursement for telemedicine services. Also, duty-to-warn notification of threatened targets of violence is required in some states but prohibited in others.

The practitioner must follow all federal and state laws regarding prescribing, especially the prescribing of controlled substances. The Ryan Haight Online Pharmacy Consumer Protection Act of 2008 was established to ensure that consumers could not obtain controlled substances over the internet without physician oversight (38). In recent years, there was some confusion over whether or not telepsychiatry prescribing was subject to statutory language limiting "obtaining controlled substances over the internet." However, the DEA did confirm that they did not intend to interfere with the legitimate prescribing of controlled substances occurring in the context of telemedicine practice (39).

It is with an examination of the fourth medical principle, justice, that the largest benefit of telepsychiatry becomes clear. Telepsychiatry allows for underserved communities to gain greater access to psychiatric care. This lack of access can increase costs to the consumer and to hospitals. In many rural communities that lack a psychiatrist, patients sometimes find themselves needing to travel to a nearby larger community that can be a few, or even several hours away. Furthermore, when faced with a patient in psychiatric crisis, a rural emergency department doctor might err on the side of caution and choose to admit a patient who might not need a psychiatric admission—and the patient might be waiting in the ED for their transfer for days. Telepsychiatry allows for rural patients and emergency departments to have the same access to psychiatrists that patients in urban centers do and can lead to decreased costs for the patient (40) and emergency departments (41).

OPPORTUNITIES AND HURDLES IN EMERGENCY TELEPSYCHIATRY

Emergency telepsychiatry has emerged as a subspecialty well suited to ameliorating certain of the problems detailed in this chapter, principally providing improved access to scarce specialists, improved quality of care, enhanced regulatory compliance, and ability to initiate active treatment promptly. In principle, equipping an emergency department with the technology necessary to provide psychiatric telemedicine consults is relatively easy. High-quality videoconference systems running on broadband Internet are readily available and affordable, providing privacy-protected, synchronous interaction between psychiatric consultants and patients. The psychiatric consultant may examine the patient from a distance, eliminating the need to be posted at the hospital or to travel to the hospital to provide services. With location eliminated as a hurdle, the consultant may be accessible to geographically distant hospital EDs as well as available to multiple hospitals from a single practice location. Near-universal deployment of electronic health records enables the ability of the psychiatric consultant to review a patient's chart and to document the consultation results for immediate availability at the ED.

However, a number of limiting factors remain. Partial easing of licensure requirements for multistate practice has been detailed above, but the practice of telepsychiatry practice remains subject to regulations and restrictions by individual state medical boards with varying telemedicine standards. Advocacy for liberalized cross-state practice hopes to ease these regulatory hurdles. In addition, telepsychiatrists must obtain and maintain medical staff privileges at hospitals for whom they provide consultations.

The provision of emergency telepsychiatry is also intrinsically complicated from an organizational standpoint. Expectations for scheduling and response time, roles of support personnel at both ends of the consultation, coordination of activities/responsibilities of the ED physician and emergency psychiatrist, and clarity regarding technical support represent only a short list of implementation tasks (24).

Financial consideration can represent a significant hurdle. In today's reimbursement climate, emergency departments rarely receive reimbursement for psychiatric consultations that even approach direct costs. In addition to care for the uninsured or underinsured, telepsychiatry has infrastructure costs including equipment and bandwidth capability for both ends, training and technical support costs, and organizational overhead for the telepsychiatry enterprise.

Salary costs for emergency psychiatrists may be driven by expectations of short response time and availability for evening, night, and weekend staffing. It is in the burden of indirect healthcare costs and on the life impact on individuals, families, and communities that the promise of telepsychiatry expansion becomes clearer. Workforce shortages in psychiatry may become even more critical as telepsychiatry growth escalates, and as programs will need to be staffed around the clock by psychiatrists willing to provide 24/7 emergency services via technology. To the positive, emergency telepsychiatry offers expanded and flexible practice options as the field moves beyond its historical territory of the practice office, clinic, or hospital. Such flexibility offers new practice options for practitioners interested in home-based or semiretirement practice options. Short of massive expansion of the psychiatric workforce and/or mandated availability of practitioners in every hospital regardless of location, telepsychiatry represents the health system's most promising solution for care of psychiatric emergencies (42).

REFERENCES

1. Owens, P. L., Mutter, R., & Stocks, C. (2010). *Mental health and substance abuse–related emergency department visits among adults, 2007; Statistical brief #92*. Retrieved from http://www.hcup-us.ahrq.gov/reports/statbriefs/sb92.pdf.

2. American College of Emergency Physicians. (2016, October 17). *Waits for care and hospital beds growing dramatically for psychiatric emergency patients*. Retrieved May 18, 2018, from http://newsroom.acep.org/2016-10-17-Waits-for-Care-and-Hospital-Beds-Growing-Dramatically-for-Psychiatric-Emergency-Patients.

3. Bloom, J. D. (2015). Psychiatric boarding in Washington state and the inadequacy of mental health resources. *Journal of the American Academy of Psychiatry & the Law, 43*(2), 218–222.

4. Joint Commission on Accreditation of Healthcare Organizations. (2012). APPROVED: Standards revisions addressing patient flow through the emergency department. *Joint Commission Perspectives®, 32*(7), 1–5.

5. Lutterman, T., Shaw, R., Fisher, W., & Manderscheid, R. (2017). *Trend in psychiatric inpatient capacity, United States and each state, 1970 to 2014*. National Association of State Mental Health Program Directors.

6. Abid, Z., Meltzer, A., Lazar, D., et al. (2014). Psychiatric boarding in the US EDs: A multifactorial problem that requires multidisciplinary solutions. Policy brief. *Urgent Matters, 1,* 1–6.

7. Bishop, T. F., Seirup, J. K., Pincus, H. A., & Ross, J. S. (2016). Population of US practicing psychiatrists declined, 2003–13, which may help explain poor access to mental health care. *Health Affairs, 35*(7), 1271–1277.

8. Nikpay, S., Freedman, S., Levy, H., & Buchmueller, T. (2017). Effect of the Affordable Care Act Medicaid expansion on emergency department visits: Evidence from state-level emergency department databases. *Annals of Emergency Medicine, 70*(2), 215–225.

9. Shore, J. H. (2015). The evolution and history of telepsychiatry and its impact on psychiatric care: Current implications for psychiatrists and psychiatric organizations. *International Review of Psychiatry, 27*(6), 469–475.

10. Bashshur, R. L., & Shannon, G. W. (2009). *History of telemedicine: Evolution, context, and transformation*. New Rochelle, NY: Mary Ann Liebert, Inc.

11. American Psychiatric Association. *Evidence base. Telepsychiatry toolkit*. Retrieved May 18, 2018, from https://www.psychiatry.org/psychiatrists/practice/telepsychiatry/evidence-base.

12. Mehrotra, A., Huskamp, H. A., et al. (2017). Rapid growth in mental health telemedicine use among rural Medicare beneficiaries, wide variation across states. *Health Affairs, 36*(5), 909–917.

13. Locatis, C., & Ackerman, M. (2013). Three principles for determining the relevancy of store-and-forward and live interactive telemedicine: Reinterpreting two telemedicine research reviews and other research. *Telemedicine Journal and e-Health, 19*(1), 19–23.

14. Meltzer, B. (1997). Telemedicine in emergency psychiatry. *Psychiatric Services, 48*(9), 1141–1142.

15. Mannion, L., et al. (1998). Telepsychiatry: An island pilot project. *Journal of Telemedicine and Telecare, 4*(Suppl. 1), 62–63.

16. Sorvaniemi, M., Ojanen, E., & Santamaki, O. (2005). Telepsychiatry in emergency consultations: A follow-up study of sixty patients. *Telemedicine Journal and e-Health, 11*(4), 439–441.

17. Shore, J. H., Hilty, D. M., & Yellowlees, P. (2007). Emergency management guidelines for telepsychiatry. *General Hospital Psychiatry, 29*(3), 199–206.

18. Pearlmutter, M. D., Dwyer, K. H., Burke, L. G., Rathiev, N., Maranda, L., & Volturo, G. (2017). Analysis of emergency department length of stay for mental health patients at ten Massachusetts emergency departments. *Annals of Emergency Medicine, 70*(2), 193–202.

19. Stone, A., Rogers, D., Kruckenberg, S., & Lieser, A. (2012). Impact of the mental healthcare delivery system on California emergency departments. *Western Journal of Emergency Medicine, 13*(1), 51–56.

20. Nicks, B. A., & Manthey, D. M. (2012). The impact of psychiatric patient boarding in emergency departments. *Emergency Medicine International, 2012,* 5, Article ID 360308.

21. Seidel, R. W., & Kilgus, M. D. (2014). Agreement between telepsychiatry assessment and face-to-face assessment for emergency department psychiatry patients. *Journal of Telemedicine and Telecare, 20*(2), 59–62.

22. Southard, E., Neufeld, J. D., & Laws, S. (2014). Telemental health evaluations enhance access and efficiency in a critical access hospital emergency department. *Telemedicine and e-Health, 20*(7), 664–668.

23. South Carolina Department of Mental Health. (2018, October 10). *SCDMH telepsychiatry program history.* Retrieved December 25, 2018, from https://scdmh.org/dmhtelepsychiatry/telepsychiatry-and-telehealth-program-history/.

24. Cuyler, R. N., & Holland, D. (2012). *Implementing telemedicine: Completing projects on target on time on budget.* Bloomington, IN: Xlibris.

25. APA Achievement Awards, 2011 APA Gold Award: A telepsychiatry solution for rural Eastern Texas. *Psychiatric Services Psychiatry Online.* Retrieved December 25, 2018, from https://doi.org/10.1176/ps.62.11.pss6211_1384.

26. Internal outcome data, 2014, 2015. Burke Mental Health Center Communication. Retrieved from www.myburke.org.

27. Webb, F. *Doc in a box: Using telepsychiatry for patrol deputies in the Harris County (TX) sheriff's office.* CIT International. Retrieved December 25, 2018, from http://www.citinternational.org/resources/Documents/Using%20Telepsychiatry%20for%20Patrol%20Deputies%20in%20the%20Harris%20County%20(TX)%20Sheriff%27s%20Office.pdf.

28. Emergency & Assessment/Mobile Crisis. Charleston Dorchester Mental Health Center. Retrieved December 25, 2018, from http://www.charlestondorchestermhc.org/services/emergency/.

29. Clark, P. A., Capuzzi, K., & Harrison, J. (2010). Telemedicine: Medical, legal and ethical perspectives. *Medical Science Monitor, 16,* 261–272.

30. Beauchamp, T., & Childress, J. F. (2001). *Principles of biomedical ethics* (5th ed.). New York, NY: Oxford University Press.

31. Fishkind, A. B., Cuyler, R. N., Shiekh, M. A., & Snodgrass, M. (2012). Telepsychiatry and e-mental health. In McQuistion, H. L., et al. (Eds.), *Handbook of community psychiatry* (pp. 125–140). New York, NY: Springer.

32. Shore, J. H., Yellowlees, P., Caudill, R., et al. (2018, April). *Best practices in videoconferencing-based telemental health.* American Psychiatric Association and American Telemedicine Association.

33. Zhu, J. M., Singhal, A., et al. (2016). Emergency department length-of-stay for psychiatric visits was significantly longer than for nonpsychiatric visits, 2002-11. *Health Affairs, 35*(9), 1698–1706.

34. Kapur, N., Cooper, J., Rodway, C., et al. (2005). Predicting the risk of repetition after self harm: Cohort study. *BMJ, 330*(7488), 394–395.

35. Damisch, M. M. (2018). Telemedicine licensure and related challenges for physicians. *Medical Economics, 95,* 7.

36. Hedman, L. C., Petrila, J., Fishman, W. N., Swanson, J. W., Dingman, D. A., & Burris, S. (2016). State laws on emergency holds for mental health stabilization. *Psychiatric Services, 67*(5), 529–535.

37. Interstate Medical Licensure Compact, 2018. Retrieved from https://imlcc.org.

38. Public Law 110-425: Ryan Haight Online Pharmacy Consumer Protection Act of 2008, 122 Stat. 4820, H.R. 6353, enacted October 15, 2008.

39. Arnold, J. Telemedicine and the Controlled Substances Act. Presentation at the Short Course, 21st Annual Meeting of the American Telemedicine Association, Minneapolis, MN, May 2016.

40. Hilty, D. M., Ferrer, D. C., Burke Parish, M., et al. (2013). The effectiveness of telemental health: A 2013 review. *Telemedicine and e-Health, 19,* 444–454.

41. Narasimhan, M., Druss, B. G., Hockenberry, J. M., Royer, J., Weiss, P., Glick, G., Marcus, S. C., & Magill, J. (2015). Impact of a telepsychiatry program at emergency departments statewide on the quality, utilization, and costs of mental health services. *Psychiatric Services, 66*(11), 1167–1172.

42. Rago, B. *Exploring cost avoidance in area hospitals: The impact of Burke's Mental Health Emergency Center.* Retrieved December 25, 2018, from https://myburke.org/wp-content/uploads/2018/12/MHEC-Cost-Avoidance-Report-2018.pdf.

49

Disaster Psychiatry and Psychiatric Emergency Services

Anthony T. Ng, Joshua C. Morganstein

"The opinions and assertions expressed herein are those of the author(s) and do not necessarily reflect the official policy or position of the Uniformed Services University or the Department of Defense."

Emergency departments (EDs) and Emergency Medical Services (EMS) are often the first to respond to a disaster or mass casualty incident. An understanding of the adverse mental health effects of disasters enhances response by healthcare personnel. Adverse psychological and behavioral effects represent a significant portion of healthcare burden, both in human suffering and financial cost (1). These effects may persist for months or years following a disaster event, long after physical injuries have healed and infrastructure has been repaired. Certain individuals are at increased vulnerability to these adverse effects of disasters and benefit from special consideration by disaster emergency planners (2). The majority of individuals that seek care following a disaster will do so in primary care and emergency settings.

WHAT IS A DISASTER AND WHO IS AT RISK FOR ADVERSE EFFECTS?

Disasters produce a predictable range of distress reactions, health risk behaviors, and psychiatric disorders for many affected individuals. Disasters can be massive events affecting a large number of people or a large area, or they can be localized. The term "disaster" is generally used to describe events that result in a predictable range of adverse psychological and behavioral effects, and the needs from the events outstrip resources. A disaster is an event that overwhelms the preexisting coping capabilities of a community whereby needs exceed available resources (see Figure 49.1).

Disasters often have direct and indirect impacts on communities. In addition to the primary disaster victims and their immediate families, the effects of disaster can extend to other family members, friends, coworkers, and caregivers, including medical professionals, through secondary traumatization. Traditional and social media transmit extensive details of disaster events instantly around the world, significantly increasing adverse mental health effects throughout the exposed population (3). It is important for psychiatric emergency services (PESs) to consider not only those in geographic proximity to the disaster event, but also the broader exposed population, in disaster preparedness, response, and recovery.

Disasters can be natural or human-generated (see Figure 49.2) with different impacts on individuals and communities. Natural disasters may bring up issues that are different from those of human-made disasters, including terrorism (4). Depending on the severity and scale of disasters, some less severe ones may necessitate a more immediate and robust response from mental health services, including PESs, with a lesser strain on the system response.

A variety of individual and community factors influence the extent of psychiatric burden following a disaster. Socioeconomic status, cognitive and mobility limitations, and gender can all be risk factors for adverse psychological and behavioral effects (5). Event factors including the direct impacts of the disaster itself may also increase risk, including physical injury, loss of home, death, or severe injury of a loved one.

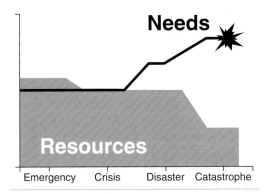

FIGURE 49.1 • Needs versus resources in various extreme events.

PSYCHOLOGICAL CONSEQUENCES OF DISASTERS

The psychological and behavioral responses to disasters are well established. These include distress reactions (insomnia, irritability, scapegoating), health risk behaviors (increased use of alcohol and tobacco, social isolation, overdedication), and psychiatric disorders (posttraumatic stress disorder [PTSD], major depression, anxiety disorders, and substance abuse disorders) (5,6). Somatic symptoms may occur and are most prominent following disasters involving exposure and contamination, including pandemics, chemical spills, and threats of bioterrorism (7). Psychological and behavioral response to disasters may also be observed in the following categories: physical, emotional, cognitive, behavioral, and spiritual. Table 49.1 lists specific examples of each category.

Disaster-induced stress reactions can influence the management of such events (8,9). Some individuals seeking postdisaster care will be directly affected physically, but many others will have physical symptoms without an identifiable source or etiology. Sudden increases in the demand for medical services may overwhelm emergency department surge capacity (10,11).

PES staff may need to evaluate and treat symptoms of insomnia, severe anxiety, and nonspecific somatic complaints, all of which may lead to secondary reactions among others. For example, providers may become upset about an individual's distress or become angry at a person for not being "in control." Over time, disaster stress reactions can lead to interpersonal problems, family strain and conflict, and erosion of social support (12). After a disaster, individuals with prior psychiatric conditions may present with exacerbation of their psychiatric disorders.

In the longer term, the psychiatric consequences of disaster that PESs may encounter include mood and anxiety disorders, new onset of PTSD, and substance abuse problems. They may also see social and family issues stemming from the event (eg, job loss, displacement, and family and relationship discords).

DISASTER RESPONSE STRUCTURE

Command and control are an important component of disaster response (13). PESs need to recognize two main disaster response hierarchies: external and internal. The external hierarchy encompasses the wide variety of responding entities in the community at large. Depending on the type and severity of disaster, various local, state, and federal agencies and coalitions may be involved, including local and state Emergency Management

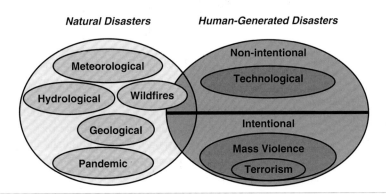

FIGURE 49.2 • Types of disasters. (Adapted from DEEP PREP at www.umdeepcenter.org.)

TABLE 49.1 Immediate Reactions to a Sudden and Violent Event

Physical Reactions
Nausea, gastrointestinal distress
Sweating, shivering
Faintness, dizziness
Muscle tremors, weakness
Elevated blood pressure
Elevated heart and respiration rates
Uncoordinated movements
Extreme fatigue, exhaustion
Headache
Narrowed visual field
Emotional Reactions
Numbness, anxiety, fear
Rapidly shifting emotions
Guilt, survivor guilt
Exhilaration, survivor joy
Anger, sadness
Helplessness, feelings of detachment
Feeling unreal
Disorientation
Feeling out of control
Denial, constriction of feelings
Strong identification with victims
Feeling overwhelmed
Cognitive Reactions
Difficulty concentrating
Racing, circular thoughts
Slowed thinking
Memory problems
Confusion, difficulty naming objects
Impaired problem-solving, calculations
Difficulty making decisions
Intrusive images of disaster
Loss of perspective
Loss of ability to conceptualize, prioritize
Behavioral Reactions
Startled reaction, restlessness
Sleep and appetite disturbances

TABLE 49.1 Immediate Reactions to a Sudden and Violent Event   (Continued)

Difficulty expressing oneself
Constant talking
Arguments, angry outbursts
Withdrawal, apathy
Exaggerated gallows humor
Slowed reactions, accident-prone
Inability to rest or let go
Increased use of alcohol, tobacco
Spiritual Reactions
Intense use of prayer
Loss of faith in self
Profound loss of trust

Agencies, the Federal Emergency Management Agency (FEMA), and nongovernmental agencies, such as the American Red Cross (ARC) and state and national VOADs (Voluntary Organizations Active in Disasters). It is important to understand the roles and functions of these entities, which may provide mass care and shelter, medical services, or financial benefits. This allows for appropriate consideration of needs assessment, interventions, and, most importantly, collaboration.

Most response agencies' responsibilities in disasters are defined by roles using a model called the Incident Command System (ICS). ICS establishes the overall command function, including logistics, planning, operations, finance/administration, safety, and public information (14,15). ICS is part of the National Incident Management System (NIMS), which is part of FEMA. It defines the responsibilities of the various agencies that may respond in a national emergency. NIMS helps to ensure a greater degree of management and coordination of resources (16).

The internal hierarchy structure refers to the institution or hospital system of which PES is a part. Every hospital should have a disaster response plan that specifies each department's responsibilities. Hospitals use the Hospital Emergency Incident Command System (HEICS), which identifies clear roles and functions and ensures coordination among all departments during a disaster response (17,18). PESs should

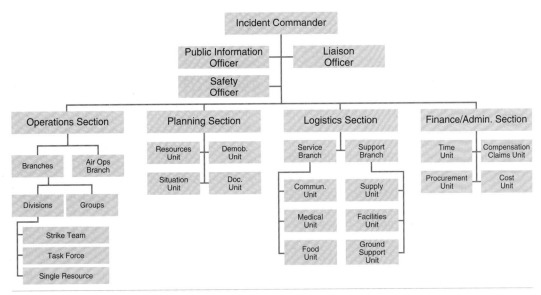

FIGURE 49.3 • Incident command system.

plan how they will work with the hospital's HEICS, as well as having their own response plan to continue functioning in a disaster. Figure 49.3 describes the roles of each ICS function.

PSYCHIATRIC EMERGENCY SERVICES IN DISASTERS

The importance of integrating behavioral health into disaster emergency planning is well established throughout the national and global community (19,20), including the role of emergency mental health professionals and, where one exists, an organized PES. (The term *PES staff* is used in this chapter to refer to any emergency mental health professional.) There was a 10% temporal increase in one study in the rate of ED behavioral and mental health diagnoses among Medicaid enrollees within a 3-mile radius of the World Trade Center site in New York City after the September 11th terrorist attack (21). In another study, it was noted that the surge in psychiatric emergency department visits persisted for 4 to 6 months after Hurricane Sandy (22). It is critical that disaster mental health services be actively integrated into emergency medicine at every stage of an organized disaster response. PESs are vital to the overall EMS response and a natural leader of a community's collaborative mental health response in part because of their close connection to EMS and medical emergency services.

In disaster planning, PES faces a variety of challenges. Similar to general medical EDs, PESs are under-resourced and overcrowded (23). Additionally, EDs and PESs are often not fully integrated, and communication and collaboration between the two services are not optimized. PES and the ED often operate as separate, distinct services. Even when integrated, the two services have distinct cultures and structures that are often not fully understood by the other. There may be stigma toward both psychiatric clinicians and patients with psychological symptoms or mental illness, who are viewed as troublesome or demanding to a system that is already stretched. Psychological and behavioral symptoms have not traditionally been viewed as a priority for both clinical care and staff wellness. Administrators may also view the needs of PES as secondary (24). However, given that both ED and PES are used to working in crisis mode and have some adaptiveness to working with insufficient resource, this may provide flexibility and even synergy in meeting postdisaster health and mental health needs of the affected community.

PSYCHIATRIC EMERGENCY SERVICE DISASTER PLANNING

PES disaster planning should address all types of disasters. It can be conceptualized in a cyclical manner that includes pre-event, acute response, and postevent phases and provide a paradigm to guide planning, policy development, and response implementation (25).

Pre-Event Phase

Preparation in the pre-event phase enhances the effectiveness of any interventions during the actual event. It begins with an all-hazards assessment to identify hazardous events that a community, including the healthcare facility itself, may face. Advance planning helps to develop a response mindset and structure to deal with other events. Senior leadership must be willing to allocate resources such as personnel and time for the development of any disaster response plan (26).

Psychiatrists, and PESs, should participate in the development of the disaster response plan within the hospital and community (4). Tabletop exercises and disaster drills help to identify a number of issues that can be expected to arise (19). For example, while the PES's staff are off responding to external emergencies, the PES needs to maintain enough staff to cover its own operation (27). Contingency planning for alternate transportation and communication needs to be addressed. Patient clinical information needs to be accessible and adequately safeguarded. PESs, working in conjunction with the hospitals, will need to establish the mechanisms for managing volunteers, including emergency credentialing.

Education is an important component of PES disaster preparedness and mitigation. In the pre-event phase, PESs play an important educational role for ED staff as well as other hospital personnel regarding the psychological impacts of disasters and essential aspects of early interventions (24). PESs can also educate their own communities and the public about normal reactions following disasters, which mitigates excessive healthcare utilization within a resource-constrained postdisaster environment.

PESs must appreciate the unique needs of the community and advocate for public participation in disaster planning with EDs and PESs. This fosters trust between the community and the ED and PES and, more importantly, the empowerment of the community to facilitate its own resilience.

Acute Response Phase

A primary responsibility for PES personnel in the acute response phase is to maintain internal continuity of services. Patient and staff safety and other staff concerns within the PES and the hospital are addressed immediately. Given the high likelihood that EDs will already have psychiatric patients, PES will need to ensure that there is rapid assessment, treatment, and disposition of these patients to increase the ED capacity to deal with the disaster surge. Once the internal response is organized, PES clinicians can turn to the external disaster response. The ED can begin by sending out a small team to assess the external situation before more hospital staff are deployed. PES clinicians need to rapidly identify who is involved in the response and the ED command structure. They also need to identify available mental health resources and assets and to set up a complementary command structure.

When it comes to individuals who present for care in a disaster setting, PES and ED staff must collaborate to develop plans to properly refer individuals who seek help, including those seeking psychological care (24,25,28). Disaster psychiatric triage may be influenced by several factors, such as patient surge (how many patients present for care), the resources the ED and PES have at the time (how many staff and how much space), and the severity of psychiatric distress and impairment, including imminent risks to self and others.

Lastly, PES staff can take a proactive role in working with ED staff in the execution of the general hospital disaster response plan. PES clinicians can aid in formulating appropriate and clear messages. Consistent, understandable, and reliable information from trusted sources can diminish public anxiety about the event (2,9).

Role of Leadership

Leaders play an important role in reducing harm and mitigating adverse impact of the event. What leaders do and say in these situations matters a great deal and can significantly influence the trajectory of recovery for those around them (29). Active listening, empathy, and a desire to help reduce the public's feelings of fear and isolation. This initial support is critical in reducing distress and promoting recovery. Leaders can also help with education efforts, for example, by reinforcing the idea that distress reactions are a normal response to extreme events.

There are effective (and ineffective) crisis communication strategies. Leaders should provide timely, accurate, updated, and repeated messages to populations impacted by an event. They should not attempt to control information to avoid "panic" or other feared behaviors. Accurate information builds trust and a foundation for partnering with members of organizations and communities in addressing important disaster-related needs.

It is important for leaders to address grief and loss. Grief leadership is the process of recognizing and giving voice to what has been lost following traumatic events, providing a sense of hopefulness about recovery, realism about adverse effects, and a positive outlook on the future.

Leaders must also pay attention to their own distress reactions and health risk behaviors. Poor sleep, failure to eat and hydrate adequately, and overdedication to the point of exhaustion or withdrawal from their leadership role will have a negative effect on coping following traumatic events. PES staff can act as confidants to leaders, buffering the inevitable extremes of stress and enhancing their effectiveness.

Effective Interventions

In the acute phase of disaster response, individuals often struggle to deal with concrete needs, such as arranging for burials or memorials, finding shelter, or navigating through the postdisaster benefit structure. The response environment is chaotic, especially in the immediate aftermath, not only for the public but also for the responders. Survivors may have anxiety, dissociation, hyperarousal, and insomnia.

To assist with emotional needs, most practitioners are currently de-emphasizing critical incident stress debriefing (CISD) in favor of psychological first aid (PFA) (30). PFA is an effective postdisaster mental health intervention by personnel with and without mental health training (31). It is a set of pragmatic interventions during the first 4 weeks after an event that promote adaptive coping and enhance problem-solving ability. PFA consists of five elements that are designed to promote realistic perceptions of physical and psychological safety; calming; social connectedness; personal and community efficacy; hope; and optimism. PFA emphasizes empathic and nondirective listening. PES staff can help to engage other behavioral and nonbehavioral health workers trained in PFA in both emergency and primary care settings.

Disasters and Psychiatric Medication

Prescribers must address two issues: medications prescribed for psychiatric conditions prior to the disaster and prescriptions for symptoms developing after a disaster. Patients on psychiatric medications may go to PES for medicine due to inability to access their own prescribers or pharmacy or loss of their supply. Patients with substance abuse disorders on a regimen of opiate replacement therapy are particularly at risk for withdrawal symptoms.

In the assessment of individuals on preexisting psychiatric medications, it is important to inquire about their level of adherence prior to the disaster. The benefit of continuing stabilizing medicine for major mental illness or substance use disorders may be straightforward. On the other hand, the benefit of restarting patients on psychiatric medications to which they had not previously been adherent may place them at greater risk because of difficulty monitoring them for efficacy and side effects. Patients should be reconnected with their prescribers as soon as possible.

Regarding the initiation of new psychiatric medications, research on the actual use of psychiatric medication in the acute management of mass casualty incident trauma and disaster victims is scarce (32). Much of what is known about the role of psychopharmacology in disaster is extrapolated from the extensive literature on medications and trauma (33,34).

Because of their intense emotional reactions, some survivors of disaster situations may have a sense of urgency about relieving their distress. Clinicians need to determine the acuity of the psychiatric distress, the level of impairment, and whether the benefit of clinical intervention with medication outweighs the risks. Postdisaster conditions such as the abuse potential of psychotropic medications, displacement issues, and the shifting priorities of survivors need to be considered. Survivors should be strongly encouraged to use behavioral interventions, including progressive muscle relaxation, guided visual imagery, and relaxation breathing techniques.

Short-term sedative-hypnotic medication may be used to relieve insomnia. Prazosin has demonstrated some efficacy in treating insomnia associated with posttraumatic symptoms as well as reducing the frequency and severity of associated nightmares and may be used at doses up to 15 mg nightly (35). For those who develop psychiatric disorders (such as PTSD, depression, or anxiety) following a traumatic event, evidence-based pharmacotherapy includes the use of SSRIs and SNRIs as first-line therapy. Mirtazapine (Remeron) shows evidence of efficacy in treatment of PTSD. Benzodiazepines (Valium, Klonopin, Xanax, and others) have primarily negative evidence and are generally discouraged (36).

Postevent Phase

PESs have significant roles in the postevent phase of disaster response. Patients may present to the EDs with ongoing and persistent psychological distress and somatic symptoms. As the postdisaster environment becomes more stable, they may benefit from additional and targeted interventions, including the use of psychotropic medications and supportive, cognitive, and behavioral interventions (31,32). These are complex issues. PESs should continue to work closely with EDs to ensure ongoing education and communication for both psychiatric and nonpsychiatric emergency staff.

SPECIAL POPULATIONS

Ensuring PES and ED staff wellness in disasters is a key component of any acute disaster response by a PES. Disaster workers are subjected to secondary vicarious traumatization that may lead to a broad range of adverse psychological and behavioral reactions (37,38). In working with this population, PES staff need to develop an understanding of the first-responder culture such as their work demands, the role of camaraderie, and organizational structure. First responders may be apprehensive about mental health interventions because of the stigma of mental illness. PES staff need to take a proactive role in engaging with ED and hospital staff, as well as other response partners, to address staff wellness and mitigate burnout issues.

In the planning of their own disaster response, PESs need to appreciate that the concepts of mental health and grief vary with culture, as do help seeking and communications (39,40). Some groups, such as immigrants, both documented and undocumented, may have concerns about seeking postdisaster care with any links to governmental entities. They may have fears of reprisals in this country or memories of negative experiences with the government in their country of origin. PESs should incorporate cultural competency, including language capability and interpreters, into their planning. Cultural brokers can provide valuable input as well as promote trust. Effective brokers are individuals who are accepted by the relevant cultures, such as community leaders and healthcare providers who have been working closely or associated with different cultural groups.

CONCLUSION

In recent years, the field of disaster mental health has evolved rapidly. It integrates crisis intervention with community resources and strengths. The psychiatric consequences of disasters are both acute and chronic; hospitals and emergency services may expect to play an expanding role in disaster response. It is important that PESs develop an understanding and recognition of the unique public health issues of disasters. EDs and PESs should continue to forge closer relationships with each other around disaster preparedness. Lastly, research should help to refine the role of PES and disaster mental health, not only in the scientific and clinical arena, but also operationally in terms of structure of response. A comprehensive model of care that is developed to promote community preparedness and resilience in disasters can also serve to enhance everyday clinical practice.

REFERENCES

1. Schoenbaum, M., Butler, B., Kataoka, S., et al. (2009). Promoting mental health recovery after hurricanes Katrina and Rita: What can be done at what cost. *Archives of General Psychiatry, 66*(8), 906–914.
2. Somasundaram, D. J., & Van de Put, W. A. (2006). Management of trauma in special populations after a disaster. *Journal of Clinical Psychiatry, 67*(Suppl. 2), 64–73.
3. Pfefferbaum, B., Newman, E., Nelson, S. D., et al. (2014). Disaster media coverage and psychological outcomes: Descriptive findings in the extant research. *Current Psychiatry Reports, 16*(9), 464.
4. Ursano, R. J., Fullerton, C. S., & Norwood, A. E. (1995). Psychiatric dimensions of disaster: Patient care, community consultation, and preventive medicine. *Harvard Review of Psychiatry, 3*, 196–209.

5. North, C. S. (2003). Psychiatric epidemiology of disaster responses. In Ursano, R. J., & Norwood, A. E. (Eds.), *Annual review of psychiatry* (Vol. 22, pp. 37–62). Washington, DC: American Psychiatric Association.

6. Pfefferbaum, B., North, C. S., Flynn, B. W., et al. (2001). The emotional impact of injury following an international terrorist incident. *Public Health Reviews, 29,* 271–280.

7. McCormick, L. C., Tajeu, G. S., & Klapow, J. (2015). Mental health consequences of chemical and radiologic emergencies: A systematic review. *Emergency Medicine Clinics of North America, 33*(1), 197–211.

8. DiGiovanni, C., Jr. (2003). The spectrum of human reactions to terrorist attacks with weapons of mass destruction: Early management considerations. *Prehospital and Disaster Medicine, 18,* 253–257.

9. Noy, S. (2004). Minimizing casualties in biological and chemical threats (war and terrorism): The importance of information to the public in a prevention program. *Prehospital and Disaster Medicine, 19,* 29–36.

10. Duclos, P., Sanderson, L. M., & Lipsett, M. (1990). The 1987 forest fire disaster in California: Assessment of emergency room visits. *Archives of Environmental Health, 45,* 53–58.

11. Hick, J. L., Hanfling, D., Burstein, J. L., et al. (2004). Health care facility and community strategies for patient care surge capacity. *Annals of Emergency Medicine, 44,* 253–261.

12. Norris, F. H., Friedman, M. J., Watson, P. J., et al. (2002). 60,000 disaster victims speak: Part I: An empirical review of the empirical literature, 1981–2001. *Psychiatry, 65,* 207–239.

13. Geiling, J. A. (2002). Overview of command and control issues: Setting the stage. *Military Medicine, 167*(Suppl. l), 3–5.

14. Maniscalco, P. M., & Christen, H. T. (1999). EMS incident management: Emergency medical logistics. *Emergency Medical Services, 28,* 49–52.

15. Londorf, D. (1995). Hospital application of the incident management system. *Prehospital and Disaster Medicine, 10,* 184–188.

16. Annelli, J. F. (2006). The National Incident Management System: A multi-agency approach to emergency response in the United States of America. *Revue Science et Technique, 25,* 223–231.

17. Zane, R. D., & Prestipino, A. L. (2004). Implementing the Hospital Emergency Incident Command System: An integrated delivery system's experience. *Prehospital and Disaster Medicine, 19,* 311–317.

18. O'Neill, P. A. (2005). The ABC's of disaster response. *Scandinavian Journal of Surgery, 94,* 259–266.

19. Flynn, B., & Sherman, R. (2017). *Integrating emergency management and disaster behavioral health: One picture through two lenses.* Amsterdam: Butterworth-Heinemann.

20. UNISDR 3rd United Nations World Conference. (n.d.). *Sendai framework for disaster risk reduction 2015–2030.* UNISDR Sendai. Retrieved from https://www.unisdr.org/we/coordinate/sendai-framework.

21. Dimaggio, C., Galea, S., & Richardson, L. D. (2007). Emergency department visits for behavioral and mental health care after a terrorist attack. *Annals of Emergency Medicine, 50*(3), 327–334.

22. He, F. T., Lundy De La Cruz, N., et al. (2016). Temporal and spatial patterns in utilization of mental health services during and after Hurricane Sandy: Emergency department and inpatient hospitalizations in New York City. *Disaster Medicine and Public Health Preparedness, 10*(3), 512–517.

23. Vieth, T. L., & Rhodes, K. V. (2006). The effect of overcrowding on access and quality in an academic ED. *American Journal of Emergency Medicine, 24,* 787–794.

24. Ruzek, J. I., Young, B. H., Cordova, M. J., et al. (2004). Integration of disaster mental health services with emergency medicine. *Prehospital and Disaster Medicine, 19,* 46–53.

25. Gurwitch, R. H., Kees, M., Becker, S. M., et al. (2004). When disaster strikes: Responding to the needs of children. *Prehospital and Disaster Medicine, 19,* 21–28.

26. Mattos, K. (2001). The World Trade Center attack. Disaster preparedness: Health care is ready, but is the bureaucracy? *Critical Care, 5,* 323–325.

27. Doyle, C. J. (1990). Mass casualty incident. Integration with prehospital care. *Emergency Medicine Clinics of North America, 8,* 163–175.

28. Van Amerongen, R. H., Fine, J. S., Tunik, M. G., et al. (1993). The Avianca plane crash: An emergency medical system's response to pediatric survivors of the disaster. *Pediatrics, 92,* 105–110.

29. Birkeland, M. S., Nielsen, M. B., Knardahl, S., et al. (2015). Time-lagged relationships between leadership behaviors and psychological distress after a workplace terrorist attack. *International Archives of Occupational and Environmental Health, 89*(4), 689–697.

30. Everly, G. S., & Flynn, B. W. (2006). Principles and practical procedures for acute psychological first aid training for personnel without mental health experience. *International Journal of Emergency Mental Health, 8,* 93–100.

31. National Institute of Mental Health. (2002). *Mental health and mass violence: Evidence-based early psychological intervention for victims/survivors of mass violence. A workshop to reach consensus on best practices* (NIH Publication 02-5138). Washington, DC: US Government Printing Office.

32. Katz, C. L., Pellegrino, L., Pandya, A., et al. (2002). Research on psychiatric outcomes and interventions subsequent to disasters: A review of the literature. *Psychiatric Research, 110,* 201–217.

33. Davidson, J. R. (2000). Pharmacotherapy of post-traumatic stress disorder: Treatment options, long-term follow-up, and predictors of outcome. *Journal of Clinical Psychology, 61*(Suppl. 5), 52–56.

34. Albucher, R. C., & Liberzon, I. (2002). Psychopharmacological treatment in PTSD: A critical review. *Psychiatric Research, 36,* 355–367.

35. Kung, S., Espinel, Z., & Lapid, M. I. (2012). Treatment of nightmares with prazosin: A systematic review. *Mayo Clinic Proceedings, 87*(9), 890–900.

36. Guina, J., Rossetter, S. R., DeRhodes, B. J., et al. (2015). Benzodiazepines for PTSD: A systematic review and meta-analysis. *Journal of Psychiatric Practice, 21*(4), 281–303.

37. Fullerton, C. S., Ursano, R. J., & Wang, L. (2004). Acute stress disorder, posttraumatic stress disorder among disaster and rescue workers. *American Journal of Psychiatry, 161,* 1370–1376.

38. Palm, K. M., Polusny, M. A., & Follette, V. M. (2004). Vicarious traumatization: Potential hazards and interventions for disaster and trauma workers. *Prehospital and Disaster Medicine, 19,* 73–78.

39. Wheat, M., Brownstein, H., & Kvitash, V. (1993). Aspects of medical care of Soviet Jewish emigrés. *Western Journal of Medicine, 139,* 900–904.

40. Lin, T., Tardiff, K., Donetz, G., et al. (1978). Ethnicity and patterns of health seeking. *Culture, Medicine, and Psychiatry, 2,* 3–13.

Index

Note: Page numbers followed by "f" indicate figures, "t" indicate tables and "b" indicate boxes.

GUIDE TO
Minimally Invasive
Aesthetic Procedures

M. Laurin Council, MD

Associate Professor of Dermatology
John T. Milliken Department of Internal Medicine
Division of Dermatology
Washington University School of Medicine in St. Louis
St. Louis, Missouri

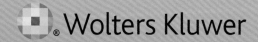
Wolters Kluwer

Philadelphia • Baltimore • New York • London
Buenos Aires • Hong Kong • Sydney • Tokyo

Acquisitions Editor: Colleen Dietzlcr
Development Editor: Eric McDermott
Editorial Coordinator: Cody Adams
Production Project Manager: Kim Cox
Design Coordinator: Steve Druding
Manufacturing Coordinator: Beth Welsh
Prepress Vendor: TNQ Technologies

9 8 7 6 5 4 3 2 1

Printed in China

Library of Congress Cataloging-in-Publication Data

ISBN-13: 978-1-975141-28-8

Cataloging in Publication data available on request from publisher.

shop.lww.com